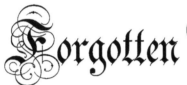 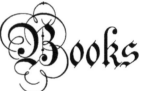

ISBN 978-1-5278-2751-6
PIBN 10893170

1 MONTH OF
FREE
READING

at

www.ForgottenBooks.com

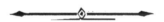

By purchasing this book you are
eligible for one month membership to
ForgottenBooks.com, giving you
unlimited access to our entire
collection of over 1,000,000 titles via
our web site and mobile apps.

To claim your free month visit:

www.forgottenbooks.com/free893170

English
Français
Deutsche
Italiano
Español
Português

www.forgottenbooks.com

Mythology Photography **Fiction**
Fishing Christianity **Art** Cooking
Essays Buddhism Freemasonry
Medicine **Biology** Music **Ancient**
Egypt Evolution Carpentry Physics
Dance Geology **Mathematics** Fitness
Shakespeare **Folklore** Yoga Marketing
Confidence Immortality Biographies
Poetry **Psychology** Witchcraft
Electronics Chemistry History **Law**
Accounting **Philosophy** Anthropology
Alchemy Drama Quantum Mechanics
Atheism Sexual Health **Ancient History**
Entrepreneurship Languages Sport
Paleontology Needlework Islam
Metaphysics Investment Archaeology
Parenting Statistics Criminology
Motivational

TRAUMATIC SEPARATION

OF

THE EPIPHYSES

TRAUMATIC SEPARATION

OF

THE EPIPHYSES

BY

JOHN POLAND, F.R.C.S.

WITH THREE HUNDRED AND THIRTY-SEVEN ILLUSTRATIONS
AND SKIAGRAMS

LONDON
SMITH, ELDER, & CO., 15 WATERLOO PLACE
1898

TO MY FATHER

RICHARD HENRY POLAND

I DEDICATE THIS WORK

JOHN POLAND

PREFACE

I venture to trust that this volume will prove of assistance in elucidating a large class of injuries which up to the present time have not been properly understood.

My warmest thanks are due to my friend Mr. Hugh A. Webster, Librarian of the University of Edinburgh, for the great labour entailed in revising the proof-sheets, and for many valuable suggestions. To Messrs. Churchill I am indebted for two blocks from Mr. T. Bryant's 'Art and Practice of Surgery,' and to Messrs. Longmans & Co. for one from Messrs. Ashby and Wright's 'Diseases of Children'; and I take this opportunity of thanking the publishers, Messrs. Smith, Elder, & Co., and the printers, Messrs. Spottiswoode & Co., for the way in which all my wishes have been carried out.

Most of the illustrations have been made for me by Dr. C. W. Hogarth and Mr. John Burman, while the engraver, Mr. T. P. Collings, has done much to enhance their value.

The kindly help of my brothers, Messrs. Charles and Ernest Poland, who have respectively assisted me with the German literature and proof-sheets, has saved me much labour.

To my old friend Mr. William Webster, one of the chief exponents of the Röntgen ray process in this country, I owe a debt of gratitude for his valuable series of skiagrams showing the normal epiphyses of the hand.

Finally, I thank the many kind friends, especially those in the profession both at home and abroad, who have conduced so much, by their interesting contributions of cases and photographs, to the completeness of the book.

J. P.

INTRODUCTION

WHILE most of the standard works on surgery mention epiphysial separations, very few give any cases or enter into any detail either as to their diagnosis or treatment. This may account for the fact that these lesions do not sufficiently occupy the attention of practitioners.

Epiphysial separations are still continually mistaken for ordinary fractures or dislocations, and in many cases suitable treatment is not adopted.

Numerous specimens of such separations now exist in museums, and clinical cases not unfrequently afford accurate data upon which an exact diagnosis may be made.

Though the literature of the subject is most extensive, it is very scattered. It has cost me some years of labour to bring together and summarise the records hitherto published. Almost all references have been verified, and, in a great number of instances, corrections have been made in the dates as well as in the pages.

My interest in the subject was first aroused when, sixteen years ago, I held for two and a half years the post of Registrar at the North-Eastern Hospital for Children, and for a time took the duties of the Acting-Surgeon. I then came across more than one complicated injury to the joints in children which perplexed me very much.

Most of the anatomical details were worked out during the years I acted as Demonstrator and Senior Demonstrator of Anatomy in the Guy's Hospital Medical School. Many are not to be found in any anatomical or surgical text-book; they are now published for the first time.

For permission to make use of the clinical cases at Guy's Hospital up to the year 1884, collected when I was Surgical Registrar to the Hospital, I am greatly indebted to the members of the surgical staff.

A very large number of cases have been under my own observation and care, more especially at the City Orthopædic Hospital and at the Miller Hospital, Greenwich.

Separation of the epiphyses, with their symptoms, mechanism, causes, pathological anatomy, treatment, and prognosis, will be considered first in general.

The symptoms, treatment, &c., special to each variety of separation will then be described in their appropriate chapters.

All separations verified by direct examination have been placed under the head of 'Pathological Anatomy,' which has also been made to include nearly all compound separations ; and throughout it has been my endeavour to place the subject upon a sound anatomical and pathological basis.

The total number of cases I have here collected is over seven hundred, though a large number of published reports have been rejected on account of their obscure nature.

I hope this work may induce hospital surgeons to publish the cases under their observation, which are numerous, if we may judge by the annual statistical reports of many of the hospitals.

DEFINITIONS

EPIPHYSIS, from ἐπί, upon ; φύσις, growth, from φύω, to grow.   An *accretion* ; something that grows *to* another.

Synonyms.—Diductio epiphysium.   Diastasis, disjunctio, divulsio, discessio epiphysium.   Traumatische Epiphysentrennung, Absprengung der Epiphysen, Trennung der Epiphysen.   Divulsion, disjonction, décollement traumatique des épiphyses, séparation des épiphyses.   Disjonction diaphysaire (Ollier).   Décollement juxta-épiphysaire.   Fracture juxta-épiphysaire.   Desépiphysation.   Distacco delle epifisi.

Various names have been applied in this country to these injuries, such as disjunction, divulsion, epiphysial detachment or separation, juxta-epiphysial fracture and separation, epiphysial diastasis.

Juxta-epiphysial separation or fracture would limit the solution of continuity to the juxta-epiphysial region, which has been called the bulb of the bone (*bulbe de l'os*) by Lannelongue, and which is a short distance from the epiphysial cartilage.

The name of diaphysial separation (*décollement diaphysaire*) has been proposed by M. Ollier, and with considerable accuracy, for in a typical epiphysial separation it is the diaphysis which is separated from the epiphysial cartilage, and not the epiphysis.   The term 'epiphysial separation' would then be reserved for those very rare cases where the epiphysis is detached from the epiphysial cartilage.

But there would be little advantage in changing a title with which all are now so familiar.

CONTENTS

———◦———

PART I

TRAUMATIC SEPARATION OF THE EPIPHYSES
IN GENERAL

PART II

*TRAUMATIC SEPARATION OF THE EPIPHYSES OF
THE UPPER EXTREMITY*

a

PART III

TRAUMATIC SEPARATION OF THE EPIPHYSES OF THE LOWER EXTREMITY

PART IV

I. *TRAUMATIC SEPARATION OF THE EPIPHYSES OF*
       THE VERTEBRÆ AND RIBS

LIST OF ILLUSTRATIONS

SKIAGRAMS

ILLUSTRATIONS IN TEXT

FIG.   PAGE

PART I

TRAUMATIC SEPARATION OF THE EPIPHYSES
IN GENERAL

———◆◇◆———

CHAPTER I

HISTORICAL

AN often quoted fable attributes to the Amazons the custom of separating the epiphyses of their male children, with the design of assuring to the female the supremacy of strength and beauty.

Among ancient writers Hippócrates has often been referred to as the first to make any allusion to separation of the epiphyses. An equivocal quotation from a passage where he treats of dislocations of the wrist has led to some discussion on the subject : ἔστι δ' ὅτε καὶ ἡ ἐπίφυσις ἐκινήθη. ' Quandoque autem et epiphysis emota est ' (*Hipp. de articulis*, 27, Littré's ed. vol. iv. p. 138). It would be useless to attempt any precise explanation of the phrase, for Hippocrates appears to have used the term *epiphysis* in a very indefinite manner. With the same uncertainty he alludes to abruption of the epiphysis or trochlea of the humerus as being a much milder form of accident than other injuries at the elbow joint.

Many centuries appear to have elapsed without any mention of this kind of injury.

Realdus Colombus (*De re anatomica*, Venetiis 1559, lib. i. p. 6), in the sixteenth century, clearly pointed out the possibility of the occurrence of epiphysial separation, alluding to it in the following passage : ' Quam luxationem nunquam, aut summa quidem certe cum difficultate, curari posse crediderim propter sinuum tuberculorum multitudinem, quibus utraque pars tam appendicis quam ossis cui adnascitur abundat & eorundem mutuum ingressum postulat.' He was the first to point out the existence of separation of the epiphyses in newly born infants.

Morgagni quotes (*De sedibus et causis morborum*, Ep. lvi. a) another passage from Colombus in the following words : ' Si les os tendres des enfants sont maniés trop fortement par leś mains d'un médecin inhabile, les ligaments s'étendent jusqu'à entraîner les appendices (epiphyses) avec eux.'

1 0

Rognetta (*loc. cit. infra*) and others have on insufficient grounds considered a case to be one of separation of the great trochanter which Ingrassias describes in his commentaries on the works of Galen (ch. xx.), but it does not appear that Ingrassias was cognisant of epiphysial injuries (J. P. Ingrassias, *In Galeni librum de ossibus doctissima et expectatissima commentaria, Panormi* 1603). It was the case of a young man who, whilst fencing with a halberd, had torn off the trochanteric process by a violent movement.

Coming to 1614 we find Ambrose Paré noticing, in two places at least in his works, the probable occurrence of epiphysial separation. In one of them he expresses himself thus : ' Nous avons vu une autre sorte de luxation qui se fait, principalement en os des jeunes, par une séparation des épiphyses, comme la tête de l'os adjutoire (humérus) et fémoris, et autres iointures, et cela se cognoist en ce qu'on voit séparation des os avec crépitation et impotēce de la partie.'   Again, with reference to dislocations, the following quotation is from Thomas Johnson's translation of the *Chirurgical works* of Ambrose Parey (London, 1634, p. 596) : ' Also that dislocation is uncurable, when-as the ligaments, steeped and swollen up with an excrementitious humiditie, are so much shortened and contracted in their length, as they have acquired in their breadth ; and thus they draw away and plucke off the *appendices* of the bones from whence they arise, and by reason the bone and the appendix doe enter and receive each other by manie cavities and prominences, therefore they cannot, by how skilfull hand soever they may be handled, be again fitly placed and put together.' Paré quotes Hippocrates as calling the upper appendix (epiphysis) of the tibia the diaphysis. He has only recorded one case of detachment of an epiphysis, that of the pelvic end of the femur, which at first had been mistaken for a dislocation of this bone.

Poupart and others about this time observed cases following small-pox and scurvy, and denied that separation could take place without some pathological condition.

Ruysch is said to have made some experiments on new-born children.

In 1632 a Neapolitan surgeon, Marcus Aurelius Severinus, drew attention (*De abscessuum recondita natura lib., de gibbis, valg. et var.*, Lugd. Bat. 1724, cap. vii. p. 428) to separation of the upper and lower epiphyses of the tibia as well as to the deformities of the knee and foot which result from such separation.

Towards the middle of the same century, Eysson specially studied diseases of the bones in children, and particularly treated of separa-tion of the epiphyses (H. Eyssonius, *De ossibus infantis*, 1625 ; also V. Coiter, 1659).   Rognetta states that the work of Eyssonius (*Tractatus anatomicus et medicus de ossibus infantis cognoscendis, conservandis et curandis*, Groningæ, 1659, vol. i.) was in 1834 exceedingly scarce in Paris.

Fabrice de Hilden about the middle of the seventeenth century

(Fabricius Hildanus, Francofurti, 1646), and Jean B. Verduc towards the end of the same century, 1696 (*Bandages et fractures*, 1696), also vaguely alluded to the separation of the upper epiphysis of the femur.

It was not, however, until the beginning of the eighteenth century that any real work on this subject appeared.

Both J. L. Petit (*Maladies des os*, Paris, 1705 ; also *Description exacte des os*, Leyden, 1709) and G. J. Duverney (*Maladies des os*, Paris, tom. i. 1751 ; also trans. by Sam. Ingham, Lond. 1762) allude to this injury in connection with fractures of the neck of the femur. While the former associated it with fractures themselves, the latter did not believe in its existence without some morbid condition of the bone (scurvy, &c.).

J. M. Schwartz mentioned the subject in his thesis (*Disputatio de ossium epiphysibus*, Lipsiæ, 1736).

Although, as we have seen, separations of the epiphyses were admitted as possible by so many writers from the earliest times, but little practical interest or importance can be attached to the published records before Reichel's special treatise in 1759, one hundred and thirty-seven years ago (M. Geo. Christian Reichel, *Dissertatio de epiphysium ab ossium diaphysi diductione*, Thesis, Lipsiæ, April 27, 1759 ; Edwardus Sandifort, *Thesaurus Dissertationum*. vol. i. Roterdami, 1768–78). He was the first author who had made a special study of these lesions and insisted upon their reality. The pathological specimens, however, brought forward by him appear to have been fractures which occurred in persons of very advanced years, for the three figures given by him as united epiphysial lesions are probably united fractures—two specimens of separation or fracture of the neck of the humerus, and one a spontaneous separation of the lower epiphysis of the femur. He was, nevertheless, the first to correctly distinguish traumatic separations from those due to disease (or spontaneous). From an examination of Reichel's plates, Delpech (*Chirurgie clinique*, 1823, tom. i. p. 246) doubted the real occurrence of epiphysial separation in these instances.

Reichel also described a case of separation of the upper epiphysis of the femur.

We then come down to Ambrosio Bertrandi of Turin, who, in an article in 1787, 'Della Separazione delle Epifisi delle ossa' (*Opere anatomiche et cerusiche : Malattie delle ossa*, Turin, 1787, tom. v. cap. xv. p. 156), noted one or two cases which he had established by dissection in infants ; but the data he gives are not very accurate, and cannot be relied upon as at all certain. He endeavoured to draw up a general description of these lesions, and was the first to direct attention to disjunction of the humeral epiphysis during delivery. He mentions instances at the upper extremities of the humerus and tibia, and at the lower extremity of the femur and ulna.

Rognetta and others also allude to another Italian surgeon,

Monteggia of Milan (Monteggia, *Instit. de chirurgie*, tom. iv., Milano, 1814), as having given some attention to this subject. Monteggia refers to cases at the upper extremity of the tibia and the lower extremity of the humerus.

J. B. Palletta, also an Italian surgeon (*Exercitationes anatomicæ*, Mediolani, 1820), likewise added a few new cases in support of the occurrence of this lesion.

Portal (in his *Anatomie médicale*, Paris, 1803, tóm. i. p. 31) says the epiphyses are sometimes detached from the body of the bones, especially in children. He believed that the upper extremity of the radius and the neck of the femur were the most frequent subjects of these disunions; and that, as they were often mistaken for dislocations of these bones, errors in their treatment took place.

De la Motte also mentions some cases of the same injury.

Petit-Radel (*Chir. encyclopéd.* art. ' Épiphyses,' tom. i. p. 433), like Bertrandi, added but little to the knowledge of the subject; while his article in ' L'Encyclopédie Méthodique ' is merely a translation of Bertrandi's work.

In 1816 M. J. Delpech, with much reason, seeing the uncertainty felt in the minds of surgeons by these first attempts at descriptions of these injuries, doubted the existence of the occurrence of detachment of the epiphyses. But some years later, in 1823 (*Chirurgie clinique de Montpellier*, tom. i. 1823), he was convinced of their occurrence after seeing the pathological specimens of separation of the lower epiphyses of the femur and of the radius described and recorded by M. Roux. In this volume Delpech describes the specimen of separation of the lower epiphysis of the femur published by M. Coural, and at that time in his possession (the first of Roux's specimens).

Boyer, about the year 1815, and likewise Dupuytren, dismissed the subject in a few words. The former only mentions (*Chir.* tom. iii. 4me édit. p. 211) the possibility of these lesions at the upper end of the femur and humerus, and asserts that they usually take the place of fractures.

In 1817 Champion (*Bull. de la Fac. et de la Soc. de Méd.*, Paris 1817) made careful observation of several cases, which he proved anatomically by examination after death (see also Champion, 'Décollement des épiphyses des os longs,' *Journal complém. du dict. d. sc. méd.*, Paris, 1818).

Laurent, in his article ' Observations pour servir à l'histoire du Décollement des épiphyses des os longs ' (*Journal complém. du dict. d. sc. méd.* Paris, 1818, tom. i. pp. 317–26), was unable to throw any fresh light upon the subject.

In England James Wilson (*Lectures on Diseases of the Bones and Joints*, London, 1820) added a few facts with regard to the mechanical production of these injuries; but he gives no description, and indeed makes no mention, of epiphysial separation as met with in the living subject. We shall allude to this again later on.

Epiphysial separations were described nearly at the same time by MM. Roux and Guéretin.

M. Roux de Brignolle wrote his thesis at Montpellier entitled *Dissertation sur la disjonction des épiphyses*, February 8, 1822. It contained a description of two specimens obtained by amputation : (1) Coural's case of separation of the lower epiphysis of the femur, which had occurred in 1816 ; and (2) a very remarkable case of disjunction of the lower epiphysis of the radius, the styloid epiphysis of the ulna, and the upper epiphysis of the first phalanges of the thumb, index, and middle fingers. This occurred in 1821. Both these cases are fully described in their proper chapters.

Roux says that his thesis was written to prove to some sceptical minds the possibility of such a lesion of the osseous system after the first few years of life. He insisted upon, 'first, the danger of ignoring epiphysial separation when its reduction ought to be possible ; secondly, the progress of the phenomena which result from such an error of judgment ; thirdly, the possibility of separation of the epiphyses occurring up to the eighteenth year ; fourthly, the possibility of such separation taking place on the largest cylindrical bones, as well as on the medium-sized and smallest.'

Writing in 1825 (*loc. cit. infra*), Jarjavay says : 'Aussi en clinique, il est bien difficile, sinon impossible dans certains cas, de déterminer si la lésion est un décollement plutôt qu'une fracture. Il ne faut pas perdre de vue, si l'on cherche à arriver à ce diagnostic, ce fait anatomique, à savoir, que les épiphyses ne comprennent généralement que les deux tiers seulement des extrémités des os longs, et que la diaphyse fournit l'autre tiers.'

Goyrand in 1836 published his first observations on separation of the lower epiphysis of the radius.

Guéretin's valuable work, 'Recherches sur le Décollement spontané et traumatique des Épiphyses' (*La Presse Médicale*, 10 Mai, 13 Mai, 17 Mai, 1837, i. No. 7, &c. pp. 290, 297, 305), was published in 1837, and added some important facts. This author collected a number of cases (forty-five) published up to this date. Many of these were fractures in adults, some were separations through disease. He also endeavoured by numerous experiments on the dead body, as well as by careful examination of clinical cases, to clear up the many obscure points with which the subject was then surrounded. But from want of sufficient material his descriptions were very incomplete, and many points of interest were not even mentioned.

Nearly a century after Reichel's thesis, M. Rognetta ('Mémoire sur la Divulsion traumatique des Épiphyses,' *Gazette Médicale*, Paris, 1834, p. 433) published an elaborate memoir upon traumatic separation of the epiphyses. To this interesting memoir we are indebted for much valuable information, and in it we find brought together everything bearing upon the subject that had been previously published. M. Rognetta has collected some instances of epiphysial separations met with in the trunk as well as in the long bones. His work is unfortunately too full of theories to the neglect of direct anatomical research, and he appears to believe in a simple separation of the epiphysial cartilage from the bone in most cases without any portion of the latter ever being dragged away.

M. Roux, fifteen years after the publication of his first work, states ('Sur le Décollement épiphysaire,' *La Presse Médicale*, Paris, 1837, tom. i. No. 55, July 12, 436–438) that on August 30, 1836, he communicated a memoir to l'Académie Royale de Médecine containing several (4) new cases of epiphysial separation occurring in his practice, but only one of these was verified by direct examination.

Sir Astley Cooper in England, in his *Fractures and Dislocations* (new edition by Bransby B. Cooper, 1842), was one of the first to clearly point out that epiphysial separations are mostly mistaken for dislocations rather than for fractures. He especially so alludes to this lesion at the lower end of the humerus. He has added one or two interesting cases.

In 1840 M. Piscart, in his inaugural thesis (Thèse de Paris, 1840, No. 219), indicated the occurrence of traumatic separation during delivery and after birth. Champmas' thesis in the same year (Thèse de Paris, 1840, No. 139) furnished no further facts for the elucidation of these injuries beyond those of his predecessors (especially Rognetta).

The distinguished Nélaton, in his *Éléments de pathologie chirurgicale* (tom. i. p. 678, sec. 3: 'Divulsion traumatique des Épiphyses'), treats the subject in the following manner :

'Bien que les décollements des épiphyses se trouvent indiqués dans les livres hippocratiques, et que depuis Ambroise Paré un grand nombre d'auteurs aient parlé de cette lésion, on peut cependant affirmer que nous manquons de documents nécessaires pour faire un exposé dogmatique de cette affection. En effet, presque tout ce que nous possédons sur ce sujet se réduit à des assertions sans preuves et à quelques observations sans valeur, à cause de l'absence complète des détails.' However, he quoted some valuable examples which were known at that time.

Voillemier, in 1842, made a special study of the mechanism of separation of the lower epiphysis of the radius.

M. Salmon's doctoral thesis on traumatic solutions of continuity of the bones during youth (P. A. Salmon, *Des solutions de continuité traumatiques des os dans le jeune âge*, Thèse de Paris, 1845) contains out of 129 cases a description of sixty-eight experiments on the upper extremity, in which he detached the epiphyses by extension of the fore-arm on the arm. They are mostly (64) of the lower end of the humerus, one of the internal epicondyle, two of the upper end of the ulna, and one of the upper end of the radius. This series of experiments contributed some details as to the anatomical character of separations. Salmon was the first to prove that when the periosteum is lacerated, the separation is accompanied by displacement. He also noted the frequency of separation, and the easy mode of its production at the upper end of the femur in newly born infants (ten out of eleven being in infants less than a month old), but he was unable to detach the upper epiphysis of the humerus. Those of the upper end of the femur were, as he describes, a detachment of the whole cartilaginous end of the bone, to which he alludes in an earlier part of his thesis. Salmon's thesis is, however, entirely without clinical cases.

Detachment of the cartilaginous ends of the bones during delivery was especially investigated by M. Pajot in his thesis *Des lésions traumatiques que le fœtus peut éprouver pendant l'accouchement*, Paris 1853.

Prof. R. W. Smith, of Dublin, showed (*Treatise on Fractures in the Vicinity of Joints*, Dublin, 1847) a very clear conception of one or two of these lesions, and paid considerable attention to the subject. His accounts of certain forms of separation of the upper and lower epiphyses of the humerus and of that of the lower end of the radius are still regarded as most trustworthy descriptions (see also, *Dublin Quarterly Journal of Med. Science*, vol. ix. New Series, 1850, p. 63).

Cruveilhier, writing in 1849 (*Traité d'anatomie pathologique*, Paris, tom. i. p. 101), says of the thirty-eight cases of traumatic epiphysial separation then known to science, that there was but little reliance to be placed on them.

E. E. Klein devoted a thesis to this subject (*De epiphys. dissolutione*, Diss. inaug., Gryphiæ, 1854; see also C. R. Zuehlke, *De diastasi epiphysium et ossium diaphysi*. Halis Sax. 1859).

Dr. J. Ludw. Thudichum appears ('Die Absprengung der Epiphysen,' *Münchener illustrirte medicin. Zeitung*, 1855, Bd. iii. s. 188) to have given some attention to fracture of the epiphyses, and furnishes a brief account of epiphysial separation of most of the long bones. Thudichum also wrote 'Ueber die am oberen Ende des Humerus vorkommenden Knochenbrüche,' Giessen, 1851.

Malgaigne admitted (*Traité des fractures*, 1855) the occurrence of epiphysial separations as proved by dissection at both ends of the humerus, femur, and tibia, and at the lower end of the radius, and ranked them among fractures because they have 'the same causes, present the same symptoms, call for the same treatment, and, lastly, cannot always be exactly distinguished from fractures properly so called.' He therefore did not attach much importance to distinguishing between them. He considered, and rightly so, that in the majority of cases there is a more or less considerable detachment of the osseous end of the shaft. Malgaigne attributed the first distinct and satisfactory notice of separation of the epiphysis to Bertrandi towards the close of the last century. He quoted several cases, and also added that he knew of no instance occurring in a female.

These lesions were also especially alluded to by Gurlt (*Handbuch der Lehre von den Knochenbrüchen*, Berlin, 1862). This author carefully collected the literature of the subject up to this date, and after the examination of anatomical specimens, experiments, and clinical cases, came to the conclusion that epiphysial separations were very rare injuries. He thought that this was to be accounted for by the fact that the epiphyses, being in relation to the diaphyses larger in infants than at a later period, were less frequently the subject of injury, and that infants were less exposed to external injury than children at puberty, when epiphysial separation very unfrequently occurred. Gurlt collected eighteen cases verified by dissection.

Bardeleben, in his 'Handbook of Surgery,' agreed with Gurlt's decision.

Another French surgeon, M. Foucher, in 1860 ('Recherches sur la disjonction traumatique des épiphyses,' *Monit. des Sciences méd. et pharm.* No. 90, 1860 ; *Annales du Congrès médical de Rouen*, 1863), added some valuable experimental knowledge of the subject, gave a clear description of the pathology of the lesion, indicated several varieties of separation, and drew up a classification which is even now more or less adhered to. His experimental work is still the best on the subject, and he summed up in a very complete manner all that was known up to that time as to the mechanism of these lesions. Nevertheless this author states that separation is effected with great difficulty even in infants. In 1863 Foucher collected a number of cases ('De la Divulsion des Épiphyses,' *Cong. méd. de France*, Paris, 1863, tom. i. pp. 63–72).

Prof. R. W. Smith, writing in 1865 and 1867 (*British Medical Journal*, August 17, 1867), believed them to be very frequent and common. This view was also held by Broca and Uffelman. Smith has described many interesting specimens and cases which still maintain their value to the practical surgeon.

Dr. A. Coulon, in 1861 (*Traité des fractures chez les enfants*, Paris, 1861), totally denied the existence of these injuries, notwithstanding the writings of M. Guéretin and Rognetta. He came to this conclusion after many years' experience at children's hospitals, and quotes (Richet, *Anatomie chirurgicale*, p. 64) M. Richet's decision in the following words: 'A l'état normal, l'union est si intime entre le cartilage de conjugaison et le tissu osseux en voie de formation, qu'on peut les regarder comme un seul organe, les vaisseaux sanguins se portant sans interruption de la diaphyse dans l'épiphyse. Howship, qui avait étudié avec le plus grand soin ce point d'anatomie, a dit, avec raison, que le cartilage épiphysaire était continu et non pas contigu à l'os. C'est donc une erreur de dire que le cartilage de conjugaison et l'os se touchent par deux surfaces, l'une osseuse et l'autre cartilagineuse, onduleuses et anfractueuses, se recevant réciproquement ; ce n'est qu'après macération qu'on trouve cette disposition, car, à l'état sain et frais, le cartilage et l'os ne font qu'un, il y a fusion intime, continuité en un mot.

'Cette remarque conduit à rejeter le décollement des épiphyses admis par quelques chirurgiens, puisque la diaphyse et l'épiphyse ne sont pas accolées, mais bien réunies par l'intermédiaire de leur cartilage de conjugaison ; et quand, par suite de violences extérieures, il y a séparation en ce point, c'est une véritable fracture comme celles qui s'opèrent dans la continuité des os. M. Guéretin (loc. cit.), MM. Cruveilhier et Bonamy (Traité d'anatomie pathologique, tom. i.), qui, dans le but d'éclaircir cette question, se sont livrés à une série d'expériences et de recherches, ont vu à peu près constamment que l'épiphyse, en se séparant, entraînait toujours avec elle une lamelle plus ou moins considérable du tissu osseux ; et les faits de disjonction des épiphyses observés sur le vivant ont présenté le même phénomène. A la rigueur, cependant, on conçoit que le cartilage de conjugaison puisse se rompre précisément au niveau de sa fusion avec le tissu osseux, et les faits observés par Bertrandi sur la tête du fémur et celle de l'humérus, par MM. J. Cloquet et Rognetta sur l'extrémité inférieure du radius, tendent à prouver que la brisure peut quelquefois avoir lieu dans ce point même et sans solution de continuité du tissu osseux ; mais, dans ce cas encore, c'est à une fracture et non à un décollement simple que l'on a affaire, puisque l'inspection anatomique a prouvé qu'il y avait fusion des deux tissus.

'Ce n'est là d'ailleurs, il faut bien en convenir, qu'une discussion sans importance pratique, puisque le pronostic et le traitement de ces prétendus décollements épiphysaires sont identiques avec ceux des fractures des extrémités articulaires complétement ossifiées.'

M. Coulon, after quoting Malgaigne's words, sums up the matter by saying that traumatic separation of the epiphyses is extremely rare, that it is recognised by the same signs as fracture in the neighbourhood of the joints, that its gravity is the same, and that it demands the same treatment.

In Russia these injuries have been studied by Michniowsky, especially by means of experiments ('Untersuchungen über den Heilungsvorgang bei gewaltsamer Epiphysenlösung,' Militärärztl. Journal (Russisch), 1864 ; Petersb. Med. Zeitschr. 1866, Bd. x. s. 300).

Richet, denying the existence of true separation, considered, from the anatomical evidence which could then be produced, that the cases brought forward by Bertrandi, Cloquet, and Rognetta of solution at the site of the epiphysial junction were really fractures.

Guersant (Chirurgie des enfants), during twenty years' service at the Children's Hospital, met with very few instances.

The injuries were the subject of a special discussion at the Société de Chirurgie de Paris in 1865, by many able surgeons, on

M. Dolbeau presenting before the society two specimens of separation of the lower epiphysis of the radius (*Gazette des Hôpitaux*, 1865, No. 145, 147; Extract in New Sydenham Society's *Retrospect*, 1865–6, p. 248). M. Marjolin believed separations of the epiphyses to be so extremely rare that their existence might almost be denied, and produced in proof of this opinion some details of fractures at the Hôpital Ste. Eugénie which showed, at any rate, that they had been very rarely diagnosed at the hospital from which his statistics were drawn. Out of 600 fractures in children, he found no cases of separation of the epiphyses. He added Malgaigne's opinion that this lesion was rarely perfect, being almost always accompanied by a fracture of the diaphysis which adhered to the epiphysis. M. Guersant also said that he had never been able to diagnose the injury with certainty, nor had he ever had occasion to verify it anatomically, but spoke in favour of its occurrence. M. Chassaignac expressed his opinion that true separation of the epiphyses hardly ever occurred ; that a small portion of the shaft almost always adhered to the epiphysial cartilage, and that it was impossible to make a special diagnosis. M. Trélat maintained that an epiphysial separation, from a surgical point of view, in symptoms and cure, in contradistinction to a fracture, was not to be accepted. M. Broca, however, reminded the Society that the injury could easily be produced in the dead subject, and therefore was very probably more frequent in the living than was supposed. In experiments on the dead subject, the cartilage was usually found attached to the epiphysis. M. Richet and M. Blot spoke in the same sense.

M. A. T. Cosseret's doctoral thesis, *De la divulsion des épiphyses* (Thèse de doctorat, Paris,. 1866, No. 141), was suggested by Foucher's work in 1860 (*loc. cit. supra*), but contains little of importance in addition to what had been previously written. He adhered to the opinion of Malgaigne, Marjolin, Coulon, and others by placing these lesions amongst fractures.

Bouchut describes (*Traité des maladies des enfants*, 1867) separation of the epiphyses in young children in his article on fractures, but gives no examples. He states that in this solution of continuity of the bone there is no rupture of the osseous tissue, and that the injuries are generally produced by. a considerable strain on the articulation, and are not as a rule the result of a direct blow. He also says that besides the pain and swelling, there is preternatural mobility, and often a dull *grating* crepitus, very different from the crepitus of bone.

The labours of Professor Ollier did much to put epiphysial separations on a well merited footing. By his researches on the regeneration of bones (*Traité de la régénération des os*, tom. i. 1867), on the unequal growth of the two extremities of the long bones, and on the physiology, anatomy, and pathology of the diaphyso-epiphysial region, a complete study has been permitted of these interesting lesions. He calls these lesions *diaphysial separations* because the separation almost always takes place between the diaphysis and the cartilage, and not between the latter and the epiphysis.

Professor Poncet, of Lyons ('Des Déformations produites par l'arrêt d'accroissement d'un des Os de l'avant-bras,' *Lyon Médical,* 1872), has also given some valuable remarks upon the arrest of development following lesions of the epiphysial cartilages, and upon the deformities which result from them, in the parallel bones of the forearm and leg.

Epiphysial separation was the subject of M. Jules Colignon's thesis (*De la disjonction traumatique des épiphyses,* Thèse de Paris, 1868, No. 226), especially as regards the lower epiphysis of the radius. Some interesting experiments on the dead body were included, and the number of published cases was brought up to seventy-nine; many, however, of these were very incomplete. This thesis was based upon those of Guéretin and Foucher, the former of which was one of the best memoirs then published.

Even up to that date the possibility of these injuries on the living subject was still doubted by certain authors. M. Colignon brought some exact clinical observations to bear upon the question, the study of which by means of post-mortem experiments had now been fairly well carried out.

From this time the pathological and clinical observations of many authors began to place the study of the lesions upon a firmer basis.

Mr. Timothy Holmes, in his *Diseases of Children,* 1868, attached some importance to these injuries, and drew some conclusions from a study of the museum specimens then existing in the London hospitals. His inquiries, he says, were due to his desire of testing the relative accuracy of M. Chassaignac's and Professor Smith's opinions on this subject. He thought the precise line of solution of continuity was the chief point of importance in the probability of suspension of growth after such injuries. 'Thus it is seen that out of the preparations from the lower end of the femur, three are uncomplicated with visible fracture—one in early infancy, the other two in late puberty; and that these are the only genuine specimens of epiphysiary disjunction which our museums contain; the two of the fibula at St. George's being somewhat doubtful, and that of the upper end of the ulna in infancy rather a fracture of the cartilaginous extremity of the bone than a separation of its epiphysis, which at that early age can hardly be said to exist, at any rate has not begun to ossify.'

Émile Barbarin, in his thesis (*Contribution à l'étude des fractures chez les enfants,* 1873), while admitting the occurrence of epiphysial disjunctions, thought, nevertheless, that they were rare in practice.

M. Alfred Leblois (*Contribution à l'étude des fractures chez les enfants et de leur traitement,* Paris, 1894) alludes to them in a cursory manner.

Manquat, in his essay ' Sur les Décollements épiphysaires trauma-tiques' (Thèse de Paris, 1877), collected 130 cases of epiphysial separa-tion—all of which had been previously published. Even at this period he believed they were rare accidents. He classed 'toute solution de continuité brusque survenant par le fait d'un traumatisme entre la diaphyse et l'épiphyse d'un os au niveau du cartilage épiphysaire' as traumatic epiphysial separation.

In the same year Professor Novaro (*Gazzetta delle cliniche*, 1877), whilst referring to a clinical case of separation of the upper epiphysis of the humerus, briefly expounded traumatic separation of the epiphyses in general.

Writing in 1878 M. E. Pingaud (*Dict. encycl. des Sciences médicales*, I^{me} sec. tom. xxi. p. 627) thought that all cases should be considered as true fractures. He says : ' Et d'ailleurs, comment une semblable séparation pourrait-elle avoir lieu, quand on considère combien est intime, à l'état physiologique, l'union qui existe entre le cartilage de conjugaison et le tissu osseux en voie de formation ? Car il n'y a pas simplement juxtaposition entre ces deux parties de l'os, mais fusion complète, continuité absolue de tissu ; à l'état frais, l'os et le cartilage ne font qu'un, et les vaisseaux sanguins se portent sans interruption de l'un à l'autre. Le périosté enfin, très dense et très adhérent au niveau de la ligne de conjugaison, ajoute encore à la solidité de l'union de l'épiphyse avec la diaphyse. Quand donc une violence extérieure paraît diviser un os au niveau de la ligne de con-jugaison dia-épiphysaire, il y a toujours une véritable fracture, le cartilage, en raison de son élasticité et de sa ténacité, arrachant toujours, plutôt que de céder, une lamelle plus ou moins considérable de tissu osseux. Il suffit d'ailleurs de considérer la forme du segment détaché pour voir de suite qu'il n'est pas uniquement constitué par l'épiphyse, et que la calotte diaphysaire qui le pénètre a été arrachée en même temps que lui.'

Professor Syme, in 1842, wrote on diastasis or separation of the epiphyses thus : ' The symptoms resemble those which would result from fracture in the same situation, and the treatment does not in any respect require to be different' (*Principles of Surgery*, p. 179, 1842).

Sir William Fergusson also wrote (*System of Practical Surgery*, 1846, p. 123) : ' No particular allusions will be made to separation of the epiphyses—diastasis, as the accident is called—a kind of injury which is occasionally met with in the young subject; and the reason for this is, that I know of no difference of treatment which such cases may require, whilst every anatomist must be aware that a solution of continuity is as likely to occur in such a situation as elsewhere. If they deserve especial comment, it is that crepitus will probably be less distinct; and also with reference to the proximity of the injury to the joint; but on the latter point, the principles of treatment for ordinary fractures are equally applicable, whilst if the symptoms are so obscure as to make crepitus essential to the diagnosis, it is evident that if there be a fracture at all, it must certainly be one of a most simple character.'

Joseph Amesbury, in his work on 'Fractures of the Trunk and Extremities,' does not even allude to the possibility of epiphysial injury.

In 1862 Gurlt was able to collect only eighteen cases of separation of the epiphyses during life, in which the diagnosis was verified by dissection; of these, five were of the humerus (four being of the upper and one of the lower end), four of the lower end of the radius, five of the lower end of the femur, and three of the tibia. Gurlt was of opinion that separation was a rare form of accident.

Writing in 1863, Stimson says that his experience of these injuries was limited to two cases, both compound, one of the proximal phalanx of the great toe and the other of the upper end of the fibula.

In a later edition of his work, Syme, in 1866 (*Principles of Surgery*, 4th edit. 1866, p. 170), dismissed the subject in the following words : 'Before the epiphyses are united to their respective shafts, they are apt to suffer separation from them by such violence as, in the adult, would occasion fracture of the bones concerned, or dislocation of their articulating extremities.'

Holmes says, in 1869 : ' The conclusion to which my experience of this injury would lead me is, that fracture occurs not very rarely at or in the immediate neighbourhood of the epiphysial line ; that the line of fracture coincides in these cases partially with that of the epiphysial cartilage, but seldom completely ; that the general symptoms are therefore the same as those of fracture, while the special symptoms must be sought for from the anatomy of each joint.'

It is thus only during the last twenty years that traumatic separations of the epiphyses began to be generally admitted, and described with any accuracy. But there can now be no doubt of their frequent occurrence ; and in this country their importance has been often alluded to for many years by Mr. Jonathan Hutchinson, Professor Sir George Humphry, and others.

Their chief exponent is Mr. Jonathan Hutchinson, who has from time to time since the forties published a number of cases and specimens bearing out the reality of these lesions, and also the not infrequent result of loss of growth in length of the bone affected.

Mr. Hilton and his surgical colleagues at Guy's Hospital were also amongst the first to point out many important details respecting these injuries.

Mr. T. Bryant, in his *Practice of Surgery* and elsewhere, has published numerous cases of separation of the various epiphyses, many of them of great value and many showing arrest of growth.

The London hospital is indebted to Mr. Nathaniel Ward for many specimens in its museum, and others have been added by Mr. Hutchinson.

As to our current works on surgery, we find these injuries are still scarcely mentioned in many of them, while only a few give any information with reference to them. Though not so common as fractures, the number of separations now recorded leads to a more careful investigation of their clinical signs.

We find, even as late as 1884, Hamilton, in his *Fractures and Dislocations*, 7th edit. p. 37, stating : ' *Epiphysial separations* we shall not hesitate to class with fractures, and to submit them to the same rules of nomenclature. These accidents rarely occur after the twentieth year of life ; since after this period, and in the case of some bones at a much earlier period, the epiphyses are usually united to the diaphyses by bone.' However, he gave a distinct heading to many of these injuries, and in a few cases considered their diagnosis from fractures. He published a number of new cases from his own observation.

Even at the present day we see that there are very contradictory opinions with regard to these injuries ; one surgeon detects them very frequently while another never does so, or only admits that they are rarely met with. This difference of opinion has been due in part to the absence hitherto of direct examination in a large proportion of cases, and in part to the ease with which epiphysial separation may be confused with dislocation or fracture of the end of the diaphysis.

Numerous cases followed by an autopsy or by amputation, others in which the presence of a wound has permitted a direct examination of the separated fragments, and many instances in which an open operation has been undertaken in simple cases for replacement of fragments, have now clearly and definitely established the frequent occurrence of epiphysial separation.

Germany has furnished us with two important monographs on the subject by P. Vogt and Paul Bruns, both of which appeared in Langenbeck's Archiv (*Archiv für klin. Chirurg.* 1878 and 1882), and proved that these injuries are by no means so rare as had been previously held by some. Vogt believed that separation without displacement was common in early life. Paul Bruns has published a large series of cases (verified by an autopsy) for statistical purposes, and in order to throw some light upon their history and after consequences. He collected eighty-one such cases and added three from his clinic at Tübingen. He believed the injury to be not at all an uncommon one, and that if he had included simple cases the number collected would have been much greater.

Some other French writers have contributed special articles on one or other of the epiphyses (Delens, *Archives générales de Méd.* 1884, p. 272 ; Farabeuf, *Bull. et Mém. de la Société de Chir.*, Paris, tom. xii., 1886, p. 692 ; Bergès, Thèse de Paris, 1890).

In 1882 Dr. Erasmo De Paoli published (*Del distacco traumatico delle epifisi*, Torino, 1882) a concise account of these injuries, adding some new cases and experiments of his own.

G. Mazziotti has also furnished some articles (' Del distacco delle epifisi, e sue differenze dalla frattura,' *Giorn. internaz. d. sc. med.*, Napoli, 1880, ii. p. 957 ; *ibid.* 1882, new series, iv. p. 371 ; also *Ann. clin. d. osp. incur.*, Napoli, 1882, viii. p. 162).

' The diagnosis of traumatic separation of the epiphyses' formed the subject of a paper read by the author before the West Kent Medico-Chirurgical Society in April 1886.* In this paper attention was drawn to the frequent occurrence of separation *without displacement*, especially at the lower end of the femur, and to the common escape from injury of the neighbouring joint in many of the more simple separations, e.g. at the lower end of the radius. Allusion was also made for the first time to the gradual displacement of the diaphysis or epiphysis subsequent to the accident in instances in which the lesion had been overlooked or not diagnosed. This want of recognition the author believed to be due to the absence of displacement at the time of the accident. Permanent deformity and pressure upon important structures, leading to disastrous consequences, resulted in several cases. After examination of the specimens in the hospital museums of London and other cities, and after collecting statistics, the fact was noted that the epiphyses of certain bones, from their anatomical peculiarities, were more liable to be broken off at particular ages than at others.

The thesis of Dittmayer deals with arrest of growth in length following traumatic separation of the epiphyses, and that of Wilhelm Stehr with arrest of growth of the radius following epiphysial separation (Dittmayer, Thèse de Wurtzbourg, 1887 ; Wilhelm Stehr, Thèse de Tübingen, 1889).

M. Joseph Curtillet has given (*Du décollement traumatique des épiphyses*, Lyon, 1891, pp. 107) the proportion of cases of epiphysial separation to those of ordinary fracture met with in children as twenty to a hundred. His figures were taken from cases under the care of M. Vincent of Lyons.

In 1891 Mr. Jonathan Hutchinson, jun., was awarded the Jacksonian Prize at the Royal College of Surgeons for his essay upon ' Injuries to the Epiphyses of Long Bones,' and he has supplemented much of his father's work in this direction.

He embodied this work in his lectures in 1893 on ' Injuries to the Epiphyses and their Results,' delivered at the Royal College of Surgeons.

* (Printed in *Pediatrics*, New York and London. Vol. iv. No. 2 July 15, 1897, p. 49).

CHAPTER II

ANATOMY

A KNOWLEDGE of the bones is imperfect without an accurate and complete acquaintance with the anatomy and connections of the epiphyses.

In his address on surgery at the British Medical Association (*loc. cit. infra*) Professor R. W. Smith said : 'When the surgeon is called upon for his opinion respecting the nature of injuries occurring in the vicinity of the larger joints in early life, he will find a knowledge of the anatomy of the epiphyses of the greatest importance.' This instruction, however, is seldom afforded to students during their anatomical course.

Very false conceptions as to the parts included in the epiphyses and diaphyses have led to many errors in diagnosis, and in many cases, it might be added, to improper treatment.

We find during the development of the bones that the boundary line between the epiphysis and the diaphysis alters its relationship very considerably with regard both to those parts, to the neighbouring joint, and to other surrounding structures.   Marked examples of this may be seen at the lower end of the humerus and the upper end of the femur.   In the latter the whole upper extremity in infancy comprises the head, neck, and greater and lesser trochanters in one cartilaginous mass, but, as age advances, the head and trochanters form separate epiphyses by the upward growth of the neck from the diaphysis.

Not only do the individual epiphyses alter their relationship with the corresponding diaphyses during the different stages of their development, but the same epiphysis will have a very different anatomical appearance at different periods—e.g. during infancy and during adolescence—at one time forming a relatively large portion of the end of the bone, and at another time a small one, as at the upper end of the humerus.

Diaphysis.—The long bones have a large epiphysis at each end of the diaphysis, with the exception of the clavicle, the metacarpus, the metatarsus, and the phalanges of the hand and foot, which have only one.

It will be seen later on that the epiphyses of the long bones in children do not comprise the whole of the end of the bone as seen in the adult, but only about two-thirds, the remaining third (e.g. the lower end of the humerus) being formed by the diaphysis (Cruveilhier).

At birth the epiphyses are almost entirely cartilaginous, with the exception of the lower epiphysis of the femur and the upper epiphysis of the tibia, and are somewhat larger in proportion to the diaphysis than they are when their ossification is complete. , By the process of ossification advancing into the epiphysial cartilage from the diaphysial end the epiphysis becomes, as a rule, relatively smaller towards its diaphysial surface. This may be readily seen on comparing the upper end of the humerus in infancy and at puberty. In the case of the long bones the whole diaphyses are ossified at birth. The bones, at first entirely cartilaginous, are invested with a perichondrium which is comparable to the periosteum of later years and which similarly consists of a superficial and a deep layer. The superficial layer, like that of the periosteum, passes over the articulations as its capsule, and the deep layer unites with the cartilaginous end of the bone, blending with it at the level which marks later on the union of the epiphysis and the diaphysis.

The long bones increase in length rather than in thickness from the time of birth up to the sixth or seventh year by the process of ectochondral ossification, precisely similar to that of a centre of ossification. The growth and ossification of the cartilage take place on the diaphysial aspect only—in fact, according to Busch, the exclusive function of this cartilage is the ossification of the shaft. John Hunter proved experimentally on animals that the increase in length of long bone took place at the epiphysis. His experiments were adopted and corroborated by Béclard.

The unequal growth of the two ends of the diaphysis has also been conclusively proved experimentally by Hales, Ollier (*De l'inégalité d'accroissement des deux extrémités des os longs chez l'homme*, Paris, 1863; *Mémoires de la Société des Sciences Médicales de Lyon*), Duhamel (*Histoire de l'Académie des Sciences*, 1743), Leser (Langenbeck's *Archiv f. klin. Chirurg.*, Bd. xxxvii. 1880), Flourens (P. Flourens, *Théorie expérimentale de la formation des os*, 1847; 'Sur le développement des os en longueur,' *Gaz. des Hôp.*, Paris, 1861, xxxiv. p. 74; also *Ann. de la Chir. franç. et étrang.*, Paris, 1844, xii. p. 170; and *ibid.*, 1845, xv. 230–39; also, *Recherches sur le développement des os et des dents*, Paris, 1842); and others have fully confirmed the experimental results obtained by these authors.

In every long bone ossification proceeds more rapidly in one direction than another; hence increase in length takes place by the growth of the cartilage continuing at the opposite end. While the elongation of the long bones is chiefly the result of addition to the

c

58

shaft at the epiphysial junctions, the growth takes place more rapidly and is continued longer at the end where the epiphysis is last united. The oblique direction of the vascular canals is due to this inequality of growth, which causes a shifting of the periosteum investing the greater part of the shaft, and so draws the proximal portion of the medullary artery towards the more rapidly growing end, and gives rise to its canal.

The newly formed bone in contact with the diaphysial side of the conjugal cartilage is exceedingly vascular. The medullary canals, therefore, run in the direction of the end in which ossification is progressing most rapidly and away from the end in which increase in length takes place. As Humphry points out, this is in order to maintain the proper relative position of the soft parts which exists during the period of growth. After piercing the shaft the nutrient artery, as seen in the cartilaginous state of the diaphysis, divides into two chief branches which extend upwards and downwards towards either end of the bone. Other branches are given off from these which finally reach the epiphyses.

In his excellent description of the nutrient canals and the growth of the long bones, Schwalbe, in 1876, has given a true account of the position of the nutrient canal in relation to the ends of the bones.

While the two ends of the diaphysis take an unequal share in the increase in length, there is a difference for each particular bone. Thus in the tibia and humerus the upper ends, in the femur and bones of the forearm the lower ends, are in this respect the most active.

Individuality plays so important a part in the rate of growth in length in the long bones and in the union of the shaft with the ends, that it has been found extremely difficult to give precise figures. According to Topinard, individual variations are numerous, and doubtless both race and sex influence the time of union of the epiphysis and diaphysis; the state of health or disease also must modify the process, seeing that the growth of bone is only the expression of the rate of ossification and renewal of calcareous material, which must be considerably influenced by a good or bad nutritive process. This increase of the diaphysis at the extremities will be found to be almost entirely due to that part of the conjugal cartilage, or disc, which is in contact with the diaphysis. Excision of the epiphysis itself, leaving this cartilage, was found by Ollier to lead only to a temporary checking of nutrition and arrest of growth of the bone. The conjugal cartilage still proliferated and produced new osseous material.

Duhamel in 1743, as regards the tibia, recognised that the upper end increased more than the lower; this was also seen by Flourens a hundred years later in 1847. The difference in the growth of the long bones according to their ends was established in 1852 by the researches of Broca who was one of the first to make experiments on this subject; and by Ollier and Humphry in 1861 (*Med. Chirurg. Transactions*, vol. xlv. 1862).

The difference in the increase in length of the ends of the long bones is manifested from birth, and does not depend upon the early or late period of union of the epiphysis with the diaphysis, although there is a relationship between these two, for it is the epiphysis which joins on last that grows the most; but they do not depend one on another—they are both the expression of a general condition (Ollier). Furthermore, experimental researches, clinical and post-mortem experience have proved conclusively that the value of each epiphysis of the long bones for the growth in length is very different in the various periods of young life.

Besides this increase in length of the long bones from their ends, it has been asserted recently by some German authors that a certain amount of increase may be met with interstitially; for in the adult an increase in length of the long bones has been noted in more than one specimen, even long after the disappearance of the epiphysial cartilage. These cases must be regarded as belonging rather to pathological than normal anatomy.

Epiphysis. *Structure.*—The epiphyses are either for the formation of the joints, for the attachment of tendons or ligaments, or for the development in length of the bone, but more frequently they fulfil all these functions at the same time. They have a sort of independent existence from the rest of the bone, being supplementary processes designed to protect the functions of the part whilst the diaphysial ossification is extending. In certain bones, therefore—the outer end of the clavicle, the metacarpus and metatarsus, for example—we see the diaphysial ossification extending to the end of the bone. The epiphyses are, proportionately to the diaphyses, larger in early infancy than later on, and at first sight this relatively large size of the joints in infancy would appear to be more favourable to receive external violence and predispose to epiphysial separation. Yet this is not borne out by facts. About the second or third year the epiphyses become less bulky and the periosteum begins to diminish in thickness, while at the tenth and on to the fifteenth year they have very much diminished in size relatively to their diaphyses.

The epiphyses, when fully formed, are somewhat similar in structure to the short bones of the body, being composed of spongy cancellous tissue, arranged in a definite and distinct mechanical manner and surrounded by a thin layer of compact bone. Their diaphysial surface is not smooth but covered with small mamillary projections and pits which accurately fit corresponding depressions and ridges on the end of the diaphysis, strengthening the union between the epiphysis and diaphysis. On the diaphysial ends of some of the long bones, as at the lower end of the tibia, these ridges and elevations are arranged in a very definite manner.

The epiphyses at the two ends of the diaphysis of the long bones at the period of maturity freely communicate by means of openings into the medullary canal, the alveoli of the spongy epiphysial tissue at this period passing into those of the diaphysis.

It is only in rickets and some other pathological conditions that the cartilaginous line is penetrated by blood vessels; the epiphysial cartilage, small though it may be, will in the normal state completely shut off the alveolar spaces of the epiphysis from those of the diaphysis.

The epiphyses obtain their blood supply from the periosteal network of arteries, large branches of which perforate the thin layer of compact tissue on their exterior, and are distributed throughout the spongy cancellous tissue. Nearly the whole of the blood supply is therefore independent of the diaphysis. Only one or two minute arteries pass into the epiphyses from the diaphyses through the conjugal cartilage. This accounts for the comparatively infrequent occurrence of necrosis of the epiphysis in traumatic separation of the epiphysis even when the diaphysis is more or less completely displaced from off the epiphysis.

According to many observers, the veins are enclosed in distinct channels formed of thin plates of bone, and have very thin walls.

Ossification.—In the ossification (endochondral) of the cartilaginous ends of the bones the cells are collected into columns, which are usually in a direction parallel to the long axis of the bone, separated by the cartilaginous matrix, which becomes granular, calcifies, and forms between the altered cartilage cells areolæ or meshes. In this calcified matrix the osteoblastic material is very soon deposited and blood vessels form. This material breaks the meshes up by absorption (chiefly through the medium of the osteoblasts) and forms secondary areolæ. These areolæ contain the osteoblasts and some giant cells. The vessels shoot from the periphery towards the centre point of the cartilaginous end. The osteoblasts become separated from one another by an intercellular matrix entering into a calcareous condition and surrounding the osteoblasts, which now become the bone corpuscles and communicate with one another by means of the canaliculi. Ossification takes place from the centre of the epiphysis towards the periphery. It commences in the cartilaginous epiphysis by one or more central points or nuclei, and extends by the same process of intracartilaginous ossification peripherally until all the epiphysis is invaded and occupied by osseous material except a narrow line of cartilage usually called the epiphysial cartilage or disc at the junction with the shaft.

For instance, in the lower end of the humerus there are four such centres, in the upper end two, at each end of the femur only one.

The principal osseous centres appear gradually in the epiphyses of the long bones up to about the eighth year, each epiphysis having its own special time for appearance, subject to some variation according to the individual, &c. The centres for the lower epiphysis of the femur and the upper epiphysis of the tibia are the first to appear.

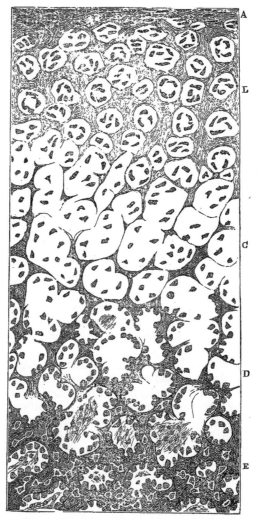

Fig. 1.—LONGITUDINAL SECTION OF EPIPHYSIS OF THE FEMUR OF A HUMAN FŒTUS
(BURDON-SANDERSON)

A and B, pure hyaline cartilage of the joint; C, layers in which the cartilage capsules are distinctly enlarged, i.e. where the intercellular substance is diminished; at D, the cell elements (derived from the cartilage cell of the cartilage capsule) begin to place themselves in regular order peripherally; the intercellular substance still further diminishes and passes over into bony trabeculæ—the embryonal bony tissue of the layer E; in this layer he cell elements of the spaces, which answer to the cartilage capsules of the previous layer D, have precisely the position of osteoblasts.

M. Arthaud says that the epiphyses corresponding to ginglymoid joints ossify much earlier than those of orbicular joints; but this rule is far from a universal one—e.g. the upper end of the humerus, corresponding to the orbicular shoulder joint, ossifies sooner than the lower end.

From a series of experiments, J. B. Sutton (*Journal of Anatomy and Physiology*, xvii. p. 479) was induced to formulate the following new and general rule: 'The centres of ossification appear earliest for those epiphyses which bear the largest relative proportion to the shafts of the bones to which they belong.' His intention was to show that the ratio of a terminal cartilage to the diaphysis being given, on referring to the table (which he arranged) the date of appearance of its ossific centre might be inferred with a tolerable amount of accuracy.

The epiphysis ossifies first at the end where the greatest increase in length takes place, but the epiphysis joins the shaft first towards the end where ossification of the shaft progresses most rapidly—that is, the end towards which the nutrient canal slants or is directed. Growth of the long bones, therefore, takes place more rapidly, and is continued longer, at the end where the epiphysis is last united to the shaft. But the direction of the nutrient canal has of itself no importance as regards the increase in length of the bone—it is only a curious coincidence in man which is not found in other animals (Ollier). Bérard, in a memoir (*Archives gén. de méd.*, févr. 1837) on the relationship which exists between the direction of the medullary canals of the long bones and the order in which the epiphyses join, was the first to enunciate the law that *of the two ends of a long bone, it is always that towards which the nutrient canal is directed which joins first with the shaft of the bone.*

Bérard also thought that this arrangement might have some influence on the consolidation of fractures, and believed that the formation of callus frequently failed in fractures of the portion of the diaphysis opposite to the direction of the nutrient canal; but this does not appear to have been borne out by the cases collected by M. Guéretin (*Presse médicale*, 1837, p. 45) and by Varris, quoted by Malgaigne (*Anatom. chirurg.* tom. i. p. 201), of non-union after fracture, which they found to be as numerous at one end as at the other. In the long bones, where there is only one epiphysis, the nutrient canal is directed towards the end which has no epiphysis, e.g. outwards in the clavicle, towards the distal end of the metacarpal bone of the thumb and great toe, and upwards towards the proximal end of the rest of the metacarpal and metatarsal bones.

Bérard and Flourens appear to think that the precocious union is due to a greater activity in the formative function of the epiphysial cartilage, an increased blood supply being directed towards it by the nutrient artery. But Ollier has proved that the earlier junction of an epiphysis with the diaphysis is the index of an exhausted nutrition, that the epiphysis joins on first where the increase in growth has almost entirely ceased, and that the end which joins on last is that which has the greatest activity in proliferation; this difference between the two ends of a bone being manifested from the time of birth and, it may be, before any of the epiphyses are joined on. Therefore, as will be seen later on, the unequal growth of the two ends is due to the unequal value of the epiphysial cartilages, and is manifested from the time of birth quite independently of the union of the epiphyses. Humphry was the first to point out, from his experiments on animals, that the increase in length of the end of the shaft in each bone where the epiphysis is last ossified is twice as great as that of the other end, or even more. As Ollier gives it: 'Ce sont là deux faits corrélatifs; quand l'accroissement cesse par épuisement des matériaux d'ossification, l'épiphyse se soude; mais la soudure est plutôt l'effet que la cause de l'inégalité d'accroissement.'

There is really less physiological activity in the cartilage at the end of the bone which joins on first and sooner completes its evolution. This is a very different explanation from that of Bérard.

In the bones of the forearm and arm the medullary canals are directed towards the elbow, and in the bones of the leg and thigh away from the knee. In the femur, ulna, radius, and metacarpal bones of the thumb and great toe and the phalanges, the medullary canal is directed towards the proximal end, whereas in the humerus, tibia, and other metacarpal and metatarsal bones the direction is towards the distal end. Therefore in the increase in length of the arm and forearm, the epiphyses at the elbow will play a much smaller part than the epiphyses at the shoulder and wrist; whereas in the lower limb the epiphyses of the femur and tibia at the knee joint are of more importance in this respect.

In bones having only one epiphysis—i.e. clavicle, metacarpus, metatarsus, phalanges—the growth in length of course takes place at this end only. In other irregular bones, such as the ilium, growth occurs chiefly in the vicinity of their epiphyses.

It is the lower end of the fibula which grows most, and hence it is the lower epiphysis of this bone which commences to ossify earlier and consolidates before that of the upper, which is in a rudimentary condition.

M. Ollier (*Traité de la régénération des os*, 1867, tom. i. p. 358) puts it in the following manner: the analogous bones in the upper and lower extremity are in an inverse relation in this respect, for the femur increases by its lower extremity inversely to the humerus, and the radius and ulna inversely to the tibia and fibula. As regards the forearm and arm, the ends of the bones at a distance from the elbow increase the most, whilst in the lower extremity the ends of the bones of the leg and thigh at a distance from the knee increase the least, thereby constituting a sort of opposition between the elbow and knee; or, in other words, in the bones of the same limb the same inverse relationship exists, the humerus increasing mostly by its upper end, the femur by its lower, the radius and ulna by their lower, whilst the tibia does so by its upper end.[1]

Sappey says that the last epiphyses to join on are the lower end of the tibia, the lower end of the femur, the upper end of the humerus, and then the lower end of the radius. By this arrangement the upper limb arrives at maturity before the lower limb.

The following table gives the times of appearance of the centres of ossification in the various bones.

Date of Appearance of the Centres of Ossification of the Chief Epiphyses of the Long Bones

Upper Extremity

Clavicle	. . . . . .		18th year
Humerus	. upper epiphysis (head) .		about 15 months after birth.
	lower ,,	capitellum	2nd to 3rd year.
		trochlea	11th year.
		external epicondyle	.13th year
,,	internal epicondyle	.	5th year (at times earlier).
Radius	. upper epiphysis .	.	at the end of 5th year.
,,	. lower ,,	.	towards end of 2nd year.
Ulna	. upper ,,	.	10th year.
,,	. lower ,,	.	4th to 5th year.
Metacarpus	. . . .	.	2½ to 5th year.
Phalanges	. . . . .	.	3rd to 5th year (1st, 2nd, and 3rd row successively).

Lower Extremity

Femur	. upper epiphysis (head) .		10th month after birth.
,,	. lower ,,	.	2nd or 3rd week before birth.
,,	. trochanter, great .	.	4th year.
,,	. ,, · lesser .	.	13th year.
Tibia .	. upper epiphysis	.	2nd week after birth.
,, ·	. lower ,,	.	at 18th month after birth.
Fibula	. upper epiphysis	.	4th year.
,,	. lower ,,	.	2nd year.
Metatarsus	1st (proximal epiphysis)		3rd year.
,,	4 outer (distal epiphyses)		about 4th or 5th to 8th year.
Phalanges	. . . . .	.	4th to 8th year.

---

[1] 'Au membre supérieur, pour les os du bras et de l'avant-bras, c'est l'extrémité concourant à former le coude qui s'accroît le moins.'

The period and order in which the consolidation of the epiphyses with the shaft takes place vary considerably in the different bones, in different individuals, and in the sexes. As Topinard remarks, the times of union have, unfortunately for comparative anthropology, been most studied among European races. They no doubt vàry in other races, and are important from an anthropological point of view. The time of union of the epiphysis to the diaphysis proceeds in an inverse order to the time of commencement of their ossification. Thus at the upper end of the femur, the lesser trochanter, whose ossification appears last, joins on first, then the great trochanter, next the head.

The first to appear of all the epiphyses of the long bones is that of the lower end of the femur, while the upper epiphysis of the radius is one of the last, and it is not a little interesting to note that the latter unites with the shaft almost the first, but the femur, as a rule, the very last. The union between the epiphysial cartilage and the diaphysis appears to be even and uniform, but the surface of union is strengthened by small interlacing prominences or projections, so that portions of the diaphysis or scales towards the periphery may be broken off in epiphysial separations. Generally, the consolidation between the epiphyses and the shaft is completed at or soon after puberty, i.e. the sixteenth to seventeenth year (Topinard). In some instances, however, the union is not perfect till a considerably later period—up to the twentieth year, and often till the twenty-fifth in the irregular bones of the body, a thin layer of cartilage existing between the epiphysis and the body of the bone even at this late period of life. In females the union takes place a little earlier than in males. Otto found none of the epiphyses united at the ages of twenty-two and twenty-three, and noted the same in the case of a man aged twenty-seven. Topinard believed that, generally speaking, the process was completed earlier in the lower than in the upper extremity. He gives (*Anthropologie générale*, 1885, p. 416) twenty-six years as the termination of this process in the male.

At the elbow-joint, injuries cannot be complicated with epiphysial separation after the eighteenth year, while in the case of the knee epiphysial separation of the tibia is possible up to the twentieth or twenty-first year.

From some observations made upon the skeleton, Dwight has come to the conclusion ('The Range and Significance of Variation in the Human Skeleton,' *Boston Medical and Surgical Journal*, August 2, 1894, p. 97) that the union of distinct parts occurs

'Au membre inférieur, pour les os de la cuisse et de la jambe, c'est l'extrémité concourant à former le genou qui s'accroît le plus.

'Les deux segments principaux d'un même membre se trouvent par cela même dans un rapport inverse entre eux; les os du membre supérieur sont aussi dans un rapport inverse relativement aux os analogues du membre inférieur.'—Ollier.

These rules are of vast importance when the operations for resection of joints are considered, as well as those for the injuries we are now concerned with.

earlier than accords with the general teaching, to the speedy disappearance of the epiphysial lines.

The site previously occupied by the epiphysial cartilage is indicated for many years after complete ossification by a thin line of osseous material.

The following table gives the

TIMES OF UNION OF THE CHIEF EPIPHYSES TO THE DIAPHYSES OF THE LONG BONES

Upper Extremity

Clavicle	. . . . . .	22nd to 25th year.
Humerus	. upper epiphysis .	. 18th to 22nd year.
,,	. lower ,, .	. 17th year.
,,	. internal epicondyle	. about 18th year.
Radius	. upper epiphysis .	. about 16th year.
,,	. lower ,, .	. 19th to 23rd year.
Ulna	. upper epiphysis .	. 16th to 17th year.
,,	. lower ,, . .	. 18th to 20th year.
Metacarpus	. . . .	. 20th year.
Phalanges .	. . . .	. 18th, 19th, or 20th year.

Lower Extremity

Femur	, upper epiphysis (head) .	19th year.
,,	. lower ,, .	. 20th to 23rd year.
,,	. trochanter, great ,	. 18th to 19th year.
,,	. ,, lesser .	. 18th year.
Tibia	. upper epiphysis .	. 21st to 22nd year.
,,	. lower ,, .	. 18th year.
Fibula	. upper epiphysis .	. 20th to 22nd year.
,,	. lower ,, .	. 19th to 21st year.
Metatarsus	1st (proximal epiphysis).	19th year.
,,	4 outer (distal epiphyses)	20th year.
Phalanges .	(posterior epiphyses) .	17th to 20th year.

Topinard gives (*Anthropologie générale*, 1885, p. 1028) the following table of individual variations of the times of union of the epiphyses. It shows the extreme variations noted by this author, and is interesting anthropologically.

TIMES OF UNION OF THE EPIPHYSES WITH THE BODY OF THE BONE

Individual Variations

Bodies of vertebræ, upper and lower epiphyses, dorso-lumbar			22nd to 26th year.
Clavicle, inner end			20th to 25th year.
Scapula	coracoid		14th to 17th year.
	acromion		17th to 18th year.
	lower and posterior marginal epiphyses		22nd to 24th year.
Humerus	upper epiphysis		21st to 25th year.
	lower epiphysis	Condyle (capitellum), trochlea, and outer tuberosity (epicondyle)	15th to 16th year.
		Inner tuberosity (internal epicondyle)	16th to 17th year.
Radius	upper end		12th to 19th year.
	lower end		18th to 25th year.
Ulna	upper end		14th to 19th year.
	lower end		21st to 24th year.
Os innominatum	union of the three primary portions		15th to 18th year.
	various supplementary centres		14th to 28th year.
	upper marginal epiphysis		15th to 16th year.
Femur	upper end		16th to 22nd year.
	lower end		20th to 25th year.
Tibia	upper end		18th to 24th year.
	lower end		16th to 18th year.
Fibula	upper end		18th to 22nd year.
	lower end		18th to 19th year.
Os calcis			16th year.

Dwight gives (*loc. cit. supra*) the following table of the times of union of the epiphyses of the long bones, but adds that the dates are somewhat too late. It is here quoted, although in several particulars the times are not quite accurate.

'From sixteen to eighteen, lower epiphyses of the humerus (except internal condyle), upper ends of radius and ulna, lesser trochanter of femur. At eighteen, internal condyle of humerus, great trochanter.

'From eighteen to nineteen, head of femur, lower end of tibia. From twenty to twenty-one or twenty-two, head of humerus, lower end of radius and ulna, condyles of femur, lower end of fibula, upper end of tibia. From twenty-two to twenty-four, upper end of fibula.

Dwight's observations offer the following as a provisional chart for seventeen years onwards :

'At seventeen years things are much as described from sixteen to eighteen, but perhaps a little more advanced. The lower end of the humerus is joined, excepting possibly the inner condyle. Subsequently the process is more rapid, so that the epiphyses of the long bones are usually firmly joined to the shaft at nineteen. At this age the lines of union about the elbow, hip, and ankle are nearly gone. At twenty all are indistinct or quite wanting. The epiphyses of the crests of the ilia and of the posterior border and inferior angle of the scapula are among the last to unite. They probably join at about twenty-one, but the lines of the crests of the ilia may be seen in parts for some years.'

Up to the present time the order of union of the epiphyses has been investigated by Béclard, Cruveilhier, Humphry, Rambaud, Renault, Sappey, &c., only in the case of Europeans; but, as Topinard says, there is probably considerable variation in different races.

The new skiagraphy by Röntgen's process will undoubtedly in the near future furnish us with very exact information as to the appearance of the centres of ossification of the epiphyses, their position and form at different ages, and, lastly, as to the time of union of the epiphyses to the diaphyses.

As to the reason for the separate centres of ossification forming the additional epiphyses or processes (apophyses), it is still a matter of speculation. These do not contribute to the increase in length of the shaft.

The epiphysial or conjugal cartilage (*cartilage de conjugaison*), cartilage of conjunction, or disc of cartilage is a very important structure. It is the cartilaginous layer or disc left by the ossification of the epiphysis between it and the diaphysis.

The epiphysial line of junction is more or less transverse in infancy, but as age advances the under surface of the epiphysis in many of the long bones becomes cup-shaped, especially projecting laterally, as at the lower end of the humerus, or anteriorly, as at the upper end of the tibia. During adolescence and almost up to the time of union of the epiphysis with the diaphysis it maintains a fairly uniform thickness. It then disappears by its complete ossification.

Broca, in 1852 (*Bulletins de la Société Anatomique*, 1852), though recognising that the different long bones increased in length more by one extremity than the other, appeared to think that this was due to the greater thickness of the chondroid layer (*couche chondroïde*) of the conjugal cartilage and to the relative height of the nutrient

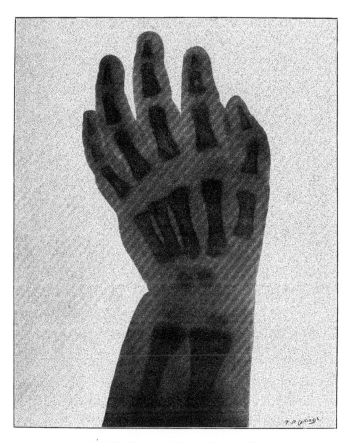

FEMALE INFANT AGED TWELVE MONTHS.
MR. T. P. COLLINGS'S GRANDCHILD. FIRST CHILD OF PARENTS.

'Snap-shot' exposure.   Taken by Mr. WM. WEBSTER.

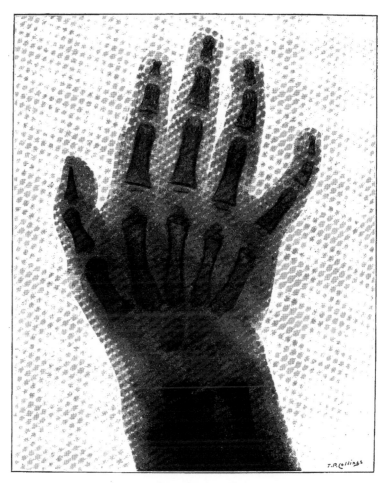

CHILD AGED TWO YEARS. THIRD CHILD.
Ossification in some respects more advanced than in the following skiagram.
Taken by Mr. WM. WEBSTER.

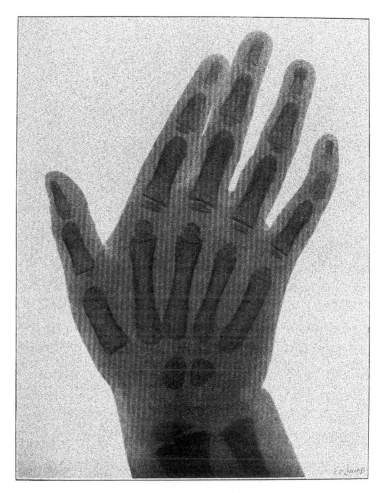

CHILD AGED THREE YEARS. EIGHTH CHILD.
Taken by Mr. WM. WEBSTER.

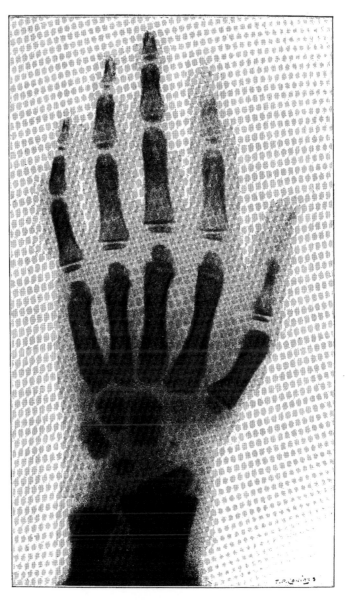

MALE CHILD AGED FOUR AND A HALF YEARS.

$\frac{1}{16}$ second exposure.

Taken by Mr. WM. WEBSTER.

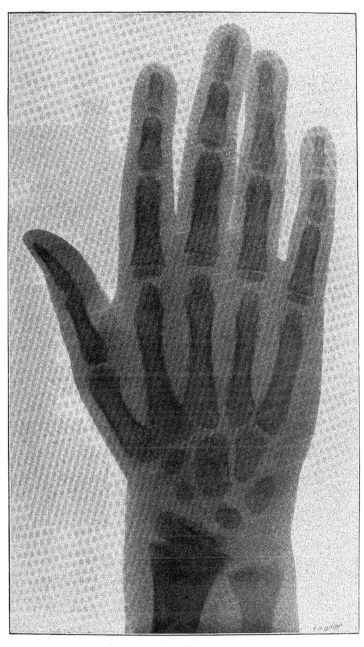

CHILD AGED FIVE YEARS. SECOND CHILD OF PARENTS.

Taken by Mr. WM. WEBSTER.

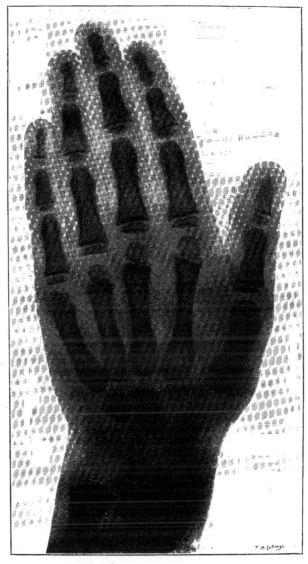

CHILD AGED FIVE YEARS. THIRTEENTH CHILD OF PARENTS.

Ossification not so advanced as in the following skiagram of a child of same age (second child), and in some respects no further advanced than in skiagram of child of three years.

Taken by Mr WM. WEBSTER.

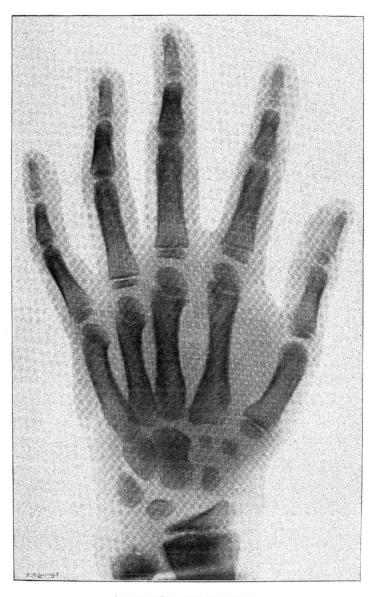

MALE CHILD AGED SIX YEARS.

$\frac{1}{12}$ second exposure.   Taken by Mr. WM. WEBSTER.

d

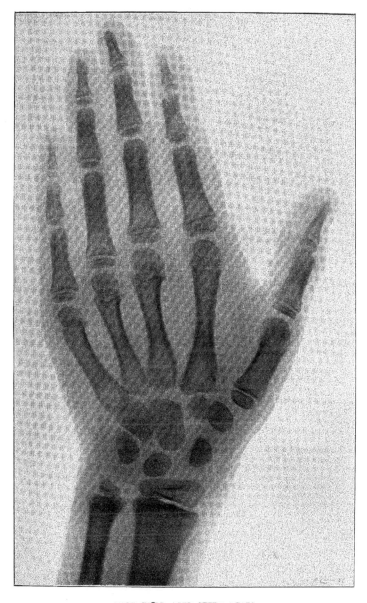

MALE CHILD AGED SEVEN YEARS.

¾ second exposure.   Taken by Mr. Wм. Webster.

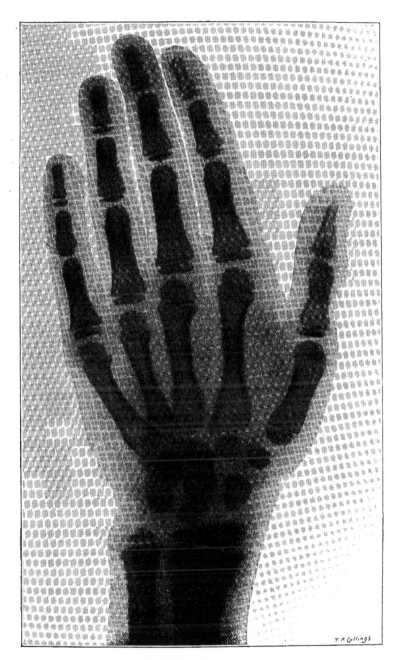

T. P. Cullings

MALE CHILD AGED EIGHT YEARS.

1 second exposure.

Taken by Mr. WM. WEBSTER.

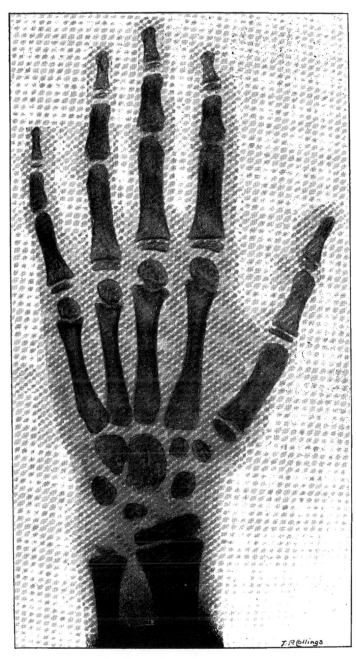

AUTHOR'S SON (R. D. T.), AGED EIGHT YEARS AND FIVE MONTHS.
Skiagram of Hard taken in April 1896 by Mr. C. SWINTON.

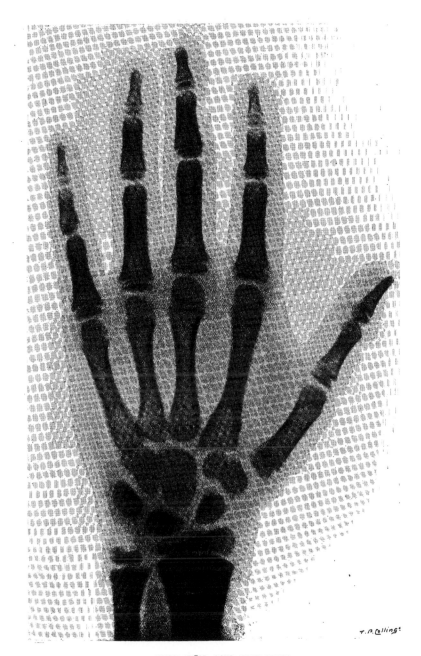

T. P. Collings

MALE CHILD AGED NINE YEARS.

1 second exposure.

Taken by Mr. Wм. Webste

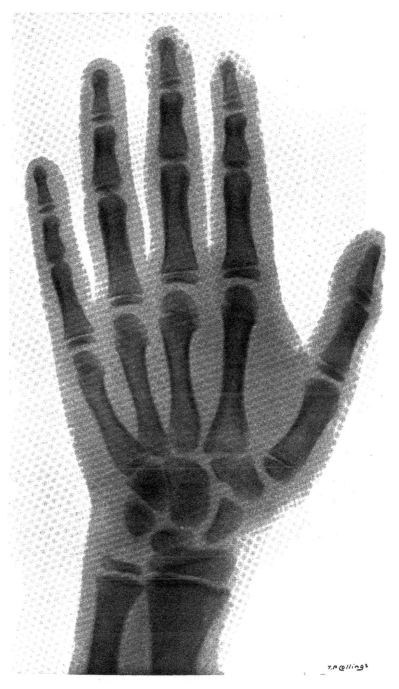

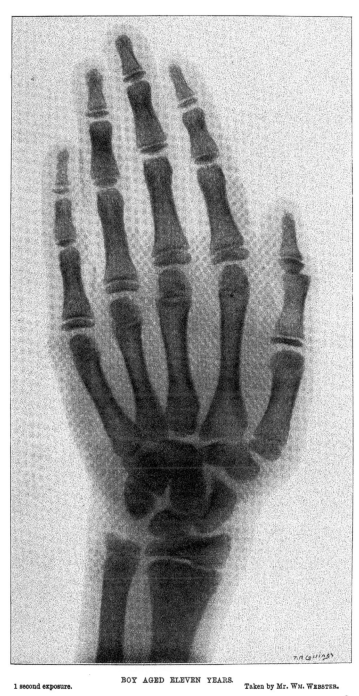

1 second exposure.   BOY AGED ELEVEN YEARS.   Taken by Mr. WM. WEBSTER.

g

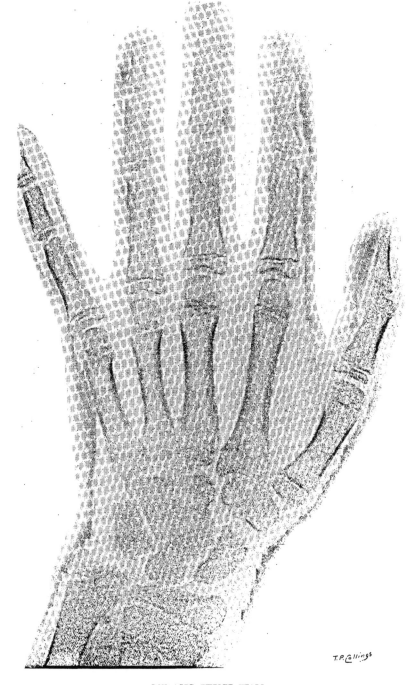

T.P. Callings

BOY AGED TWELVE YEARS.

1 second exposure.

Taken by Mr. Wm. Webster.

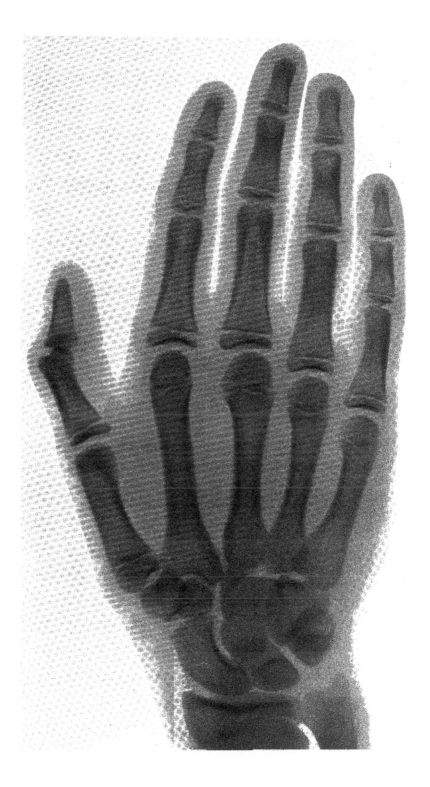

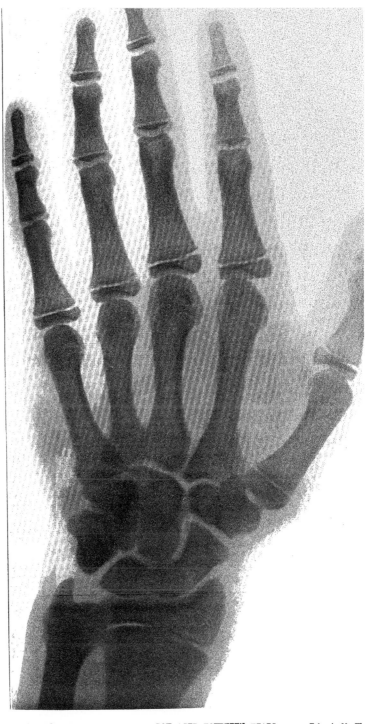

2 seconds exposure.   BOY AGED FOURTEEN YEARS.   Taken by Mr. W

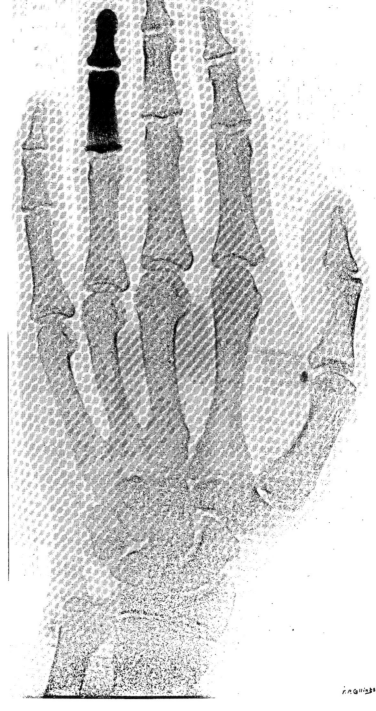

3 seconds exposure.   BOY AGED FIFTEEN YEARS.   Taken by Mr. WM. WEBST

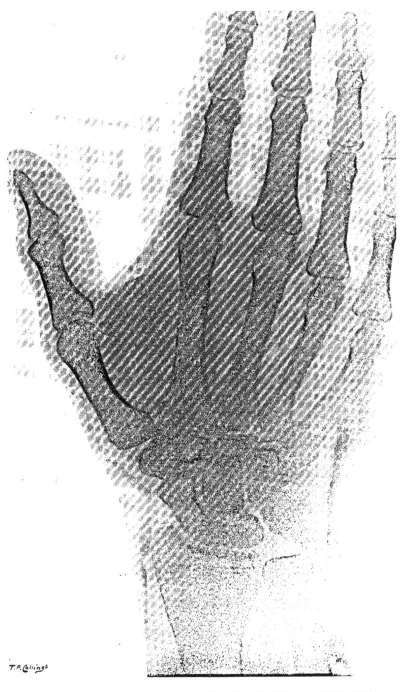

T.P. Collings

BOY AGED SIXTEEN YEARS. MR. T. P. COLLINGS'S YOUNGEST SON (SIXTH CHILD).

seconds exposure.

Taken by Mr. WM. WEBB

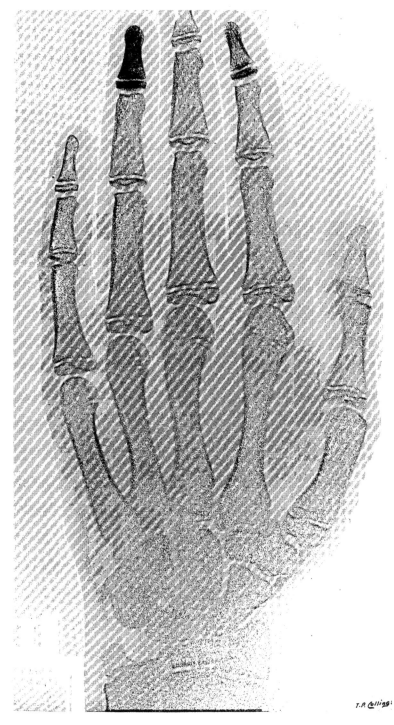

T.P. Collins

1 second exposure.   BOY AGED SEVENTEEN YEARS.   Taken by Mr. WM. WEBSTE

canal at the different ages. He laid considerable stress upon the fact that the thickness of the chondroid layer is proportionate to the activity of the local growth.

Ollier agrees in a general way with Broca in his theory that 'l'activité de l'ossification est proportionnelle à l'épaisseur de cette couche chondroïde.' This is verified by his experiments on animals.

According to Ollier, fourteen-fifteenths of the length of a bone is due to the activity of the diaphysial surface of the epiphysial discs. This diaphysial surface has an osteogenic power twelve times greater than that of the epiphysial surface, the ratio of growth being therefore as twelve to one. The growth in length of a long bone takes place in this layer of cartilage between the end of the shaft and the epiphyses by the proliferation and successive ossification of the layers of the cartilage at their diaphysial surface. Physiological activity is greatest in this situation, the epiphyses taking a very small part in this process, so that we may say that the growth in length of the long bones is the exclusive function of the epiphysial line of cartilage.

The layer—disc or bar—of cartilage between the epiphysis and the shaft varies with the age of the patient. As youth advances, the epiphysial or conjugal layer of blue hyaline cartilage becomes thinner, while in infancy there is a considerable mass of cartilage intervening between the ossifying centre or centres of the epiphysis and the shaft. As its surface, however, is encroached upon by its undergoing ossification in the part nearest to the diaphysis, an interstitial fresh zone of cartilage is produced by proliferation of the pre-existing cartilage, and a constant cycle of changes goes on uninterruptedly so long as the growth of the bones continues—the growth of the epiphysial cartilage always being, so to speak, in advance of the ossifying process.

The circumference or peripheral margin of the conjugal cartilage projects over the outer aspect of the end of the diaphysis, and becomes blended with and forms the deep or under layer of the periosteum.

This overlapping of the circumference of the conjugal cartilage more or less accounts for the cup-shaped appearance of many of the epiphyses into which the diaphysis is received at the age of puberty, when the conjugal cartilage is fully formed.

The increase in length at the diaphysial ends of the same bone is, as stated above, very unequal, so that all extremities of the long bones have not the same importance.

Ollier (*Traité de la regénération des os*, tom. i. and tom. ii. 1867) has fully discussed the increase of the long bones generally, the relationship of the unequal growth with the order of union of the epiphysis, and with the direction of the nutrient canals. He has investigated this unequal growth with reference especially to the unequal thickness of the chondroid layer of the conjugal cartilage, at the same time giving in detail many experiments. (See also 'De la part proportionnelle qui revient à chaque extrémité des os des membres dans leur accroissement en longueur,' Ollier, *Journal de la physiologie de Brown-Sequard*, 1861 ; 'Recherches expérimentales sur la mode d'accroissement des os,' Ollier, *Archives de physiologie*, 1873 ; ' De l'accroissement normal et pathologique des os,' Ollier, ' Congrès de l'Association française pour l'Avancement des Sciences, Session de Lyon, 1873 '·&c.)

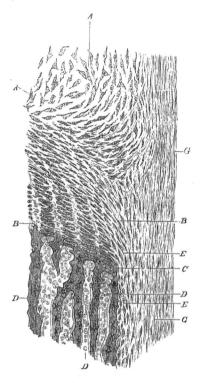

FIG. 2.— SECTION OF EPIPHYSIS THROUGH LINE OF GROWING BONE AND PERIOSTEUM
· (MACNAMARA)

A A, cartilage cells: some of them are seen to be undergoing fibroid changes ; B B, cartilage cells rapidly proliferating and becoming arranged into rows continuous with the medullary spaces in the newly formed bone ; D D, nuclei of cartilage cells passing into the medullary spaces of the bone. Along the sides of these spaces some of the round cells are seen to be transformed into bone corpuscles. C C, cartilage cells passing into and forming the deep layers of the periosteum. Some of these cells are undergoing changes into bone corpuscles ; E E, the inner layers of the periosteum ; G G, the outer layers of the periosteum.

It is conclusively shown by this observer and others that when two metal nails are inserted—at a given distance apart, but nearer to the upper epiphysis than to the lower—into the diaphysis of the long bone of an animal, the distance between the nails is the same after the bone has grown, but that the upper nail is now further from the upper epiphysis than the lower nail is from the lower epiphysis, thus proving conclusively that the chief growth in length of the bone is at the upper epiphysis.

Flourens erroneously supposed that all long bones increased more by their upper than by their lower epiphyses.

The difference in the various epiphyses as regards the growth in length of the bones has also been investigated by Kölliker, Vogt, Humphry, Schwalbe ('Ueber die Ernährungskanäle der Knochen und des Knochenwachsthums,' *Zeitschrift für Anatomie und Entwicklungsgeschichte*,' 1876, i. s. 307), Strelzoff, and others.

The rate of growth, as well as the value, of each of the epiphysial cartilages of the long bones is very exact on the opposite sides, although so unequal at each end of the same bone. All this is more fully alluded to under the head of 'Epiphysis.'

What we know of the function of the epiphysial cartilage from experiments is corroborated by pathological as well as clinical experience. Conical stumps are continually found in the arm and leg, after amputation, from continued growth at the upper epiphysial lines of the humerus, fibula, and tibia. The radius, ulna, and femur mainly depending upon their lower epiphyses for increase in length, such stumps in the forearm and thigh from this cause are seldom found in children. See discussion at the Société de Chirurgie in 1858 (*Bulletin de la Société de Chirurgie*, 1859).

Humphry has also made experiments on the limbs of animals and proved the same thing (*Medico-chirurg. Transactions*, 1861, xliv. p. 117), but, as he truly states, this elongation frequently falls short of the proper amount and is not in precise proportion to the corresponding bone of the opposite healthy limb. Again, the indirect irritation of a long-continued osteo-myelitis or chronic endostitis may stimulate the conjugal cartilage to increased growth and increased length of the bone. Excessive elongation from such a cause must therefore not be looked upon as a healthy growth.

Mr. Bryant (*Practice of Surgery*, vol. viii.) describes the case of a boy aged seven years, whose leg was amputated. Subsequently, on two occasions, at intervals of three years, it became necessary to remove a piece of the tibia an inch long; the tibia grew faster than the fibula, so that at the second operation the fibula required no shortening. Mr. Bland Sutton, in a lecture on 'Amputation Stumps' (*Lancet*, December 8, 1888), alludes to a similar case in a girl aged thirteen years under his care at the Middlesex Hospital. She had had amputation of the leg performed, for injury, at the age of two years.

It is a question whether it would not be justifiable intentionally to destroy the central layer of the epiphysial cartilage, and so arrest the growth at the epiphysial line at the time of amputation.

The cartilaginous line between the epiphysis and the shaft is more or less transverse, but is much altered in its direction by processes of the epiphysis in certain directions; e.g. in the upper end of the tibia there is a tongue-shaped process extending from the epiphysis downwards in front, forming a part of the anterior tubercle ; and in the lower end of the humerus, on the inner and outer side, a bending upwards (up to a certain period) to form the inner and afterwards the outer epicondyle. It is more often concavo-convex on its surface and sinuous, as is well seen in the case of the lower end of the femur (very marked in the lower animals), and affords a remarkable reciprocal socket between the epiphysial cartilage and the diaphysis.

This sinuous appearance is but little marked at birth, when the surface of the epiphysis is more distinctly cup-shaped, but is more and more characteristic as the time of union of the epiphysis with the diaphysis is approached.

Although by reason of its softness the conjugal cartilage predisposes to epiphysial separation, and to certain inflammatory diseases —viz. acute epiphysitis, ulceration, &c.—yet it must not be forgotten, as Sir George Humphry says (*A Treatise on the Human Skeleton*, 1858, p. 42), ' that advantages, more than outweighing these inconveniences, accrue to the young subject from this subdivision of its skeleton and the interposition of cartilaginous plates between its segments. Besides the greater facilities for growth thus afforded, its flexibility is thereby greatly increased, and its escape from injury during the many falls incidental to this time of life is, in no small degree, attributable to this cause.'

The epiphysial discs also act as barriers to the articulation and for a time prevent inflammation of the diaphysis and medulla spreading to and invading the joints. All round their circumference they are, like the epiphyses, intimately connected and blended with the periosteum. On the side next the epiphysis continual proliferation takes place, while on the diaphysial side there is a production of osseous material which is permanent, the process of ossification being identical with that of the cartilage of the epiphyses themselves.

To the naked eye the division between the diaphysis and epiphysis— viz. the passage of the cartilage into the osseous tissue—appears very abrupt, but on closer examination it looks less so. In infancy the separation between the diaphysis and epiphysis is more decided and abrupt than in adolescence, when it becomes a little less distinct. In reality the gradation of cartilage into bone is imperceptible. Broca was one of the first to distinguish *two layers or zones* in this region, and his description has been generally accepted by histologists, such as Todd and Bowman, Ranvier and Robin.

The *first zone* or proliferating layer (*couche chondroïde*, Broca) is composed of the normal cartilage, and is of a light bluish colour and translucent. Its thickness varies from one to two millimètres. The cells have lost their angular foetal shape, and have become enlarged, more numerous, rounded, and arranged in columns or linear series which are less regular as the unossified part is reached (*cartilage sérié*). These columns are separated by longitudinal intervals.

This chondroid zone is said to be more distinct in some bones than in others; it is very distinct at both ends of the tibia, the upper end of the humerus, the lower end of the fibula, and the lower ends of the bones of the forearm; very thin at the upper end of the femur and at the lower end of the humerus, and almost completely absent at the upper end of the fibula, ulna, and radius.

The *second zone* or osteoid layer of Ranvier (*couche ostéoïde; couche spongoïde*, Broca) is of a yellowish grey colour, granular, and opaque. Here there is a simple calcareous deposit which without any formation of true osseous tissue takes on an appearance somewhat resembling it. In this manner a reticulated calcified cartilage is produced (*cartilage calcifié*, Gegenbauer; *la zone granuleuse*, Robin). The cartilage cells are still present. The areolæ are more delicate than those of the ordinary spongy osseous tissue and are more friable.

The blood vessels are dilated and form loops or sinuses springing from the already formed medullary cavities of the bone, which invade and cause absorption of the calcified cartilage. The rows of cells disappear towards the osseous tissue and the cartilage cells become dissociated.

It is into these meshes of the calcified substance that the osteoblastic tissue penetrates. These last procedures constitute the commencement of true ossification.

The osseous layer (*couche osseuse*, Ranvier) is that portion beyond, where some osseous cells are found deposited in the cartilaginous arches separating the first medullary spaces, and is therefore composed of temporary and brittle bone.

From the fact of a partial absorption of the cartilage, and the weak and dilated condition of the vessels in a part where the true osseous tissue is not found, we can fully realise the comparatively weak nature of this region.

The important physiological *rôle* of this cartilage will be found under PROGNOSIS, but we can readily see that the irritation or destruction (partial or complete) of this structure will very materially modify this function.

It is unnecessary here to reproduce the experiments of Ollier upon animals; the reader must refer to his work *De la régénération des os*, Paris, 1867, pp. 394-396; also fig. 27, p. 395. He found that simple incision of the conjugal cartilage retards the growth, whilst lesion of the same produces complete want of development of the bone. In Germany the subject has been studied by Bergmann, Billroth, Langenbeck (1869), Weinlechner and Schott (1869).

The direction of the conjugal line of cartilage, its relation to the neighbouring joint, and its precise distance from the interarticular line can be best studied on the living subject by means of the new skiagraphy. By this method the position of the lines of cartilage of the various epiphyses at different ages can be determined; and it will

D

doubtless supplement the information here given in our several chapters.

The juxta-epiphysial region of Ollier at the end of the diaphysis is the soft spongy layer of the bone uniting this latter with the conjugal cartilage, and in it the most active processes take place. The epiphysial line is here of a reddish colour and very vascular.

This region is the weakest part of the bone, and the one which gives way first to external violence, so that, as M. Rollet remarks, the lesions under consideration are not strictly epiphysial but juxta-epiphysial. The layers of new bone adjoining the cartilaginous layer are soft and spongy. Ollier, in his experimental researches on the growth of bones, has clearly demonstrated the importance of the juxta-epiphysial region (Ollier, *Encyclop. internationale de chirurgie :* ' Maladie des os,' tom. iv. 1885 ; *Traité des résections*, tom. i. and ii., Paris, 1885 and 1888).

The periosteum in young subjects is a thick, vascular, greyish-white, fibrous structure, and forms the external covering of the diaphysis, except where the tendons and aponeuroses are attached. It becomes continuous with the periarticular ligaments at the articular ends or epiphyses, and forms one of the principal bonds of union between the epiphysis and the diaphysis. Many experimentalists have found that if the periosteum be removed the epiphysis may be very readily detached from the diaphysis. It is a most important structure owing to the part which it takes in reproducing osseous tissue, and contains vascular plexuses which, together with some delicate fibrous tissue, enter the foramina on the surface of the bones and help to bind the periosteum to the bone. But in young subjects it can be readily separated from the diaphysis. It is composed of *two layers*, the one consisting of connective and elastic fibres, with adipose tissue, in which the vessels and nerves ramify, the other of osteogenic tissue. The *outer layer* is a fibrous membrane, in which the elastic fibres become more numerous as the inner part is reached. The *inner* layer in contact with the bone comprises a network of very fine elastic fibres, in the meshes of which are found cells which form bone during the active time of development, and add to their thickness externally. This is known as the osteogenetic layer. The cells of which it is composed are osteoblastic.

Epiphysial separations are of less frequent occurrence than they might be, not so much on account of the firmness with which the epiphysis adheres to the shaft, as in consequence of the great support given at the epiphysial lines of junction by the periosteum. At this part the periosteum is very thick and strong, becoming thinner and more loosely attached to the bone as it passes along the shaft. The periosteum is tougher and more resisting during the first few years of life than later on. At this early period it forms the chief bond of connection between the epiphysis and diaphysis. The great cartilaginous mass of an epiphysis is intimately connected with the periosteum and appears to be, as it were, a massive expansion of the periosteum of the diaphysis on which it is placed and grows. Duhamel, indeed, regarded the epiphyses as formed by such an expansion or enlargement of the periosteum, on account of this intimate connection of the periosteum with the conjugal cartilage and cartilaginous ends of the bones. The periosteum proper does not reach beyond the cartilage; it has therefore no part in the ossification of the epiphysis. This function of the periosteum, serving to unite the epiphysis with the diaphysis, is well illustrated in Wilson's experiments, in which the epiphysis was much more readily detached from the diaphysis after the removal of the periosteum.

As we shall see hereafter, the tough periosteum by its intimate connection with the epiphysis will very frequently prevent any displacement when epiphysial separation has occurred, and will often (by its swelling &c.) effectually mask the nature of the lesion even when slight displacement has occurred.

During adolescence the periosteum becomes thinner and more adherent. It is then more likely to be lacerated, and to a less extent stripped off the diaphysis in traumatic epiphysial separations.

In some situations, as over the great trochanter, the olecranon process of the ulna, and part of the acromial process of the scapula, the periosteum becomes very thin, if not entirely deficient. The dense tendinous fibres which are present in these instances are almost directly attached to the osseous tissue itself.

In such instances the periosteum is more likely to be torn across in epiphysial detachments if the violence be sufficiently great to lacerate the powerful tendinous fibres covering these processes and to allow of displacement.

The periosteum is also the principal factor in the production of callus for the union of the fragments after epiphysial separation.

From the second or third year onwards the periosteum begins to diminish in thickness; by the tenth to fifteenth it is so much thinner that many of the older writers believed that the periosteum at this later age was more liable to be lacerated than to separate off from the diaphysis, as usually occurred in younger life. After the union of the epiphysis with the diaphysis, and therefore after the growth in length of the bone is complete, the growth in thickness is still carried on by the periosteum.

Ollier has proved that if the whole surface of a periosteal layer is scraped after being detached, new osseous material will not be reproduced under the portion so treated. His experiments on animals have recently (1892) been entirely confirmed by Matchinsky's observations on the human subject.

The nerves and vessels and lymphatics ramify in the periosteal membrane before entering the diaphysis, which they do by the large orifices freely scattered over its surface.

The nerves mostly belong to the sympathetic system, and are not very abundant in number.

The **articular cartilage** capping the layer of compact tissue at the extremity of the epiphysis is composed of hyaline cartilage with its characteristic cells, or chondroblasts, and its homogeneous intercellular substance. This permanent articular cartilage is the remains of the original cartilage forming the epiphysis, so that the ossification of the epiphyses may be said to be never completely accomplished.

The synovial membrane extends for a short distance over the cartilage to which it is strongly adherent, but is absent where the articular cartilage is in apposition with its articular fellow.

In the encrusting or articular cartilage of the epiphyses the cartilage cells are arranged at their deeper parts in columns at right angles to the surface of the bone, while the superficial ones lie parallel to its surface.

It is sufficient to allude to this point in Prof. Sir George Humphry's words (*A Treatise on the Human Skeleton*, 1858, p. 41) :

'It is remarkable that, although the cartilage of an epiphysis presents throughout the same characters, ossification takes place in a part of it only ; a thin portion next the surface of the joint remains unossified, and forms the articular cartilage. This becomes in course of time somewhat more opaque and more dense ; but I am not aware that it has ever been known to be converted into true bone, even in morbid states or in old age.'

In its deeper portion, however, near the bone, this cartilage frequently calcifies in old age. Ollier, Busch, Ogston, and others think that in later years, besides their mechanical function, the articular cartilages are connected to a slight extent with the production of new bone, repairing the constant loss of this tissue from pressure at the articulation.

Relation of articular capsule to conjugal cartilage.—Another most interesting anatomical condition is the exact relationship or attachment of the capsule of the joint with regard to the limit of the epiphysis. If the capsule be attached beyond this boundary, a separation of the epiphysis will be an intra-capsular one, and the synovial membrane of the joint will probably be opened.

The relation of the capsule to the epiphysial cartilage in many instances alters with the age of the individual.

Relation of synovial membrane to conjugal cartilage will be discussed along with each individual epiphysis. It is of great importance in certain epiphyses which may be considered as intra-articular. During infancy the osseous centre of the cartilaginous epiphysis of several of the long bones is wholly surrounded by the synovial membrane. This relationship has been the subject of some investigations by Schwegel in 1858, who has written a work on the development of the epiphyses (*Die Entwickelungsgeschichte der Knochen*

des Stammes mit Rücksicht auf Chirurgie, &c. ; Wien, 1858), by Sésary
('Recherches sur les synoviales considérées dans leurs rapports avec
les extrémités des os longs,' *Lyon Médical*, 1870, p. 227 ; and *Bull.
Soc. Anat. de Paris* (1870), 1874, xlv. pp. 104–9), by J. Uffelmann
(*Anatomisch-chirurg. Studien oder Beiträge z. d. Lehre von den
Knochen jugendlicher Individuen*, Hameln, 1865), and by Dr. A.
V. Brunn (*Das Verhältniss der Gelenkkapseln zu den Epiphysen*,
Leipzig, 1881).

Projecting processes which have special nuclei forming separate
epiphyses have little to do with the increase in length of the bone.
They are intended rather for the greater strength and the firmer and
more extensive attachment of the powerful tendons, muscles, or
ligaments with which they are connected, e.g. great and lesser
trochanters of femur, inferior angle of scapula, iliac crests, &c.

The exact size, form, and situation of these are important details
to the surgeon.

CHAPTER III

ETIOLOGY, AGE, SEX

ETIOLOGY.—GURLT thought the rareness of these traumatic separations was due to the fact that children are seldom exposed to sufficient violence to produce them. In the eighteen cases he was able to collect it was clear that the violence was much greater than that which is the usual cause of fracture at the corresponding periods of life.

He believed that, with the exception of the cases produced on infants during delivery, the amount of force required was very considerable. Thus in three of the cases the fracture was produced during the delivery of the child by traction upon the foot, arm, or axilla; in seven, it was the result of severe falls; in five the limb was caught by machinery or between the spokes of a waggon wheel; and in one, separation of the upper epiphysis of the humerus was produced in a child three years old by jerking its arm.

Boyer says 'que, dans les jeunes sujets, les causes capables de produire la fracture du col de l'humérus peuvent donner lieu à la séparation de l'épiphyse supérieure d'avec le corps de l'os' (Boyer, *Traité des maladies chirurgicales*, tom. iii. p. 211, 4ᵉᵐᵉ éd.).

Taken as a whole the causes which produce these lesions are the same as those of fracture, but as a rule they are more severe. This is especially true as regards such severe forms of separation as have been examined anatomically (see under PATHOLOGICAL ANATOMY). There are, however, differences according to the epiphysis involved, and in many of these cases the violence is less than what would produce fracture of the same bone—e.g. hyperextension at the knee.

The precise mechanism of these lesions has also now been pretty well established by numerous experiments on the dead subject.

An injury which would be sufficient to produce a dislocation in an adult will in the child produce a separation of the epiphysis; epiphysial separation in the child may indeed be called the analogue of dislocation in the adult.

Children at the age of puberty are more exposed to injuries by reason of the games they play, and of their erratic tendency and generally thoughtless doings; in this way some have attempted to prove the greater frequency of epiphysial separation in them than in children during the first few years of life, when they are more under protection and guidance.

Pathological separations.—A slight violence applied to an epiphysis in a young subject with some constitutional affection is often sufficient to cause its separation, without producing any displacement. (See SEPARATION OF EPIPHYSIS OF HEAD OF FEMUR.)

Rickets so alters the normal condition of the end of the diaphysis and the epiphysial structure that separation under these conditions is entirely different from that occurring in healthy subjects. According to M. Ollier, it is not, in rachitic children, that the cartilage has a greater tendency to separate from the diaphysis (for it is, on the contrary, more adherent than in healthy children); but that bending and solution of continuity take place in the bulbar region of the bone (*région bulbaire*, Lannelongue) between the limit of the medullary canal and the spongy layer. The weak spongoid material produced from the epiphysial cartilage, though irregularly formed and with wide meshes, is true osseous tissue.

Other conditions, such as starvation, septicæmia, pyæmia, tubercle (Maisonneuve), scurvy, congenital syphilis, prolonged mercurial treatment (Lobstein), &c., which produce more or less grave alterations in the skeleton, must be placed in the same category as rickets.

Iscovesco describes (*Congrès français de chirurgie*, tom. v., Paris, 1891, p. 596) four cases of epiphysial fracture produced by forcible attempts at straightening for white swelling of the hip and knee.

In certain cases, then, it is exceedingly difficult at first sight to express a very decided opinion as to the separation. The diseased or unhealthy condition of the child may have been entirely overlooked by the parents, or a previous illness been intentionally kept from the notice of the surgeon. In such cases the slight degree of violence causing the injury is always a suspicious factor. Where the violence appears to be inadequate for the production of separation, a careful examination of the general condition of the child should be made in order to determine the existence of any of the above-mentioned conditions.

Suppuration of a single epiphysis causing separation is frequently detected, and distinguished from a true traumatic separation by the presence of a fistula. This must not be confounded with suppuration due to traumatism; the former is usually more acute, the latter chronic.

At first sight it might be supposed that on limbs affected with infantile paralysis or paralysis from cerebral disease, separation of the epiphyses would occur from slight violence, but in the author's experience such is not the case. Separation may take place in a child so affected but not more easily than in one in a healthy condition. This seems strange, but nevertheless it is a fact.

Indirect violence is the most frequent cause of detachment of the true or osseous epiphysis, and it is generally of a severe character. In this respect these injuries are much more like dislocations than fractures—being occasioned by such violence as a fall from a height (as, for example, out of a second or third story window, or from a mast-head to a ship's deck or into the hold ; from a tree, or from crags) or by a fall whilst running—such falls being on to the extremity of the limb, which transmits the shock to the epiphyses.   Or again, a child may have fallen with one of its joints doubled beneath it, the joint being thus fixed in position and receiving the. weight of the body. Another frequent cause is the entanglement of the limb in the revolving wheel of a vehicle, in the revolving wheel or strap of machinery, or in a ship's rope ; or the patient may have been rolled round by the band of a machine.   All these are examples of the greatest indirect violence to which a limb can be exposed, and combine traction with torsion.   Violently lifting the child by its limbs is also a not infrequent cause.   Reichel believed this to be a very common mode of injury, resulting in the separation of the humeral head.

In other cases the limb, or part of the limb, may be fixed and the rest of the body violently thrown in one or other direction : in climbing over a fence, for instance, the foot may be caught in the rails at the top and the child fall to the opposite side ; or the leg may be caught in a hole or between the joists of a floor, or otherwise fixed, and the child fall forwards ; or the toe may be pushed under a door, and an attempt be made to withdraw it.

The less severe forms of epiphysial separation, in which the displacement is not complete and which are diagnosed clinically as belonging to this class of injury, are found to be caused by a proportionately smaller amount of violence.   A fall from a short height—for example, off a tree a few feet high—is sufficient to separate the upper epiphysis of the humerus, but not to completely displace the fragments.   Or a fall on the palm of the hand whilst walking may suffice to separate the lower epiphysis of the radius.

In infancy the cartilaginous and elastic condition of the epiphyses assists materially in preventing separation.

Direct traction on the axis of the limb.—Violent traction of the limbs at birth has frequently produced separation, but many of these cases may have been associated with disease and cannot be considered as authentic; moreover, they were doubtless combined with some torsion of the limb.   It is certain that direct traction, however forcible, will less readily detach an epiphysis than force applied obliquely or at right angles to the axis of the bone.   Thus M. Champion in 1810 observed (*Journal Complémentaire*, tom. i. p. 317) separation of the lower epiphysis of the left tibia in a child at birth by violent pulling on the foot.

Madame Lachapelle gives (*Pratique des Accouchements*, tom. ii. p. 225, and tom. iii. p. 180) a similar case from a like cause ; and another in which the traction on the foot separated at the same time the inferior epiphysis of the femur and the superior epiphysis of the tibia.   In both these instances, as well as in that quoted by Bertrandi of separation of the humerus, the children were born dead.

A similar separation was observed by Chapelain Durocher (*Thèse Inaugurale*, Paris, 8 Frimaire, an xii.) in a child which survived fourteen months; the midwife caused it by hooking her finger in the attempt to assist the delivery. Obstetric physicians have from time to time noted cases of separation of the epiphysis of the femur and tibia from traction on the lower limbs during pelvic version or in delivery by the breech.

Bailly (*Nouveau Dictionnaire de Médecine et de Chirurgie pratique*, 1872, xv. p. 33) briefly notes the possibility of these injuries.

Dr. Carl Ruge has also (*Zeitschrift für Geburtshülfe und Frauenkrankheiten*, Berlin, 1876, s. 86) alluded to the same amongst the frequent and unsuspected injuries to the fœtus produced during delivery.

Pajot thought that epiphysial separations, as a consequence of obstetrical manipulations, were more frequently met with than fractures or dislocations.

Dr. Sam. E. Milliken, of New York, records (*Archives of Pediatrics*, vol. xii. 1895, p. 611) a case of separation of both ends of the humerus during delivery. The labour had been a tedious one. The separation of both epiphyses was complete.

Forcible torsion.—M. Champion (*loc. cit. supra*) has given two remarkable examples due to twisting in boys from eleven to thirteen years old. One had his arm caught in the spokes of a wheel, and the other had his forearm entangled in a carding machine. In the former there resulted separation of the superior, and in the latter of the inferior, epiphysis of the humerus.

M. Ricard has recorded (S. Duplay et P. Reclus, *Traité de chirurgie*, tom. ii. 1890, p. 346) a very clear case in a lad aged nineteen years, who had the upper epiphysis of the left humerus separated by his arm being seized and violently twisted.

Reichel mentions *forcible rotation* of the upper extremity as a cause of disjunction of the upper epiphysis of the humerus.

Direct violence.—Direct violence, such as the passage of a cartwheel over the limb, or severe violence applied directly to the epiphysis (or in the situation of the epiphysial cartilage), as from the fall of a wall or heavy weight upon the part, is the common cause of separation of the epiphyses at all periods as well as of detachments of the cartilaginous ends of the bones in infancy. Ordinary direct blows and injuries, however, do not so frequently give rise to separations of the epiphyses as they do to fractures. The rarity of injuries produced by direct violence is dependent upon the small size of many of the epiphyses.

Malgaigne expresses the opinion that epiphysial separation could only be due to indirect causes, and states that there are no examples of such results from direct blows. The number of cases of undoubted separation of the upper end of the humerus from blows or falls on the shoulder nowadays conclusively refutes such a statement.

Violence applied in the neighbourhood of a joint in children is much more likely to be followed by an epiphysial separation than a fracture, although it may be only partial or complete, with or without displacement of fragments.

Compression separations of the epiphyses are a constant accompaniment of severe crushings of the limbs in the neighbourhood of joints in children, and they often occur in hospital practice.

Muscular violence.—Gross (*System of Surgery*, vol. i. p. 935, 5th edit. Philadelphia) asserts that there is no example in which muscular action alone has ever determined the detachment of any epiphysis ; and Nélaton expresses a doubt on this point (*Traité de pathologie ext.* tom. ii. p. 235, 1867) ; yet many instances are now recorded of epiphysial separation by muscular action, and several have been verified by an autopsy. Van Swieten attributed separation of the femoral head to the muscular action of a child in arms throwing itself violently backwards. The cases described by Ingrassias (great trochanter) and Foucher (upper end of humerus), which have been often quoted, are very doubtful. The latter case of Bouchut's was probably one of acute epiphysial osteomyelitis. A girl, aged thirteen, on taking an embroidery frame down from a wall, felt a crackling and acute pain in the left shoulder. Suppuration and signs of acute infective fever supervened, followed by death at the end of the sixth week (see UPPER EPIPHYSIS OF THE HUMERUS).

A case is related by Mr. Christopher Heath (*loc. cit. infra*) of a boy who separated the epiphysis of his clavicle whilst raising his arm violently to bowl at cricket.

The lesser trochanter of the femur, the anterior iliac spine, and anterior inferior spinous processes have been detached by muscular violence. Strong action of the biceps has occasionally torn off the upper fibular epiphysis. (Stanley Boyd, *Treves' System of Surgery*, vol. i. 1895, p. 734.)

Violent movements, acting directly upon an articulation or upon the contiguous bones themselves, which in an adult produce stretching and laceration of the ligaments, or even detachment of portions of bone into which these are inserted, produce in young children lesions of the spongy juxta-epiphysial region of the diaphysis. The bulbous portion is the most yielding and least consistent part of the bone, and gives way rather more easily than the ligaments or the cartilaginous epiphyses, which escape injury by reason of their elasticity. This yielding of the bulbous region (Lannelongue) of the diaphysis, giving rise to ecchymosis, crushing, and laceration of its substance, is of common occurrence in infancy, and very frequent in rachitic children. The epiphysial cartilage being relatively more adherent to the diaphysis in them than in healthy children, the slightest force only is sufficient to lacerate the soft tissues at the juxta-epiphysial line. Injuries of the juxta-epiphysial region present various lesions of the spongy and compact peripheral layer of the bone, and are grouped by Ollier (*Revue de Chirurgie*, 1881) under the name of *juxta-epiphysial sprains* (*l'entorse juxta-épiphysaire*). Although not apparent from the outside, they are yet important lesions, since they are the immediate or remote cause of various inflammations of the bone or joints. Such lesions are of especial importance in children predisposed to tubercle, or who have suffered from septic poisoning. Many of the pains called 'growing pains' are due to juxta-epiphysial sprains or injury. A juxta-epiphysial sprain is often nothing but the first degree of an epiphysial separation, in the same way that an articular sprain is nothing but the first degree of dislocation.

AGE. Intra-uterine separation of an epiphysis.—The occurrence of this injury apart from disease appears to the author to be extremely doubtful. M. Piscart was one of the earliest authors who considered intra-uterine separations possible. Rognetta says that a fall upon the abdomen in the ninth month of pregnancy, or a violent blow can give rise to this injury. Guéretin doubted the reality of such cases. There is no authentic case recorded in this country, such cases as that described by Carus (*Archives gén. de médecine*, tom. xvi. p. 288) in a six-months-old fœtus, where the lower epiphysis of the tibia was found separated, and the projecting bone necrosed at the delivery at full term, being extremely rare. The mother had fallen from a height upon the abdomen ; she immediately felt the fœtus violently move, but soon these movements ceased. Reduction was unsuccessfully tried, and the child died on the thirteenth day. Other instances have been described by Velpeau (*Lancette française*, tom. v. p. 368), Monteggia, Rognetta, and Chaussier (*Journal de Médecine*, No. 43).

Devergie relates the case of a woman who had struck herself against the corner of a table at the sixth month of pregnancy and gave birth to a child having a separation of the lower epiphysis of the tibia, the upper fragment projecting through a wound.

Epiphysial separation during childbirth.—Many cases are recorded by Bertrandi (upper epiphysis of the humerus and femur from traction on the arms or feet by the midwife), also by Bitot, Volkmann, Moldenhauer, De la Motte (upper epiphysis of the humerus), Champion (lower end of the tibia), Dubroca (upper epiphysis of the humerus), and others, as occurring *during childbirth* from excessive or awkward traction by the accoucheur ; but it is questionable whether many, if not all, were not due to a diseased, or at any rate an altered, condition of the bones.

Cruveilhier, in 1849, declared with much veracity that these were due to putrefactive changes following the death of the child before birth. In Bitot's case (*Gaz. Médicale de Paris*, 1860, p. 361) the infant lived twelve days, and on section the epiphysis appeared to be uniting to the diaphysis by soft, spongy bone.

It is true that attempts to produce dislocations, as at the hip, by traction on the limbs of the fœtus only separate the cartilaginous ends of the bones.

Guéretin and Champmas were never able to produce dislocations in the newly born.

The case of separation of the lower epiphysis of the tibia related by M. Champion in 1816, caused by the violent tractions of a midwife, is open to great doubt, inasmuch as the infant was dead before delivery. The foot was displaced forward with the epiphysis, and parallel with the leg.

Many of the cases of separation of the cartilaginous ends of the bones which have been recorded as occurring in the first few years of infancy have been due to disease. Some are less doubtful but still open to criticism, as in the case of a male infant, thirteen months old, who fell out of the cradle and was believed by Hamilton to have separated the upper epiphysis of the humerus. It is unlikely that a separation of the *healthy* cartilaginous end in infancy will readily take place from indirect violence.

The cartilaginous epiphyses at this early age may readily be crushed off by severe direct violence—as by the passage of a cart-wheel over the limb.

Hutchinson mentions a separation of the lower epiphysis of the femur in a child aged eighteen months, who had been run over in the street.

The force of violent traction upon the limbs during delivery, or a few days after birth, will be expended rather upon the epiphysis than upon the articulation itself, the resistance of the uniting material between the cartilage and the bone being much less than that of the ligaments and articular capsule.

Periods of age.—Up to the time of Roux's dissertation in 1822, epiphysial separations were very generally believed to occur only in infancy or the first few years of childhood. Malgaigne states that separation had been observed mainly during the period from birth up to fifteen years of age, and that, although separation might be possible up to twenty-five years of age in subjects in whom the epiphyses were as yet unconsolidated, he knew of no instance of its occurrence above the age of fifteen.

Although the possibility of separation of the epiphyses of bones after the first few years of life was doubted by many eminent surgeons, M. Roux, in 1837, related (*La Presse Médicale*, No. 55, July 12, 1837; extract in *British and Foreign Medical Review*, vol. v., January 1838, p. 250) a number of cases which proved that it may occur as late as the eighteenth year.

He relates an instance of separation of the condyles of the femur in a boy of eleven years; of the inferior extremity of the radius, the styloid process of the ulna, the head of the first phalanx of the thumb, and of the fore and middle fingers of the left hand in a boy of eighteen years of age; of the humerus in a boy of twelve years; of the lower extremity of both radii in a boy of seventeen; of the head of the humerus in a boy of fifteen; and of the lower extremity of the radius in a man of twenty-two years of age. None of these, however, appear to have been clearly established.

According to Colignon's estimate, the majority of traumatic epiphysial separations occurred between the ages of twelve and thirteen years.

This is greatly at variance with the results arrived at by many experimentalists on the dead subject. Guéretin found experimentally that at the age of nine months separation was produced in about one case out of four, the other three being true fractures; from two to seven years of age, one separation out of nine cases, the others resulting in fractures or dislocations; from seven to fourteen years out of ten attempts not a single epiphysial separation was produced, but fractures or dislocations in every case. In many recent works the first decade of life is still given as the usual period. Thus M. A. Leblois, in 1894, says (*Des fractures chez les enfants et leur traitement*, Paris, 1894, p. 17) that the first years of life up to the age of ten are the times when epiphysial separations most frequently occur, and that the nearer the time of birth the more easily is this lesion produced. Ricard (*Traité de chirurgie*, Duplay and Reclus, tom. ii. 1890, p. 343) also says that separations are almost always met with in the first few years of life, before the twelfth or fifteenth year, and that the younger the subject the more easy it is to separate its epiphysial ends experimentally.

From statistics the author has given in each chapter it is clearly proved that these accidents are less common in early childhood than after the age of eleven or twelve. This is contrary to what has commonly been conjectured by former writers and those just mentioned -- viz. that young children are the most frequently affected with traumatic epiphysial separations. The belief probably arose from the fact that the epiphyses at this early age are considerably larger in proportion to the diaphyses and less strongly united to them than they are at a later period. In reality, the period of eleven or twelve to eighteen years of age is the one in which these injuries are most likely to be met with, which fact is largely due to the circumstance that children at this age are more exposed to severe injuries, such as are likely to cause epiphysial separations.

Knowing that the osseous union of the epiphysis to the diaphysis may be delayed beyond the twenty-first year, we may expect to find occasionally an epiphysial separation at a more advanced age than that just given. Voillemier experimentally separated the lower epiphysis of the radius in a powerful muscular male subject aged twenty-four years.

The *precise age* of the child is therefore one of the most important points in the consideration of separations, for not only are particular bones more liable to be separated at a certain period of life, but the separations are also more likely to be purer in character at the same period.

Again, many of the epiphysial processes—for instance, those at the lower end of the humerus, internal and external epicondyles, &c.—are only distinct epiphyses from the rest of the lower end of the humerus at a particular period, and often for only a few years. A pure separation of such processes can, therefore, only occur at this particular period of childhood. Age has, consequently, a very marked influence in determining the anatomical character or variety of the separation.

We may now state that the various epiphyses have certain periods in which they are most liable to separation, although there is still great discrepancy among authors as to the comparative liability to separation of the various epiphyses at the different ages. Allowance must also be made for the diversity in the period of coalescence of the epiphysis with the diaphysis which is found to exist in individuals.

Another difficulty experienced in detecting these lesions is the want of precision in fixing the exact date of union of the individual epiphyses. The same epiphysis may have some years' difference in different subjects before it is finally blended into the diaphysis.

Uffelmann states (*Deutsche Klinik*, 1864, p. 183) that he found the epiphyses still dis-united in subjects beyond thirty years of age.

CHRONOLOGICAL TABLE OF THE
DATES OF APPEARANCE OF THE CENTRES OF OSSIFICATION
OF THE EPIPHYSES

At Birth . .	The centre of ossification of the *Lower epiphysis of the femur* already exists.	
At the 1st year .	*Upper epiphysis of the tibia* appears, and *Upper epiphysis (head) of the femur.*	
At the 15th month	*Upper epiphysis (head) of the humerus.*	
At the 18th month ,,	*Lower epiphysis of the tibia.*	
At the 2nd year .	*Lower epiphysis of the radius, Lower epiphysis of the fibula, and Capitellar portion of lower end of humerus.*	
Between 2½ and 5 years ,,	*Epiphysial heads of the metacarpus.*	
At the 3rd year .	*Great and small tuberosity of the upper end of the humerus, Epiphysis of the first metatarsal bone, Epiphysis of first metacarpal bone, and Great trochanter of femur.*	
Between the 3rd and 5th years ,,	*Epiphyses of phalanges of the fingers.*	
At the 4th year .	*Internal epicondyle of humerus.*	
Between the 4th and 5th years ,,	*Upper epiphysis of the fibula and Lower epiphysis of the ulna.*	
Between the 5th and 6th years ,,	*Head of the radius and Four outer metatarsals.*	
About the 7th year	*Epiphyses of phalanges of the toes.*	
About the 10th year ,, ,,	*Olecranon epiphysis.*	
At the 11th year .	*Trochlea of the humerus.*	
At the 13th year . ,,	*Lesser trochanter of the femur and External epicondyle of the humerus.*	
At the 18th year .	*Epiphysis (sternal) of the clavicle.*	

The union of the epiphyses to the diaphyses commences during the period of puberty. The last to unite are the lower epiphysis of the femur and the upper epiphysis of the tibia in the lower extremity, and the upper epiphysis of the humerus and the lower epiphysis of the radius in the upper extremity; those of the lower extremity, as a rule, unite before the upper, the tibia before the femur, the humerus before the radius.

THE TIMES OF THE UNION OF THE EPIPHYSES TO THE DIAPHYSES
OF THE LONG BONES

At the 16*th year* . . .	. *The upper epiphysis of the radius.*
Between the 16*th and* 17*th years*	. *The olecranon epiphysis of the ulna.*
At the 17*th year* . . .	. *The lower epiphysis of the humerus.*
At the 18*th year* . . .	. *The internal epicondyle of the humerus.*
Between the 17*th and* 20*th years*	. *The epiphyses of phalanges of toes.*
Between the 18*th and* 20*th years*	. *The epiphyses of phalanges of fingers, and lower epiphysis of ulna.*
About the 20*th year* . . .	. *The metacarpal epiphyses.*
Between the 18*th and* 22*nd years*	. *The upper epiphysis of the humerus.*
Between the 19*th and* 23*rd years*	. *The lower epiphysis of the radius.*
Between the 22*nd and* 25*th years*	. *The epiphysis of the clavicle.*
At the 18*th year* . . .	. *The lesser trochanter.*
Between the 18*th and* 19*th years*	. *The great trochanter.*
Between the 19*th and* 20*th years*	. *The metatarsal epiphyses.*
At the 19*th year* . . .	. *The epiphysial head of the femur.*
Between the 18*th and* 19*th years*	. *The lower epiphysis of the tibia.*
Between the 19*th and* 21*st years*	. *The lower epiphysis of the fibula.*
Between the 20*th and* 22*nd years*	. *The upper epiphysis of the fibula.*
Between the 21*st and* 22*nd years*	. *The upper epiphysis of the tibia.*
Between the 20*th and* 23*rd years*	. *The lower epiphysis of the femur.*

In the female the union takes place, as a rule, a little earlier than in the male; in the former about the twenty-second year, in the latter at the twenty-third, or even as late as the twenty-fifth.

The frequency of each separation varies considerably according to the age of the patient in whom it is produced.

M. Curtillet gives the following statistics of twenty-one cases of epiphysial separation occurring in children from one to ten years of age, in the practice of M. Vincent :

Humerus {	Upper epiphysis .	.	.	.	2	
	Lower epiphysis .	.	.	.	11	
Radius, lower epiphysis		.	.	.	2	
Femur, lower epiphysis		.	.	.	2	(doubtful)
Epitrochlea .	.	.	.	.	3	
Epicondyle .	.	.	.	.	1	

Separations of the femur and radius, usually considered amongst the most frequent, are here in the minority, and M. Curtillet explains this preference for epiphysial separations of the lower extremity of the humerus by the assumption that these very young children, being as yet unacquainted with protective movements such as carrying the hands forward during a fall, come to the ground in a clumsy manner, fracturing the elbow or the two bones of the forearm, instead of falling on the hand and injuring the wrist.

He remarks that, from a large collection, the most common injuries of the upper extremity in quite young children were fractures of both bones of the forearm, somewhere in the shaft, and fracture or epiphysial separation of the lower end of the humerus.

It is probable that the comparative immunity from these injuries in early childhood is due to the fact that these very young children are less exposed to the various sources of injuries which produce separations in older children—such as falls, games, and other violent exercises; at the same time, the muscular system is much less developed.

Colignon rightly recognised that epiphysial separations were more frequent during adolescence than in the first years of life.

Among Gurlt's collected cases (1862) verified by dissection, with the exception of the three newly born children, only one of the patients was less than nine years old ; the oldest was eighteen.

In Bruns' statistics the frequency of epiphysial separations based on anatomical grounds in the different periods of childhood and youth is tabulated as follows.

The most frequent period noticed was between the ages of ten and nineteen years, for in sixty-one cases in which the age was known forty-four belonged to this period. The greatest frequency observed was between the sixteenth and seventeenth years (fourteen cases), twelfth to fourteenth years (fifteen cases), eighteenth to twentieth years (nine cases), and tenth to eleventh (six cases). The least frequent period was from one to nine, with a record of only eight cases.

Out of seventeen cases verified by an autopsy which Gurlt collected in 1862, with the exception of three in the newly born infant, only one of the patients was less than nine years old. The oldest was eighteen (the lower end of the radius) ; all the others were below the age of $16\frac{1}{2}$, the majority occurring between nine and fifteen years of age. Gurlt knew of no case of pure separation, confirmed anatomically, after the twentieth year.

Separation may, however, occur in certain individuals after the twentieth year.

Dr. Jetter records two cases of separation of the upper epiphysis of the humerus (verified by operation) in a woman in her twenty-third year, and in a man in his twenty-first year.

In an old separation of the upper epiphysis of the humerus, operated upon by P. Bruns for great loss of power and utility of the limb, the age of the patient was twenty-four, so that, as he says, the limit of the age up to which these injuries may occur must be extended beyond the twentieth year.

As a rule, epiphysial separation can only occur before the

twentieth to twenty-first year, the time of osseous union of the epiphysis with the shaft, or body of the bone. Several cases have been recorded of separation at the twentieth year, but their true nature is somewhat doubtful.

It must be remembered, however, that in certain epiphyses consolidation is not complete until the twenty-fifth year, or even later.

Gurlt quotes Platner (J. M. Schwartz, *Diss. de ossium epiphysibus*, Lips. 1786, and J. Z. Platner, *Opuscula*, tom. i., Lips. 1788, 4, p. 174) as being able to show the skeleton of a big fully grown man in which most of the epiphyses were still attached by cartilage to the diaphyses. Nanula (of Naples), according to Rognetta, had possession of a skeleton of a man, aged 26½ years, in whom most of the epiphyses were still visible.

. Twenty-four or twenty-five must be the extreme limit of age at which these exceptional cases can occur, although the usual highest limit for the epiphysial junction is, according to Sappey, from the eighteenth to twentieth year.

SEX.—In all the cases diagnosed during life, and also in those verified by an autopsy, which were known to Malgaigne, the lesions were all in male subjects.

The author's statistics, showing the enormous difference in frequency of occurrence between the male and the female sex, are as follows.

Total number of separations occurring in the three most frequent situations, viz. :

Lower epiphysis of femur.—Out of 114 cases, the sex is stated in 96—83 males and 13 females, all the latter below fourteen years of age.

Lower epiphysis of the radius.—Out of 112, the sex is given in 89, as 79 in males and 10 in females ; the whole of the latter being at or below fourteen years of age.

Upper epiphysis of the humerus.—Out of 119, the sex is given in 104. Of these, 85 were males and 19 females (16 being at thirteen years and below, three above).

Cases verified anatomically. *Lower epiphysis of femur.*—Out of 80 (age stated in 68) the sex is given in 55 as 46 in males and 9 in females. All the latter were from fourteen years of age downwards, none above.

Lower epiphysis of the radius.—Out of 60 cases, the sex is given in 45—viz. 41 males and 4 females ; all the females at or below five years of age.

Upper epiphysis of the humerus.—Out of 21 the sex is stated in 12—all males.

Simple cases. *Lower epiphysis of femur.*—34 cases ; sex stated in 32, as 28 males and 4 females ; all the latter were from thirteen years downwards.

Lower epiphysis of the radius.—52 cases ; sex stated in 44, as 38 males and 6 females ; all females were below fourteen years.

Upper epiphysis of the humerus.—Out of 98 cases, the sex is

E

stated in 92 ; 19 only of these of the female sex (16 at thirteen years and below, 1 at fifteen, 1 at sixteen, and 1 at twenty-three).

In 231 cases of the upper extremity represented by the lower epiphysis of radius and upper epiphysis of humerus, the sex is given in 193 as 164 males and 29 females ; all the females except 3 were at or below fourteen years of age.

Out of the total number of cases (345), the sex is stated in 289 as 247 males and 42 females ; all except three of the latter being at or below the age of puberty.

Sex in the different epiphysial injuries.—Delens states, as regards the lower epiphysis of the femur, that the injury has almost always been observed in boys. Out of 23 cases where the sex of the patient had been noted, 20 were boys and only 3 girls. In the lower and upper extremity the percentage of males and females is very similar.

In the lower extremity, as represented by the lower epiphysis of the femur, 86·44 per cent. of the cases were in males, and 13·52 per cent. in females ; all the females were at or below fourteen years of age.

In the upper extremity, represented by the upper epiphysis of the humerus, 81·76 per cent. were in males, 18·28 per cent. in females ; and by the lower epiphysis of the radius, 88·6 per cent. were in males, 11·2 per cent. in females. This makes a total percentage of 84·8 in males and 15·5 in females.

Sex in the different periods of age.—Before puberty the vast excess of males over females is somewhat less than after this period ; this is particularly marked in the earlier years of childhood. Under the conditions of external surroundings, in their games, &c., girls are exposed to injury almost equally with boys, whereas in later years they isolate themselves more and are not exposed by their occupation to severe injuries.

As we have just seen, out of 289 instances only 42 were in females, and with three exceptions all occurred at or below the age of puberty.

The so-called equality of the sexes, and the modern tendency for females to undertake the work of the male sex and imitate their habits, may in the remote future considerably modify the statistics of the past and present.

CHAPTER IV

FREQUENCY OF THE VARIOUS SEPARATIONS

THE frequency of epiphysial separations varies not only with the different ages but also with the various epiphyses involved. The epiphyses of the long bones are far more frequently detached than those of other bones—e.g. iliac crest, tuberosity of os calcis, or of ischium.

It is probable that in infancy many cases of separation without displacement, and juxta-epiphysial sprains are often overlooked.

The true osseous epiphyses are more frequently separated than the unossified cartilaginous epiphyses, or cartilaginous ends of the diaphyses.

DATE OF OSSIFICATION OF THE CHIEF EPIPHYSES OF THE LONG BONES

At birth	Lower end of the femur Upper end of the tibia
At 1 year . . .	Upper end of the femur Upper end of the humerus
At 1½ years . . .	Lower end of the tibia Lower end of the humerus
At 2 years . . .	Lower end of the radius Lower end of the fibula
At 3 years . . .	Great trochanter of femur Great tuberosity of humerus
At 4 years . . .	Upper end of the ulna Upper end of the fibula
From 5 to 6 years . .	Upper end of the radius
At 8 years . . .	Lower end of the ulna Lesser trochanter of femur

The epiphyses of certain bones appear to have never been detached during life.

The epiphyses of some of the long bones are found to be much more frequently affected than others, which is explicable to a great extent on anatomical grounds, but partly also by physiological as well as mechanical reasons. Thus the lower end of a femur, which ossifies at the same time as the upper end of the tibia, will give way rather than the epiphysis of the tibia in a fall upon the knee.

It might be supposed from the longer period in which separation is possible that the epiphyses of the long bones which joined on later to the diaphyses—and which, as a rule, begin to ossify first—would be the most commonly affected, and it has been pointed out that this agrees with the order of frequency of separations given by previous surgeons.

This, however, according to the large number of cases collected by the present writer, is not strictly accurate. It would seem that a joint which has very free mobility with a large unprotected epiphysis will be more frequently the seat of separation than one whose epiphysis is small and well protected. Again, the lower ends of the radius, femur, and humerus are, from their situation, most liable to be affected by injury.

The cause of the frequency of separation of particular epiphyses will be considered under the head of each epiphysis.

Many French and German writers have collected cases of epiphysial separation, but they lack the importance which is attached to Bruns' cases from the fact that the greater proportion were very doubtful, and only a few verified by direct inspection.

Thus Manquat in 1877 (*Essai sur les décollements épiphysaires traumatiques,* Thèse de doctorat. Paris, 1877) collected 130 cases, the majority of which were of the lower epiphysis of the radius (twenty-three) and of the lower epiphysis of the femur (twenty-three); while the upper (thirteen) and lower ends (eighteen) of the humerus were the next most frequent; the upper end of the femur following with ten, and the upper and lower ends of the tibia with seven each.

To these P. Bruns added, in 1886 (*Deutsche Chirurgie,* Billroth and Luecke, 1886; 'Die Lehre von den Knochenbrüchen,' p. 119), ten cases, mostly of the lower epiphysis of the radius and of the upper epiphysis of the humerus.

C. O. Weber also published a number of cases in 1859.

Again, with regard to the lower epiphysis of the radius, some writers regard the injury as very common, while others believe it to be quite exceptional.

Malgaigne claimed that as fractures of the lower end of the radius were the most common, so separation of the corresponding epiphysis was most frequently met with, in children.

Gurlt's tables show a vast preponderance of fractures at the lower end of the humerus over those at the upper in the first two decades of life; indeed, he found that up to the tenth year the lower portion of this bone was considerably more than twice as often fractured as the upper end and shaft together. It can readily be understood that a great number of these cases were probably epiphysial separations of one or other variety.

Other surgeons (Reeve, &c.) consider separation of the lower epiphysis of the humerus to be the most frequent.

Packard says that 'the epiphyses of the humerus are far more often separated by violence than those of the femur.'

Professor E. de' Paoli, of Perugia, states (*Communicaz. della Clinica Chir. Propedeutica dell' Univ. di Perugia*, 1891, p. 52) that out of 105 cases of epiphysial separation proved by anatomical examination, fourteen were of the upper end of the humerus.

Such complications as gangrene and hæmorrhage from injury to the vessels or the presence of a wound, especially noticeable in separation of the lower epiphysis of the femur, have necessitated surgical interference and led to a complete examination of the injury. We see, therefore, that separation of the lower epiphysis of the femur has been most frequently confirmed by direct examination of the fragments.

Other epiphysial separations are usually less complicated and less liable to secondary complications, or to complications which call for surgical interference, so permitting an inspection of the fractured surfaces. Probably, also, in many situations such separations are often overlooked.

Pick says (*Fractures and Dislocations*, 1885, p. 14) that 'separation of the epiphysis appears to occur more commonly in the lower end of the femur than in any other situation. After this the lower end of the radius, the lower end of the tibia, and the extremities of the humerus are the bones most frequently affected.'

As regards the lower end of the femur, M. Delens has written (*Archiv. gén. de méd.* 1884) a very complete monograph on this form of epiphysial separation.

Champmas (*Thesis*, Paris, 1840) gives the following order:

Divulsion of the upper epiphysis of the humerus			.	12 cases
,,	inferior	,,	radius .	.	7 cases
	upper	,,	femur .	.	5 cases
	inferior	,,	humerus	.	4 cases
,,	inferior	,,	femur .	.	3 cases

In Colignon's figures, of fifty-nine cases of traumatic separation of the epiphyses of the long bones, thirty-five were of the upper and twenty-four of the lower extremity ; of these, twelve were of the upper end of the humerus, fifteen of the lower end of the radius, ten of the upper, and seven of the lower end of the femur. From his experiments and collected cases, Colignon believed that the lower epiphysis of the radius separated most easily and most frequently, next the upper epiphyses of the humerus and the femur, and lastly the lower epiphyses of these two latter bones.

Guéretin gives, out of thirty-seven cases, ten of the upper end of the humerus, four of the lower end of the radius, five of the upper, and three of the lower end of the femur.

Gurlt, in 1862, only collected eighteen cases verified by autopsy.

Humerus	Upper epiphysis .	.	.	.	4 cases
	Lower epiphysis .	.	.	.	1 case
Radius	Lower epiphysis .	.	.	.	4 cases
Femur	Great trochanter .	.	.	.	1 case
	Lower epiphysis .	.	.	.	5 cases
Tibia	Upper epiphysis .	.	.	.	1 case
	Lower epiphysis .	.	.	.	2 cases

Bruns collected in 1882 (*Archiv für klinische Chirurgie*, Langenbeck, Bd. xxvii. 1882, S. 240) seventy-eight published cases, and three of his own from his Tübingen clinic, in which the diagnosis had been confirmed by direct examination of the seat of injury, either through an accompanying wound, or after amputation or death. In eleven instances the injury was double or multiple (2 to 4), the total being 101.

The division of cases was as follows:

Humerus	Upper epiphysis .	.	.	.	.	11
	Lower epiphysis .	.	.	.	.	4
Ulna	Upper epiphysis .	.	.	.	.	1
	Lower epiphysis .	.	.	.	.	2
Radius	Lower epiphysis .	.	.	.	.	25
Ossa pubis	.	.	.	.	.	3
Femur	Upper epiphysis .	.	.	.	.	3
	Lower epiphysis .	.	.	.	.	28
Tibia	Upper epiphysis .	.	.	.	.	4
	Lower epiphysis .	.	.	.	.	11
Fibula	Upper epiphysis .	.	.	.	.	3
	Lower epiphysis .	.	.	.	.	4
Metatarsus	.	.	.	.	.	2
					Total	101

Bruns says that, although it had hitherto been customary to believe that separation of the upper epiphysis of the humerus was the most frequent, his statistics proved that the lower epiphysis of the femur stands first in order of frequency, then the lower epiphysis of the radius, and, thirdly, the upper epiphysis of the humerus. The first two mentioned together comprised more than half of all the cases.

He accounts for this frequency by the large size of the lower epiphysis of the femur, its late union, and the great strain which is thrown upon the conjugal cartilage by the powerful leverage of the leg ; but at the same time he is of opinion that probably separation of the lower epiphysis of the radius will be found to be as frequent, or even more so, when we consider how often these separations are without complication, and unite without any direct examination of the lesion having been made.

Several other writers have endorsed Bruns' statement.

For instance, in 1892, Dr. Joseph Prochnow (*Pest. Med. Chir. Presse*, Budapest, 1893, xxix. S. 389) states that separation of the lower end of the femur takes the first place in regard to frequency.

Coming to the latest paper by Dr. C. A. Sturrock (*Edinburgh Hospital Reports*, vol. ii. 1894), we find the same statement (p. 598) : 'As regards the relative frequency of epiphysial injury in different situations, separations seem to occur most often at the lower extremity of the femur, and at the lower and upper extremities of the humerus.' And this is repeated by Mr. D'Arcy Power (*The Surgical Diseases of Children*, 1895, p. 163) when he says that 'it occurs most frequently at the lower end of the femur, next at the upper and lower ends of the humerus, at the lower end of the radius, and at the lower end of the tibia.'

Putting the statistics of previous writers together, the order of frequency with regard to the long bones would be as follows : (1) Lower epiphysis of femur ; (2) lower epiphysis of the radius ; (3) upper epiphysis of the humerus ; (4) lower epiphysis of the humerus ; (5) lower epiphysis of the tibia ; (6) upper epiphysis of the tibia.

Although the cases verified by direct examination afford the best data for statistical purposes, the many hundreds of clinical cases cannot be ignored ; yet here also a large number are even at the present time often overlooked or mistaken for dislocations.

Nevertheless in Bruns' 100 cases, verified by autopsy, the upper end of the humerus only took the third place (11 per cent. of the cases) ; indeed it must be placed first if we include, as we should, the many clinical cases which have of late years been so accurately recorded.

Dr. G. Jetter states the order of frequency from cases observed at the Tübingen clinic (*Beiträge zur klinischen Chirurgie*, 1892, S. 362) during ten years : First, the upper epiphysis of the humerus ; secondly, the lower epiphysis of the radius ; and thirdly, the lower epiphysis of the femur, which in Brüns' statistics is placed first (28 per cent.).

With reference to the relative frequency of the different varieties of fractures or separations about the elbow-joint, M. Guedeney has collected sixty cases from the clinic of M. Vincent at Lyons (*Du traitement des fractures du coude chez l'enfant, &c.*, Lyon, 1893) extending over a period of about seven years. Twenty-seven are classed under the heads of juxta-epiphysial disjunctions, fractures of the lower extremity of the humerus, *fractura disjunctiva humeri* (Hueter), supra-condyloid fractures (Malgaigne), &c. Amongst these, T, ⅄ and Y-shaped fractures were perfectly made out seven or eight times. Fourteen were fractures of the epicondyle (external epicondyle), but two were accompanied by detachment of the capitellum (condyle), six were fractures of the epitrochlea (internal epicondyle), five of the olecranon, and four fractures of the upper part of bones of the forearm, mostly accompanied by dislocation backwards of the elbow ; two of the latter being diagnosed as separation of the upper epiphysis of the radius.

From practical experience one is led to the belief that separations of the lower end of the humerus in their various complicated forms are perhaps the most frequent.

The epiphyses of the upper limbs are much more often involved than those of the lower. The author's figures are 423 in the upper extremity and 253 in the lower extremity.

Mr. Hutchinson, junr.'s, collection consists of about 350 cases, of which nearly 150 were not previously published (*British Medical Journal*, July 8, 1893, p. 53, &c.) :

Clavicle	3	Upper epiphysis of femur	26
Upper epiphysis of humerus	66	Epiphysis of lesser tro-	
Lower epiphysis of humerus	52	chanter	1
Internal epicondyle	38	Lower epiphysis of femur	75
Upper epiphysis of ulna	2	Great trochanter of femur	11
Lower epiphysis of ulna	6	Upper epiphysis of tibia	10
Upper epiphysis of radius	2	Epiphysis of tubercle of tibia	6
Lower epiphysis of radius	54	Lower epiphysis of tibia	27
Epiphyses of phalanges and		Upper epiphysis of fibula	4
metacarpal bones	10	Lower epiphysis of fibula	2

The author's statistics of separations of the epiphyses of the long bones are as follows :

UPPER EXTREMITY

—	Pathological anatomy	Compound cases	Simple	Tota
CLAVICLE	1	1	3	5
HUMERUS, upper epiphysis	33	7	80 (including nine operation cases)	120
„ lower end (before puberty)	13	18	44	75
„ lower epiphysis (at and after puberty)	1	1	4	6
„ internal epicondyle	5	—	56 (including five operation cases)	61
„ external epicondyle	3	—	6	9
RADIUS, upper epiphysis	2	—	5	7
„ lower epiphysis	46	14	52	112
ULNA, upper epiphysis	4	2	3	9
„ lower epiphysis	6	—	5	11
PHALANGES OF FINGERS	1	—	2	3
METACARPUS	—	—	8	8
Total	115	43	268	426

LOWER EXTREMITY

—	Pathological anatomy	Compound cases	Simple	Tota
FEMUR, epiphysis of head .	4	—	31 (including two opera-tion cases)	35
„ great trochanter .	11	1	2	14
„ lesser trochanter .	1	—	—	1
„ lower epiphysis .	72 (including many com-pound, which were ampu-tated)	12 (terminat-ing in re-covery)	41	125
TIBIA, upper epiphysis .	12	1	11	24
„ epiphysis of tubercle	—	—	10 (including two opera-tion cases)	10
„ lower epiphysis .	11	11	24	46
FIBULA, upper epiphysis .	3	—	—	3
„ lower epiphysis .	3	2	—	5
PHALANGES OF TOES . .	—	1	1	2
METATARSUS	—	—	2 .	2
Total	117	28	122	267

From the total number, 426, of separations in the upper extremity, and the total 267 in the lower extremity, a grand total of 693 [1] exists.

After the lower epiphysis of the femur, the lower epiphysis of the radius stands next in order of frequency in the number of specimens which pathological anatomy can show, whereas at the upper end of the humerus there are few specimens compared with clinical cases. The fallacy lies in the fact that in the lower end of the femur the injury is more frequently followed by serious complications, amputation, or death.

[1] The grand total has been considerably increased since these figures were drawn up.

CHAPTER V

EXPERIMENTS IN PATHOLOGICAL ANATOMY AND THEIR HISTOLOGICAL ANATOMY. MECHANISM

Experiments in pathological anatomy and their histology.—Ollier found that pure epiphysial separations could only be effected with difficulty in animals on account of the periosteum, which is intimately blended with the conjugal cartilage; but if the periosteum were divided round the cartilage, separation was readily effected. Many experiments on the human subject have given the same results.

Wilson, in some experiments on the bodies of infants in 1820 (*On the Bones and Joints*, London, 1820), found in one instance that it required the weight of 550 lbs. to detach an epiphysis from a growing bone from which the periosteum was not removed; whereas when the periosteum was removed from the corresponding bone of the other side, 119 lbs. detached the epiphysis, showing the great strength of the periosteum in binding the epiphysis to the diaphysis.

The true osseous epiphyses (*ostéo-épiphyses*, P. Vogt) are far more readily separated in experiments on the dead subject than those epiphyses (*chondro-épiphyses*) which are still entirely cartilaginous. This is due to the elasticity of the latter, which presents less resistance to the force of the violence acting upon them. Pure separations were the rule in the latter case, whereas in the former they were usually accompanied by fracture of the diaphysis in the immediate neighbourhood.

Foucher believed that, if the separation did not take place in the spongy bone itself, it sometimes occurred between the chondroid and spongy layers, and sometimes between the spongy layers and the spongy bone.

Michniowsky, in his experiments on living animals, by forcibly separating the epiphyses by means of hyper-extension found that the separation never took place in the epiphysial cartilage itself, but always between its calcareous layer and the most recently formed osseous layer of the diaphysis.

Similar experiments by Ollier gave the same result, so that he termed these lesions 'juxta-epiphysial.'

Gurlt, in his experiments on newly born children and infants a few months old, found that epiphysial separations were at the same time accompanied by a tearing away of pieces of the diaphysis, notably in the case of the epiphyses of the larger bones. On the contrary, in Colignon's experiments on the bodies of newly born infants the cleanly separated surface of the epiphyses of the femur, tibia, and bones of the upper extremity presented no osseous particles to the eye or touch; it was exactly at the level of the conjugal cartilage. Experiments on animals led to similar results.

The more recent experiments of Barbarin on the bodies of children one to twelve years of age gave the same results at the lower end of the femur.

Lateral flexion at the knee-joint, as in straightening for knock-knee, has produced the same effects.

Ollier found separation through the epiphysial cartilage to be frequent in his experiments on the bodies of children, a portion of the cartilage remaining with the diaphysis. This agrees with the actual condition found at times in the living subject.

Vogt finds on microscopical examination of the separated epiphysial cartilage, in true epiphysial separations, numerous pieces of already ossified epiphysial flakes, separated by well-marked intervals, clinging to the cartilaginous area.

Salmon's experiments in 1845 were principally on the elbow-joints of children's bodies. He divided them into (1) complete, and (2) incomplete separations of the epiphysis, and (3) incomplete separations both with and without simultaneous fracture.

Most of his experiments were undertaken on children under three years. At the elbow-joint in 129 cases he found that a clean and smooth separation of the cartilage from the osseous end of the diaphysis is very uncommon, while perfect separations of the epiphysis are combined with partial detachment of the osseous substance, traces of which were perceptible on the cartilaginous epiphysis. He also found that it was still rarer for fragments of the cartilage to partially cling to the rough end of the diaphysis.

In Guéretin's experiments on bodies of children from one to fourteen years of age, he only once obtained a pure separation of the epiphysis in four instances of children one year old. In subjects of two to seven years old the comparison was one to nine of fracture of the diaphysis at a distance from the epiphysial cartilage. In ten cases between the ages of seven and fourteen years not one case of pure epiphysial separation occurred, but in nearly all there was dislocation or fracture at a short distance from the epiphysis.

M. Cruveilhier, in 1849, considered that the subject of epiphysial separations should be studied afresh, and at his request MM. Jarjavay and Bonamy made some experiments on five subjects from eight to ten years of age, but they were able to separate only the lower epiphysis of the radius—and once only the lower epiphysis of the femur and the olecranon epiphysis. MM. Cruveilhier,

Jarjavay, and Bonamy (*Traité d'anatomie pathologique*, 1849, tom. i.) also found in their extensive experiments that the epiphysis almost always dragged away a more or less considerable layer of the osseous tissue. These last observers do not mention the various means employed by them to effect the separations.

M. Broca, in his experiments on the dead body, always found that the epiphysial cartilage remained adherent to the epiphysis.

Richet, in similar investigations, ascertained that the cartilage was frequently attached to the epiphysis (*Gazette des Hôpitaux*, 1865, p. 147).

Ménard always found separation of the periosteum on one side of the diaphysis in his post-mortem experiments on the bodies of children from two to sixteen years of age. In complete separations it was torn through 2 to 4 centimetres distant from the conjugal cartilage.

M. Foucher, in his 'Recherches sur la disjonction traumatique des épiphyses,' 1860 (*Moniteur des Sciences Méd. et Pharm.* 1860, July 31, p. 743), relates in detail the results of his numerous experiments on the dead body. He says that these separations can be produced 'with difficulty;' but one of the conclusions he came to—viz. that 'separation never takes place in the middle of the cartilaginous layer'—is certainly erroneous and not confirmed by later experience.

Most of his experiments were undertaken to ascertain the mechanism by which epiphysial separations were produced. Direct traction and forcible movement at the articulations were carefully studied by him, and his experimental researches are doubtless some of the best which have been made on the subject. This author termed it an epiphysial fracture when the epiphysis dragged away with it a finely granular layer.

MM. J. Bret and J. Curtillet ('Du décollement traumatique des épiphyses,' *La Province Médicale*, Jan. 23, 1892; No. 4, p. 40) have worked out the histological features of epiphysial separations which up to that time had only been examined macroscopically.

In microscopical sections of the epiphyses detached experimentally in a fœtus immediately after death at full term, M. Curtillet graphically describes (*Du décollement traumatique des épiphyses*, Lyon, 1891) the appearance of the articular cartilage succeeded by the thick layer of fœtal cartilage with its angular cells. Lower down, these are seen flattened and arranged in columns, separated by the formative substance which also intervenes between them; still lower, these cells become rounded. Below, the cartilage abruptly ends in the osseous substance, osteoid layer (*couche ostéoïde*), where the detachment always occurred. This layer without cartilage cells appears to be implanted on the cartilage (*cartilage sérié*) by a number of perpendicular tooth-like processes, and in direct continuation with the formative material between the columns of cartilage cells. The layer is not true bone, for no osteoblasts exist at any part, but it is pervaded throughout by blood vessels (blood globules). The trabeculæ are here thin. This layer is, on the one hand, less resistent than the compact cartilage, and, on the other, more fragile than the bone which is more calcified. Sometimes the separation in these experiments was effected a little lower, just at the junction of the spongoid (*couche spongoïde*) and spongy (*couche spongieuse*) layer; but the long, needle-like processes which project from the conjugal cartilage contained no osteoblasts at their borders, which are festooned, and have their ends large and toothed, indicating the site of rupture. In one case of the lower end of the humerus the separation took place even in the midst of the spongy tissue, where the osteoblasts exist.

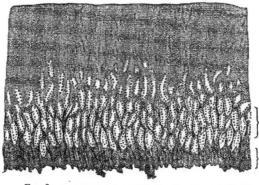

Cartilage with cells arranged in rows (chondroid layer)

Normal spongoid tissue (osteoid layer)

Fig. 3.—EPIPHYSIAL SEPARATION IN A NEWLY BORN INFANT
(CURTILLET)

Specimens such as these are very much the same as those obtained in infants where separation has been due to disease or ante- or post-mortem maceration.

In similar sections taken from a separation in a child three years old, M. Curtillet found the appearance absolutely different. The separation, when viewed under the microscope, had taken place in the midst of the osseous tissue. To the cartilage (*cartilage sérié*) there succeeded a very thin but uniform layer, which, on account of its thinness at this period (in the fœtus it is of a considerable thickness), is probably often overlooked by the naked eye. This is the osteoid layer destitute of osteoblasts (*couche ostéoïde*, Ranvier). It appears like a series of gaping spaces below the cartilage filled with blood globules, and limited by trabeculæ of a homogeneous refracting substance destitute of osteoblasts; and on this are placed a few fine medullary spaces.

This latter osseous layer (*couche osseuse*), which is dragged away by the epiphysis, is very thick in comparison with the former layer, forming the true intermediary zone between the cartilage and the true bone, presenting a form of osseous tissue in an imperfectly constructed and transitional state. The trabeculæ limiting the medullary spaces show a clear yellow colour in the centre and are bordered by an edge containing a large number of osteoblasts. The spaces between the trabeculæ are filled with blood globules and embryonic cells. The layer is consequently less resistent to injury than the completely formed bone of the diaphysis. The spaces here are larger, the trabeculæ more slender, and the embryonic cells less numerous than one finds lower down in the diaphysis. In the latter the osteoblasts are numerous, with long, slender prolongations; but in the former angular in outline, or slightly star-shaped, with feebly developed prolongations.

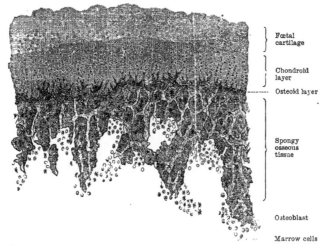

Fœtal cartilage

Chondroid layer

Osteoid layer

Spongy osseous tissue

Osteoblast

Marrow cells

Fig. 4.—TRAUMATIC SEPARATION OF AN EPIPHYSIS IN A CHILD THREE YEARS OF AGE
(CURTILLET)

'The separation has taken place further off the epiphysial cartilage than in the fœtus, and beyond the thin osteoid layer in the true intermediary zone between the cartilage (*cartilage série*) and the perfectly formed spongy tissue of the diaphysis; in the specimen the edge of the layer is formed by a number of irregular fractures of its small osseous lamellæ, detached from the trabeculæ and filling up the medullary spaces. The osteoid layer of Ranvier at this period is very insignificant, but, on the contrary, in the fœtus it is of considerable thickness.

In two children, aged thirteen and sixteen years, M. Curtillet detached almost all the epiphyses and found that the lesions presented to the naked eye appearances precisely similar to those just described. So that from the histological (or microscopical) point of view pure separation does not exist according to M. Curtillet. Although in the fœtus the epiphysial cartilage appears to the naked eye to be destitute of any osseous layer, there is a minute layer over its surface which, while it is not bone, as it does not contain osteoblasts, is not cartilage ; for it has blood-vessels and on the surface of its trabeculæ some osseous formative material. In older children the separation does not pass, as Foucher believed, through the spongoid zone, which is now extremely thin, but through true osseous tissue, and.it may therefore be definitely considered as a true fracture when viewed by the microscope, and not merely macroscopically.

But Curtillet thinks that for other reasons these separations should not be classed with ordinary fractures—viz. from the fact of their close relation with the line of ossification, the special signs which they present, the consequences which may follow from the developmental aspect, and lastly from the special treatment which is often called for ; and he therefore places under the heading of traumatic epiphysial separation ' all fractures occurring between the conjugal cartilage and the bulbar region of the diaphysis.'

Detachment of the periosteum.—The detachment of the periosteum from the diaphysis, which occurs to a variable extent, will be discussed under the head of pathological anatomy. The periosteum remains connected with the epiphysis and epiphysial cartilage.

On its under aspect, especially in very young children, there is to be seen a portion of its osteogenic layer, in which the process of ossification has already commenced. It is therefore very similar to the conjugal cartilage, which has clinging to it some of the ossifying tissue of the diaphysis (*couche spongoïde*).

Salmon, in his experiments on the dead subject, came to the conclusion that the periosteum might or might not be lacerated, but, if it were, displacement was generally present—that is, no displacement could occur without laceration of the periosteum, and displacement was in the same direction as laceration.

Besides the constant occurrence of separation of the periosteum which Colignon noted in his experiments on infants' bodies, he also carefully remarks upon the frequent laceration existing at one part or other of its extent, and explained in this way some of the displacements which he had observed.

The periosteum is more or less extensively stripped from the diaphysis, especially when displacement has been effected ; in the latter case it is also lacerated to a greater or less extent, while it remains untorn when there is little or no displacement. These results agree with the anatomical conditions found in the postmortem experience of recorded cases.

Mechanism and experiments.—In the first place it must be remembered that all violent movements of the joints in young children do not usually produce appreciable articular lesions, but expend themselves upon the bones, or rather the weakest part of them, the immediate neighbourhood of the conjugal cartilage, or the juxtaepiphysial region of the French writers. This portion of the bone is, as we have now seen, the one least able to resist twists, great pressure, or violent movements.

A natural question is : Are epiphysial separations more readily produced by some forms of violence than others ?

Numerous experiments have been made to ascertain the degree and direction of the force requisite to produce epiphysial separations. Hitherto the scanty clinical data have added but little to their pathology. They contrast very forcibly with dislocations, which are very difficult to produce experimentally at this age; but this is easily understood when the comparatively weak conjugal neighbourhood in these young subjects is fully appreciated. The violence producing the two forms of injury—epiphysial separation in children and dislocation in the adult—is frequently of the same character. The mechanism is often precisely similar, being exaggerations of certain movements ; in the former injuries, however, muscular action is of a rather secondary importance. Gurlt, in his work on fractures, gives abstracts of the results obtained by different experimentalists.

Ruysch was one of the earliest experimentalists (1713) to find that considerable force was required to separate the epiphyses from the diaphyses, as these were firmly connected externally by means of the periosteum, and internally by the mamillary processes existing between the two. In Guéretin's experiments on the bodies of infants he found that the head of the humerus was more often separable than any other epiphysis.

Another question to be answered is this. Does the character of the violence bear any relation to that of the epiphysial separation ?

The purity of the separation, its complication with a fracture of the diaphysis, or the occurrence of juxta-epiphysial separation will rather depend upon the age of the subject than upon the character of the violence. The latter, however, has very great influence in this direction, as numerous experiments prove.

In the first place, we may say generally that violent movements of all sorts applied to a joint in childhood produce separation. Their numerous forms and efficacy in producing separation will vary according to the joint upon which they act.

The author himself made many experiments, both on animals and on the dead bodies of children from two to seventeen years of age, which essentially agree with the results obtained by previous writers.

Indirect violence is a much more frequent cause than *direct violence.* Kustner's experiments (Simpson, *Edinburgh Med. Journal,* June 1880) ' showed that in the lower extremities of infants the epiphyses that yield most easily under a strain are those at the lower end of the tibia and fibula. In one experiment the application of a weight of ten kilograms for two minutes produced a diastasis of these bones, with laceration of the periosteum. The weight having been kept on for four minutes, there was found besides to be great loosening of the upper tibial epiphysis, and rather less in the upper fibular epiphysis. The lower epiphysis of the femur was only slightly movable, the upper quite firm.   Küstner quotes an experiment of Pajot, who found the upper epiphysis of the femur intact after a strain of sixty-three kilograms had been applied; but in his own experiments he found that a weight of thirty-two kilograms left it unaffected, and doubts whether it can be injured under simple traction in a full-time fœtus. He finds, however, that this epiphysis very easily gives way from within outwards when the thigh is placed at right angles to the trunk and then moved strongly outwards.'   Simpson believed this was the mechanism of separation of this epiphysis produced during version.

In experimenting upon the bodies of three infants aged respectively seventeen days, a month, and two months, Colignon in the first instance produced with the greatest ease separation of almost all the epiphyses of the long bones. But in the second instance the employment of the same force gave no result; although very energetic traction was made in the axis of the limb, Colignon was only able to obtain an incomplete separation of the lower epiphysis of the radius.   On the third infant (who died of cholera) he was quite unsuccessful in causing epiphysial separation; pre-epiphysial fractures were alone produced.

Traction in the axis of the limb.—Traction alone, although it may be considerable, will rarely be sufficient to produce separation beyond the age of infancy.   Foucher, Wilson, and some others, as stated above, obtained separation in infants from one to twelve months old by considerable traction in the axis of the limb—viz. from 200 to 250 kilograms.   Foucher in this manner detached the epiphyses of the femur and humerus, the lower epiphysis of the humerus usually giving way first.   Gurlt, in his experiments on the dead bodies of infants, was unable to separate any of the epiphyses of the upper or lower extremities by *direct traction,* as many other experimentalists have done; at the ginglymoid joints he readily effected separation by over-extension or by lateral movements while the epiphysis was fixed, and at the enarthrodial joints by excessive abduction of the diaphysis, because in this position the epiphyses were most easily fixed in the articular cavity.   He found it more difficult to effect separation in older children.

In an experiment on traction alone by James Wilson (*Lectures on Diseases of the Bones and Joints,* London, 1820, p. 45) it was found that it required the weight of 550 lb. to detach an epiphysis from a growing bone from which the periosteum was not removed; whereas when the periosteum was taken off from the corresponding bone of the other side, 119 lb. detached the epiphysis.

Pajot proved the same by his experiments, with some appreciable difference from those of Wilson ('Des lésions traumatiques, que le fœtus peut éprouver pendant l'accouchement,' *Thèse de Concours,* Paris, 1853, 8), on the bodies of newly born children, showing that

F

the soft parts materially increased the connection between the epiphysis and diaphysis. He found that at the upper end of the humerus, separation could be effected by a weight of nineteen kilograms after division of the muscles, the capsule and periosteum being preserved; whilst on the opposite limb, all the soft parts being preserved, separation only occurred with a weight of thirty-five kilograms. Thirty-eight kilograms were necessary to separate the lower epiphysis of the humerus.

Pajot's experiments on the lower limbs of infants at full term, which were of average development and weighed three to four kilograms, gave the following detachments:

1. The upper epiphysis of the humerus with 19 kilograms (the soft parts being removed).

2. The lower epiphysis of the humerus with 35 kilograms (the soft parts being preserved).

3. The lower epiphysis of the humerus with 38 kilograms.

4. The lower epiphysis of the femur with 63 kilograms during nine minutes.

5. The lower epiphysis of the tibia with 16 kilograms.

Foucher had to employ a much greater weight than 100 kilograms to produce separation in newly born infants; 200 to 250 kilograms to detach the upper epiphysis of the humerus in children one year old.

MM. Petit Radel and Salmon could not in their experiments separate the upper epiphysis of the humerus. Salmon separated the upper epiphysis of the femur in ten instances out of twelve; in eleven children, of whom nine were less than a month old—four of the latter cases being on the two sides.

The diversity in all these experiments made on the newly born is explained by the amount of force necessary to separate the epiphysis varying with the different bones, by the variation both in the subjects and in the manner in which the traction was applied.

Although Pajot, Wilson, Foucher and others have employed heavy weights in order to detach the epiphyses, we must remember that traction was employed only in the direction of the axis of the bone; whereas during life the violence also acts in more or less perpendicular direction to the bone, and usually with a sudden jerk or shock.

Direct traction, as in dragging a child by the arm, may separate one of the epiphyses of the upper extremity.

Separation of the epiphyses during delivery of an infant may be produced by the same cause.

The force required is at all times considerable; if we find the epiphyses detachable by a slight amount, some nutritive change about the epiphysial line of cartilage at once suggests itself as the reason.

Forcible hyper-flexion and hyper-extension of a joint, especially of the ginglymoid articulations of the elbow and knee, where the normal range of movement is limited, will readily effect a separation of the epiphysis of the humerus, femur, or tibia, especially if combined with a certain amount of rotation.

The articular ligaments, by these forcible movements of extension, are placed in their greatest state of tension ; at the ankle joint it is common to find the foot fixed and the joint over-extended or flexed, as when a boy, in climbing over a fence, gets his foot fixed in the railings and falls over, hanging by a leg.

Colignon could nearly always separate, by forcible extension, in very young children, the lower epiphysis of the humerus, but never the olecranon epiphysis.

Gurlt's experiments of forcible extension and flexion easily produced the same results on the same joints.   Such movements will have no effect upon the articulation of the shoulder.

Out of 129 cases of separation of the epiphyses at the elbow joint produced by hyper-extension, Salmon found sixty-four were of the whole lower epiphysis of the humerus.

Voillemier in a few instances produced separation of the lower radial epiphysis by hyper-extension, ' par arrachement,' and by hyper-flexion of the wrist ; Colignon, by hyper-extension, easily obtained the detachment of this epiphysis, but only in young subjects ; also that of the lower femoral epiphysis, though seldom that of the upper tibial epiphysis, by hyper-extension of the knee-joint in newly born children.   Hamilton separated the olecranon while reducing a dislocation of the elbow in a child.

Salmon, in his experiments, separated the lower epiphysis of the humerus as a whole sixty-four times by employing forcible extension at the elbow-joint in 129 bodies of infants.   In one other case the internal condyle was detached, in two the upper epiphysis of the ulna, and in one the upper epiphysis of the radius.

Foucher was always able to separate the lower femoral and upper tibial epiphyses in children less than a year old by over-extension or over-flexion of the knee.

At the ankle-joint Colignon only once separated the lower tibial epiphysis by this means ; in another case of a child aged three months he produced a *pre-epiphysial fracture.*

The epiphyses, having a broad and more or less flattened surface of union with the diaphyses—e.g. the lower end of the femur and radius and lower end of the tibia—are more easily separated on the dead body than those which have an irregular reciprocal surface.

During life we mostly find that epiphysial separations are produced by the violence acting perpendicularly or obliquely to the axis of the bone. . The bone is usually fixed somewhere in the neighbourhood of the epiphysis, and gives way closely at the epiphysial line— its weakest point.   A good example of this is afforded by Fontanelle's case.   A boy, aged eleven years, whilst running caught his leg in a hole, into which it was plunged to above the knee. The child's body being carried on by the force acquired in running, the femur broke at its weakest part and at a place nearest to its fixed point—viz. at the level of the epiphysial line of cartilage. The lower epiphysis was thereby separated.

It is quite unnecessary to describe the experiments already alluded to of Ollier, Vogt, Michniowsky, and others upon living animals, the anatomical conditions differing so vastly in them from those of the human subject that they can only have a relative value.

Forcible abduction and adduction, combined with torsion or rotation, act very powerfully in separating the lower epiphyses of the femur, tibia, fibula, and radius.

Abduction of the limb with a certain amount of rotation outwards is the chief and the most easy way of producing separation of the upper epiphyses of the femur and humerus.

Separation of the internal epicondyle may also be readily effected by abduction of the forearm at the elbow.

Fixing the epiphysis and forcibly flexing or extending the shaft, or moving it in a lateral direction, readily effects a separation. Gurlt easily produced separation in this manner. Terrillon, Ménard, and Barbarin produced separation of the epiphyses at the knee-joint by powerful lateral flexion.

Torsion of the limb is most effectual when combined with flexion or extension. It is more powerful in its action in older children, where the articular ligaments are more resistent and rigid, than it is in infants with laxer articulations.

Colignon easily produced separation of the upper epiphysis of the humerus and femur by violent abduction and rotation outwards.

Ricard quotes the following case (*Traité de chirurgie*, Duplay and Reclus, tom. ii. 1890, p. 346) as an illustration of epiphysial separation by torsion. An altercation having sprung up between a boy aged nineteen and his master, the latter seized him by the middle of the left arm and violently twisted him in order to push him outside. Although the youth had not received any direct blow, he experienced very acute pain at the shoulder, and found himself unable to use his arm. He was admitted to the Hôpital de la Pitié, and the next day there was found to be a fairly considerable swelling of the shoulder and upper half of the arm. The elbow was a little away from the side, but could be brought to it, though this caused some pain. Active movement could not be effected, and passive movements were painful. There was great effusion into the sub-deltoid bursa and joint. The swelling extended to the infra-clavicular region and rendered its exploration more difficult; however, it was found that there was no abnormal projection either here or in the axilla. The clavicle and scapula were intact. Very acute pain was caused by direct pressure on the humerus; it was limited, and situated two fingers' breadth below the acromion; it was also produced when pressure was made from below upwards on the elbow. On seizing the lower part of the arm and rotating it slightly round the axis of the humerus, smooth and muffled crepitus could be distinctly felt by the other hand on the shoulder, and appeared to be situated at the same painful spot above. This smooth crepitus was quite characteristic. The next day the swelling of the shoulder was more marked, and the inner aspect of the arm was extensively ecchymosed. Careful measurement of the two arms did not show any appreciable shortening. Firm union took place, but with some displacement of the humerus forwards, so that the head formed an angle with the axis of the shaft, being situated at its posterior and inner side, while all movements were perfectly free.

Forcible extension and abduction, combined with rotation or torsion, are then, as a general rule, the most potent means of separating the epiphyses.

During life this form of mechanism is brought about when, say, a child's leg is caught in the revolving spokes of a carriage wheel, and the lower epiphysis of the femur separated; or when the arm is seized by the revolving strap of a machine, and the lower epiphysis of the humerus detached.

Direct violence.—Malgaigne did not admit direct violence as a cause of separation, but the numerous cases quoted later on in this work are sufficient to disprove this opinion and to clearly establish its frequent occurrence. The smallness of the epiphyses in general often permits of their escape from injury in direct violence. However, a fall or blow on the great trochanter is sufficient to separate this epiphysis, as in Aston Key's case.

Direct blows on the lower end of a limb more often produce a fracture than a separation.

In many instances violence applied to the lower end of a limb, though appearing direct, acts only indirectly upon the epiphysial junction or the epiphysis.

M. Delorme has carefully studied, by means of experiments, the form and situation of fractures of the epiphyses by gunshots.

The author has gone at some length into the causes and mechanism, experimental and otherwise, of epiphysial separation, as a knowledge of them is of great assistance in forming an accurate diagnosis, especially when they are considered with the symptoms present.

CHAPTER VI

PATHOLOGICAL ANATOMY

SITE OF SEPARATION

THE pathology of epiphysial separation still affords some obscure points of interest.

The epiphysial junction line of cartilage is the weakest part of a bone in infancy and youth, and consequently the part most likely to give way when violence is applied in the neighbourhood of an epiphysis.

When a child meets with an accident, by twisting or dragging of a limb, the violence will be transmitted to the elastic epiphysial junction cartilage. The greatest strain will, however, be manifested at the junction of the more rigid diaphysis with the junction cartilage, which as a rule will yield.

In illustration of the epiphysial junction being the weakest part of the bone, Mr. Hutchinson mentions that he had made an autopsy where there were five detachments of the epiphyses with only one fracture, that of the clavicle, and he could recollect another where there were nearly as many in one limb.

The same author, in a clinical lecture at the London Hospital, says (*Medical Press and Circular*, Nov. 18, 1885, 461) that separations of the epiphyses occur not unfrequently in the lower animals. 'In pigs it is not very uncommon, so I have been informed, that, in copulation, when a heavy boar is put to a young sow, his weight may be sufficient to detach the upper epiphysis of the femur. I have, too, a preparation showing this accident both in pigs and rabbits.'

Separation at or soon after birth.—Separation of the epiphyses from the shaft of long bones in consequence of violence inflicted at the time of birth or in very early infancy is of frequent occurrence, although Guéretin in 1837 could not find any recorded case of intra-uterine separation.

J. K. Hornidge (Holmes' *System of Surgery*; 3rd edit. 1870, vol. ii. p. 40) states that separation of an epiphysis may occur during intra-uterine life from blows received by the mother, and that it has been not unfrequently produced during birth by violent attempts at delivery.

O. Küstner has given a full account (*Die typischen Verletzungen des Extremitätknochen des Kindes durch den Geburtshelfer*, Halle, 1877) of the literature of this subject.

Since the anatomical conditions of a cartilaginous end.of a bone at the time of birth are very different from what they are later on, and since the greater number, if not all, of these separations in this early condition of the bones are really the effect of disease, but little importance can be attached to many of them as true examples of epiphysial detachment.

Dr. A. Russell Simpson related to the Obstetrical Society of Edinburgh (*Edinburgh Medical Journal*, June 1880, p. 1057) a case of diastasis in the bones of the lower extremity of a fœtus produced by the accoucheur. 'It was a case of multiparal placenta prævia, and the right leg that was seized and brought down. The child was dead before being fully delivered. The limb presented nothing special in its external appearance beyond a slight abrasion over the internal malleolus. There was no swelling or distortion of the limb; and except that the foot seemed somewhat more loosely jointed to the leg, as if some of the ligaments had been torn, it might have been thought that no injury had been sustained. Certainly there was no deformity that the eye could detect, or crepitations that the finger could produce. Yet at three different points fractures were found on dissection. They were all fractures of the kind known to surgeons as " diastases "—the shaft of the bone, that is to say, had become detached from the epiphysis. The seats of the diastases in the right leg were: first, the upper end of the femur below the trochanters; second, the lower end of the tibia; and third, the lower end of the fibula. There had also been some separation of the epiphysis of the lower end of the femur of the same (right) leg, for the epiphysis was slightly movable on the diaphysis; but the upper ends of the tibia and fibula were quite firm. In the left leg the epiphysis of the lower end of the tibia was loosened, but the epiphyses at both ends of the femur were firm.'

Pure separation.—According to the majority of authors, true separation only exists where the lesion is characterised by a clean separation between the osseous tissue and the epiphysial cartilage, and in the larger proportion of cases the disjunction is effected by means of a fracture, the cartilage dragging with it a more or less appreciable portion of the osseous tissue of the diaphysis.

The writer in the *British and Foreign Med. Chirurgical Review* (1862, vol. ii. p. 149) quotes as follows from M. Coulon (*Traité clinique et pratique des fractures chez les enfants*, Paris 1861, p. 15): ' We find that the united experience of Marjolin and Coulon has not enabled them to produce a single example of true separation of the epiphyses, notwithstanding the frequent occurrence of fracture near the large joints—a striking example of the rarity of the accident. We may also add that after examining a good number of specimens we have found in most of those in which the accident was recent that the fracture, if it traversed the epiphysial line at one part of the bone, generally left it at another part.'

Richet sums up the question of true epiphysial separation in the following words:

' Ce n'est là d'ailleurs, il faut bien en convenir, qu'une discussion sans importance pratique, puisque le pronostic et le traitement de ces prétendus décollements épiphysaires sont identiques avec ceux des fractures des extrémités articulaires complètement ossifiées.'

In the discussion at the Société de Chirurgie, Paris, in 1865, some speakers, in particular M. Chassaignac, appeared to admit as separations only those which were absolutely pure—namely, those in which there is a complete separation of the epiphysis and diaphysis just at the level of the junction of the cartilage and bone.

Taken in this way, it is true, separations are exceedingly rare, inasmuch as it is a true fracture of the spongy tissue of the shaft in proximity to the epiphysial cartilage, for the cartilage is usually found covered with thin granular particles which have been detached from the diaphysis.

Every solution of continuity near the epiphysial cartilage, or between it and the bulbar region (*région bulbaire*) of the diaphysis, must be considered as a separation.

R. W. Smith, of Dublin, maintained that separations follow exactly the line of the cartilage. Some few authors still declare dogmatically that such separations do not exist, but that in all cases the line of separation passes through the osseous tissue. In many the solution of continuity undoubtedly takes place through the spongy tissue of the diaphysis near the epiphysis (*fracture pré-épiphysaire,* Foucher). We must also admit with Foucher that a large majority partake of the characters of all forms, and yet, from numerous specimens now in existence, the question of the reality of pure forms of separation can no longer be doubted.

The frequent presence of an associated fracture is a matter of secondary importance; the principal lesion is the epiphysial separation.

Foucher (*Annales du Congrès médical de Rouen,* 1863), who was one of the first to carefully study the pathology of epiphysial separations, divided them into three classes:

1. Pure separation of the epiphysis from the diaphysis (*divulsion épiphysaire*) without any osseous tissue adhering to it.

2. Separation of the epiphysis with a thin, finely granular layer of osseous material attached to it (*fracture épiphysaire*).

3. Solution of continuity of the diaphysis in the midst of the osseous spongy tissue near the epiphysis (*fracture pré-épiphysaire*). In instances in which this occurs ossification is fairly well advanced, the epiphysis being almost joined to the diaphysis.

Foucher adds: 'It sometimes happens that the solution of continuity is not so uniform, its surface presenting these three characteristics at the same time.'

The third kind mentioned is a true fracture of the diaphysis near the epiphysial line, the ends of fragments being irregular, with large pointed processes; the medullary spaces are opened, and the oily red marrow fluid oozes out.

In speaking of separations of the lower radial epiphysis, M. Anger terms 'epiphysial fractures' those taking place at the epiphysial line after union of the epiphysis.

Since Foucher's researches, pure separations of the epiphysial cartilage from the diaphysis have been generally admitted.

Bruns expresses his opinion that simple, uncomplicated cases of epiphysial detachment are much more common than is generally believed.

There are *three kinds of pure epiphysial separations* (macroscopically):

1. The separation takes place through the cartilaginous layer itself, so that more or less of this cartilage still adheres to the diaphysis as a thin layer: a rare and quite exceptional form. The conjugal cartilage is the only part involved.

2. The separation takes place exactly at the epiphysial line, the epiphysial cartilage clinging entirely to the epiphysis: the common form. The two fragments are separated exactly above the line of junction of the epiphysis and diaphysis without any portion of bone remaining on the epiphysis. All authors who have doubted the reality of traumatic separations have laid particular stress upon the rarity of this lesion in its pure form. This is the *divulsion épiphysaire* of Foucher.

3. Juxta-epiphysial separation. The tract of separation passes below the spongy layer of Broca. More or less of the osteoid layer remains attached to the conjugal cartilage. This is the *fracture épiphysaire* of Foucher, and is the most frequent variety of pure separation.

Notable examples of pure separation passing, partly at least, through the midst of the cartilage itself are given by A. Broca in the case of the lower end of the femur and by Esmarch in a case of compound separation of the upper epiphysis of the humerus, quoted by Gurlt in his *Handbuch der Lehre von den Knochenbrüchen*.

In one case reported by M. Richet the diaphysial extremity was said to be covered with cartilaginous projections, and in another there was a compound separation of the lower epiphysis of the tibia with the same existing condition.

In sixty-one out of eighty-one of Bruns' cases in which exact details of the separated surfaces were given, twenty-eight were pure epiphysial separations without any fracture of the bone, and in five of these the separation was through the cartilage itself, both separated surfaces being covered with cartilage. Thirty-three cases were partly diaphysial—that is, were associated with a more or less extensive fracture of the diaphysis.

A pure separation of the epiphysial cartilage from the diaphysis is more frequent in young children. The diaphysis presents a slightly convex or undulating surface, which has been already alluded to in the anatomy of this region. Its surface is covered with small projections and excavations, which look like small granulations, and to the finger it has a soft oily sensation, as though it were smeared with some greasy substance.

The surface of the epiphysis, on the other hand, is concave, presents corresponding small depressions and hillocks, with a pinkish grey colour and the appearance of soft vascular cartilage. To the naked eye not a particle of osseous material (spongoid layer), excepting perhaps a little here and there at the edges, clings to it. If, however, a very thin section of it be held on a sheet of glass up to the light, a very fine layer of this material may be distinguished, which appears of a yellowish opaque colour placed on the transparent and bluish chondroid layer indistinguishable by any rougher method of examination (Curtillet).

In the more common injury (Foucher's second class) the separation taking place through the juxta-epiphysial region, the surface of epiphysial cartilage is covered with a layer, or more usually small patches or particles of the osteoid layer or true osseous tissue, which is quite evident to the naked eye.

The diaphysial surface is rougher, more dry and spongy in appearance, and presents numerous holes.

The general outline of both separated surfaces is the same as in the last class.

Foucher and others have thought that each of these varieties occurred more or less readily according to the different ages. In infants from birth up to about one year, pure and simple separations ; from one to four or five years of age, epiphysial fracture, so called ; from five to ten years and above, pre-epiphysial fracture.

Bruns also thinks that pure separations are most commonly met with in early childhood. This classification cannot be accepted with our present knowledge of anatomical facts.

Gurlt, too, says that after the age of two years the separation is seldom a pure one, and nearly always a more or less considerable fragment is separated from the diaphysis, and remains adherent to the epiphysis.

The author's own opinion is that the limit of period for the ordinary cases of pure separations (Foucher's second class) is much more extended than is usually supposed, and may be met with even up to the eighteenth year.

Anatomy of the epiphysial region.—There are two distinct periods in the growth of the bones before the final blending of the epiphysis and diaphysis, in which the various parts have a somewhat different relation to one another.

Clinically these two periods are now recognised not only in connection with traumatic separation of the epiphyses and cartilaginous ends of the bones, but also with regard to acute periostitis, rickets, syphilitic epiphysitis, acute pyæmic arthritis of infants, abscess of bone, tuberculous and cancerous disease, &c. Some of these are clinically confined to one or other of these periods.

As Uffelmann has pointed out, separation of the cartilaginous epiphysis (*chondro-epiphysis*), which presents a continuous mass of cartilage, is to be distinguished clearly from separation of the osseous epiphysis (*osteo-epiphysis*), in which the osseous centres in the epiphysis have united, and the whole of the epiphysis is for the most part ossified, leaving the thin but more or less broad cartilaginous layer between the diaphysis and ossifying epiphysis.

The causes of the separation and the manner in which it is produced in the two classes are somewhat different ; the disjunction itself (i.e. the injury) varies also.

Vogt believes, from experiments he has made, that separations of the cartilaginous ends of the bones or epiphyses are mostly pure in character, and that separations of the osseous epiphysis are mostly associated with fracture of the diaphysis. In the former case he thinks that the cartilaginous epiphysis yields somewhat to the pressure of the firmer diaphysis, and that in the latter case no such compressibility, or only a slight one from the pressure on the junction cartilage, is allowed.

First period.—Although the diaphysis is rapidly ossifying, the end of the bone is entirely cartilaginous, and the cartilage forming the epiphysis cannot be distinguished from the articular cartilage.

In the bones forming the elbow-joint, this period lasts till about the third year.

Second period.—This extends to the twenty-first and twenty-second year, or even a little later.

The vascular supply of the epiphysis is now quite distinct from the diaphysis.

The cartilaginous junction-disc is non-vascular, but firmly blended with the deeper layer of the periosteum at its circumference. In some situations, as at the head of the femur, it is entirely intra-articular, in others entirely extra-articular. It is rapidly proliferating on both surfaces, and a layer of soft embryonic tissue adjoins it, situate between the medullary canal of the diaphysis and the cartilaginous disc. This layer of embryonic or nearly ossified tissue is called the *juxta-epiphysial layer*.

Broca was the first to lay down the rule that in epiphysial separations the cartilage remains with the epiphysis, and this is now very generally accepted by authors, and is well established from the number of authentic specimens now in existence. The surface of the separated epiphysis is formed of cartilage over its greater extent; here and there, more often in the centre of this smooth and slightly excavated surface, a few granules of osseous material are to be found. In the newly born and in infants the separation takes place a little lower through the spongoid layer of Broca without involving the spongy osseous tissue.

Hence M. E. Rollet thinks (*Lyon Médical*, March 29, 1891) that the title of 'juxta-epiphysial detachment' is the best one for the injury usually known as epiphysial detachment, inasmuch as it is really the diaphysis of the shaft of the long bone, and not the epiphysis, that is separated from the intervening cartilage.

Guéretin says that there are no epiphysial separations in the proper sense of the word, and that they are always accompanied by fracture; and from the histological aspect this is really true, the separation taking place directly above, in the spongy osseous tissue, some of which is nearly always dragged away.

This agrees with the opinion of many surgeons that the separation most frequently occurs immediately above the epiphysial line, and that the injury is really a fracture of the extreme portion of the diaphysis, a thin layer of the ossifying tissue (*couche spongoïde*) of the diaphysis still clinging to the cartilage.

From this anatomical point of view, juxta-epiphysial separation closely resembles separation of the diaphysis in infective osteo-myelitis, of which M. Lannelongue (*De l'ostéomyélite aiguë*, p. 43, Paris, 1879) has given so clear a description.

In this disease a layer of osseous tissue of variable thickness remains attached to the epiphysis.

M. Ollier, in discusssing epiphysial separations (*Traité de la régénération des os*, tom. i. p. 220, 1867), says that 'la disjonction ne se fait jamais sur la limite même du cartilage, c'est au niveau de la couche spongoïde normale. Cette particularité est importante au point de vue de la cicatrisation, car ces décollements se réparent comme des plaies osseuses et non comme des plaies cartilagineuses.'

Fracture oblique or transverse of the diaphysis, immediately above the epiphysial line, may occur at the same age and from the same causes as epiphysial separation, which it very closely simulates.

Several specimens are now on record of transverse fracture of the lower end of the humerus immediately above the epicondyles, and on a level with them.

The question whether epiphysial separations of the more common type are really true fractures is of interest also from the *jurisprudential aspect*.

A curious instance in which this question was raised, in the case of a separation of the great trochanter from a kick, is related by John Hilton (*Guy's Hospital Reports*, 3rd series, vol. xi. 1865, p. 342). According to the medical report of the post-mortem examination, the boy's death was produced by '*fracturing the thigh bone.*' 'The counsel for the defence took advantage of this verbal inaccuracy in the indictment, and used it successfully in his client's favour, proving satisfactorily that it was not a fracture, but a simple separation of portions of bone from disease ; and so the prisoner got off. The thigh bone, trochanter, and adjacent parts were sent up to Mr. Hilton in order to verify the separation of the epiphysis ; and as no doubt could be entertained about the character of the accident, the indictment for murder failed from the inaccuracy of the designation of the injury to the bone.'

INCOMPLETE SEPARATIONS. JUXTA-EPIPHYSIAL SPRAINS

Incomplete separations, without displacement, are often entirely overlooked. Clinically, as Gurlt pointed out in 1862, although they are exceedingly difficult of diagnosis, their frequent occurrence is undoubted. Experiments amply prove this. Gurlt says that in these the mobility may be very slight, or not to be noticed at all on account of the soft parts covering in the end of the bone.

Foucher says that he had never seen an incomplete separation— that is, where the diaphysis and epiphysis have still some points of continuity.

Incomplete fractures or sprains occurring in the juxta-epiphysial region have been recently studied by M. Ollier, and are called by him juxta-epiphysial twists or sprains (*entorses juxta-épiphysaires*) (Ollier, *Revue de chirurgie*, tom i. 1881, p. 785).

He describes the following lesions of the juxta-epiphysial osseous tissue : incomplete fracture of the juxta-epiphysial region, characterised by crushing, fracture of the trabeculæ of the bones, and separation of the periosteum and of the epiphysial cartilage, indicated externally by a juxta-epiphysial notch.[1]

The greatest crushing takes place eight or ten millimètres below the conjugal cartilage.

The following are the conclusions arrived at by M. Ollier in his memoir on juxta-epiphysial sprain, *l'entorse juxta-épiphysaire.*

I. Juxta-epiphysial sprain is the lesion commonly produced in the juxta-epiphysial region of the diaphysis of long bones by violent manipulations at the articulations.

[1] Écrasement du t:ssu spongieux juxta-épiphysaire, masqué d'abord par la fracture incomplète sous-périostéale de la couche compacte périphérique, fractures trabéculaires du tissu spongieux ; expression du suc médullaire à travers les orifices vasculaires et les déchirures du périoste. Si l'effort continue, tassement plus prononcé de la substance aréolaire juxta-épiphysaire, séparation d'esquilles du tissu spongieux (Ollier).

II. Such violence at the articulations, especially in young children below the age of three, gives rise to lesions in the osseous tissue of the juxta-epiphysial region, and not to any notable injuries to the articulation.

III. These lesions of the osseous tissue consist of incomplete diaphysial separations and of incomplete fractures of the juxta-

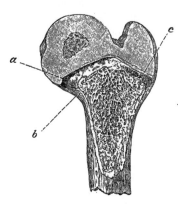

epiphysial region, and are very readily brought about when the bone has been considerably altered in its structure by rickets or by some other acute or chronic affection disturbing the proper nutrition of the bone.

IV. These lesions, occurring in the deeper parts of the bone beneath the periosteum, often pass unobserved, not only by clinical but also by experimental observers, although they are of necessity present in all their experiments on the so-called epiphysial separation.

Fig. 5.—LESIONS PRODUCED BY FORCIBLE ABDUCTION OF THE FEMUR IN A CHILD AGED TWENTY-TWO MONTHS. Oblique section of specimen. *a.* Commencement of diaphysial disjunction on the inner side. *b.* Periosteum intact. *c.* Compression of the spongy tissue on the outer side below the trochanter. (Ollier.)

V. The lesions comprise crushing, compression or fracture of the trabecular processes of the spongy tissue; inflexion, twisting, and fracture of the thin compact peripheral layer; and consequently exudation of the medullary fluid, extravasation of blood into the spongy tissue and under the periosteum, which is more or less separated.

VI. If the violence be continued, permanent depression of the compact layer is produced on the side of flexion, forming the juxta-epiphysial notch, while rupture (*fracture par arrachement*), stretching, and laceration of the periosteum occur on the side of extension. Now is the time that fracture or separation of the diaphysis is on the point of occurring, along with its displacement outside of the periosteal sheath.

VII. Juxta-epiphysial sprain is not usually serious, and is limited to a painful loss of power which soon disappears of itself; but if the child is not looked after, if it is scrofulous or has any hereditary tendency to tubercle, the lesion will often be the starting point, early or late, of some form or other of osteomyelitis, which is directly explained by the bending and fracture of the tubercular processes of the spongy osseous tissue.

VIII. Juxta-epiphysial sprain gives rise to a more or less painful but very distinct swelling of the juxta-epiphysial region, while the neighbouring joints remain free. *This is the characteristic symptom of the lesion,* and is due to the swelling of the separated periosteum and to the hyperplasia of its osteogenic layer.

IX. What has been called ' painful pronation' (*pronation forcée douloureuse*), painful loss of power (*torpeur douloureuse*), may in great measure be explained by juxta-epiphysial sprain. The former is a juxta-epiphysial sprain of the lower end of the radius or ulna.

X. In order to prevent the dangers of juxta-epiphysial sprain, the limb need only be immovably fixed for a sufficient length of time. It is necessary, therefore, in young children to carefully examine the limbs which have been subjected to violence, or which have been injured by a fall, and if juxta-epiphysial swelling is noticed, whether painful or painless, to look carefully after those children until the bone has regained its normal size.

These incomplete separations have been recognised by the author for many years as the origin of a large proportion of cases of hip, spinal, and other diseases, such as articular ostitis and diaphysial ostitis, produced by violence in the neighbourhood of the joint, or by falls, which are so frequent at an early age.

OTHER LESIONS

Fracture of the diaphysis.—The separation passes not unfrequently for a greater or less extent through the level of the epiphysial cartilage, and then runs vertically or obliquely upwards through a portion of the diaphysial end, detaching a large or small portion of this, which remains with the epiphysis.

Epiphysial separations are frequently complicated by a true fracture or fractures of the end of the diaphysis, but very rarely or never of the epiphysis; in fact, the form of separation, with more or less splintering of the shaft, is the rule, and pure separation the exception.

Splinters of the diaphysis, especially if denuded of periosteum, will add greatly to the severity and risks of the injury.

Under this heading some authors place those instances of pure separation where a portion of the ossifying layer remains in contact with the epiphysis.

Malgaigne believed that beyond the age of two years separation was rarely perfect; there being nearly always a fragment, greater or smaller, detached by actual fracture from the diaphysis and remaining adherent to the epiphysis.

M. Richet, in his *Traité d'anatomie,* says that separation is never simple, but ' il est accompagné d'un arrachement plus ou moins étendu de la substance osseuse, ce qui constitue en définitive une véritable fracture.'

Foucher thought that pure separation occurred in very young children up to one year of age, that there was fracture of the diaphysis, and at any rate a considerable portion of the osseous tissue clinging to the epiphysial cartilage, when the accident occurred from one to four or five years of age.

After examining the museum specimens of epiphysial separation contained in the London hospitals, and the recorded cases of compound separation in which the condition of the separated fragments

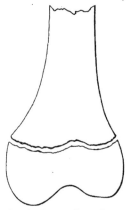

Fig. 6.—Pure and complete separation

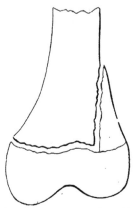

Fig. 7.—Partial separation, with fracture of the diaphysis

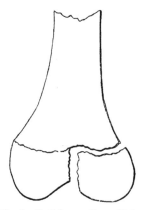

Fig. 8.—Partial separation, with fracture of the epiphysis

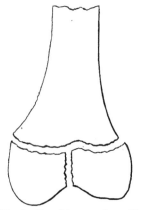

Fig. 9.—Complete separation, with fracture of the epiphysis

DIAGRAMS OF THE COMMON FORMS OF EPIPHYSIAL SEPARATION

could be clearly seen, the author came to the conclusion that as a bone approaches a certain period in its development the traumatic separation would be of a more simple character.

In each long bone there is a *certain period* peculiar to its epiphysial ends in which traumatic separation of the epiphysis is of a pure character, uncomplicated by fracture ; *below this period*, but more especially *above*, the liability of the separation being accompanied by fracture becomes manifest.

In numerous experiments on the dead subject, the author arrived at a precisely similar conclusion with regard to all the epiphyses of the long bones ; a period is reached in each end of a bone when the epiphysis is fairly ossified and developed, and likewise the end of the diaphysis, leaving a weak point along the epiphysial line of cartilage. The separation is then a pure one. When, however, the epiphysis is approaching the time of its complete union with the diaphysis, the separation will most probably be accompanied by a fracture of a portion of the diaphysis. Professor Vogt has expressed a somewhat different opinion (*Archiv für klinische Chir.*, Langenbeck, 1878, S. 343)—that true separations along the epiphysial line predominate in the case of the chondro-epiphyses, and that in the osteo-epiphyses fracture of the diaphysis more commonly occurs.

We find other writers stating the same opinion, that the earlier the separation occurs the more likely is the injury to be limited to the epiphysial line. The older the patient the greater the probability of its involving the diaphysis.

Ricard (1890) also says that in the newly born pure separations which involve only the epiphysial cartilage are the rule, while in later years the epiphysial region acquires greater strength on account of the ossification of the cartilage, and that then they are rarely pure, but accompanied with fracture.

In Bruns' sixty-one cases, thirty-three were associated with fracture of the diaphysis, and almost all of these were between the ages of ten and twenty years.

The diaphysial end has been observed to be much splintered or even comminuted in severe separations.

The existence of a few fragments of the diaphysis does not alter the characteristics of epiphysial separations, which are situated in the neighbourhood of a joint, at a part of the bone which has an important physiological function. The fractures are in some instances produced by special conditions, and the peculiarity of the fragments, their displacement, and treatment must, therefore, demand careful attention.

Detachment of periosteum is one of the most important concomitants. Epiphysial separations are always accompanied by stripping of the periosteum from a portion of the end of the shaft, as is, to a greater extent, observed in fractures in the same position. The periosteum is separated with ease from the shafts of the bones in children, but still remains in nearly every case attached to the epiphysis, with which it is intimately connected. This happens on account of the thickness, the great vascularity, and the loose connection of the periosteum with the shaft, and the intimate connection of the periosteum with the perichondrium of the epiphysis. Much of the danger of epiphysial separations is due to this circumstance.

G

Malgaigne was the first to point out the extensive stripping of the periosteum from the diaphysis.

Foucher also strongly indicated the same fact, as he had found it so constantly in his experiments.

The extent of the stripping up is very variable, according to the displacement of the epiphysis—often more than half the length of the diaphysis, sometimes the whole length of the bone (Foucher).

It is questionable whether this stripping will interfere with the proper union of the fragments by delaying the formation of the uniting callus. If it be not extensive, there is no reason to suppose that it will interfere appreciably with the length of time of union.

Even in cases where *there is no displacement* of the fragments, the periosteum may be detached for a certain extent, but yet remain untorn, and by reason of its toughness it tends to keep the fragments in position and prevent displacement. This is likely to be the case in rickets and other diseased conditions of the bones as well as in the juxta-epiphysial sprain of Ollier (*l'entorse juxta-épiphysaire*). This must be the case whenever there is the slightest gaping or separation of the epiphysis from the diaphysis.

The periosteum may be separated from the whole circumference of the diaphysis, or only for a short distance on one or other aspect of the bone. This arises from its loose connection with the shaft and its peculiar toughness. It still retains its connections with the soft parts. This adhesion of the periosteum is especially noticeable in children below fifteen years of age (Ollier).

It is only torn and lacerated in cases of separation accompanied by displacement; a rent is then made in the periosteal sheath on the side towards which the diaphysial end is displaced. In more severe injuries the laceration takes place some little distance from the epiphysis, through which rent the end of the diaphysis protrudes in amongst the muscles of the limb, and offers one of the chief obstacles to reduction.

The end of the diaphysis is seen thus to be embraced by a sheath of periosteum clinging to the epiphysis, which Hutchinson has likened to a sleeve.

Incomplete displacements, or separations *without displacement*, are much more common than cases where the epiphysis is completely displaced from the diaphysis.

In a considerable number of cases displacement is very incomplete at the time of the accident—the epiphysis being merely loosened from the shaft; for the violence which is requisite in severe separations to separate and completely displace the fragment is only sufficient to loosen the union or to produce a slight overlapping of the epiphysis.

These separations without displacement will be found to be very common, especially in younger children; they are usually looked upon as sprains, and treated accordingly. The history of many examples of arrest of growth of bones is that the injury had been considered as that of a sprain.

As far as concerns the upper humeral epiphysis, Moore (*Trans. Amer. Med. Association*, 1874) believes that the displacement is almost always incomplete.

Separation without displacement is often the starting-point, in strumous subjects, of osteo-myelitis.

Complete displacement.—The displacement of the epiphysis may be completely off the diaphysis, displaying an extreme amount of deformity.

The liability to displacement varies not only with the direction and amount of the violence, but with the epiphysis involved. Some have powerful muscles or tendons attached to them, or have the same structures acting upon them, whilst others have no such anatomical relations. Again, the anatomical shape of the diaphysial and epiphysial surfaces contributes very largely to the character and amount of the displacement. In some cases these surfaces—as at the lower end of the tibia—are more or less flattened, and permit the gliding of one surface upon the other; whilst in others the concavity and convexity of the two surfaces may, as in the upper end of the humerus, become so locked or impacted in one another as to prevent complete displacement, unless a very severe amount of injury be present.

Those epiphysial surfaces which have an oblique as well as flat surface will be still more disposed to displacement.

Multiple separations.—Not unfrequently several epiphyses are detached at the same time, as in Holmes' case of separation of the lower epiphysis of the femur, of the tibia, and of both epiphyses of the fibula.

Fischer and Hirschfeld diagnosed separation of both epiphyses of the fibula and the upper epiphysis of the tibia in one leg, and separation of the lower epiphysis of the opposite femur; the former was verified by dissection. The lower epiphysis of each radius is frequently separated in falls from a height.

Mr. Hutchinson also mentions a case of separation of the lower epiphysis of one humerus, and of both epiphyses of the other, in a sailor boy, aged fourteen, who fell from a masthead.

COMPLICATIONS. **Fracture of the epiphysis.**—It occasionally happens that the separation is complicated with a fracture of the epiphysis passing into the joint itself. This most often takes place at the lower end of the femur, next in frequency at the lower end of the humerus (before puberty), and least commonly at the lower end of the radius.

It very often occurs in gunshot fractures, while a comminuted separation results from direct crushing violence. It is improbable that the articulation should entirely recover its normal functions after such an injury.

Dislocation.—Displacement of an epiphysis from its articular relations is very rare ; there are few dislocations or fractures in the neighbourhood of a joint in early life which may not be complicated with a partial separation of the epiphysis from the shaft, but in its complete form it is occasionally seen at the upper and lower end of the humerus, while in other situations it is exceedingly rare. At the elbow a dislocation is commonly complicated by a separation of the internal, or more rarely of the external, epicondyle.

Contusion and laceration of muscles, fasciæ, and other soft parts are often greater than in fractures in the same position.

Injury to blood vessels.—These are much more frequently injured through pressure or laceration by the displaced end of the diaphysis than in fractures at the corresponding part.

This is especially marked in separation of the lower epiphysis of the femur, and next in frequency in that of the lower end of the humerus.

Articular lesions.—No definite rule can be said to exist on this point.

Separations of some epiphyses might be divided into intra-articular and extra-articular classes ; for particular joints are very liable to be involved in detachments of the neighbouring epiphysis, since the capsule in these more or less entirely includes the epiphysis and epiphysial line of cartilage.

Moreover, at the different periods of infancy and puberty the particular joint may be more or less likely to be opened, and its synovial membrane torn in epiphysial separation—e.g. the upper end of the humerus and upper end of femur.

Sir John E. Erichsen, in the tenth edition of his *Science and Art of Surgery*, 1895, vol. i. p. 555, says : 'In these cases of separation of an epiphysis with protrusion of the end of the shaft through the skin, although the fracture is in close vicinity to the joint, the articulation is not affected, and careful examination will always prove its sound condition. . . . In two instances I have sawn off the projecting end of the shafts, in lads ; in one near the shoulder, in the other near the ankle. An excellent result, without impairment of the joint, followed the operation.'

Teno-synovitis. – The sheaths of the tendons, muscles, and other tissues of this region are often the seat of effusion of blood as well as of serous fluid from synovitis. Teno-synovitis is not so persistent as in adults.

Effusion of blood occurs to a greater or less extent in every case of epiphysial separation.

It may be superficial, extending along the limb and towards the joint, the outline of which is rapidly obscured, but is more constant and abundant in the deeper parts, from laceration of muscles, and from the detached or lacerated periosteum.

The space between the detached periosteum and the diaphysis is constantly found to be occupied by blood clot.

Injury to nerves.—Paralysis, due to pressure upon or laceration or partial division of a nerve, is not very common. It has been observed at the lower end of femur, and at the upper and lower end of the humerus.

For later complications see under SEQUELÆ.

SEPARATIONS THE CAUSE AND CONSEQUENCE OF DISEASE

Separations the cause of disease.—It is highly probable that separations without any displacement of the epiphysis, or partial separations, are the very frequent cause of strumous disease of a joint—e.g. hip disease, caries of the spine, or suppurative disease of the bone or periosteum. This is very likely in weakly or strumous children ; whereas in children of a strong and healthy constitution such lesions— which are very frequently overlooked from their difficulty of diagnosis, or are only treated as sprains—will get well quickly and unite firmly without any untoward consequences.

M. Fournier relates (*Bulletin de la Soc. Anatomique*, xxx. 1855, p. 50) a well marked example of ostitis and acute disease following slight injury to the epiphysial line. The ostitis affected the lower two-thirds of the femur, and was accompanied by sub-periosteal abscess and separation of the lower epiphysis of the femur.

Other instances are too numerous to be mentioned here.

Separations the consequence of disease, although of very considerable interest and perhaps too little studied, cannot be considered in this place.

Separations the result of slight injury, or spontaneous separations occur in diseased conditions of the region of the conjugal cartilage, osteo-myelitis, periostitis, congenital syphilis, scurvy, hæmorrhagic periostitis.

Some of these separations—e.g. those due to osteo-myelitis—have been known to reunite without suppuration having taken place.

Separation in syphilitic infants is of common occurrence.

Bouchut records (*Diseases of Children*, translated by Bird, 1855, p. 693) a well marked instance of separation of several epiphyses of the long bones in a newly born female child which was considered by M. Valleix as due to *syphilis*. M. Valleix (*Bulletin de la Soc. Anatomique*, ix. 1834, p. 169) also noted in this interesting case the occurrence of subperiosteal abscess and remarkable production of bone, which rather pointed to pyæmic infection than to syphilis.

Macnamara has reported (*Diseases of the Bones and Joints*, third ed. 1887, p. 165) the case of an emaciated infant in whom the epiphyses of the right elbow- and knee-joints were separated and movable. The child died two months after birth. There was no history of syphilis in this case, nor any sign of inflammation in the part, but simply molecular disintegration of the tissues at the line of junction between the diaphysis and epiphysis of the affected bones.

Another case of separation of the lower femoral epiphysis, produced by osteo-myelitis, is related by A. H. Meisenbach (*Annals of Surgery*, Feb. 1895, p. 159).

A well marked instance of separation of the articular epiphyses in an idiot child aged ten with symptoms of *scurvy* is related by Dumont-Pallier (*Bulletin de la Soc. Anatomique*, xxvii. 1852, p. 421). Two interesting cases of separation of the lower epiphysis of the femur associated with *tuberculous disease* of the knee-joint in children aged 6½ and 3¼½ years are recorded by Mr. Edmund Owen (*Lancet*, Jan. 28, 1893, p. 194).

Separation from tuberculous disease in the latter situation is seldom observed, yet the same process in the neighbourhood of other joints is far from rare—viz. hip-joint, spine, &c.

Compound Separations

Considering the violence of the injury which produces compound separation, and the ease with which the periosteum is at all times detached, it is not surprising that the end of the diaphysis is always completely stripped of this membrane.

In Bruns' 100 cases, confirmed by direct examination, 24 were compound separations.

In the author's own analysis of 692 cases, 71 were compound separations terminating mostly in recovery, although in not a few the limbs were amputated.

Compound separations occur with greater frequency in the case of epiphyses of certain bones. Compound separation of the lower epiphysis of the humerus, for example, is a much more common accident than the same lesion at the upper end of the same bone, while in the lower extremity compound separation of the lower epiphysis of the femur greatly preponderates.

Maunder says : ' Compound separation of an epiphysis is a more grave injury than compound fracture, both as regards the present and the future. By reason of the separation of the periosteum from more or less of the shaft of bone, necrosis must be anticipated and suppuration will be profuse and prolonged, while the secondary consequence, supposing the limb to be saved, will very probably be arrest of development of the injured bone and permanent shortening of the limb.'

Suppurative periostitis, followed by necrosis of the diaphysis, is of more frequent occurrence after compound separations in certain of the long bones than in others. At the lower end of the femur it is a common result, while at the lower end of the humerus it has seldom been recorded.

Hæmorrhage may occur from the diaphysial surface, if, as is often the case, the shaft is extensively fractured, and may be an important factor in determining the question of primary amputation.

It is also probable that the occurrence of hæmorrhage may interfere with the process of union in these as well as in simple cases.

CHAPTER VII

SYMPTOMS AND DIAGNOSIS

SEPARATION WITH DISPLACEMENT.—Professor R. W. Smith, in his address in 1867 (*British Medical Journal*, August 17, 1867, p. 122) to the British Medical Association on ' epiphysiary disjunctions,' says :

' I may mention the numerous instances in which I have seen errors of diagnosis committed regarding them ; the serious results of such mistakes ; their being either but slightly noticed or altogether omitted in our systematic works on surgery ; the absence of any special treatise on the subject ; and the ignorance respecting them displayed by continental writers. Even Nélaton, who may be truly said to wield at present the sceptre of surgery in France, has said that the materials of a complete exposition of these injuries are wanting ; that we have nothing to deal with but assertions unsupported by proofs—cases destitute of value, because destitute of details ; and he sums up his brief remarks by the erroneous assertion that the signs which attend them are the same as those which indicate the existence of fractures in their immediate vicinity.

' Moreover, in the *Gazette des Hôpitaux* for the year 1865 there is recorded a discussion at the Surgical Society of Paris in which some of the most distinguished members stated that these injuries could not be diagnosed with certainty, while others (including Chassaignac) doubted that they ever occurred. In my opinion, they constitute a class of injuries the diagnosis of which can be formed (by the surgeon familiar with the anatomy of the epiphysis) with more facility and a greater amount of certainty than that of any other variety of fracture. Moreover, they possess this special peculiarity (at least as regards the shoulder, elbow, wrist, and ankles), that, although they are accompanied by many signs and symptoms the aggregate of which establish the nature of the injury which the bone has sustained, there is a single sign which, by itself, is pathognomonic of the disjunction of the epiphysis.'

Even as late as 1882 we find Gross giving little attention to the subject. He says (*System of Surgery*, vol. i. 1882, p. 927) :

' The symptoms of this lesion do not differ essentially from those of fracture properly so called. Its existence may generally be suspected when an accident affecting a bone occurs in a young subject and in the neighbourhood of a joint ; when the ends of the fragments are transverse or nearly so ; when the articular piece retains its position while the other moves about ; and, lastly, when the crepitation produced by rubbing the ends of the fragments against each other is of an unusually dull, rough, grating character. Moreover, it will commonly be found that the parts when once reduced are less likely to be dragged asunder by the action of the muscles than in an ordinary fracture. The prognosis is generally favourable, union commonly taking place very promptly, especially in young subjects. The accident, if neglected or unskilfully treated, is liable to be followed by severe inflammation, abscesses, erysipelas, and more or less deformity. The treatment is the same as in ordinary fracture.'

Nélaton observed that separations of the epiphyses are in almost all cases accompanied with fracture, and therefore present identical symptoms with those of fracture in the neighbourhood of the epiphysial junction.

Malgaigne likewise said that the symptoms do not differ from those of simple fracture in the vicinity of joints.

In 1862 Gurlt expressed his opinion that symptoms characteristic of epiphysial separation alone did not exist, and that diagnosis was always obscure, but more especially when no displacement was present.

The difference of opinion held by surgeons up to recent times as to the occurrence of these lesions has now been permanently set at rest by the large number of examples proved by dissection which now exist. These have served the useful purpose of assisting in forming a diagnosis in other cases during life.

Clinically they are distinct from ordinary fractures for many reasons.

Apart from cases of compound separation, when the wound permits of a direct examination of the lesion, there have been at the present day so many clinical cases published that their symptoms can be fairly established, at any rate in certain of the epiphyses.

It is true that nearly all the signs of ordinary fractures may be observed in separations, yet there are a few which, although not often found together, will help very considerably in diagnosis, or even be quite characteristic of these injuries.

Pure separations, it need scarcely be stated, are much more easy of diagnosis than the partial separations complicated with a fracture of part of the diaphysis, while in some instances the signs of epiphysial separation are so little marked that it is hardly possible to suspect the true nature of the injury unless we are cognisant of all its forms.

In their symptoms epiphysial separations have more resemblance to dislocations than fractures.

The history of the injury is of great importance. The exact mode of occurrence will often suggest to a surgeon's mind at once an epiphysial separation, some epiphyses being more easy of detachment with certain forms of violence, e.g. lower epiphysis of femur by entanglement of the leg in the revolving wheel of a vehicle.

Age of the patient has already been fully discussed in Chapter III.

Mobility.—The only symptom upon which reliance can be placed is the existence of unnatural mobility in the bone at the point where anatomy informs us the epiphysis is united to the shaft, in the immediate neighbourhood of the conjugal cartilage, always recollecting that this line in the same bone alters its position in the different periods of infancy and puberty. This mobility of a limb after obstetrical manipulations or rough handling of an infant should suggest at once an epiphysial separation. When the periosteum has been stripped up or lacerated, and permits displacement, the mobility will be even more marked and easier of detection in certain cases than in ordinary fractures, by reason of the regularity of the separated surfaces and the absence of all tooth-like projections.

In other cases mobility will be less distinct from the impaction or locking of the fragments, or from the mixed character of the separation, being complicated with a greater or less fracture of the diaphysis.

Sometimes, after a fall or blow, a child is brought by the parents for examination on account of *loss of power* in the limb only, when the surgeon will often detect unnatural mobility, pain, and other signs leading to detection of the injury.

There is often **great swelling** of the soft parts in ordinary cases of epiphysial separations, so that the outlines of the bones about the joint are completely masked, and the diagnosis without other aids is rendered impossible.

Distension of the articulation is very great when the epiphysis is an intra-articular one, and gives rise to acute pain, which often prevents complete exploration of the part without chloroform.

Pain as a symptom of separated epiphysis is of great practical use, as it indicates the precise spot where the solution of continuity exists—viz. at the diaphysio-epiphysial line. It is especially valuable in separations caused by indirect violence or muscular action, rather than by direct violence, where there is great contusion and consequently great pain over a considerable area. In fractures near the joints or in separation of the epiphyses the pain is generally greater than in fractures elsewhere.

It has been stated, somewhat theoretically, that the pain in separations in very young children or in the new-born is very slight, and due to the absence of bruising of the soft osseous tissue of the diaphysis and medullary tissue which is found in older children. This does not appear to be supported in any way by clinical facts.

Ecchymosis and extravasation of blood in the neighbourhood of the juxta-epiphysial ends of the bones are often very excessive and dependent upon the rich vascular supply to all the structures involved—viz. at the epiphysial and diaphysial junction.

A circular ecchymosis round the limb has been noted by Bertrandi in the case of separation of the lower epiphysis of the femur, a sign more fanciful than real.

Deformity.—The deformity will vary in each case according to the displacement of the diaphysis near the joint affected, the amount and mode of application or direction of the violence applied to the limb, and according as the separation is a pure one or complicated with fracture.

Malgaigne stated that, if there is displacement, in proportion to the extent of it we easily recognise the fracture or confuse it with dislocation; but he did not believe that it was possible to determine whether it was a fracture or a separation of the epiphysis.

The form of the displacement is very largely dependent upon the characteristic and complete separation at the conjugal line, just as we find in adults that the direction of the fracture often determines the form of displacement. In epiphysial separation the detached surface is often more regular, without any projection, and more easy of displacement that in ordinary fractures.

In many separations the tendency to displacement is very slight, due to the great breadth of the bone at the epiphysial junction, the integrity of the thick periosteum, the more or less transverse direction of the opposed surfaces, and the smaller amount of violence required than in separation accompanied by displacement.

The projection caused by the diaphysial end may be made to appear or disappear during certain movements of the limb.

The osseous projection of the end of the diaphysis often appears as a *distinct ridge.*

Its border or surface felt beneath the skin is more or less smooth, regular and uniform, unlike the rough and irregular projection of true fractures. Sometimes it is distinctly rounded, like the articular end of a bone.

The characteristic appearance of each diaphysial end differs in each particular bone. The anatomical characters which each epiphysis possesses as to size, form, and extent at different periods of age are therefore of the greatest importance in diagnosis.

In partial separation associated with fracture, although the projecting fragment may be more irregular, the angular form is often not altogether lost.

A depression or hollow on the epiphysial side of the separation has been noted in a few rare cases, but more usually it is obscured by the swelling of the soft parts.

In the case of the upper epiphysis of the humerus, a cup-like hollow has been felt on the under aspect of the epiphysis.

In some instances where there is but little swelling, *a gap* has been noted between the epiphysis and the diaphysis, whilst the limb has been adducted or abducted.

In separation of an epiphysial process, the exact form of the normal epiphysis may be recognised in the detached fragment, but in many instances the outline of the process is entirely obscured by the surrounding extravasation of blood.

Crepitus.— Great importance is to be attached to this sign.

There is no true bony crepitus. The sharpness, roughness, loudness, or distinctness which is found in true fracture of bones is absent.

It is described as dull, indistinct, cartilaginous, soft, ' grating,' ' mortary,' ' of a muffled character,' and is produced by the passage of the diaphysis over the epiphysis. It can be felt during the reduction of the diaphysis, or after the fragments have been reduced, by a slight gliding movement of one surface upon the other, as at the lower end of the humerus, rather than by the rubbing of the ends.

In younger infants, where the separation is unaccompanied by fracture, the diaphysial end of the bone covered by the greasy layer glides over the conjugal cartilage and produces a very typical crepitus ; whereas in older bones, where ossification has advanced farther, the crepitus of a juxta-epiphysial separation will approach nearer to that of true bony crepitus.

It will therefore be more or less decided or sharp, according as the separation involves the spongy tissue of the diaphysis. When this rough kind of crepitus is present Gurlt believed it to be almost impossible during life to distinguish between an epiphysial separation and a fracture.

In many cases it is absent, as frequently happens with separation of the lower extremity of the radius, from the interposition of a portion of the torn periosteum, or from the peculiar position of the fragments.

Nélaton says that 'apart from the inability to use the limb—the unnatural mobility and the deformity being signs which closely resemble fractures in the same position—crepitus is the only distinguishing sign ; but then even here the modified crepitus may be overlooked ; besides, this sign is wanting in a great number of cases of fracture in the vicinity of the joints, and separation is seldom perfect, but is accompanied by a greater or less extent of fracture of the diaphysis.'

Bouchut (*Maladies des nouveau-nés*) says that ' a dull crepitus like rasping may be felt, very different from the clear, dry crepitus which indicates a solution of continuity of the bones.'

Holmes remarks that in early infancy, when the end of the bone is entirely cartilaginous, fracture may no doubt traverse the epiphysial cartilage ; here there would be no crepitus, and, he would suppose, little possibility in most cases of diagnosing the injury.

In separations associated with fracture of the diaphysis, so frequently present in older children, crepitus, as in an ordinary fracture, will be more of an osseous character.

In experiments on the dead body it is very easy to distinguish these differences in the character of the crepitus, and to determine by this means the form of the lesion produced.

Holmes says (*loc. cit. supra*) : ' The diagnosis of separation of the epiphyses rests, then, not on any supposed peculiarity of the crepitus, but on the age of the patient, and the anatomical characters which will be found in each particular case.'

He adds with regard to the specimens from the St. George's Hospital Museum : ' This collection, then, favours the opinion expressed by the French surgeons so far as that it shows that the line of fracture seldom runs accurately through the epiphysial cartilage in its whole course ; and therefore that the descriptions of the symptoms of this accident in which we are told that crepitus is absent, or is less distinctly felt in consequence of the fractured surfaces being covered with cartilage, are probably imaginary.'

Malgaigne says : ' Doubtless, when the accident occurs before the age of fifteen, when the solution of continuity is on a level and in the same direction with the epiphysial cartilage, the presumption is in favour of separation, but certainty can be arrived at only by an autopsy. It has been thought that absence of crepitus was characteristic of separation ; but in many fractures near joints crepitus is wanting, as, for instance, it often is in those of the lower extremity of the radius.'

Other evidences of a separation being very distinct, no search for this modified crepitus should be undertaken.

Inability to use the limb is a marked symptom when the separation is accompanied by displacement.

Other complications.—Epiphysial separation accompanied by a *dislocation* or displacement of the epiphysis is very rare.

It may be readily mistaken for a simple dislocation unless great care be exercised.

Separations of the epiphyses, such as the upper epiphyses of the radius and femur, which are intra-articular, are especially important, inasmuch as they may involve *serious articular lesions* and their consequences.

There will be many of the same symptoms as in intra-articular fractures : extensive effusion of blood, with effusion into the joint, great ecchymosis, and acute pain.

SEPARATION WITHOUT DISPLACEMENT.—The symptoms are but few, uncertain, and equivocal, often overlooked or regarded as sprains, there being no deformity present ; the epiphysis being held in position by the muscles, periosteum, the extent of the epiphysial surfaces, and their reciprocal adaptation. It is owing to the thickness and integrity of the periosteum, especially in very young children, that displacement is absent, and abnormal mobility exceedingly difficult of detection.

On account of the attendant dangers from stripping up of this membrane we should not be too determined in seeking for the latter sign.

The existence of epiphysial separation should always be suspected, even though there be no displacement (Malgaigne).

These lesions are common in rachitic children and in other morbid conditions of the epiphysial ends of the bones, and are brought about by slight violence.

The signs are:

Pain about and along the epiphysial line, and upon moving the limb.

Tenderness or pressure along the epiphysial line.

Contusion or ecchymosis about the joint (a most important factor).

Mobility, often slight, from the fact of the periosteum not being lacerated.

Loss of power over the limb.

Immobility of the limb by the patient and the difficulty of passive motion on account of pain experienced (equivocal signs).

EPIPHYSIAL SPRAINS IN INFANCY.—Owing to the absence of displacement and the actual lesions being masked by the surrounding periosteum, which is intact, the injuries often pass unobserved, especially in mild cases; but they often lead to acute or chronic ostitis, or even to inflammation of the neighbouring joint.

The following is what generally happens, according to Ollier, in simple cases after a fall or violent wrench. The child cries and holds its limb fixed; but the suffering appears to be lessened after some rubbing and movement, and the child can then use its joints, although a little tardily. The joint on examination is found to be movable, and, with the exception of a little bruising or slight swelling, nothing abnormal is distinguishable. There are, however, already some spots painful on pressure at the level of the juxta-epiphysial region, yet even these in milder cases have to be sought for in order to be distinguished. At the commencement there is only pain at the level of the juxta-epiphysial region; but at the end of two or three days there is more or less marked swelling in this region, while the joint always remains intact. In most cases this characteristic swelling spontaneously disappears at the end of a few days, in others it persists, and the child, who has retaken to its play after the first pain has passed away, again complains, and the limb is more or less swollen. In very severe cases acute periostitis, with intense fever and consecutive necrosis, results. At other times it is only at the end of some weeks or months that swelling above or below the injured joint may be perceived; this is accompanied by more or less dull pain, when the age of the patient allows it to be complained of. Symptoms of chronic osteo-myelitis are then present. An abscess forms, and a sinus results, leading to a small sequestral cavity.

Ollier says that these juxta-epiphysial sprains are doubtless the explanation of the numerous cases of the affection of the elbow described by Goyrand, Bourguet, and Chassaignac under the name of '*pronation douloureuse des jeunes enfants.*'

Where the separation is more complete, some *mobility* at the epiphysial line may be expected, slight though it may be.

DIAGNOSIS.—There is no doubt whatever that numerous instances of epiphysial separation are overlooked—a great many cases treated without any attempt at an exact diagnosis being made. Separated epiphyses, especially of the ends of certain of the long bones, are extremely common, as most surgeons know who take the trouble to diagnose between these and ordinary fractures; but all recognise that certain of them are among the most obscure forms of injury in the vicinity of joints.

It is especially with regard to injuries about the elbow in children that the greatest difficulty in diagnosis exists.

Fergusson, in his *Practical Surgery*, says: 'In my notices of fractures no particular allusions will be made to separation of the epiphyses—*diastasis*, as the accident is called—a kind of injury which is occasionally met with in the young subject; and the reason for this is, that I know of no difference of treatment which such cases may require, whilst every anatomist must be aware that a solution of continuity is as likely to occur in such situations as elsewhere.' He treats the subject as though it were only a question of diagnosis between epiphysial separation and fracture.

Also Packard, in Ashhurst's *Encyclopædia* (vol. iv. 1884), says that epiphysial separations do not differ materially from fractures, although the tissue which gives way is not true bone, but the cartilage-like, osteogenetic matrix.

A separation presents in certain particulars the characters both of a dislocation and of a fracture.

Its occurrence is liable to be overlooked on account of the absence of crepitus.

Hitherto the data for distinguishing a separation from a fracture at the same point have been insufficient for the purpose of obtaining statistics of the relative frequency of these two injuries in the different periods of infancy and youth.

Epiphysial separations must frequently be mistaken for sprains, especially in young children, where there is either no displacement or the displacement is incomplete.

Partial separations are at times only suggested to the surgeon by slight mobility, it may be by slight deformity, and perhaps by the presence of a greenstick fracture of the shaft above.

Fracture.—Epiphysial separations differ from fractures in many important particulars.

The *situation of the solution of continuity* in a pure example of separated epiphysis is exactly in the line of the epiphysial cartilage.

The *shape* of the displaced epiphysial fragments in a long bone is often quite unmistakable.

The *deformity* in many instances of epiphysial separation is very characteristic, e.g. when occurring at the upper end of humerus.

Crepitus in a pure separation is of the soft, smooth kind described above.

Where the separation is accompanied by a greater or less fracture of the diaphysis, the character of the crepitus approaches more or less exactly to that of true fracture, and renders the diagnosis exceedingly obscure.

Under certain circumstances, however, especially at the lower end of the humerus, the diagnosis is extremely difficult.

Dislocation.—Dislocations are among the rarest of accidents in young subjects, particularly in infancy; and in experiments on the dead body they can with difficulty be produced.

Until recent years almost all disjunctions of the epiphyses were regarded as dislocations. In young patients under twenty years of age, where a dislocation is said to exist, a careful examination in most cases will reveal the presence of an epiphysial separation.

It is on account of the proximity of the seat of injury to the joint that we have to distinguish epiphysial fracture with displacement from dislocation. Moderate traction will usually be sufficient to restore the displaced fragments to their natural position, which will, however, only be maintained as long as the extension is kept up; in fact, in many instances of epiphysial separation it is a matter of extreme difficulty to maintain thorough co-aptation; but to this there are exceptions. In dislocation there is but little tendency for the displacement to recur.

The deformity of separation is frequently that of dislocation; yet on careful examination of the projecting diaphysis it may be seen to differ from that of the articular end. The unnatural mobility is a very distinguishing feature in separation, while the epiphysis, if it be that of a long bone, occupies its normal relations with the joint.

The shortening in separation is generally much less than that in dislocation.

The reduction of the displaced diaphysis is not effected with the very perceptible jerk met with in reducing dislocation, although in some instances it is carried out suddenly and with a 'jump.'

The pain and discomfort after reduction is not so greatly relieved as in dislocation.

In many of the joints the epiphysis will be found to be still connected with the joint, and to retain its normal relations with the surrounding articular structures.

Separation also differs from dislocation in the fact that the articulation is nearly always intact, and movements are frequently free.

In all cases where the swelling is so great that a definite lesion cannot be clearly made out, an anæsthetic should be at once administered and the diagnosis cleared up.

The manipulation must be a systematic and careful one ; indeed, any indiscriminate or rough examination will only add to the bruising and laceration of the injured soft parts.

As a rule, under the influence of an anæsthetic the necessary manipulation for diagnosis, as well as for co-aptation, reduction, and immobilisation of the fragments, should be effected all at the same time. The plan of waiting till the swelling has subsided is most fallacious, for not only are the osseous projecting fragments in these young subjects less distinct after even a short interval of time (the gaps between the fragments being rapidly filled up by new osseous material poured out by the periosteum), but the immediate replacement of the fragments in their normal position produces a more rapid union of the fragments, and also tends to diminish the amount of effusion between the fragments and in the soft parts around the seat of fracture.

Both these latter points were well shown in a case of separation of the lower epiphyses of the radius and ulna with considerable displacement which has been mentioned in its appropriate chapter.

The clinical application of the new skiagraphy by means of Röntgen's rays is of great value in the diagnosis and elucidation of epiphysial lesions. The achieved and practical utility of this method of producing diagnostic photographs has been lately fully demonstrated by Mr. Sydney Rowland (*Archives of Clinical Skiagraphy*, 1896) ; and it is of very great importance to obtain skiagraphs of certain forms of recent complicated injuries to the epiphyses (*Brit. Med. Jour.*, Mar. 7, 1896, p. 620). At the lower end of the humerus, for example, there are but few anatomical specimens in museums to guide the surgeon in making an exact diagnosis of the numerous and complicated lesions which from daily experience must exist during life. If this knowledge be obtained by Röntgen's method, it will materially assist the surgeon in giving a decision as to immediate operative measures in elbow-joint injuries of children, and in removing some of the many instances of subsequent severe deformity and loss of function of the joint and limb now so little creditable to surgery.

As Mr. Sydney Rowland observes (*Brit. Med. Jour.*, April 11, 1896, p. 933), there seems reason to anticipate that in this rather difficult and hitherto unsatisfactory class of injuries and affections the new process will prove of considerable use as an auxiliary to surgical practice.

Compound dislocation.—Even in compound separation the diaphysial end has been frequently mistaken for a dislocated end of the bone. The articular cartilage covering the end of the bone forming the joint should alone, with its characteristic features, be sufficient to distinguish it from the end of the diaphysis.

H

CHAPTER VIII

PROGNOSIS AND RESULTS

<small>UNION—NON-UNION—DEFORMITY—IMPAIRED MOVEMENTS OF JOINT AND ANKYLOSIS —ATROPHY OF LIMB FROM DISEASE—EXUBERANT CALLUS—ARREST OF GROWTH : PARTIAL AND COMPLETE—SUPPURATION FROM OSTITIS —PERIOSTITIS—NECROSIS OF SHAFT AND NECROSIS OF EPIPHYSIS—ANEURYSM—DISEASE DUE TO PARTIAL SEPARATION--PYÆMIA—PROGNOSIS IN OTHER SEVERE LESIONS—PROGNOSIS IN COMPOUND CASES—GANGRENE</small>

Union.—Malgaigne believed that these injuries united as well and as rapidly as ordinary fractures in the neighbourhood of the joints, and mentions the case of a child, aged six, whom he treated for a separation of the lower end of both radii, which rapidly united in the usual time without deformity ; also in a case of separation of the head of the humerus with great displacement at an early age, the union, although faulty, was very firm, though the arm was atrophied and hung almost powerless by the side of the body.

In Ollier's experiments upon animals he found that reunion takes place, the spongoid tissue blending with the corresponding surface of the diaphysis, the layer nearest the cartilage continuing to proliferate and undergo osseous transformation.

As regards Bruns' autopsy cases, union was found in five cases— two of the lower end of the femur, one each of the upper end of the tibia, of the humerus, and of the radius.

In six other cases consolidation took place after re-section of the displaced diaphysial end.

Dr. Edward Borck, of Saint-Louis, Mo., in a paper before the American Medical Association, June 1889 (*Archives of Pediatrics,* vol. vi., Jan. to Dec. 1889, p. 574), makes the following astonishing statement which is quite at variance with facts :

'Separation of the epiphyses I see much more frequently in late years than formerly, in all shapes and forms, at all stages ; sometimes directly after the injury has occurred, at other times weeks, months, and years afterwards. My observation has taught me that separation of the epiphyses of the humerus and femur are the most frequent, and no matter at what time the injury is recognised, nor how carefully it is treated, the results are never very satisfactory. The separated epiphysis is partly or completely absorbed and therefore will have only partial or no union at all, and the limb will have a dangling motion, though time may improve the usefulness of the limb; but the patient never recovers as well as after a fracture in other parts of the bone.'

Dr. Borck's words are quoted in order that a most emphatic denial may here be given to his assertions, more especially to that contained in the first clause of the last paragraph.

In more severe cases associated with other lesions the prognosis is doubtless grave, but it is very favourable in a very large majority of simple cases where the fragments are not displaced. It is a well-known fact that these injuries generally do well, and consolidation takes place without any further trouble or permanent deformity. Whatever the ultimate result may be to the bone, reunion takes place in the most rapid and satisfactory manner.

Nélaton believed that separations of the epiphyses united in all probability like a fracture of cartilage.

When completely reduced they unite by the same process as fractures of the bones, taking place in the large majority of cases in the soft osseous tissue of the diaphysis, flakes of which adhere to the cartilage and assist the periosteum and the separated surface of the diaphysis in the formation of callus, whilst the cartilage in its immediate neighbourhood continues to proliferate and carry on the process of normal ossification; an outer sheath of callus is formed as in fractures, the inner callus, produced especially from the diaphysis, blending with the calcifying layer of the epiphysial cartilage.

These opinions are confirmed by Michniowsky's experiments on living animals in order to ascertain the precise mode of union in these lesions.

It is in some respects a regrettable as well as a remarkable fact that no specimen is in existence showing the normal process of union in epiphysial separation, after reduction of the displacement or where no displacement has taken place.

The physiological difference in the times of union of the epiphyses at the elbow and knee from those at the other ends of the bones led M. Guéretin to inquire (*La Presse Médicale*, No. 37, 10 Mai, 1838, p. 290) whether a separated epiphysis would unite more quickly at the elbow than at the shoulder or wrist, or more slowly at the knee than at the hip or ankle.

Guéretin came to the extraordinary conclusion that union took place very rapidly, and was more frequently met with in the upper than in the lower extremity.

The error of such a statement will be at once appreciated, although as a broad rule it is clear that the smaller bones require less time for healing than the larger ones.

Union takes place by callus even where displacement is present and has not been reduced; this is formed through the bridge of periosteum uniting the two fragments.

In every case of fracture in the neighbourhood of a joint in young subjects, and in all cases in which it is presumed that a separation of the epiphysial ends of the long bones has occurred, it is most desirable that the responsibility of the case should not rest with a single surgeon. However skilful he may have been in the treatment of the injury, he is liable to be unjustly blamed afterwards by the parents or friends for some untoward result for which he was in no way responsible, and which probably could not have been avoided. Ankylosis of the joint, deformity, a certain loss of power, or a crippled condition of the joint, rendering the proper function of the limb less than was anticipated, arrest of growth of the limb, suppuration, and even death from pyæmia, are all possible contingencies. They should be carefully guarded against by a timely warning to the parents, a proper explanation of the serious character of the lesion, and by taking the precaution of obtaining a second opinion. The prosecution of medical men for malpractice after these injuries, especially at the elbow-joint, appears (from the accounts given by Hamilton and others) to be a not uncommon occurrence in America; and instances of a like kind are not unknown in our own country.

Non-union.—In none of the numerous museum specimens has the author been able to find any absolute evidence of non-union after any epiphysial separation diagnosed during life. No authentic case of non-union of the separated entire end of a long bone has been recorded. Malgaigne alludes to a case of non-union of the head of the fourth metacarpal bone after an injury thirteen years previously, but the diagnosis of separation in this case was not clearly made out, and it has even been suggested that rachitic enlargement of the epiphysial cartilage led to the traumatic separation of the epiphysis.

Reichel figures another doubtful specimen (of Ludwig's) at the upper end of the humerus. Guéretin did not consider it a true epiphysial separation on account of the shortening of the bone portrayed by Reichel. Bruns alludes to one of the upper epiphyses of the humerus mentioned by Bertrandi (*Opere anatomiche e cerusiche*, tom. v. Torino, 1787, p. 168), and also quoted by Gurlt. The preparation then said to exist in Paris was taken from the body of a child in whom, after detachment three years previously, the head of the humerus had united to the scapula, but was hollowed out and had formed a false joint at the point of separation, and took the place of the glenoid cavity. The movements were not impaired.

The separation in this case was probably the result of disease— a not uncommon condition already alluded to.

A similar case in an infant at birth is recorded by Durocher.

Guéretin thought that non-union could only be met with at the upper end of the humerus and femur; he attributed it not only to the want of fixation and to the slight nutrition of these epiphyses, but also to the rotation of the epiphysis, so that its articular surface came more or less in contact with the diaphysis, and prevented the due formation of callus.

Hamilton has seen one case in a child thirteen months old of epiphysial separation of the upper end of the humerus, which had not united five months after the accident, and the child had not the power to lift the arm.   It had been' treated by an empiric, who regarded it as only a sprain.

Should non-union occur, the author is strongly of opinion that it will be found to be due to imperfect fixation, or to the injury being overlooked and treated as a sprain, and mobility of the fragments being permitted.

A skiagraphic representation of an ununited condylo-capitellar detachment of the humerus is given in a later chapter.

Deformity.—The modelling process, after union has occurred, is effected so rapidly and completely, even in many instances in which the reduction has not been quite perfect, that within a few months after the injury it is almost impossible to.detect the precise situation of the lesion.

A more or less considerable enlargement of the diaphysial end as compared with the sound side is always present, and is especially noticeable when the periosteum has been detached to any extent.

This increase in volume of the injured. bone remains for a year or two, but disappears more rapidly the younger the age of the patient.

Deformity and shortening have hitherto been unfortunately too frequent.

The displacement may be so great that, the vessels of the diaphysis being no longer in contact with the epiphysial cartilage, the nutrition and function of the latter may be seriously interfered with; it should, however, only be a temporary derangement until the subsequent absorption of callus, which rapidly unites the separated ends.

As a rule, the surface of the diaphysis still in contact with the epiphysis is quite sufficient to carry on the vascular supply in a very short period of time.

Ollier, in experiments on animals producing epiphysial separations —or, as he terms them, diaphysial separations—viz. detachment of the diaphysis from the conjugal cartilage of the epiphysis with protrusion outwards from the periosteal sheath—found that this periosteal sheath, which always accompanies the conjugal cartilage, ossified and formed a new diaphysis by the side of the old one.   This new diaphysis gradually formed the future shaft, whilst the old one tended to disappear by degrees, taking little or no part in this work.

The diaphysial end in these circumstances often lacerates and penetrates the periosteal sheath, and, being irreducible, undergoes atrophy and partial absorption, while a greater or less portion of the diaphysis, according to the extent of the displacement, is reproduced by a new shaft formed by the periosteum.

Permanent deformity, with vicious union and impaired movements of the joint from displacement of the fragments, is usually the result of imperfect reduction—it may be from want of care in reduction or proper appreciation of the exact form of the lesion, or from the injury having been mistaken for a dislocation, an attempt made at reduction, and no splint applied.

Even with the most skilful treatment and careful attempts at replacement of the fragments, some irregularity or ridge of bone close to the epiphysial line must be expected, scarcely amounting to deformity. In other cases the lesion is so near to the articulation that complete reduction is very difficult, the epiphysial fragment affording so little hold for the more ordinary splints.

The projecting edge is moulded down in a very few weeks' time if the displacement has not been great.

At times the deformity is due to the smallness of the epiphysis, and to the difficulty experienced in grasping and retaining it with a proper apparatus.

Many of these old deformities, persisting after separation, have been mistaken for neglected dislocations, and attempts made to reduce them. In some instances the diagnosis between the two after this interval of time is somewhat difficult.

Dr. G. Jetter (*Beiträge zur klinischen Chirurgie*, 1892, S. 361) states that during the ten years previous to 1892 twenty-one cases of traumatic separation of the humerus had been observed at the Tübingen clinic. Out of seventeen cases of which accurate records had been kept, seven treated outside the hospital had united with great displacement and loss of function of the arm, necessitating operative measures.

Impairment of neighbouring joint.—Traumatic arthritis is acute when the epiphysis is intra-articular, and, if intense, may be the forerunner of stiffness and loss of function of the limb, of irregularity, misshapen or exuberant callus, or, on the other hand and very rarely, of a defective fibrous callus, or even absence of consolidation.

The joint may be left stiff, or even deformed, the result of inflammatory extension from the epiphysial injury in its neighbourhood. Foucher has correctly described intra-articular epiphysial separations as having the same prognosis as a true intra-articular fracture.

In epiphysial separations about the elbow-joint, incomplete recovery of the function of the limb is especially of very common occurrence. But in other separations this loss of function and shape of the limb is not so apt to occur.

In cases of permanent stiffness of a joint following an injury, in which a ridge of bone or some irregularity is to be felt about the conjugal line, it is highly probable that the original lesion has been an epiphysial detachment, and not a dislocation, for which it may have been mistaken.

Although union is always effected, the neighbouring joint, from one of the reasons just mentioned, may be functionally impaired ; indeed, in the most simple cases this may be the result. It is therefore of the greatest importance that the patient's friends should in all cases be early forewarned against such an occurrence, before treatment is commenced.

Ankylosis due to arthritic inflammation may be occasioned not only by the injury to the joint at the time of the accident—viz. an intra-articular fracture, &c.—but also by the displaced fragments, if they are not properly reduced, keeping up the inflammatory process.

This point is of especial importance in the case of the elbow-joint, where so much controversy has arisen as to keeping the fragments in position, and shows that ankylosis may occur if special precautions be not taken to guard against it, whatever be the position the limb is placed in.

Displaced fragments, if not reduced, not only keep up the inflammatory process and serous effusions, but also lead to the production of much irregular and vicious callus.

Exuberant callus, leading to impairment of the joint, is often due to the extensive stripping up of the periosteum from the shaft.

Suppurative inflammation of the neighbouring joint is rarely met with. It occurred in Fischer and Hirschfeld's case of suppuration and necrosis following separation of both epiphyses of the fibula and the upper epiphysis of the tibia.

Muscular atrophy is often very marked and obstinate, but disappears as the limb regains its proper functions.

Muscular atrophy may be brought about by sero-sanguineous effusion into the substances of the surrounding muscles from laceration of the synovial membrane.

Epiphysial separations at the lower end of the humerus and femur are very liable in this way to be followed by atrophy of the triceps or crureus.

In other severe instances the limb may remain in an ill developed condition, the muscles having undergone atrophy and fatty degeneration from disuse.

Exuberant callus.—An excessive amount of callus is unfortunately too often met with in cases of incomplete reduction of the displacement.

In many situations, as at the lower end of the humerus, it limits to a very great extent the movements of the joint.

Paralysis of nerve, due to inclusion by callus, has been noted in a few instances at the lower end of the humerus.

Arrest of growth.—The prognosis, as regards the subsequent growth of the bone after separation of its epiphysis, is of the greatest importance to the practical surgeon. For reasons which will be stated presently, this growth is not of necessity interfered with, because the epiphysial cartilage performs its function in many cases as perfectly as before the injury.

A proper study of interference with the growth of the bones appears to have commenced about the middle of this century, at the same time that experiments were being made to discover the normal growth of bones.

Rognetta, in 1834, clearly describes shortening of the arm, deflection of the hand, displacements of the foot and knee, and shortening of the leg, as being most often the result of an undetected epiphysial separation.

This surgeon wrongly attributed congenital dislocation of the hip to epiphysial separation, whereas, as we shall see, these consequences are rarely met with in separation.

As a rule, in a simple case of separation the callus is more quickly formed and leaves less trace than in the case of a similar fracture.

The epiphysial cartilage of union, apart from any other structure, is alone responsible for the development of the bone; and any interference with its function, the proliferation and ossification of its layers, will necessarily be immediately followed by some alteration in the growth of the bone.

The function of the epiphysial cartilage has been fully investigated by Duhamel ('Mémoires divers sur l'accroissement des os,' 1739–1743, *Mém. Acad. des Sciences*, Paris), Hales, Flourens, L. Ollier, Humphry, Broca, Hunter, Stanley, and others, and is fully described in Chapter II.

Stanley is usually credited as having been, in 1849, the first to draw attention to the disturbances in the growth of bones; it is, however, certain, as has already been stated, that they had been observed many years previously.

In Germany, Uffelmann was the first to point out, in 1865, the occurrence of a case of shortening of the limb after traumatic separation of its epiphysis.

In 1873 Bidder ('Experimente über die künstliche Hemmung des Längenwachsthums,' &c., *Archiv f. experimentelle Path. u. Pharm.* 1873, S. 248) made many valuable experiments on animals in artificially arresting the growth in length of the long bones.

The growth in length of the tibia in rabbits he found to be dependent on the integrity of the epiphysial cartilage. In the cases where arrest of growth occurred, this cartilage was degenerated or replaced by bands of fibrous tissue or osseous processes, which directly united the epiphysis and diaphysis. He also found that arrest did not take place when the needles which he inserted in the epiphysial line in order to produce local irritation had not penetrated the epiphysial cartilage, but passed beneath the same into the bone.

Ollier arrested the growth of the limbs of animals by removing the conjugal cartilage, by lacerating it, by crushing it up, or by incising it (*Traité de la régénération des os*, 1867, tom. i. p. 386). He also came to the conclusion that immediately reduced separations, not followed by inflammation, recover without appreciably impeding the ulterior growth of the limb, whereas this effect is produced if severe lacerations or subsequent inflammation have occurred. He observed the same results in man.

In 1874 O. Telke described many experiments he had made for ascertaining the growth of bones; and Thiel, in 1876, made many on the lower epiphysis of the radius of dogs to determine this same question.

In 1877 Helferich confirmed by numerous experiments and preparations the results obtained by Bidder and others on the increase in length of bones.

In 1878 Prof. Paul Vogt, of Griswald (*Archiv für klin. Chirurgie*, 1878, B. xxii. S. 343, 'Die traumatische Epiphysentrennung,' &c.), discussed at some length traumatic separation of the epiphyses and its influence on the growth in length of the long bones.

Stimson says: 'Another fact, which is a reason why the interference should not be noticed rather than why it should not occur, is that the injury is by far most frequent at an age when the growth of the skeleton is almost completed, and when the result of an arrest of growth, in the upper extremity at least, might easily pass unnoticed.'

It is certain that separations are much less frequent during the first ten years of life than during the second decade, and the separation more likely to be followed by arrest of growth in the former than in the latter, when the bone is more developed and less under the influence of the epiphysial cartilage.

Many instances of dwarfing of the limbs have been recorded as the result of epiphysial injuries, but the most marked cases have occurred after injury to the upper epiphysis of the humerus. In this instance, as in other epiphysial separations, the wasting and diminished growth of the limb are in part dependent upon the loss of the natural function or diminution in the use made of it, the result of ankylosis of the joint.

As might have been supposed, arrest of growth occurs most often at the upper epiphysis of the humerus, and at the lower epiphyses of the femur, tibia, and radius, by reason of the late period of their union with the diaphysis, and their being the most frequent seats of separation.

It is probably correct, as Ollier states, that the reason why these injuries are so seldom followed by arrest of growth is that the separation seldom occurs in the conjugal cartilage itself, but rather in the ossifying or ossified spongy tissue (*couche spongoïde*) which immediately adjoins the cartilage, and a certain amount of which always clings to the cartilage; again, that these injuries often occur still further towards the diaphysis—viz. in the juxta-epiphysial spongy tissue.

In this connection we may remember that premature ossification or destruction of the function of the epiphysial cartilage may be brought about by true fracture of the diaphysis (cases recorded by Bryant and others).

Bryant mentions a case of arrest of growth of the humerus, amounting to 3½ inches, following fracture of the shaft at the age of eight years, which he attributed to injury of the nutrient artery, and the author recently (1896) had under his observation at the City Orthopædic Hospital a well-marked arrest of growth of the lower end of the tibia following transverse fracture of the diaphysis.

The relative value of each epiphysis in continuing the growth in length of a bone must be taken into consideration in determining the question of arrest of growth after injury—e.g. being more marked in detachment of the upper than of the lower end of humerus, &c.

At whatever age the arrest of growth is produced, the end at which the most rapid disturbance of growth ensues is always that which joins on last, and which has the greatest function in the process of the development of the bone ; but it must be borne in mind that the influence of the injury upon the growth of the bone will be in proportion to the age of the patient.

Professor P. Vogt reported (loc. cit. infra ; Langenbeck's Archiv, Bd. xxii. 1878, S. 343) an instance in which the left humerus had become thirteen centimetres shorter than its fellow in consequence of an injury received at the age of ten years, which was probably a separation of the upper epiphysis. Bruns relates another in which the shortening of the humerus in an adult, following separation of the upper epiphysis of the humerus at the age of two years, was fourteen centimetres.

Bryant mentions a similar shortening of the same bone which amounted to five inches, and another of one inch in two years in the tibia of a child aged eight.

P. Bruns (Allgemeine Lehre von den Knochenbrüchen) succeeded in collecting 100 cases of traumatic separation of the epiphyses, amongst which thirteen only had brought about an arrest of the proper growth of the bone—eight times in the lower epiphysis of the radius, three times in the upper epiphysis of the humerus, once in the lower epiphysis of the femur, and once in the lower epiphysis of the tibia.

Curtillet, in his Thèse de Lyon, 1891, has collected all the published cases known to him, which only amounted to twenty-four.

It is probable that non-interference with the growth of the bone is due, in most cases at any rate, to the fact that the point of separation is most frequently through the layer of partly formed bone next to the cartilage (the spongy layer of Ollier), and not actually through the cartilage itself, so that the greater portion of this layer usually adheres to the cartilage, and thus there is in reality a fracture of the bone at its junction with the cartilage. The osteogenic layer remains, therefore, in most cases uninjured, and its function is not thereby interfered with.

Again, separations are frequently accompanied by fracture of the diaphysis, so that some portion at any rate of the epiphysial cartilage is not damaged. The arrest may under these circumstances only occur at the injured part, producing most irregular increase of the end of the bone.

Arrest of growth will probably not occur if the separation takes place between the epiphysis and the epiphysial cartilage, which, however, is very rare.

From the cases here recorded it is manifest that arrest of growth is rare in comparison with the number of cases of epiphysial separation. Epiphysial separations are not so frequent during the first ten years or so of life, when the functional activity of the conjugal cartilage is the greatest, but are oftener met with up to the eighteenth year, when injury to the conjugal cartilage is not likely to be so serious, the growth of the bone having already much advanced. The cases of arrest of development reported in the present volume are 56 in number, and, though relatively few in comparison with the frequency of these injuries, yet suffice to put us always on our guard against such an event : 17 are of the lower epiphysis of the radius ; 6 of the lower epiphysis of the ulna ; 14 of the upper end of the humerus ; 10 of the lower end of the tibia ; 7 of the lower end of the femur ; 2 of the upper end of the tibia. The possibility of the occurrence is quite sufficient for the practitioner to have it ever present to his mind, as well as to lead him to attempt to protect against it by appropriate treatment and to forewarn the parents or friends of the serious consequences which may attend epiphysial lesions.

Émile Barbarin (*Les fractures chez les enfants*, Thèse de Paris, 1873, No. 206, p. 41) states that in about two hundred operations, in which M. Delore separated the lower epiphysis of the femur for genu-valgum, in no case, even after the lapse of many years, was there any shortening of the limb observed.

In a discussion at the Royal Academy of Medicine in Ireland, Section of Pathology, November 30, 1888 (*British Medical Journal*, December 15, 1888), on a specimen of congenital malformation and stunted growth of the humerus taken from an Egyptian mummy, and another from a dissecting-room subject, exhibited by Professor Bennett, it was suggested by Mr. Lentaigne that the deformity might have been due to epiphysiary fracture and arrest of growth.

Professor Bennett said that Mr. Jonathan Hutchinson was the leading authority for arrest of development after epiphysiary fracture. He did not know of a single recorded case of arrested development following epiphysiary separation ; epiphysiary separations always united with great accompanying deformity ; but there was not a single trace of any such deformity on either of the bones he had exhibited.

There is still great difference of opinion as to the clinical conditions under which we find these disturbances of growth of the bones. The influence which traumatic lesions have is mostly known as the result of experiments. The period of full activity of the affected cartilage, as a rule, coincides with the occurrence of arrest of growth. The practical importance of this subject in articular and diaphysial resections has been fully investigated by M. Ollier (*Traité des résections*, tom. i. & iii.)

Ollier concluded in 1867 that arrests of growth are not due to premature union of the epiphyses, but arise from disturbance of the ossification, so that the evolution of the epiphysial cartilage, far from being accelerated, is on the contrary diminished.

That elongation is not due to exaggeration of the activity of the cartilages, nor arrest of growth to their premature disappearance, has lately been proved by G. Nové-Josserand's microscopical investigations (*Thèse*, Lyon, 1893) undertaken at Ollier's instigation. These show that it results from disturbance of the ossifying process after injury.

Causes of arrest of growth.—Vogt, Bidder, Wegener, Maas ('Ueber das Wachsthum und die Regeneration der Röhrenknochen,' *Langenbeck's Archiv*, Bd. xx.) and others have conclusively proved that growth in length in a bone is no longer possible after epiphysial separation in the midst of the conjugal cartilage.

In many of the recorded cases the precise nature of the original injury about the epiphysial line is far from having been clearly ascertained; moreover, premature ossification of the epiphysial cartilage can be produced by a fracture of the shaft.

M. Ollier found by incising, puncturing, lacerating, or excising a portion of the cartilage that the growth of the bone was apparently lessened, and by removing the whole of the cartilage the arrest of growth was complete; so that, theoretically, every case in which a separation passes *through the midst of the cartilage* should be followed by arrest of growth. However, as has been mentioned above, these cases are practically very rare.

He also found that by removing a portion or the whole of the epiphysis, or by removing the juxta-epiphysial region of the diaphysis, he produced an arrest of development, which, however, was less than in the case where the cartilage itself was removed. Theoretically, therefore, it is possible to get, temporarily at any rate, an arrest of growth in all forms of epiphysial separation in which any of the structures in the neighbourhood of the cartilage are involved.

Holmes says: 'The importance of the question about the precise line of fracture is this: if the fracture be really a laceration of the epiphysial cartilage, this structure may be expected to be more or less altered by the inflammatory process necessary for the cure of the injury. The ossifying tissue may be permanently damaged, and loss of growth may result. On the other hand, if the injury be confined to the diaphysis, no such consequence seems likely to follow.'

But it is possible that arrest of growth may be due to *lesions of the structures in the immediate neighbourhood of the cartilage.*

The assertion that the most frequent form of traumatic separation of the epiphysis is really a fracture of the ossifying line on the diaphysis, and not likely to be followed by arrest of growth, is certainly a fallacy.

Vogt thinks that a temporary stoppage or delay may be produced by the formation of callus, stopping the advance of the endosteal vessels, but that when normal absorption has taken place in the solid callus abundant connections are formed by the vessels, and the growth normally established again. Hence there will only be a delay, and not an abolition of growth in length. The new osseous material thrown out by the two fragments as well as by the periosteum, crowding the meshes of the spongy tissue and practically obliterating the medullary canal, forms a provisional osseous bar, as it were, which later on undergoes rarefaction, and the parts return rapidly to their normal state.

Ollier thought that the normal increase in length in a bone was often a little impeded.

If the injury to the epiphyses of the long bones be inflicted during the period of life when their integrity is essential to their proper growth, much shortening and dwarfing of the limb may possibly be the after-result, and of greater importance compared with the other result just mentioned.

Though this arrest of growth is rare, it is impossible to make even a guess at its proportionate occurrence until the frequency of separation in the cases of the different epiphyses has been approximately determined.

Mr. Hutchinson and others believed that it is chiefly in cases in which periostitis follows the injury that arrest of growth is the consequence, and that the cartilage between the epiphysis and the shaft is damaged by the inflammation, and its further process of growth and ossification arrested.

Fractures involving the conjugal cartilage, diaphysial separations, and penetrating wounds implicating both the epiphysis and the conjugal cartilage, may either arrest or disturb the proliferation of the cartilage, provided enough irritation has been caused by the injuries. Generally speaking, all injuries of the conjugal cartilage which are followed by acute inflammation, and especially by suppuration, arrest more or less the growth of the bones (Ollier).

Although often only of a transient nature, it may possibly result from the very common form of separation, as it passes through the osteoid layer. The callus which unites the divided ends in the neighbourhood of the cartilage (like the gold leaf and layer of indiarubber inserted between the diaphysis and epiphysis in Vogt's experiments on animals) shuts off from the diaphysis the endosteal loops of vessels which preside over the phenomena of ossification, and are essential to the transformation of the cartilaginous tissue into bone, bringing the materials to the cartilage necessary for the building up of the new osseous tissue, and causing absorption of the cartilaginous tissue ; the cartilage, though preserving its vitality and structure, thus loses its active formative power—at any rate, for a time.

With the natural and rapid process of absorption of the callus, the vessels will penetrate it and regain the surface of the cartilage. The interference with the function will therefore be but small or inappreciable.

Others think that the checking of the growth of the limb is occasioned by *premature ossification* of the cartilage due to the inflammation which ensues after the injury and to the rapid welding to the shaft. But Ollier has clearly established (by his experimental laceration of the cartilage, &c.) that this ossification is not thus produced ; but that it is the result of a disturbance of nutrition, of a diminution or arrest in the proliferation and evolution of the cartilage cells, which do not undergo their proper process of ossification. He found that repair takes place by fibrous tissue, and that ossification is thus retarded rather than accelerated ; at any rate, it is clear that the epiphysial junction cartilage is particularly disposed to become inflamed.

In the foregoing circumstances the elements of growth themselves are involved or destroyed, but destruction of the juxta-epiphysial region may also affect the nutrition of the same part and lead to partial arrest of growth, although it may not have actually involved the conjugal cartilage (Ollier).

In infancy the injury to the juxta-epiphysial region may be of the character so well described by Ollier, and may be considered at this time as a simple sprain, and yet be followed by arrest of growth of the bone. Mr. Mansell Moullen has observed an instance of impaired growth of the lower epiphysis and lower part of the shaft of the tibia in a lad who five years previously had caught his foot in a wheel, where it was severely twisted. The case was treated for some weeks in bed as a simple sprain. The extraordinary malleolar projection had thrust the foot into a position of false talipes varus. (See Lower Epiphysis of Tibia.)

In operations, such as re-sections, we find generally the same results, arrest of development frequently following at the upper end of the humerus and the lower extremity of the radius, also at the ends of the bones of the leg in the neighbourhood of the knee-joint.

It is a noteworthy fact that few cases of detachment of the epiphysis from suppuration, or even complete necrosis of the shaft, are followed by arrest of growth, showing that the epiphysial cartilage has great power of resisting suppurative processes. Removal of the diaphysial end, moreover, in compound traumatic separations has not invariably led to shortening or arrest of growth.

Many authors think that partial or complete arrest of growth of the long bones is associated with great displacement of the epiphyses, and. occurs in cases of severe local injuries. This is notably the case in experiments (Ollier).

But this does not appear to be borne out by the recorded cases of arrest of growth. In many of them there has been no displacement, in several but little local injury; in fact, in some previously narrated the injury had been regarded as a sprain.

On the other hand, very many cases of severe injury, with great and even permanent displacement of bones, are recorded where there has been no permanent arrest of growth of the bone, the periosteal vessels being sufficient to carry on the blood supply to the cartilage until consolidation is established. Neither does it appear to be dependent upon the stripping up of the periosteum which is so constantly found in all separations.

Ollier also believes that diaphysial separations, as he terms these injuries, cause arrest of growth if reduction has not been effected or if the wound suppurates, and that in cases of immediate reduction, where inflammation has been prevented, no appreciable arrest of growth takes place as a rule.

Gurlt holds that simple separations without displacement have as good a prognosis as fracture, and that union is, like the physiological union between the diaphysis and epiphysis, an osseous one.

Histologically nearly all separations, Curtillet reminds us, are in fact fractures; the union is effected by means of callus, which, being in the immediate vicinity of the conjugal cartilage, must have some influence on its function.

It is more probably associated with the exact seat of the separation, and dependent upon certain circumstances.

Partial arrest of growth.—It is also possible to get a partial arrest of growth, or slight diminution in length (if only two or three centimetres), though the inflammatory condition which has affected the epiphysial cartilage is of a milder character, insufficient to destroy the proper function of cartilage. In fact, in all cases the process of repair must affect the growth, if only for a very short time. The disturbance of the process of normal ossification is a transient one; it is probable that this occurs more frequently in juxta-epiphysial detachments—the common form of injury. It will not be a permanent condition provided the normal process of union by callus occurs. No great loss of length from deficient growth is noticeable, as the ossifying tissue is not permanently damaged.

The amount of this transient interference with growth will be in direct proportion to the particular epiphysis involved—that is, as regards its importance in the growth of the bone.

Such a small amount of arrest of growth occurring at the time when the growth of the bone is almost completed might easily be overlooked by the surgeon as well as the patient. This is very likely to be the case if it be the upper end of the humerus, or other bone of the upper extremity, instead of one in the lower extremity, where the shortening is more noticeable.

Vogt believes that if the epiphysial cartilage is not materially injured, and no hindrance offered to the complete inosculation of endosteal vessels by incomplete apposition of the separated surfaces by such complications as severe contusion, displacements, or inflammation produced by subsequent movements of the parts, no arrest of growth is to be considered likely to occur. So that he believes that certain primary or secondary complications must accompany the typical epiphysial separation in order to produce, directly or indirectly, the condition requisite to arrest the advance of growth.

Slight stoppage or interference with growth is seen in re-sections of joints in children, in which the portion of the epiphysis removed does not approach the epiphysial disc; yet slight interference ensues, inappreciable though it may be in amount.

In certain cases of fracture of the diaphysis in children arrest of growth has occurred, and it is interesting to note that Tillmanns, Schott, and others have recorded cases in which this shortening has diminished or disappeared in the course of one or two years.

A fracture of the diaphysis might have a fissure from it involving the epiphysial disc, and lead to arrest of growth, but the author does not know of any such case.

While some think that if the epiphysial cartilage be injured, and the union of the fragments be slow or have not taken place, its nutrition may be interfered with, and therefore an arrest of growth may result, it would appear from the history of the published cases that *mobility of the fragments*, by irritating and causing inflammation or destruction of the growing cells of the conjugal cartilage, is the most important factor in the production of arrest of growth.

Others have thought, as already stated, that arrest is chiefly met with in complete displacement of the epiphysis, but this does not appear to be borne out by the recorded cases.

Want of union by callus, unassociated with want of immobility, has also been given as a cause of arrest of growth, but is rarely met with under healthy conditions.

Anything which causes undue inflammation, destruction, or degeneration of the conjugal cartilage must be followed by cessation of its function.

It is interesting to note that the few instances of true separations through the middle of the cartilage, while occurring but seldom, did so in the recorded cases between the tenth and seventeenth years. Ossification having at this period well advanced, arrest of growth cannot be at all considerable.

The risk of arrest of growth will also be proportionately influenced as the separation is complicated by a more or less extensive fracture of the diaphysis. Where the separation takes place through only a small portion of the epiphysial line and a considerable portion of the diaphysis, principally in older patients, the risk of total arrest will be almost *nil*.

To sum up the views of the authors quoted, a shortening of the affected limb is not necessarily to be expected in all cases, provided immediate reduction has been made, immobility maintained, and inflammation avoided.

Jahn has lately made (*Schwab's Morphologisches Jahrbuch*, 1892) some experiments on wounds of the conjugal cartilage, in which he has especially endeavoured to ascertain the *rôle* played in the regeneration of the conjugal cartilage by its different layers (*couche sériée, couche de prolifération*). They showed that, after excision of the proliferating zone, growth is arrested almost as completely as after ablation of the whole, the cells of this 'layer being alone capable of self-multiplication, and consequently of permitting the formation of new cartilaginous material in front of the ossific vessels.

M. G. Nové-Josserand has also recently (*Des troubles de l'accroissement des os par lésions de cartilages de conjugaison*, Thèse de Lyon, Déc. 1893) undertaken some experimental histological work with the object of proving the truth of Ollier's opinion—viz. that arrest of growth is the consequence of a disturbance in the evolution of the conjugal cartilage, and is not due to premature union of the epiphysis resulting from an acceleration of the normal process of ossification. Nové-Josserand, whilst carefully preserving asepsis to exclude suppuration of the wounds, effected the simplest possible and most limited injuries of the epiphysial cartilage of young rabbits; after noting the arrest of growth he made a careful histological examination of the changes occurring as the result. He found that two different processes were present. *First*, a disturbance in the normal development of the cartilage cells, fibrillation of the ground substance, and atrophy of the cartilage cells. These processes may be confined to the seat of injury, but if the latter be considerable the nutritive changes will invade the whole conjugal cartilage. Moreover, as M. Ollier has already observed, the diaphysial ossification may be diminished in the injured zone so that the arrangement of the cells in parallel series is much less marked. *Secondly* (but this occurred only when a simultaneous injury was inflicted upon the adjoining epiphysial bony layer), an ossifying process developed and extended forwards through the cartilage to meet the line of ossification, and then beyond into the diaphysis, so that, as it were, an osseous 'nail' joined the diaphysis to the epiphysis. Some good microscopical drawings of the sections are given by this author. They well illustrate the histological appearances of arrest of growth due to interference with the growth of the conjugal cartilage.

C. Ghillini has also made (*Archiv für klin. Chir.*, Berlin, xlvi. 1893, S. 844) some experiments in the mechanical irritation of the epiphysial cartilage in animals. Contrary to the usual belief that ivory pegs remain unabsorbed, he finds that, although this may be true if they are inserted into the osseous substance, yet when inserted in the epiphysial cartilage they may, after a very short space of time (two months), disappear entirely. He describes, and gives some microscopical drawings of, the changes in the epiphysial cartilage and the pegs. The whole of the epiphysial cartilage disappears more rapidly than on the uninjured limb. As the result of the arrest of growth of the tibia from destruction of part of the epiphysial cartilage, he finds that deformity of the diaphysis of the bone operated on, and deformity of the knee are developed, whilst lessened growth of the condyles of the femur is brought about by increased pressure. These researches agree with Volkmann's (*Virchow's Arch.*, Bd. xxiv. 1862, S. 512).

To conclude, the causes which may produce loss of function of the cartilage may be classified as:

1. Injury to cartilage itself through crushing or bruising.
2. Callus from separation through osteoid layer stopping proper blood supply. (*a*) Transient (probably common); (*b*) complete.
3. Entire destruction or serious impairment; inflammatory complication from infection of seat of lesion by external wound, or destruction by inflammation of the epiphysis and necrosis (rare), as in Poncet's case.
4. Deficient nutrition from (*a*) imperfect reduction of diaphysis; (*b*) displacement of diaphysis (rare). The epiphysis being completely separated from the diaphysis, the latter ceases to provide it with the proper elements of growth.
5. Deficient nutrition (1) from excessive callus, or (2) from retarded consolidation due to mobility of the fragments (probably common).

Consequent deformity.—The diminution in length of a long bone from diminished growth means loss of symmetry, and in many cases loss of the proper function of the injured extremity. There is also a certain correlation between the growth of the bones and the soft structures of the limb; when the increase of the bone is arrested there is a corresponding decrease in that of the muscles and other soft parts of the limb.

Great reproach may be cast upon the surgeon at the occurrence of deformity, although, in most instances, it will have been due to no fault on his part. In all injuries near the joints in young children, it is most necessary, as has already been said, that he should protect himself against any ulterior imputations which may be cast upon his management of the case by clearly putting before the friends the statement that an imperfect result may follow the treatment.

These deformities have been carefully studied by M. Poncet, especially in the parallel bones of the forearm and leg (Poncet, ' De l'ostéite envisagée au point de vue de l'accroissement des os,' *Gazette*

hebdom., 1872 ; 'Des déformations produites par l'arrêt d'accroissement d'un des os de l'avant-bras,' *Lyon Médical*, 1872), as well as by
Vogt and some other German authors.

Bouchut was the first to notice deformity following injury to
one of the parallel bones of the extremities. In a case of separation
of the lower epiphysis of the tibia he observed an arrest of growth
of this bone whilst the fibula continued to increase in length and
produced a varus position of the foot.

When the arrest of growth involves one of the two parallel bones
of the forearm or leg, deformities which are progressive up to the
time of union of the epiphyses of the
neighbouring bone are often seen and
are of great interest, the retardation of
the growth in the one bone, with the
pressure from the continued growth of
the other, leading to considerable devia-
tions in the contour of the articular
surfaces and the peripheral parts of the
limb. For instance, when the radius is
involved the ulna continues to grow
and, obtaining its fulcrum from the
humerus, gradually drives the hand outwards. So again with regard to the
ulna, the radius, being intact and bound
to the ulna at each end, will develop and
grow curved or bowed and somewhat
flattened, as in M. Poncet's and Mr.
Hutchinson's cases, the deformity being
well marked although in an opposite
direction. The hand inclines to whichever side the arrest of growth has
taken place on. In the lower extremity
talipes valgus or varus may follow
arrest of development of the tibia or
fibula.

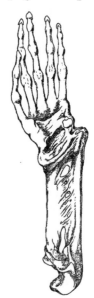

Fig. 10.—VALGUS POSITION OF HAND
PRODUCED BY ARREST OF GROWTH
OF THE RADIUS

From a dissecting-room specimen.
The elbow was also in a valgus
position (Nicoladoni)

In some cases only part of the epiphysial cartilage may be injured and
impaired, the rest of the cartilage escaping the inflammatory
change.

The hindrances to which these deformities give rise may at any
time become very considerable and serious.

Prof. Nicoladoni has shown (*Wiener medizin. Jahrbücher*, 1886,
S. 266) that not only may obliteration or premature ossification of
the epiphysial cartilage after injury take place gradually from the
inner to the outer side, or *vice versâ*, with their attendant deformities,
as in cubitus varus and valgus, but that this obliteration after injury
may also gradually occur from behind forwards, as in the case of the

lower end of the femur, and give rise to remarkable deformity of the knee-joint.

It is highly probable that many asymmetrical deformities of the trunk, such as those in the skull, the pelvis, and the vertebral column, are brought about by arrest of growth on one side, from premature ossification or impaired function of the epiphysial cartilage on that side, the result of injury.

Lengthening.—While any direct injury to the conjugal cartilage or its immediate vicinity may arrest the growth at this end of the bone, it has been demonstrated, both clinically and experimentally, that indirect irritation to the bone or medullary canal and periosteum at a distance from this cartilage may, if the irritation be sufficient and long continued, produce *overgrowth and hypertrophic lengthening of the end* of the bone. The irritation and increased growth of the cartilage cells are here more indirect and occur through the medium of the tissue of the bone marrow or periosteum, whereas the functions of the cells are arrested if directly irritated. In the human subject certain cases of central ostitis of the tibia (with quiet necrosis) have produced a lengthening of six to seven centimetres of the bone (Ollier).

There is sometimes, though rarely, seen a lengthening of the bone after fracture of the shaft in children, produced by the same cause. Ollier has mentioned the case of a child eight to ten years of age, in which the femur was found to be lengthened by two centimetres, forty days after a fracture of the diaphysis.

Max Schüller has recently (*Berliner klin. Woch.* 1891) asserted (in disagreement with Ollier) that irritations in the immediate neighbourhood of the epiphysial cartilages produce sometimes a lengthening, sometimes a shortening, according to their quality and intensity.

But we must all believe that Ollier is right in stating that it is rather a question of the seat of the irritation ; in general terms, lesions of the diaphysis, if long continued, produce lengthening, those of the epiphysial cartilage and juxta-epiphysial region a greater or less stoppage and arrest of development.

Bruns has collected (*Deutsche Chirurgie*) six cases of excessive growth in length after fracture of the femur.

May this not explain the fact that fractures of the femur in children so frequently unite without any shortening, although a little overlapping of the fragments has been present ? May not, in these rare instances, lengthening of the femur due to the irritation of the fracture have compensated for the slight shortening due to the overlapping ? However, the lengthening must be very small and only occur during consolidation. Ollier says that it cannot exceed $\frac{1}{15}$ or $\frac{1}{20}$ of the total length of the bone—e.g. in the case of the femur or tibia in a child of six years, one centimetre.

The after-results of all epiphysial separations should be more carefully recorded than they have been hitherto. The separations should be carefully examined and the limbs measured from time to time. Until this is done a proper estimate cannot be made as to after-effects in all the varying conditions.

Arrest of growth from ostitis, &c., due to epiphysial sprain or contusion. Ollier has shown that arrest of growth is frequently due to juxta-epiphysial sprain (*l'entorse juxta-épiphysaire*) or contusion producing ostitis in the rapidly developing bones of infants. He points out that the more active the proliferation of a tissue the more susceptible is it to morbid changes at any particular time, and that this is especially true of the growing bones. Consequently in infancy the effects of injuries to the rapidly developing bones are especially to be feared.

Ollier, in his memoir ('De l'entorse juxta-épiphysaire,' *Revue de Chirurgie*, 1881, p. 787), relates as an example the following case of arrest of growth of the humerus, following a fall upon the arm without the occurrence of abscess or acute inflammation.

The case was observed by him eighteen years previously, being given in his memoir presented to the Société des Sciences médicales de Lyon ('De l'inégalité d'accroissement des deux extrémités des os longs chez l'homme,' 1863; *Mém. Soc. des Sci. méd. de Lyon*). A girl of fifteen entered the hospital in March 1863 suffering from a contusion of the knee, and took the opportunity of inquiring if nothing could be done for her right arm, which was shorter and weaker than the other. She said that at the age of seven or eight she had fallen from a carriage, and that the shoulder remained painful for some time. She had often been told that *nothing had been done for it*. There was no trace of old suppuration, no cicatrix of the skin, or any adhesion of the deeper parts. The humerus was seven centimetres shorter than that of the opposite side, but freely movable without pain in both active and passive movements. The arm was weaker and smaller in size, except at the level of the neck, where it was somewhat larger than its fellow. The two forearms were equally developed. Ollier did not think that there had been an epiphysial separation, inasmuch as there was no trace of any deformity from protrusion of the diaphysial end, nor any change in the direction of the shaft. He says that he had met with a similar, though less marked (22 millimetres), arrest of growth of the radius due to the same cause.

Stanley also alludes (*A Treatise on Disease of the Bones*, 1849, p. 9) to the case of a child in whom the formation of an abscess upon the upper part of the tibia, accompanied by a partial separation of its epiphysis, was followed by so slow a growth of the tibia that, several years afterwards, it was found to be an inch and a half shorter than the tibia of the opposite limb.

Suppuration, periostitis, and necrosis of bone.—Injury to the epiphyses is apt to be followed by inflammation, which frequently passes on to suppuration, periostitis, and even osteo-myelitis.

The periostitis, starting in the inflammatory action at the

epiphysis, may affect the whole shaft, and cause partial or complete necrosis.

Suppuration and necrosis of bone are certainly more frequent consequences of epiphysial separation than is the case with true fractures. They are more likely to occur in feeble and weakly children, the pyogenic organisms finding in them a more favourable nidus in which to develop, while similar injuries in the strong and healthy would heal rapidly without being followed by any such untoward results.

Suppuration round the diaphysis which has been denuded of its periosteum, may be cast off in a necrosed condition as a sequestrum, as in a case described by Hutchinson and also in Curtillet's case.

In Esmarch's case a large abscess formed after epiphysial separation of the upper end of the humerus, which had been mistaken for a dislocation, and two attempts made to reduce it; this necessitated the removal of the epiphysis and a portion of the diaphysis.

These inflammatory complications are the most frequent causes of arrest of growth after epiphysial injury.

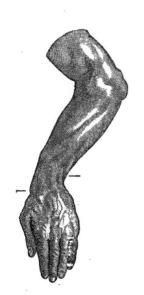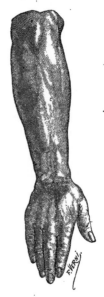

FIG. 11.—DEFORMITY FOLLOWING TRAUMATIC SEPARATION OF THE LOWER EPIPHYSIS
OF THE ULNA, WITH SUPPURATION AND NECROSIS (CURTILLET)

(See Part II. Chapter XIII.)

Periostitis and abscess.—It has been thought that the frequency of suppuration is due to the extensive separation of the periosteum always met with; although this is, no doubt, an important factor, yet it will be found to occur more often in certain sites than it does in others—viz. at the great trochanter, lower end of femur, &c.

In the extremities of the long bones it occurs more frequently at that end which is the seat of the greatest active growth.

Packard mentions a case, communicated to him by Dr. R. S. Huidekoper, of separated lower epiphysis of the femur in a foal, followed by the formation of a large abscess. The animal, five months old, in rushing through a gateway struck the stifle of the near hind leg against a heavy post. When seen by Dr. Huidekoper, there was excessive lameness; but as the animal limped the leg swung with an unnatural motion, and there was found to be looseness and slight crepitus in the neighbourhood of the femoro-tibial articulation. The exact nature of the injury could not be determined on account of the swelling of the parts, abscess ensued, the animal wasted rapidly and was destroyed. The autopsy showed a separation of the lower epiphysis of the femur with laceration of the surrounding tissues, and a large abscess.

Acute periostitis is one of the peculiar dangers attending epiphysial separation. It differs from the same complication in a fracture of the shaft on account of the thickness, strength, and vascularity of the periosteum, and the amount of the violence which it sustains in these injuries. Moreover, many muscles, ligaments, and other structures are intimately attached to it in the neighbourhood of the joints.

We find (as mentioned above) that the periosteum is seldom torn across, except where complete displacement of the epiphysis has taken place, owing to the stripping up of the membrane from the diaphysis; but it always remains firmly attached to the epiphysis, and hence there is great risk of suppuration about the end of the bone.

This stripping of the periosteum from the end of the diaphysis occurs even in cases where there is incomplete displacement or mere loosening of the epiphysis.

In this connection should it not also be recalled to mind that the end of the bone which contributes most to its increase in length is also the most frequent seat of inflammatory affections during the period of growth (Ollier), and of new growths at all ages (Ollier)?

In association with the occurrence of inflammatory mischief in the conjugal cartilage after epiphysial separation, Roux has made (*La Presse Médicale*, July 12, 1837) some curious statements which cannot be wholly accepted at the present day. Belonging to history, they may be reproduced here. '*In the neighbourhood of the larger joints,*' he says, 'when the displaced epiphysis has not been reduced, troublesome symptoms are apt to arise: inflammation, rapidly passing on to suppuration, intense pain, high fever, extensive and deep abscesses, sometimes gangrene—leading to amputation. *In the neighbourhood of the medium-sized joints* the displacement of the articular surfaces is only at times at all considerable; but consolidation in this position results in deformity of the limb, hampering and weakness of its movements. *In the small joints*, the displacement of the extremity of the bone is never great; but if retentive apparatus is neglected subsequent movements of the limb are almost impossible and the deformity is "shocking." ' Roux adds that the consolidation of the fragment even in a bad position is very rapid, but that subsequently it will be found impossible to straighten the limb.

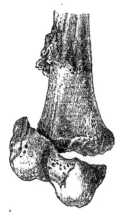

Chas. Bell's case (fig. 12) is a good example of periostitis and incipient necrosis following separation of the lower epiphysis of the femur.

Acute osteo-myelitis after epiphysial injury to the lower end of the radius in Page's case led to amputation of the limb.

Necrosis of both epiphyses of the fibula occurred in the tenth week in Dr. Fischer and Dr. Hirschfeld's case of separation of these epiphyses.

Humphry, in his article on the 'Growth of Epiphyses' in vol. xlv. of the *Roy. Med. Chirurgical Transactions* (p. 295), has collected many instances of arrest of growth of the long bones after acute epiphysitis and acute necrosis of the diaphysial and other inflammatory affections in the neighbourhood of the epiphysial junction cartilage, which we need not discuss in this place, although in many of these the suppuration and necrosis were undoubtedly due to injury, or incomplete separation at the epiphysial line.

FIG. 12.—SUPPURATIVE PERIOSTITIS AND COMMENCING NECROSIS AFTER EPIPHYSIAL SEPARATION

(Museum of the College of Surgeons, Edinburgh)

Marjolin, Stanley, Ollier, Helferich, Fischer, Paget, Birkett, Bryant, Bruns, Hutchinson, and others record similar cases, too numerous to mention here.

In a few the ostitis or osteo-myelitis has led to lengthening of the bone.

Arrest of growth is also frequently seen in operations on the ends of the bones, such as excision, interfering with the epiphysial line, although this may not have been actually injured at the time of operation.

Disease due to partial separation. *Hip disease.*—A large number of cases of arthritic diseases of the hip and of other parts of the body—e.g. caries of spine, &c.—are due rather to traumatic than constitutional causes, at any rate in the first instance. The tendency of late years has been to attribute all such joint affections to the scrofulous or tubercular diathesis quite irrespective of any mechanical injury.

In the large majority of such cases, as has been already mentioned in Chapter VI., there has been a partial separation of the epiphysis, or, as Ollier terms it, a juxta-epiphysial sprain or separation.

Pyæmia has unfortunately been the final result in too many cases in the past. Convulsions or rigors may indicate the commencement of general infection.

Other concomitant injuries.—The prognosis of many of the severer forms of injury is rendered very grave from the accompanying injuries to other parts of the body (brain, &c.).

The number of deaths in 100 cases verified by autopsy as collected by Bruns was nineteen from complications arising from injury to the soft parts, fractured skull, and other severe lesions; four from causes unknown, and five from accessory causes; two from re-sections of joint made for preserving limb; and twenty-two from amputations of the limb to preserve life.

Compound separations, unless treated with every antiseptic precaution, are liable to be followed by serious consequences, such as pyæmia, septicæmia, suppuration of the articulation, absence of consolidation, and necrosis of the diaphysis or epiphysis. It is more common in some compound separations—e.g. the lower end of the femur—than in others. At the lower end of the humerus it is of very infrequent occurrence. Again, the seat of lesion being infected, the conjugal cartilage may be destroyed, or seriously altered in its structure; and an arrest of growth may result, as occurred in many recorded cases.

Gangrene may be confined to the neighbourhood of the separation, and in these instances is due to the crushing or bruising of the part by direct violence; in others it may be due to the pressure upon the skin by the displaced diaphysis.

The whole limb below the seat of separation may become gangrenous from the arrest of circulation, due to complete or partial laceration of large vessels in the immediate neighbourhood of the diaphysial end, or to the pressure of the displaced end upon these vessels, commonly met with at the lower end of the humerus and femur.

This compression of the vessels has unfortunately in too many cases been the result of an improperly applied splint, especially at the lower end of the humerus and radius.

Tetanus is a very uncommon complication. It has occurred a few times after compound separation, very seldom after simple separation from pressure upon the neighbouring nerve by the end of the displaced diaphysis, or by excessive callus, as in Brunner's case of separation of the lower end of the radius.

Aneurysm.—Pressure of the displaced diaphysis of the femur has three times caused an aneurysm to develop in the neighbouring popliteal artery after separation of the lower epiphysis. The brachial artery at the elbow escapes this complication in a remarkable manner, although often severely pressed up by the lower diaphysial end of the humerus in separations.

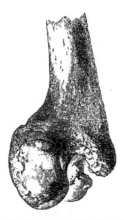

FIG. 13.—LOWER EPIPHYSIS OF THE FEMUR UNITED WITH GREAT DISPLACEMENT UPWARDS. THE PROJECTING DIAPHYSIS PRODUCED AN ANEURYSM OF THE POPLITEAL ARTERY

(Royal College of Surgeons Museum, Edinburgh. After Charles Bell. ½ size.)

CHAPTER IX

TREATMENT

In the year 1822 M. Roux laid down in his dissertation (*Dissertation sur la disjonction des épiphyses*, Feb. 8, 1822, p. 16, quoted by him in *La Presse Médicale*, No. 55, July 12, 1837, vol. i. p. 436) the following principles of treatment, which, had they been more generally known and acted upon, might have prevented the too frequent unfortunate results which occurred in so many instances in these injuries at the early part of the present century. Roux also remarks upon the brevity of description of treatment of these injuries before his time. As these rules are of historical interest, I reproduce some of them here in the form in which they are given by Roux :

'IV. The fragments of bone should be restored as soon as possible to their natural position by means of well directed traction ; the same apparatus as for fractures should then be employed to hold the fragments in position. But a shorter time will be required for their retention than in the case of fractures.

'V. It is necessary to extend the limb beyond its normal length, and direct with the hands the fragments into position in cases in which the epiphysis has been dragged on to the diaphysis by the action of the muscles.

'VI. The reduced fragments are maintained with little difficulty in position on account of the very feeble action of the muscles in young subjects.

'VIII. If the displacement of either of the fragments produces compression of the neighbouring structures, and threatens to produce tetanus, paralysis, or gangrene, it will be necessary to replace the separated epiphyses ; when this is found to be impossible by simple traction, then deep incisions should be made, or the separated epiphyses removed.

'IX. When the end of the diaphysis protrudes through the skin, incision should be made as in VIII., or resection of the end.

'X. Ensuing tetanus, paralysis, or gangrene should be treated without delay by amputation of the limb.

Nélaton and other surgeons state that the treatment does not differ from that of fractures of the ends of long bones.

The general method of treatment of traumatic epiphysial separations does not differ from that of true fractures in the neighbourhood of joints, except that they require greater attention to details and more care in preventing undue inflammation and mobility, more especially in the earlier periods of childhood.

There are, nevertheless, certain separations with displacement which differ very widely from fractures in the same situation, and which if treated in the same way would lead to most disastrous results.

With regard, e.g., to the lower end of the femur, Mr. Mayo Robson has recently called attention to the mischievous advice given in many of the modern text-books on surgery. Other instances might be mentioned here, but these will be fully discussed under the head of each epiphysis.

Separation without displacement.—There being often slight swelling of the soft parts, little or no articular inflammation, and comparatively trifling injury to the periosteum, it will suffice to fix the joint and limb in a suitable, immovable splint—as plaster of Paris, poroplastic felt, &c.—always taking the greatest care in application that it does not press injuriously in these young subjects. At the end of from ten to fourteen days the apparatus should be removed, for consolidation has already well advanced by this time, and passive motion should be commenced.

In juxta-epiphysial sprain in infancy it is sufficient to keep the child perfectly at rest and to fix the limb; any great exercise or excessive use of the limb may easily transform an insignificant lesion into a very serious disease, and one or other of the consequences of juxta-epiphysial sprain be the result.

Separation with displacement. *Deformity.*—The deformity with its symptoms and complications varies so much in the different separations near the joints that no definite treatment can be advocated for all cases.

Reduction of the displaced fragments is the first point to be aimed at, which in some few cases is readily effected with perfect co-aptation of the fragments; but in most others there is great difficulty in reduction, a point in which epiphysial lesions differ very greatly from fractures. The broad epiphysial end of the shaft having penetrated the periosteal sheath is held by it in a button-like manner.

Though the more simple cases may be treated without the use of an anæsthetic, it should always be administered in patients who are advancing towards the later years of puberty, at which period epiphysial separations are most frequently met with, especially in certain long bones and when very large surfaces of bone are involved in the injury, as in the upper end of the humerus and the lower epiphysis of the femur.

If the displacement be complete, it may be quite impossible to reduce the deformity; in incomplete separation the diaphysial end is often locked, as in the cup-like epiphysis at the upper end of the humerus, and the deformity to a large extent is maintained by power-ful muscles, so that an anæsthetic must be administered. On the other hand, it should be clearly understood that, as damage is sure to be the result, the administration of an anæsthetic is strongly to be deprecated as a means of employing force to reduce a displaced epiphysis.   Apart from the difficulty of reduction, it would be necessary for diagnostic purposes alone to give an anæsthetic where there is great swelling of the soft parts, and distension of the articulation with blood and fluid.

The greatest difficulty often attends treatment of injuries to the elbows in young subjects in whom an exact diagnosis has not been made, and it has frequently been followed by a more or less deformed and stiffened limb.

It may be summarily stated that reduction of all cases ought to be effected *at once,* and should be exact.   It is a great mistake to put up an epiphysial separation temporarily with the idea of doing so again a little better later on.

Maintenance in the normal position.—The effort to maintain cer-tain parts of the injured skeleton in their normal position is often the cause of great anxiety to the surgeon.

Plaster of Paris, in the form of Croft's lateral splints, is very efficient, with plenty of soft padding over the skin.   The immediate application of the plaster is especially useful in the milder forms of separation, where there is little displacement or swelling.

It is composed of ordinary coarse household flannel cut out to the shape of the limb and joint, and soaked on the outer side with plaster of Paris, with a gap left front and back to prevent too great pressure.

Plaster of Paris bandages should never be applied in young sub-jects, on account of the danger of gangrene, for their soft, tender, skin should ever be present to the surgeon's mind.

Gutta-percha, poroplastic, and other forms of felt splint (Hyde's &c.), carefully moulded to the part, are all useful ; all moulded and accurately fitting splints have now to a large extent replaced wooden ones.   Wooden splints in their angular form are highly useful, how-ever, in some of the less severe separations at the elbow joint.

Epiphysial processes which are small can with difficulty be com-pletely restored to their proper position or maintained there when once detached.

Owing to the smallness of the epiphysial end of a long bone there is often very little to assist in retaining the separated surfaces in position.   Ordinary wooden or other straight splints so often adopted in the case of adults render the treatment of these cases both difficult and unsatisfactory.

With respect to the ease with which the separated fragments in other instances are retained in position, epiphysial separations more resemble dislocations than fractures.

Although it is easier to effect complete reduction of the diaphysis, it is as a rule much more difficult to be quite sure of its accomplishment than in the case of a dislocation. This is in great measure due to the fact of pure separations being quite exceptional, but in the larger proportion of cases complicated by a larger or smaller fracture of the diaphysis, which remains attached to the epiphysis. However, it is most important to obtain as accurate a co-aptation of the fragments as possible ; in proportion as the reduction is perfect, the sooner will the fragments unite, and consequently passive motion become the sooner possible.

After the application of the apparatus, the condition of the circulation in the limb (especially the upper extremity) should be carefully watched for the first twenty-four hours.

All these injuries, but more especially those in the neighbourhood of the joints, ought to be carefully examined from day to day. The surgeon cannot be too careful in the treatment of all cases of separation, even the most simple ones. The retention apparatus may be removed after some days to see if the displacement has not recurred.

Happily these injuries unite more rapidly in children than similar injuries in the adult, for children are restless, and require greater and more constant supervision by the surgeon.

When the separation is *intra-articular* it is prudent to fix the limb for a shorter time, viz. for seven or eight days, provided the adaptation of the fragments has been well maintained. Careful massage and slight passive movements, such as are now often carried out in the intra-articular fractures in adults, may then be commenced if they do not give rise to great pain.

Massage and early passive motion are to be most carefully practised ; in some cases it may be necessary, after the first application of these, to re-apply the splint for a further period of eight days. In the more simple cases passive motion may be carried out daily and the splint re-applied.

Muscular wasting may thus be diminished, the absorption of inflammatory effusion, both inside and outside the joint, assisted, and the consequent usefulness of the limb greatly enhanced.

Prolonged fixation, though it may not cause ankylosis, produces atrophy of the muscles from disuse, the small blood vessels of the part are reduced in size and number, the bones themselves become softer and more spongy, and the normal development of the limb is much retarded.

Ankylosis of a joint after intra-articular fracture is the result of the injury or of the character and duration of the inflammation, but not of temporary fixation.

The greatest care should be exercised in guarding against inflammatory complications.

As to whether the flexed or extended position should be adopted in injuries extending into the elbow-joint, the reader may be referred to the chapters on the various injuries in this situation. It will depend upon whether the displaced fragments may be more accurately and completely replaced or retained in their normal position by one method or the other. Each lesion must be judged according to its suitability for treatment in either position.

As a general rule the joint should not be confined longer than two to three weeks.

Numerous papers have of late been published on the *immediate massage* treatment of fractures of the epiphysial ends of the bones by the French surgeons Jeannel, Terrier, Reclus, Kirmisson, and others since the discussion at the Société de Chirurgie introduced by Lucas Championnière.

It has been held that these injuries are to be regarded as advanced degrees of sprains, and should be treated in the same way by massage without the use of any apparatus. Ankylosis, stiffness of joints and tendons, loss of function, and atrophy of the segment of the limb below the fracture are quoted as evidence of the evil effects of putting up the limb in immovable apparatus.

It need scarcely be pointed out how harmful such treatment must be in children from the possibility of further stripping up and bruising the periosteum, and of producing the periostitis or suppuration to which these injuries are so prone. The reader may be referred to a paper by MM. Bauby and Bardier on 'Considérations sur le traitement des fractures épiphysaires,' *Le Midi Médical*, Toulouse, October 8, 1893, p. 473, where this treatment was carried out in some epiphysial fractures of the lower end of the radius in children without any harm having apparently resulted.

For a complete exposition of this subject reference may be made to Lucas Championnière's recent work, *Traitement des fractures par le massage et la mobilisation*, Paris 1895.

Leblois (*Des fractures chez les enfants et leur traitement*, Paris 1894, p. 49) advocates massage and early movement for epiphysial separation on account of the abundant callus produced in these lesions. This method, he thinks, gives superior results as regards both the duration of the treatment and the restoration of the function of the limb.

Passive movement should, as a rule, be commenced on the tenth day, and carried out gently each day, the range of movement being gradually increased.

If swelling and heat, or distension of the joint, or other signs of *inflammatory action*, have supervened before the patient has been seen, evaporating lotions or an ice-bag may be applied over the affected part, and the limb placed as far as possible in its normal position until the swelling has subsided. Reduction should then be effected at the first opportunity.

A careful and moderate use of massage has been recommended under these circumstances to hasten the process of absorption.

If **suppuration** takes place it must be treated in accordance with the general principles of surgery.

Incisions should be made at once into boggy parts. It is not necessary to wait for fluctuation.

Compound separations are frequently the most serious of epiphysial injuries. In the past they have involved, if not the death of the patient, often primary amputation. Primary amputation is now very rarely necessary. Fortunately, in compound separation of some epiphyses, e.g. the lower end of the humerus, the injury is not so severe as to require it. Antiseptic surgery permits us to save many limbs which would formerly have been sacrificed. In the milder cases, where the injury is caused by indirect violence without protrusion of the diaphysis, the wound may be disinfected, closed, and treated like a simple separation, especial care being directed to the subsequent course of the case and the temperature of the patient.

When the diaphysis is protruded and cannot be effectually reduced, or when its end has become soiled with dirt or exposed to the air for a long time, although it appears to be perfectly clean, it is necessary to carefully disinfect the wound, and remove all traces of the soiled or apparently soiled soft tissues with scissors. It is imperative to remove the protruding end of the diaphysis with a saw — a most simple procedure—and to replace the bone in position; other damaged or soiled portions of the surface of the bone in its longitudinal length may be easily cut away by means of a stout knife. Its reduction must be effected after disinfection of the wound, even though it has been extensively stripped of its periosteum; but it is often more prudent to remove a portion of the diaphysial end, for by this means subsequent necrosis and suppuration may be avoided.

A drainage is usually required, but the drain or tube should be away from the periosteal sheath, and more especially away from the opening through which the shaft has protruded (Ollier).

The fragments are easily maintained in position after reduction.

Union in the more simple cases rapidly takes place between the epiphysis and the sawn end of the diaphysis, and a good result ensues.

Resection of the diaphysial end has been performed by Esmarch in the case of separation of the upper epiphysis of the humerus (*Arch. f. klin. Chirurgie*, 1863. iv. S. 585); by Richet and by Péan at the lower end of the radius; by Gay and many other surgeons at the lower end of the femur; and by Erichsen, Spillman, and others at the lower end of the humerus.

Comminution of the diaphysis is far less common than in compound fractures in adults; the fragments should not be removed unless they are interfering with the reduction of the displaced epiphysis.

The fragments, after being accurately brought into apposition, may be held immovably together by wire or by metal or ivory nails.

The chief success in these cases lies in rendering the wound aseptic—often a very difficult matter, requiring the greatest care and patience on the part of the surgeon in the removal of all septic and contaminating material. Every such undertaking should be looked upon in the light of an important, skilful, and deliberate surgical operation in all its details.

Pressure upon the nerves or main vessels, fracture of the epiphysis into the joint, and even comminution of the fragments in compound cases, are insufficient grounds for amputation in these days of careful antiseptic measures.

So much may be effected even in apparently hopeless cases where the tissues are soiled with dirt, that primary amputation for compound separation is only necessary in complete rupture of main vessels or nerves of the limb or other extensive laceration and destruction of the soft parts.

Ollier lost a case of juxta-epiphysial fracture of the lower end of the humerus in a child from severe hæmorrhage twenty-eight days after resection of the end of the bone. Whether the brachial artery had been wounded subsequent to the operation by a projecting splinter of bone during the movements of the patient, or by something that had occurred previously, was not ascertained, as no autopsy could be made.

The protruding portion of the diaphysis, denuded of its cartilage, may be easily removed with a strong knife when the separation has only involved the ossifying layer of the epiphysial cartilage.

It is a fortunate circumstance, from the resection point of view, that the cartilage almost always remains with the epiphysis, so that the growth of bone will not be arrested in this operation.

Moreover, the articulation so often escapes by reason of the blending of the conjugal cartilage and epiphysis with the periosteum that but little danger is to be feared from articular complication.

More often the injury is a complicated one, the separation of the epiphysis being only partial, and accompanied by a fracture of the diaphysis of a greater or less extent. This diaphysial fragment attached to the epiphysis will require to be re-united to the rest of the shaft by pegs or other means.

Ligature of veins for infective thrombosis.—The timely ligature of one of the main venous trunks for thrombosis, due to injury or pressure upon them by displaced epiphysis or diaphysis, may arrest an incipient pyæmia and save a patient's life. This is particularly true in the case of compound separations.

Primary operations for irreducibility.—In many cases of epiphysial fractures, where the fragments are so locked together that they cannot be restored to their proper position, or where a fracture or comminution of the epiphysis extending into the neighbouring joint is

K

likely to interfere permanently with its normal function, or where the separation is accompanied by a dislocation impossible of reduction and by pressure upon important surrounding structures, it is certain that immediate incision under strict antiseptic precautions and replacement of the fragments is called for. This would be imperatively demanded if Ollier and other authors were correct in their belief that arrest of growth in the limb is usually the result of want of proper co-aptation of the separated surfaces.

Mr. Watson Cheyne has recorded (*British Medical Journal*, March 7, 1891, p. 516) several cases in adults and children where he had successfully and with great benefit to the patients operated for recent fracture extending into the joints.

Irreducibility may also, as has been seen in several instances, be due to the presence of a portion of muscle, or fibrous or ligamentous tissue, between the fragments. Again, it may be brought about through the penetration, in a button-hole manner, of a muscle by the diaphysial end.

Before the present days of aseptic and antiseptic surgery the surgeon was content with putting up these fractures in children in as good a position as possible. We have now to consider the advisability of immediate operation in irreducible separations, especially those involving an articulation. It must, however, only be undertaken after due consultation with the child's friends. The operation should be performed by a skilled surgeon, by one who has a thorough and practical knowledge of aseptic and antiseptic methods as well as of operative measures in general. The ' technique ' should be carefully carried out in the smallest details. Otherwise the patient and surgeon may find themselves stranded in grave disaster.

Replacement of diaphysis by operation.—In 1884 the author recommended operation in recent cases of epiphysial separation when, owing to the locking of the fragments or from other causes, the deformity could not be reduced, or when it has been found impossible to keep the fragments in position by the use of splints or other dressings—any of which are potent causes of permanent loss of function of the joint. An incision should be made down to the separated epiphysis under strict antiseptic precautions, the diaphysis loosened, replaced, and its end wired to the epiphysis if necessary.

Soon afterwards the author found that Bruns recommended precisely the same operation under similar conditions.

In some it will be found necessary to resect a portion of the diaphysial end.

Wiring the fragments together has been successfully performed at the upper epiphysis of the humerus and at the lower epiphysis of the femur, great difficulty being experienced in maintaining the fragments in their proper position.

Secondary amputation has been considered necessary for threatening gangrene from pressure of one or other fragment upon the vessels, for suppurative periostitis, and for necrosis.

Refracturing in recent cases for deformity.—A grave question is that of refracturing and resetting the bone when union is found to have taken place with some amount of deformity, and when all swelling has subsided, displaying the actual condition of the fragments. The operation should only be undertaken where the deformity is very great. The lower end of the radius, more especially, may require this treatment.

From such procedure, periostitis, acute suppuration, or severe local inflammation, may result, and at a later period arrest of growth of the bone from disturbance of the epiphysial cartilage.

These badly united separations must therefore be treated in this manner only in the early condition, viz., two or three weeks after the injury—an anæsthetic always being administered.

Loss of function and utility of the limb.—Loss of function of the limb from *stiffness of the joint or muscular atrophy*, the result of prolonged fixation, usually disappears if careful and systematic movement is daily carried out.

Massage and electricity will also render considerable service in causing the absorption of inflammatory exudation and adhesions, besides improving the quality of the muscles and hastening convalescence. Massage of the limb should be made, day by day, very gently at first, and afterwards more vigorously, but pain must never be caused.

Active movements of the limb should also be encouraged, and the child taught to make as much use of it as possible, or special exercises, such as carrying a weight for the purpose of extension in injuries of the elbow, will prove of great assistance.

Massage has of late years been advocated by many surgeons, both here and in Germany, to hasten the process of repair after fracture, and to diminish the risk of permanent stiffness in separation of the epiphyses in the vicinity of the joints.

Landerer's method of treatment of cases in which there is no comminution, or in which there is no great tendency to displacement of the fragments, is to replace the fragments in position, and 'to fix them in a firm dressing, such as plaster of Paris, until the disappearance of the swelling due to the injury. When the soft provisional callus is fully formed (which takes place in from eight to fourteen days in the case of the adult, and earlier in children), it and the surrounding muscles are to be massaged twice a day—at first gently, but later more energetically, and the mobility of the neighbouring joints is to be kept up by active and passive movements.'

Massage in the after-treatment assists very much in the absorption of the effused blood and infiltrated material around the injured bone, nerves, and other structures : for much of the muscular atrophy met with is due to the reflex irritation of this effused tissue upon the peripheral nerves, and may therefore be kept up by the too long fixation of the injured part.

The loss of function of the limb may be the result of irregular union, of displacements which have not been properly adjusted, or of the excessive formation of callus at the epiphysial line close to the articulation. Each and all of these may considerably hamper the movements of the joint and obstruct the muscles in their action, even after the completion of the modelling process.

The crippled condition of the limb and joint may under these circumstances demand *resection* of the joint.

The dangers of operative measures on the bones in these days of antiseptic surgery are slight compared with the great advantages which accrue from them.

Resection and replacement of diaphysial end, and removal of any irregular osseous projections, in *old separations* accompanied with *great deformity*, in which the natural function of the limb is greatly impaired, have been advocated and carried out by Bruns and others. This operation should be attempted in all cases in which the anatomy of the part permits such interference, but the precise details must vary with each case.

Sometimes the displaced diaphysis appears to be ready to penetrate the skin, as at the upper end of the humerus, yet the natural moulding process is often sufficient to ultimately remove even considerable deformity.

In two cases of old separation of the upper end of the humerus, Bruns successfully cut down on the epiphysis and detached the two fragments by means of a small saw, resected a portion of the diaphysial end, and replaced the fragments in their natural position.

Mr. Johnson-Smith, in the same injury, pegged and wired the fragments together after re-section of the diaphysial ends.

M. Poncet in two cases of the same lesion removed a portion of the projecting diaphysial end which had separated the fibres of the deltoid, and obtained good results.

Projecting portions of bone which are left after the moulding down of the parts, and tend to cripple the limb, should be chiselled away. The author has done this on many occasions, with the result of considerable restoration of function and symmetry of the limb.

Vicious union in the later stages, if very extreme, may require osteotomy.

Neglected cases, or cases that have fallen into the hands of bone-setters, when seen after the lapse of some little time, are very difficult of treatment if the fragments are still unreduced. Excessive callus, articular ankylosis, &c., are often advanced when seen by the surgeon, and require *resection* of the joint.

Operations for deformity due to arrest of growth.—The deformities of the leg or forearm arising from arrest of growth of one of the bones and progressive increase in the other, from injury and other causes, have been specially dealt with by Ollier (*Traité des résections*, tom. ii. 1888, p. 440).

When the deformity due to the lesion of one of the parallel bones is commencing (radius and ulna in forearm, tibia and fibula in the leg) it must be treated immediately by some form of *apparatus* which will correct the deviation or *by incising the conjugal cartilage* of the sound bone (*chondrotomie*).

If the deformity is of longer standing, the growth of the bone which is relatively too long may be checked by the operation introduced by Ollier of *removal of one or both of the conjugal cartilages* (*chondrectomie*) (Ollier, *Traité des résections*, tom. i. 1885, p. 110) ; the other bone then continuing to grow, however slightly, will correct the deformity, although the limb may be shortened. Up to the present, surgeons have been content to resect a portion of the bone.

After Ollier's operation the sound bone will cease to grow, although the limb will be permanently shortened—but straightened —that is, if the shortened bone regain the length it has lost. Much will depend upon this growth of the shortened bone, if its end still retains enough elements for growth—i.e. if the cartilage is not entirely destroyed, which, unfortunately, is usually the case.

In the choice of either of these operations, a careful consideration of the patient's age, the amount of the deformity, and the relative importance as regards the growth of the particular cartilage have to be taken into consideration.

On the other hand, indirect irritation of the cartilage by introduction of a foreign body into the medullary cavity and by lacerating the periosteum, at a distance, under antiseptic precautions may increase the growth and length of a long bone during its period of growth. The irritation set up need not be intense, but it must be long continued.

In the fully developed, adolescent youth or adult, *sub-periosteal resection* of the end of the sound bone may suffice to correct the deformity.

M. Ollier (*Traité des résections*, tom. ii. 1888, p. 445, fig. ; Ollier, *Revue Mensuelle de Médecine et de Chirurgie*, Mars 1877 ; 'De l'excision des cartilages de conjugaison pour arrêter l'accroissement des os et remédier à certaines difformités du squelette '), by removing a slice of the conjugal cartilage of the ulna in a youth whose hand was distorted after suppurative ostitis of the lower end of the radius, succeeded in checking the deformity, so that arrest of growth of the ulna took place, and the radius was able in five years to increase up to its proper relationship with the ulna. The growth of the two parallel bones developed afterwards at a regular and equal rate.

The lower epiphysis of the ulna is subcutaneous and easily reached ; as regards the radius Ollier says that it should be reached from the dorsal aspect, between the extensor tendons, and that the operation is a very simple one.

A small knife is introduced parallel to the cartilage which is incised, and a second cut made somewhat obliquely to the first, and another portion of cartilage removed. This is repeated several times until enough—either a third or a fourth of the whole—has been removed to ensure the amount of arrest of growth required to be produced. Ollier recommended, however, several partial operations repeated at intervals of some months, since such great difficulty is experienced in ascertaining exactly the amount of cartilaginous-growing elements left in the sound limb, and therefore the requisite amount to be removed from it. The effects of the first operation should, therefore, be carefully watched.

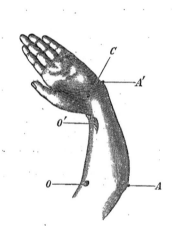
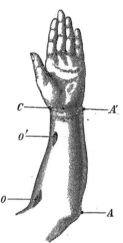

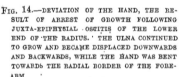

FIG. 14.—DEVIATION OF THE HAND, THE RESULT OF ARREST OF GROWTH FOLLOWING JUXTA-EPIPHYSIAL OSTITIS OF THE LOWER END OF THE RADIUS. THE ULNA CONTINUED TO GROW AND BECAME DISPLACED DOWNWARDS AND BACKWARDS, WHILE THE HAND WAS BENT TOWARDS THE RADIAL BORDER OF THE FOREARM

FIG. 15.—APPEARANCE OF THE HAND AFTER EXCISION OF THE CONJUGAL CARTILAGE OF THE ULNA. THE GROWTH OF THIS BONE HAS CEASED, WHILE THAT OF THE RADIUS CONTINUED TO A SLIGHT EXTENT, PLACING BOTH BONES ON A LEVEL. (AFTER OLLIER)

A, olecranon ; A', styloid process of the ulna projecting backwards ; o, o', sinuses through which necrosed bone was removed ; c, radio-carpal fold, very oblique before operation, transverse afterwards.

Ollier has also proposed the irritation of the injured bone by means of nails, cauterisation, &c., applied to the diaphysis, to cause increase in the growth of the epiphysial disc.

Helferich and Max Schüller have also carried out similar attempts with success.

Some surgeons think it more advisable in such cases to await the full development of the bones before performing resection of the sound diaphysis.

PART II

SEPARATION OF THE EPIPHYSES OF THE UPPER EXTREMITY

———•◦•———

CHAPTER I

SEPARATION OF THE EPIPHYSIS OF THE CLAVICLE

ANATOMY.—Although the clavicle begins to ossify at the fifth week of intra-uterine life before any other of the long bones in the body (immediately after ossification has commenced in the lower jaw), yet the small epiphysis which is developed in the cartilage of its sternal end does not begin to ossify until the eighteenth year. But this may be a little sooner or later in different subjects. It is remarkable that the clavicle—the first of the long bones to ossify in its shaft—has its epiphysis commencing to do so the last of all. At thirteen years of age the cartilaginous end is 15 mm. wide vertically by 12 mm. antero-posteriorly; at twenty years, 22 mm. vertically, and 18 mm. antero-posteriorly. Up to this time the cartilaginous end is extremely thin. A number of granules appear first in the cartilaginous disc, which is only about 3 mm. thick at the eighteenth year, 2 centimetres antero-posteriorly, and $2\frac{1}{2}$ centimetres vertically, and these soon coalesce to form a thin epiphysial plate. This lamellar epiphysis does not occupy quite the whole of the sternal end of the bone, but is mostly confined to the surface articulating with the sternum. About its centre it is slightly convex or raised to a point externally, and is about 3 mm. in thickness.

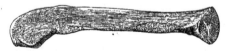

FIG. 16.—CLAVICLE AT THE NINETEENTH YEAR. THIN EPIPHYSIAL PLATE AT STERNAL END

The epiphysial plate joins the diaphysis from the twenty-second to the twenty-fifth year, the centre of the epiphysis being the first part to weld on to the shaft. Even in the fully developed state at the twenty-fifth year it does not seem much more than 4 mm. in thickness,

It is not an uncommon thing to find this epiphysis the only one still ununited to the shaft while all the rest of the epiphyses in the body have joined on.

The capsular ligament of the sterno-clavicular joint is attached to this end of the clavicle ; and from the upper and back part of the same, just beyond the epiphysial level, spring the inter-clavicular ligament and the intra-articular fibro-cartilage. The whole of the epiphysis is covered by the synovial membrane of the menisco-clavicular portion of the sterno-clavicular joint.

The epiphysial cartilage is overlapped by the synovial membrane, especially at the lower part.

The acromial end has no epiphysis.

ETIOLOGY.—There must be some particular mode of application of the violence to account for fracture of the inner end of the clavicle or separation of the epiphysis, which are both of such rare occurrence.

The author has collected five cases and one doubtful one (Lonsdale).

M. Polaillon, in his article (*Dict. Encyclop. des Sciences Médicales*, 1875, Tome dix-septième), has collected twenty-eight cases of fracture of the inner end of the clavicle. To these M. Delens has added three more (*Arch. Gén. de Médecine*, Mai 1873). Twelve of the total were from muscular, and sixteen from traumatic causes, while in three the cause was unknown. Delens has pointed out how completely they differ from fractures of the shaft proper.

Indirect violence, such as a fall or blow upon the apex of the shoulder, driving the bone inwards and forwards, will be found to be the most common cause. Even a fall on the elbow, while it is away from the side, might produce this injury in the same manner.

In Verchère's and Lonsdale's cases the violence was applied indirectly.

Direct violence.—Although it is stated in Maunder's case of compound separation that it was not evident in which direction the force had been applied, and although it might easily be imagined that the injury was caused by direct violence, through the cart wheel passing over the inner end of the bone, yet it is more probable that the force was applied more indirectly, and that the wound in front and below the separated epiphysis (the usual situation of the end of the shaft in fractures from indirect violence) was produced by the end of the diaphysis, which afterwards slipped back into its normal position.

Muscular action.—The end of the clavicle has twice (in Le Gros Clark's and Heath's cases) been detached by muscular violence. Mr. Heath believes that the entirely cartilaginous end, in his case, at the age of fourteen, must have been torn from the thoroughly ossified shaft by violent muscular action. He says : ' This does not imply, as has been erroneously supposed, a rupture of the strong, costo-clavicular or rhomboid ligament, which acted as the fulcrum upon which the bone rotated, the weight of the arm and shoulder drawing the outer end of the clavicle backwards and throwing the inner end forward beneath the skin.'

In Le Gros Clark's lad, who, performing on a trapeze, was hanging by two feet and trying to raise himself so as to seize the bar with his hands, the clavicle gave way during the effort.

The powerful clavicular fibres of the pectoralis major and deltoid are most effective factors in producing separation and causing displacement of the inner end of the bone forwards and downwards, by drawing on this portion of the clavicle whilst the humerus is fixed. This direction of displacement forwards is that usually found in fracture of the inner end of clavicle, as in separation.

AGE.—There is only a short period of time during which a true epiphysial separation of the clavicle can occur ; from the time, that is, of commencement of ossification to the time of union with the shaft—viz. from about the eighteenth to the twenty-second year or a little later. Some give the twenty-fifth year as the limit of the time of union, while Sappey says the epiphysis does not appear till towards the twentieth year.

Of the three examples of separation of the ossifying or completely osseous epiphysis, Verchère's specimen was obtained from a young man aged twenty.

The clinical cases comprise Le Gros Clark's, aged eighteen years ; and Mr. Rivington's, aged seventeen.

The examples of separation of the cartilaginous end are no more numerous : Mr. Christopher Heath's, aged fourteen ; Mr. Maunder's, aged eleven ; and Mr. Lonsdale's, aged three years.

The latter case of Lonsdale's was probably a fracture of the inner end of the bone.

SEPARATION OR FRACTURE OF THE CARTILAGINOUS STERNAL END. Before the existence of the epiphysis at the eighteenth year a true fracture or detachment of the cartilaginous sternal end of the clavicle may occur at any age.

Maunder's case of compound separation of the cartilaginous inner end occurred in a lad aged eleven years.

PATHOLOGICAL ANATOMY.—Separation of the epiphysis of the clavicle is one of the most rare of epiphysial detachments.

M. Delens, in the *Archives de Médecine* in 1873, has collected thirty-one cases of fracture of the inner end of the clavicle, without recording one of epiphysial separation.

The following case described by M. Verchère (*Le Progrès Médical*, 2ième Série, vol. iv. No. 50, December 11, 1886, and *Bulletins de la Société Anatomique*, 1886, p. 484) is the only one in which an autopsy has been made. The separation of this epiphysis was accompanied by a wound of the pleural sac on the same side, and extensive emphysema—rare complications even in fractures of the clavicle.

A young man (D., a mason), aged twenty, was brought on June 22 to the Hôpital de la Pitié, under the care of M. Verneuil. Whilst working in a refinery he was caught by his clothes in the transmission strap of some machinery and carried round three times, being finally hurled against the neighbouring wall and on to the ground. He was admitted in a collapsed and insensible condition, with rapid breathing and violent dyspnœa, skin pale and cold, temperature 35°·2 C. Subcutaneous emphysema was found occupying the whole of the upper part of the thorax, the neck, and the lower half of the face, completely effacing the natural depressions at the lower part of the neck. Some crepitation was perceived as far as the lower part of the thorax. There was no hæmoptysis. It was found to be impossible to determine the exact cause of the injury on account of the extensive swelling from the emphysema. The patient could not move the upper extremities, which did not present any signs of fracture.

There was very extensive contusion and extravasation of blood in both legs and feet, pulping of both calves, and the skin was completely stripped from the right heel. Injections of ether and morphine were administered. By the following day the breathing had become more quiet, and the emphysema had not increased to any notable extent; but there was great pain in both legs, and threatening gangrene of skin of the right calf as far as the knee and of the skin of left leg. The threatened gangrenous condition of both legs having spread, sloughs of the skin coming away in large pieces, and the whole of the right foot looking gangrenous, incisions and punctures were made on June 28 with the thermo-cautery in both feet and legs. On June 29 amputation was performed through the right thigh, and was followed by death the same evening.

At the autopsy the day after death emphysema of the face, neck, and chest was still present. No fracture of the ribs was to be seen on either side, but there was an epiphysial detachment of the inner end of the right clavicle. The periosteum was detached from the whole inner third of the bone, whose smooth, rounded, and regular end projected forwards; in the centre of this extremity two or three small cartilaginous particles still adhered to the bone. The sterno-clavicular articulation was uninjured, a disc remaining about five millimetres thick formed by the cartilage and the epiphysis of the clavicle. This fragment was firmly held by the ligaments of the articulation, and was crossed in front by the sternal head of the sterno-mastoid muscle. In the damaged cellular tissue at this level a cavity had been produced by the displaced end of the clavicle, and in the post-clavicular region at the same level an extensive perforation of the pleural sac was found, about the size of a two-franc piece. The pneumothorax which was present on this side communicated freely with the subcutaneous emphysema. The right lung was uninjured, but yet emphysematous; the left, adherent to a slight extent in front, was in a state of hepatisation. Death ensued from septicæmia, following gangrene of the lower extremities. The specimen of the separated epiphysis was placed in the Dupuytren Museum.

Mr. C. F. Maunder describes (*London Hospital Reports*, vol. iv. 1867–8, p. 227) a case of compound separation of the epiphysis of the clavicle in a lad aged eleven years who was knocked down by a cart, but it was not evident in what direction the force was applied which effected the injury. There was a loss of continuity near the sternal end and a small wound in the integument just below, over the first rib, but there was no displacement of the fragments.

The clavicle could be moved to and fro independently of its epiphysis, and instead of the hard crepitus of fracture a soft grating was felt. Unlike dislocation of the sternal end of the bone, there was no tendency to displacement. Rest in bed with a figure-of-eight bandage was the treatment adopted. The bone remained in good position, but the wound healed slowly. Twelve months afterwards the injured clavicle was found to be three-eighths of an inch shorter than its fellow.

Notwithstanding the intimate relations of the inner end of the clavicle with the subclavian artery and vein, there is no recorded case of injury to either, or to the brachial plexus, as *complications* of the separation of the epiphysis of this bone.

SYMPTOMS.—*Displacement forwards of diaphysis* has occurred in all the cases at present published.

Deformity.—Upon the anterior part of the sternum there is an abrupt and striking projection on a level with the sterno-clavicular joint, and it is found to be continuous with the diaphysis. This closely simulates a dislocation forwards.

If the case has been seen before any great amount of swelling has taken place, the flattened diaphysial end may be felt, quite unlike the pointed end of a fracture, but more like the articular end of the bone dislocated forwards. Separation of the epiphysis differs from the latter in that the supra-sternal notch remains intact.

The clavicular head of the sterno-mastoid is carried forwards and stands out prominently, so that the head of the patient may be drawn to the affected side.

If the shoulder be drawn forwards, the end of the diaphysis falls into its place, and the tumour then entirely disappears, or nearly so.

The thin osseous plate, of which this epiphysis consists, may be discovered, if there is not much effusion of blood, towards one side of the supra-sternal notch, or between it and the end of the displaced diaphysis. The supra-sternal notch is intact. In Heath's case it was 'quite distinct and equally defined on both sides.'

In Verchère's patient the extensive swelling from emphysema

due to injury of the pleura prohibited any diagnosis being made before death.

Mr. Le Gros Clark mentions (*St. Thomas's Hospital Reports*, vol. xvii. 1887, p. 1) the case already referred to of a gymnast, aged eighteen years, who was performing on the trapeze, and whilst hanging by his feet and trying to draw up his body between his legs, felt something give way on the left side of his neck. This injury was at first diagnosed as a dislocation of the sternal end of the clavicle, and unavailing attempts were made to reduce the displacement. When Mr. Le Gros Clark saw the patient the swelling had abated, and he was satisfied that the sternal epiphysis was separated from the shaft of the bone. The inner end of the shaft rested upon the sternal epiphysis of the bone, the latter occupying its normal position in relation to the sternum. The case was treated as one of ordinary fracture of the clavicle. An interesting feature in this case is the mode in which the accident occurred. There was no evidence of violence having been directly applied to the injured part; the accident was produced by muscular action during the violent effort made by the patient in performing his gymnastic feat.

Mr. Christopher Heath has put on record (*Clinical Society's Transactions;* vol. xvi. 1883, p. 37, and *Lancet*, vol. ii. 1882, p. 851) the following case of separation of the epiphysis of the clavicle by muscular action. On May 9, 1882, he was asked to see a boy, aged fourteen, who that morning, whilst forcibly raising his arm to bowl ' over-hand ' at cricket, felt something give way at his collar-bone, causing great pain. The inner end of the right clavicle was found to be unduly prominent, and presented a sharp edge beneath the skin, quite unlike the smooth end of a bone covered with articular cartilage. The supra-sternal notch was quite distinct and equally defined on both sides, and a thin lamella could be felt on the right side intervening between it and the gap caused by the starting forwards of the inner end of the clavicle. On the patient being laid flat on a mattress the bone at once slipped into place, and the deformity and pain disappeared. The arm was subsequently secured to the side with a plaster of Paris bandage and kept fixed for a month, after which gentle movement was allowed. In October the boy was reported to be quite well, there being only a little thickening left over the seat of injury.

A case of Mr. Rivington's at the London Hospital is mentioned by Mr. Hutchinson, jun., as having occurred at the age of seventeen.

Shortening.—On very careful measurement some slight shortening of the diaphysis will be found from the diaphysial end to the acromion process, as compared with the whole length of the clavicle on the other side. There will be, as in dislocation, shortening on the affected side, measuring from the acromion to the median line.

Crepitus of the usual muffled character may be felt during the reduction of the displaced diaphysis by raising the arm and drawing it backwards with the diaphysis of the clavicle. 'Soft' grating is especially noted in Maunder's case.

Crepitus was felt in Lonsdale's case, and pointed rather to fracture than epiphysial separation; however, attempts should never be undertaken to discover this sign on account of the serious damage that may be done to the periosteum and soft structures.

Mobility has only been noted in one case—that of Mr. Maunder; some amount of movement between the epiphysis and diaphysis, if the former can be distinguished, must, however, be present.

Lonsdale mentions (Lonsdale, *Practical Treatise on Fractures*, 1838, p. 206) a case, in a child (J. C.) three years old, which came under his observation at the Middlesex Hospital in 1835, and which he believed to be a separation of the epiphysis, the point of fracture being half an inch from the sternum. Crepitus could be felt, and the end of the bone moved from its natural position. The injury was caused by the child falling while at play and striking his shoulder against the edge of some steps. The other clavicle had been broken about a fortnight previously.

It is difficult to believe that this was really any other injury than a fracture of the inner end of the clavicle, for it is improbable that the cartilaginous end of the bone could be as thick as half an inch even at this early age.

Le Gros Clark has also recorded a similar case in a young child.

Swelling, from extravasated blood over the separated diaphysis, may obscure the outline of the fragments.

Mr. Edmund Owen (*The Surgical Diseases of Children*, third edition, 1897, p. 382) has met with separation of the sternal epiphysis of the clavicle on one occasion, but has given no details of the case.

EPIPHYSIAL SEPARATION WITHOUT DISPLACEMENT occurred in Maunder's patient. The injury was a compound one.

DIAGNOSIS. *Dislocation forwards of inner end of clavicle.*—Dislocation of the clavicle is rarely caused by muscular action, but more usually is produced by great violence applied to the shoulder. Moreover, great difficulty is experienced in keeping the bone in position after it has been reduced. On the hold being relaxed, the bone nearly always slips out again from its proper position, and in some cases reduction has been found to be extremely difficult, and in many a certain degree of deformity is sure to exist afterwards. The bones of the sides are almost of equal length, although in dislocation the thin intra-articular fibro-cartilage remains with the sternum. In epiphysial separation, on the other hand, at least in the recorded cases, the bone has been replaced in position with great ease, and no difficulty was in most cases experienced in maintaining the bones in their natural position.

The age of the patient is a most important point in the diagnosis of these two lesions, at any rate as regards the true osseous epiphysis

—viz. from the seventeenth to the twenty-fifth years, which are the extreme limits of commencement of ossification and final union given by anatomists.

Fracture on the inner side of the costo-clavicular or rhomboid ligament.

The *age* of the patient helps but little in distinguishing between fracture and epiphysial separation, inasmuch as fracture of the inner end of the clavicle generally occurs in early life.

Position of the fracture is a somewhat better guide ; for fracture takes place, as a rule, from three-quarters to one inch from the sternal articulation.

RESULTS, PROGNOSIS, &c.—Non-union in fractured clavicle is a very rare event, and is still more unlikely to occur as the result of epiphysial separation, which unites with great rapidity.

Shortening and deformity from malposition and displacement of the fragments will be very rare, if we regard the ease with which the diaphysis is replaced and maintained in position.

Shortening from arrest of growth is a possible though unlikely occurrence after separation of the osseous epiphysis. But it may occasionally occur as the result of fracture of the inner end of the bone or of the cartilaginous extremity.

Mr. Maunder draws a very gloomy picture of the possible consequence of arrest of growth of the clavicle after epiphysial injury. He says : ' The clavicle is the only osseous means by which the trunk and upper extremities are connected ; it suspends the arm, as it were, holds it off (after the fashion of the milkman's yoke) that it may have full play and not press down upon the ribs and interfere with respiration, but if it cease to grow while the rest of the body is still undeveloped, its good offices towards the corresponding extremity and half of the chest fail, and with this failure I should fear an enfeebled extremity, a curved spine, diminished chest capacity, partially developed lung, ill aërated blood, feeble circulation, and an ill nourished body generally—a state of things likely to engender serious disease hereafter.'

The recorded instances of non-union after fracture of the clavicle do not bear out Maunder's opinion ; in some, indeed, little or no disturbance of function or inconvenience has been experienced.

TREATMENT.—In mild *cases without displacement*, should such an injury be supposed to have occurred, it will be sufficient to support the elbow in a sling and fix the arm to the side by means of strapping to prevent any subsequent displacement of the diaphysis.

Reduction of the diaphysis when displaced is easily effected by the surgeon standing behind the patient and drawing both shoulders backwards ; in some cases it may be necessary to place the knee between the scapulæ before the reduction can be effected.

Pressure by means of the fingers or thumb upon the diaphysial end will assist in replacing the bone in position.

In Mr. Heath's case, as already stated, reduction took place on simply placing the patient on his back, the bone immediately slipping into position.

From the records of published cases it is evident that placing the patients upon their backs with the arm in a sling or fixed to the side by a plaster of Paris bandage over a jersey is quite enough to retain the bone in position.

If the patient is obliged to move about, the arm should be placed in a sling with a bandage round the elbow and body to keep the arm at rest, or the triangular bandage, applied in Mayor's fashion, may be employed.   No pad in the axilla is requisite.

Union ensues very rapidly, but the upper extremity should be kept at rest for at least two weeks.   At the end of this time passive motion may be commenced.

Should it be found impossible to keep the diaphysis in position, or should there be evidence of pressure upon the subclavian artery or vein, or upon the brachial plexus of nerves, the surgeon may feel justified in cutting down on the fragments and fixing them in position.

COMPOUND SEPARATION.—In compound cases like Maunder's, unaccompanied by any displacement of the fragments, it will be necessary to thoroughly cleanse the wound, and if the periosteum be torn (which is unlikely without displacement of the diaphysis), it should be united with carbolised silk, and the wound dressed with the strictest antiseptic precautions on account of the important blood vessels and other structures in close proximity to it.

Reduction of the displaced diaphysis and suturing of the ends with wire or stout Chinese silk, and uniting the lacerated periosteum, should be undertaken under the most careful antiseptic measures in all instances of compound separation with displacement.

CHAPTER II

SEPARATION OF THE EPIPHYSES OF THE SCAPULA

SEPARATION OF THE *GLENOID AND CORACOID CARTILAGE*—SEPARATION OF THE EPIPHYSIS OF THE BASE OF THE SCAPULA, *SUPRA-SCAPULA*—SEPARATION OF THE EPIPHYSIS OF THE *CORACOID PROCESS*—SEPARATION OF THE EPIPHYSIS OF THE *ACROMION PROCESS*

CARTILAGINOUS PARTS OF SCAPULA AT BIRTH

ANATOMY.—At birth the scapula is formed of a principal osseous piece—comprising a body and spine—and a cartilaginous mass—consisting of the coracoid and glenoid processes and two secondary cartilaginous processes (which do not ossify until late in puberty), the acromion and the supra-scapula (including the base and inferior angle). The edges of the spine are also cartilaginous.

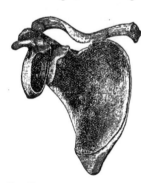

FIG. 17.—SEPARATION OF THE CARTILAGINOUS OUTER PART OF THE SCAPULA, COMPRISING THE GLENOID CAVITY AND CORACOID PROCESS, FROM A CHILD TWO YEARS AND NINE MONTHS WHO HAD BEEN RUN OVER BY A WAGGON.

There was also a greenstick fracture of the clavicle, and many other fractures of the body.

Although the coracoid process commences to ossify during the first year (sometimes at the ninth month of intra-uterine life), for the first few years of life it remains connected with the glenoid cartilaginous process, until the extension of the coracoid ossification has advanced, which it does fairly rapidly; and almost up to the time of the ossification of the intermediary (sub-coracoid) cartilage placed between the base of the coracoid and the upper part of the glenoid, it is possible for the coraco-glenoid mass to be detached by severe violence. In fig. 17 is represented an instance which (through the kindness of Dr. Fullerton) came under the author's observation in 1892 at the Miller Hospital.

The symptoms in the following case, also at the Miller Hospital (April 1896), suggested to the author the possibility of partial separation of the cartilaginous glenoid from the body of the scapula without displacement. F. P., aged 1½ years, had been violently lifted by the armpits by his sister, and had since been unable to use the left arm, keeping it close to his side.   There was no swelling or external contusion, and the head of the humerus rotated freely, smoothly, and without pain.   By steadying the clavicle, coracoid, and shoulder in front with the left hand, and pressing with the right over the spine and body of the scapula downwards and forwards, slight movement could be felt accompanied by soft crepitus ; with the left hand in the axilla and by forcibly rotating the humerus forwards, the same crepitus could be felt behind over the scapula.

EPIPHYSIS OF THE BASE OF THE SCAPULA— SUPRA-SCAPULAR EPIPHYSIS

ANATOMY.—The cartilaginous base of the scapula or epiphysis corresponding to the supra-scapular bone in many animals ossifies at the inferior angle at the sixteenth year, and also higher upwards as a line of osseous material along the posterior border of the bone at the seventeenth to eighteenth year.

An osseous frame or border along the inferior angle and posterior or spinal border is thus formed.

This epiphysis unites about the twenty-fifth year, and is the last one to join on to the body of the bone.

Although it is much exposed to such injuries as might detach it from the body of the scapula, and also to the action of powerful muscles, the author is not aware of any case of traumatic separation to which he can refer.

SEPARATION OF THE EPIPHYSIS OF THE ACROMION PROCESS

ANATOMY.—Two nuclei, one at the base, the other at the apex, and sometimes three, appear between the fourteenth and sixteenth years, often a little later.   Frequently one appears at the fifteenth and the other at the sixteenth year.   Humphry and others give only one nucleus for the apex of the acromion, but state that it varies in the size to which it attains, in some cases constituting the chief part of this process.   These nuclei soon coalesce, and form one epiphysis about the nineteenth year.

The epiphysis is united to the outgrowing spine from the twenty-second to twenty-fifth year.

The extension from the spine varies very much in different subjects.

This epiphysis generally includes the oval articular facet for the clavicle, and has attached to its apical piece the acromio-clavicular and coraco-acromial ligaments.   The junction of the epiphysis with the rest of the acromion is therefore immediately behind the acromio-clavicular joint.   In many instances it includes much more of this process, extending sometimes as far as the outer limit of the spine of the scapula, i.e. the whole of the acromion, surgically speaking.

One or other of these centres is said to remain ununited with the spine of the scapula throughout life, the junction with the spine being represented by fibrous tissue only.

This has led to the belief, which is not without much in its favour, that this process has been fractured and not reunited.

The tardy union of the acromial epiphysis has undoubtedly led to its being mistaken after death for fracture, but during life such a condition of separation of the bones has not been absolutely made out.

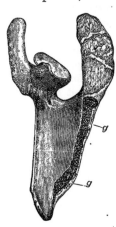

FIG. 18.—SCAPULA ABOUT THE SEVENTEENTH YEAR, SHOWING TWO CENTRES OF OSSIFICATION, ONE AT APEX AND ONE AT BASE. (AFTER RAMBAUD AND RENAULT)

A few osseous granules, *g, g*, are seen in the cartilaginous posterior border of the spine.

The following description by Professor Alex. Macalister of the development of this process will be found to differ in many respects from the accounts given by other authors (*Journal of Anatomy and Physiology*, N.S. 7, 1892–3, p. 248).

'The first trace of ossification I have found consists of a number of bony points on the surface of the cartilage from the metacromion (hindermost tubercle) forward to the middle of the deltoid edge. These rapidly coalesce into a bony strip, narrow behind, wider in front, corresponding to Uffelmann's osteo-epiphysis posterior. Almost simultaneously there appears a middle portion, consisting at first of a number of nuclei.   Those ossifying points which lie along the outer margin of this area coalesce and form the most of the remainder of the outer edge.   The ossification of this part extends gradually inwards, the clavicular facet portion of it being the last to develop.   Anteriorly a single large nucleus forms, from which the anterior tubercle is ossified.   All these nuclei are more extensive on the upper than on the lower surface of the acromion, the portion of the process formed by them on the lower surface being that bounded by a line drawn from the middle of the clavicular facet to the metacromion.   I have counted in all five large and eight small nuclei in the scapula of a boy of seventeen.   These have coalesced in a boy of eighteen into three large and four small centres.

'It is extremely probable that the number of these ectosteally ossifying nuclei is irregular; but in all cases which I have examined of acromia under eighteen there are three sets of these which fuse into three independent parts—the *metacromial* epiphysis, very slender; the *mesacromial*, which is always the most complex in formation; and the *preacromial*.

'The order of ossification is also variable. In six cases the metacromial strip had united to the base, while yet the others were detached. In all the apical preacromial portion had united with the mesacromial before the final consolidation of the latter with the spine. I have only twice seen the metacromial joined to the mesacromial before consolidation had begun. I have never found a

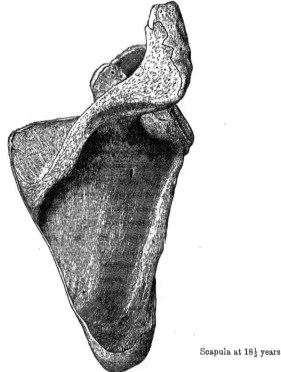

Scapula at 18⅓ years

FIG. 19.—EPIPHYSIS OF THE ACROMION EXTENDING TO THE SPINE OF THE SCAPULA
The scale-like epiphysis at the trapezoid ridge of the coracoid process is also seen.

central ossification in the cartilage like that figured by Quain or Gray. I can, however, believe that such may occur, but it must be the exception, not the rule, as in the twenty scapulæ which I have seen in this stage of growth I have detected no trace of this condition.'

The condition of the persistently separate os acromiale which Professor Macalister has found in fifteen out of a hundred scapulæ taken at random is due to the consolidation of the preacromial and mesacromial centres, and the persistence of their separation from the base of the spine and from the metacromial centre which always consolidates with the base.

This is probably too high a degree of frequency of occurrence, as many of the specimens were museum ones, among which cases of such an anomaly were naturally numerous.

Out of forty-five instances of this condition which he had examined he had never found the metacromial element attached to the ossicle. 'It is very rare,' he says, 'to find the partition of the preacromial and mesacromial centres except in young bones.' He had seen it once, but this was, he believed, only a transitory condition.

In the cases where the real os acromiale persists as a permanent condition, its union has ceased to be a true synchondrosis, and the uniting material is generally fibro-cartilage. Professor Macalister has once seen a true synovial joint with a surrounding capsule, but he had at least five times found a cavity in the uniting medium comparable, as far as the histological structure of its wall is concerned, with that of the sacro-iliac joint.

Macalister believes the order of ossification to be normally :

' 1. Many bony nuclei, forming about the fifteenth year.

' 2. Consolidation of these into three marginal centres, about seventeen.

' 3. Extension of the mesacromial centre inwards towards the clavicle, between seventeen and eighteen.

' 4. Consolidation of the metacromial centre with the basis, and of the preacromial and mesacromial with each other, about eighteen.

' 5. Consolidation of this element with the spine.'

In all cases it has been only the aspect of the metacromial angle toward the outer side that has originated from the metacromial epiphysis, here diminishing to a superficial crust, and it never extends on the hinder aspect of the process, which invariably is ossified along with the base of the scapula. (See figures 5, 7, and 8 of Professor A. Macalister's paper, *Journal of Anatomy and Physiology*, N.S. 7, 1892–93, pl. xv.)

Professor Macalister refers to a good account of observations on this process given by Uffelmann (*Anatomisch-chirurgische Studien*, Hameln, 1865).

In some instances the epiphysis of the acromion is more obliquely placed, and it usually then runs forwards into the articular surface of the acromio-clavicular joint—about its inner third. This articulation will necessarily be opened in this case, should separation occur.

ETIOLOGY.—The epiphysis may be detached by a *direct blow* or fall upon the shoulder, or, more *indirectly*, by violence applied through the humerus, as in a fall upon the elbow.

PATHOLOGICAL ANATOMY.—There is no real specimen of traumatic separation of this epiphysis known.

The number of museum specimens in existence of separate acromial process are considered by most authors as examples of traumatic separation of the epiphysis, or of incomplete ossification from the time of birth, and in this way the rarity of true fracture of the acromion has been accounted for.

The line of separation is just behind the joint, but in some instances it passes into the acromio-clavicular joint.

Mr. Lizars was one of the first to point out that 'in some individuals the acromial process continues an epiphysis during life' (*System of Practical Surgery*, John Lizars, Edinburgh, 1847).

Hamilton quotes Fergusson, who remarks 'that he had dissected a number of examples of apparent fracture of the end of this process, but in such instances it is doubtful if the movable portion had ever been fixed to the rest of the bone.'

Before the Anatomical Society of Great Britain and Ireland, in November 1887, Professor Curnow showed specimens of un-united acromial epiphyses. In January 1888 Dr. Struthers also exhibited before the same society a series of specimens of permanently separate acromion process, simulating fracture. On November 27, 1889, Professor Windle showed before the same society (*Lancet*, December 7, 1889) another series of specimens, which, he maintained, proved that the separated portions of the acromion were ununited epiphyses, and not fractures. The main evidence for this belief was that the separate parts were always symmetrical, and that there was no callus, but an intervening layer of cartilage.

At the annual meeting of the British Medical Association in Birmingham, July 1890, Dr. A. E. Mahood likewise exhibited a very interesting collection of scapulæ, showing non-union of the acromial epiphysis in advanced age on one or both sides.

Professor J. Struthers read a paper on 'Separate Acromion Process simulating Fracture' before the Medico-Chirurgical Society of Edinburgh, June 6, 1894 (*Lancet*, June 16, 1894, p. 1506; *Edinburgh Medical Journal*, September 1894, p. 253; also *ibid.* October 1895, p. 289; *ibid.* April 1896, p. 900; *ibid.* June 1896, p. 1088; *ibid.* August 1896, p. 97), in which he gives a complete account of this condition and the whole literature of the subject. He maintains that the condition is a much more common one than was generally believed, and that its existence frequently leads to errors of diagnosis in injuries about the shoulder-joint.

'The condition,' he says, 'comes (possibly) within the category of fracture in the sense that it may, in some cases, have begun as a fracture of the layer of cartilage between the basi-acromion and the ossified epiphysis, and, in that event, the movements of the acromion against the clavicle might be sufficient to prevent union and to establish a joint between the two parts of the acromion. That, however, is not likely to have been the history in cases in which the separation exists on both sides.'

Dr. Struthers adds that, while fractures of the acromion may occur at any part, the usual place of separation is at, or close to, the post-clavicular line, the point of union of the epiphysis (just behind the acromio-clavicular articulation). This is the locality for all of the thirteen cases described, and he has not seen a specimen of its occurrence at any other part of the acromion. While not doubting that true fractures of the acromion occur at and in front of the clavicular connection, and that they may remain in the ununited condition, he thinks that the fact, that the usual locality of separate acromion is at the post-clavicular region, remains for some anatomical explanation.

He arrived at the following considerations for and against the non-union or separation of the epiphysis theory :

'The place of junction of the epiphysis corresponds to the post-clavicular line. But although the epiphysial line thus corresponds to the weak point of the acromion, it is not the cause of the weakness, as after the union is completed (between the twenty-second and twenty-fifth year) there is no difference in the internal structure and no special thinness exactly at the line of union. The correspondence of the two lines is incidental except in so far that the extent of the epiphysis appears to be in adaptation to the clavicular connection. But the fact of the correspondence of the two lines introduces the element of doubt in the interpretation as between fracture and epiphysial separation when the separation occurs, as it usually does, at the post-clavicular line.

'*In support* of the epiphysis theory may be given: (*a*) That the usual place of separation corresponds to the place of epiphysial meeting, expressed generally. (*b*) It is conceivable that union may be delayed beyond the twenty-fifth year, and that if union does not occur at the usual period non-union may be permanent, as seen occasionally in the case of the inter-frontal suture. (*c*) If the specimen has been from a subject under the twenty-fifth year, the intervening layer of cartilage may have been broken by an accident to the shoulder, and the synarthrodial connection thus converted into a diarthrodial joint by the movement of the parts, as after fracture of the ossified acromion followed by non-union. That, of course, brings the case into the category of fracture (diastasis), but the line is determined by the epiphysis.

'*Against* the theories of non union or detachment of the epiphysis, as occurring in the living body, may be put: (*a*) There is a source of fallacy in regard to the interpretation of some specimens met with, in that they are but normal scapulæ just under the age at which the acromial epiphysis (the last of the epiphyses of the scapula to unite) is consolidated, the separation having taken place during maceration. Such scapulæ, wanting the epi-acromion but otherwise full-grown, are to be seen in museums. But, in regard to specimens undoubtedly beyond that age, (*b*) the line of post-clavicular separation is not exactly what would be expected had the cause been non-union or detachment of the epiphysis. Among the thirteen specimens described the separation begins, on the inner side, in some exactly at or very close to the posterior end of the facet, in some a little in front of that point, in some a little behind.

'These moderate variations in the starting-point of the separation on the inner side do not, perhaps, go against the epiphysis theory, as we do not know that normally the posterior limits of the epiphysis and of the facet correspond precisely to each other; but the outward course of the line of separation is not much, in some the opposite, of what we should expect when we bear in mind that epiphyses have a very definite shape. As seen in four specimens, the epiphysis meets the basi-acromion in a line curving outwards and very much backwards from the posterior end of the clavicular facet. Even should the posterior nucleus not unite with the main body of the epiphysis, the line of union is still curved, with the concavity backwards. But in some of my specimens, as described, there is very little backward direction of the outer part of the line ; in some the outward direction is even a little forwards. Two figures show the direction to be different on the two sides in the same person, though symmetrical in regard to beginning on the inside just behind the facet. On the whole, the general direction of the line of separation, while somewhat undulating, may be regarded as transverse or nearly so.

'Allowance must, no doubt, be made for any changes of form during perhaps many years of active working at a false joint after a supposed epiphysial detachment; but, on the whole, when the line of separation usually seen is considered, the epiphysial theory, whether by delayed union or by detachment, fails to satisfy, while the line of separation, as usually seen, with its minor variations at the post-clavicular region and its general transverse direction, tends to support the fracture theory.

'The occasional occurrence of *symmetrical* separate acromion appears at first to be a difficulty in accepting the view that in all cases the condition is one of fracture, while it is intelligible on the theory of delayed union of the epiphysis, or as a result of advanced rheumatoid disease of both shoulder-joints. Of the three cases above referred to, in two (those by R. W. Smith and J. G. Smith) there was rheumatoid disease, while in my case, a female æt. eighty-two, there was no disease. These two theories, however, when critically examined as above, must be regarded as improbable, as inapplicable to at least the great majority of the specimens. It remains only to inquire whether the seemingly not very likely occurrence of fracture of both acromions can be believed as, after all, not so very unlikely to occur. This difficulty will disappear when we think of the occasional occurrence of dislocation of both shoulder-joints, a result implying a much more forcible cause than would suffice to fracture the acromion.

'With such examples of symmetrical injury, in two of them both sides dislocated simultaneously, we need have little difficulty in believing in the occurrence of symmetrical fracture of the acromion process.

'The epiphysis theory is attractive to the anatomical mind, but, when the evidence is critically examined, has to be abandoned for the fracture theory. The explanation above given of the frequency of the locality in which the fracture is found to have occurred, the post-clavicular line, giving the family likeness to the great majority of the specimens, is, however, no less an anatomical one, and appears to me to be the true interpretation.'

In the discussion which followed, Mr. Joseph Bell said that he thought Professor Struthers had achieved a very distinct point by bringing out the fact how common it was that the terminal portion of the acromion only had separated. He thought that fracture of the acromion was not common. Reflecting on the cases he had seen, he could recall one in which he thought that he had not succeeded in curing a fracture of the acromion, but the patient was no worse. No doubt it was a case of separation of the terminal end of the acromion. Dr. Ronaldson stated that he had seen two cases in father and child of separate acromion process on both sides. He believed that when it was congenital it would always be found on both sides. Mr. David Wallace said that the subject was one that had interested him and others in the surgical department at the university for some time. Professor Chiene happened to possess at least three, if not four, specimens of the condition. It had been pointed out for a long while that fracture of the acromion process was rare, and it had always been referred to in the books as one of the instances where a persistent epiphysis might simulate fracture. Mr. W. A. Lane said that, examining in the dissecting rooms for fracture, he had found that fractures of the acromion process were the most common in the body. They were in all probability really examples of the condition to which Professor Struthers had alluded—persistent epiphysis. With regard to the diagnosis between fracture of the acromion and persistent epiphysis, in the former they would get crepitus. Further, as Hamilton pointed out, in fracture of the acromion they would have displacement downwards of the fractured portion by the fibres of the deltoid attached to it. In the specimens in the Surgical Museum there was evidence of chronic rheumatoid arthritis, but this was due, in all probability, simply to the too free movement of the head of the humerus upon the under surface of the acromion process, because the osteophytic projection and the so-called porcellanous deposit, which was really simply a burnishing of the bone, were chiefly situated on the under surface. The complete destruction of the long tendon of the biceps to which Professor Struthers had referred was further marked evidence in support of this view. Mr. Wallace had seen two such cases.

Nearly all the London hospitals contain specimens in their museums of non-union of the acromial epiphyses, the epiphyses having been loose from the time of their formation. They have probably not been separated in later life, for there exists little evidence of an epiphysis failing to unite.

Some surgeons think that the non-union of this epiphysis is an example of ununited fracture of the acromion, and that it is readily developed on account of the position and muscular attachments of this process, as well as of the difficulty in maintaining the detached fragment in a fixed position when the injury has been recognised, which they say is seldom done.

Hamilton, in discussing (*Fractures and Dislocations*, 1884, p. 244) the question of the rare occurrence of fracture of the acromion process in the adult, quotes a number of museum specimens in his own and other collections in which it was considered doubtful whether the detached portion had ever been fixed to the rest of the bone, and this fact, he believed, illustrated the lateness of the period to which bony union is sometimes delayed. In one specimen the acromial process of each scapula was fully formed, but had no osseous union whatever with the bone itself, the union being ligamentous but strong and close.

He says : ' There is some reason to believe that a true fracture of the acromion process is much more rare than surgeons have supposed, and that in a considerable number of the cases reported there was merely a separation of the epiphysis, the bony union having never been completed. If such fractures or separations occurred only in children, very little doubt might remain as to the general character of the accident; but the specimens which I have found in the museums, and the cases reported in the books, have been mostly from adults. It is more difficult, therefore, to suppose these to be examples of separation of epiphyses, but I am inclined to think that in a majority of instances such has been the fact.

'It is very probable, also, that in the case of many of the specimens found in the museums, called fractures, the histories of which are unknown, they were united originally by cartilage, and that in the process of boiling, or of maceration, the disjunction has been completed. The narrow crest of elevated bone which frequently

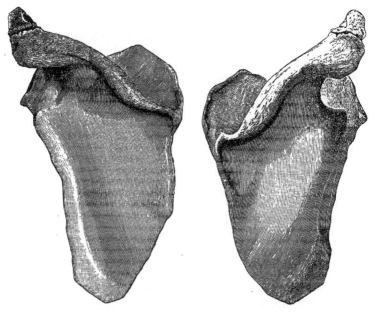

FIGS. 20 AND 21.—SYMMETRICAL SEPARATE ACROMION PROCESS

The clavicular facet is limited posteriorly by the line of junction

surrounds the process at the point of separation, and which Malgaigne may have mistaken for callus, is found upon very many examples of undoubted epiphysial separations which I have examined; and this circumstance, no doubt, has tended to strengthen the suspicion that these were cases of fracture.

'I wish to mention, also, that in the case of my own specimens of epiphysial separation, as well as most of the specimens which I have examined, the ends of the fragments were closed with a compact bony tissue.'

Besides his own specimens, Hamilton mentions a number of similar specimens in the Massachusetts Medical College Museum (reported to him by Dr. J. B. S. Jackson, of Boston, U.S.A.), the Mütter, the Jefferson Medical, and other museums in America.

Fergusson, Jackson, and others have also considered that specimens put up in museums as fractures are really delayed union of this epiphysis, separated by maceration.

The specimen here represented was obtained from the dissecting-room of Guy's Hospital when the author was Senior Demonstrator of Anatomy. It shows very clearly the separate condition of the epiphysis on the two sides in an old subject. There is no appearance of callus, and the process on both sides is united to the rest of the bone by a layer of cartilaginous-looking tissue. There was no history obtainable.

There appears to exist some connection between the absence of osseous union in these cases and osteo-arthritis of the shoulder-joint, with which it is often associated. With regard to the co-existence of these two conditions, the reader may be referred to Professor J. Struthers' exhaustive paper already quoted. He says: 'The supposition that the rheumatic tendency has had the effect of delaying the union of the acromial epiphysis would imply that the rheumatic tendency had shown itself in early life, by the age of about the twenty-fifth year, and it is not evident why that tendency should single out the acromial epiphysis among all the epiphyses of the skeleton.'

SYMPTOMS.—No case has been recorded in which the diagnosis has been absolutely established during life.

Displacement will be usually absent, as in fractures of this process, rendering the diagnosis extremely difficult; its detection will be quite impossible if any swelling has taken place.

In SEPARATION WITHOUT DISPLACEMENT from the periosteum remaining untorn, there will be merely some dropping of the shoulder, pain, and some loss of power to raise the arm.

In SEPARATION WITH DISPLACEMENT the edge of the separation may be felt with the finger, or *slight irregularity* or depression at the line of separation; and *muffled or soft crepitus* may be detected in replacing the fragments by elevation of the arm, the humerus being pressed upwards against the acromial arch by one hand, while the other hand is placed over the shoulder, or the arm being rotated, one hand is kept in the same position over the shoulder.

Mobility at the epiphysial junction may be felt whilst the epiphysial fragment is replaced in position by abducting and elevating the arm, or by pushing up the humerus, if displacement be present.

Pain and tenderness will exist at the epiphysial line of a fixed character, which may be increased on moving the arm.

Slight flattening of the shoulder will occur from dragging downwards of the epiphysial fragment by the weight of the upper extremity through the attachment of the deltoid muscles. While the spine of the scapula may be drawn up by the action of the trapezius and levator anguli scapulæ muscles, the head of the humerus retains its normal position.

Inability to use the arm will always be noticeable, especially in abduction; while in others the head may be observed to be drawn towards the affected side.

The *age* of the patient is an important factor. From the fourteenth or fifteenth to the twenty-second year is the period when separation of the ossifying epiphysis is most likely to occur.

DIAGNOSIS. *Simple contusion.*—The contusion and swelling around a separated epiphysis may entirely obscure the signs due to the injury, even when some displacement is present. The pain on pressure over the epiphysial line, and mobility and crepitus, are, however, distinguishing signs.

PROGNOSIS.—It is unlikely, from the absence of displacement and the small amount of muscular fibres attached to this process, that the muscular power in the upper extremity will be interfered with to any appreciable extent.

When there is but little displacement, separations of the acromial epiphysis will probably unite by bone. The union may, in other instances, be ligamentous, especially when the injury has not been recognised and the scapula allowed to move constantly on its epiphysis.

TREATMENT.—In all cases, even where there is little displacement, a good-sized cushion should be placed between the elbow and the side of the body, and the arm bandaged to the chest in this position, which relaxes the fibres of the deltoid and prevents displacement.

If displacement be present it may be reduced by pressure of the humerus against the acromial arch, and, to maintain the natural position, the elbow should be elevated and supported in this position by means of a sling.

It is not advisable to place a pad in the axilla, as in fractured clavicle, since it tends to displace the upper end of the humerus too much outwards, and may therefore drag the separated process out of position.

The simple roller bandage and sling may be conveniently replaced by a plaster of Paris dressing round the chest and over the opposite shoulder.

Passive movement should be commenced in about a fortnight.

SEPARATION OF THE EPIPHYSES OF THE
CORACOID PROCESS

ANATOMY.—During the first year of life ossification of the coracoid process commences in the middle of the cartilaginous process, which is rapidly invaded by it.

The coracoid process rests by its base upon the upper part of the glenoid cavity, but between its base and the circumference of the cavity at the part corresponding to the posterior half of the coracoid an intermediate cartilage is placed. The centre of ossification of the latter appears between the seventh and tenth years. This small epiphysis, sometimes called the *subcoracoid bone,* is pyramidal

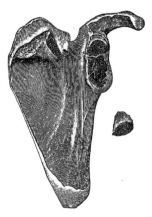

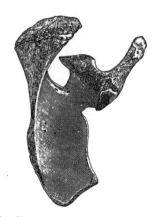

FIG. 22.—OSSIFICATION OF CORACOID PROCESS, SUB-CORACOID BONE, AND GLENOID CAVITY
(RAMBAUD AND RENAULT)

FIG. 23. — SCAPULA SEEN FROM ABOVE, SHOWING THE TWO CORACOID EPIPHYSES AND THE MORE EXTENDED FORM OF ACROMIAL EPIPHYSIS BETWEEN THE EIGHTEENTH AND NINETEENTH YEARS

in shape when fully ossified, and placed between the coracoid process and the glenoid cavity, the apex of which it assists in forming by its articular aspect.

The coracoid, as seen about the tenth year, is therefore separated from the body of the scapula by an epiphysial line of cartilage, which thence extends outwards and divides into two lines limiting the pyramidal subcoracoid.

In a short time after its appearance the subcoracoid bone joins at first behind with the body of the scapula, and afterwards a little later with the coracoid epiphysis, and finally with the bottom of the glenoid cavity. Sometimes the union is delayed till the seventeenth year.

The glenoid cavity is formed of four pieces : (1) that from the body of the scapula ; (2) a portion of the coracoid process internally ; (3) the subcoracoid bone ; (4) a thin glenoid or epiphysial plate at the margin of the glenoid, thicker at the edge and very thin towards the centre, resembling the epiphysial plate of the body of a vertebra. The glenoid cavity in its primitive state is somewhat convex ; it afterwards becomes flat, then angular, and at last concave, by the appearance of the new portions. The epiphysial margin of the glenoid joins the body of the bone from the twentieth to the twenty-fifth year.

According to Béclard, the coracoid process joins the body of the scapula from about the thirteenth to the sixteenth year, but it may take place, though rarely, as early as the fourteenth year, or be delayed till the seventeenth—usually about the time that the other epiphyses of the scapula (the acromial and suprascapular epiphyses) are making their appearance.

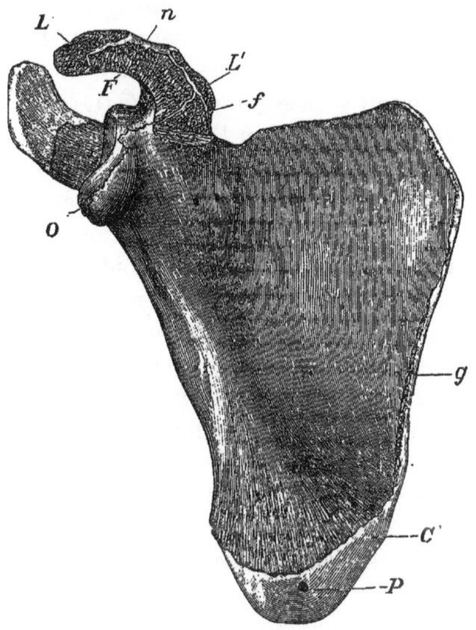

A scale-like epiphysis appears on the upper and posterior aspect of the coracoid process at the convex trapezoid ridge about the fourteenth year,

FIG. 24.---SCAPULA OF A SUBJECT AGED SEVENTEEN (AFTER RAMBAUD AND RENAULT)

f, Line still separating coracoid process from body of bone. L, L', Apical and basal epiphyses of the coracoid process, separated by a cartilaginous space, n ; the latter epiphysis overlaps the junction with the body. F, Body of coracoid process. g, Osseous granules in posterior border. O, Ossific plate of glenoid cavity. C, Inferior angle. P, Osseous centre in inferior angle.

and joins on at the eighteenth year, or even a little later—that is, after the rest of the coracoid process has been joined on to the body of the scapula.

In some instances the apex of the coracoid process has an additional point of ossification, which at the seventeenth year is seen to cover the apex like a cap. This centre never unites with the scale-like epiphysis just mentioned, but joins the body of the process from the twentieth to the twenty-fifth year.

The synovial membrane of the shoulder-joint covers the outer aspect of the subcoracoid bone, and is in close relation to a small portion of the base of the coracoid process on the inner side.

It is quite possible between the first and the fourteenth years to get detachment of this process without the shoulder-joint being opened, the process being separated from the body of the scapula and the subcoracoid epiphysial mass.

From the tenth to the seventeenth year, especially towards the latter end of this period, separation of the coracoid process, together with the subcoracoid bone, from the body of the bone is likely to occur in one piece. The upper part of the glenoid cavity will necessarily be torn open. This may also happen while the subcoracoid mass is still cartilaginous.

ETIOLOGY.—This separation may be produced by *severe direct violence*, such as the passage of a wheel over the shoulder, as in Bennett's case (*loc cit. infra*), or it may be caused by *a fall upon the shoulder*, as in the author's case narrated below. It is probable in the latter case that the direct pressure of the head of the humerus upon the coracoid and upper part of the glenoid was sufficient to cause an incomplete separation of this process. Mr. Lane believes that fracture of the coracoid process is caused by indirect violence, as in a fall with the arm fully flexed at the shoulder-joint, so that the coracoid process is pressed against the under surface of the clavicle; it may also be produced and the coracoid forced against the clavicle by a person falling from a height and suddenly seizing some object and arresting his fall.

Mr. R. Clement Lucas, in an article (*Guy's Hospital Reports*, vol. xlvii. 1890, p. 45) upon fracture of the coracoid process, draws attention to the various ways in which this process may be fractured in adults, and alludes to two cases mentioned by Bryant which he thought ought to be regarded as epiphysial separations. Both were caused by direct violence, and occurred in girls of fifteen (or sixteen) and fourteen years of age. He says: 'It is evident that as mobility and crepitus were the two symptoms by which these cases were diagnosed, there could not have been any great displacement. Judging by the time the coracoid epiphysis unites, these cases ought, however, to be classed as separations of the epiphysis.'

Muscular action.—It is possible for the apical epiphysis of the coracoid process to be torn off by the violent contraction of the muscles attached to it. No instance has as yet been recorded.

AGE.—Separation can only occur up to the seventeenth year of life.

PATHOLOGICAL ANATOMY.—Separation of the coracoid epiphysis is an extremely rare form of injury. It is possible that separation of the coracoid epiphysis alone may occur before its junction with the *subcoracoid* bone or portion of the coracoid cartilage—that is, before the tenth year—and the joint escape injury. It is, however, most probable, that, as in Bennett's case, the whole of the coracoid epiphysis, including the subcoracoid bone, will be detached, and the upper part of the glenoid cavity thus torn away with the capsular ligament and tendon of the biceps. The line of separation is on the scapular side of the epiphysial cartilage which remains with the coracoid process, and quite internal to the attachments of the powerful ·conoid and trapezoid ligaments to the under surface of the clavicle. The transverse ligament also attached to ·its base behind, and the coraco-humeral ligament to the process in front, will likewise go with. the epiphysis. The ligaments, together with the coraco-acromial ligament along the outer border, will tend to prevent any large amount of displacement, and hence but little deformity will probably be met with.

E. H. Bennett (*Transactions Roy. Acad. Med., Ireland*, vol. vi. 1888, p. 408, and *Dublin Journal of Med. Science*, August 1, 1888, vol. lxxxvi. p. 97) read a paper at the Royal Academy of Medicine in Ireland on June 1, 1888, on the following case of separation of the coracoid process produced by severe direct violence, accompanied by other serious injuries.

A boy (J. C.), aged six, was knocked down by a tramcar, and picked up from beneath its guard-board. A large flap of skin was found torn up from the front of the right side of the chest, and a second rent of the skin passed backwards beneath the axilla from the point of the anterior wound. The axillary vessels and most of the nerves were also torn through, and the upper limb all but torn off. The right forearm and many of the ribs on the right side were broken. No operation was performed for forty-eight hours on account of the collapsed condition of the patient; gangrene of the whole limb had then commenced, and amputation at the shoulder-joint was performed. Death ensued on the eighth day from tetanus. At the autopsy the second to the ninth ribs were found to be fractured (the eighth and ninth incompletely) and the coracoid process of the scapula separated. There was no injury of the lung or pleura. Professor Bennett continues : ' From the character of the wound, particularly that of the skin, it is clear that the force which inflicted the injury of the axilla was directed from below and in front, upwards and backwards, and its action ceased a little below the clavicle, which was intact. The lesion of the coracoid confirms this view. It is detached at its base, the line of separation passing through the proximal side of the cartilage, and at the upper and back part taking off a scale of bone from the supra-spinous fossa of the scapula. By misadventure the ligament of the scapular notch was cut away in making the early investigation of the injury, but the posterior margin of the notch bears incontestable proof of the quality of force that produced the lesion. A partial fracture of the scapular border behind the notch extends into the supra-spinous fossa for half an inch, and its anterior border has been sprung backwards, so that the thin layer of bone has overlapped the opposite side of the fracture and remains fixed in its displacement. This shows that the ligament of the notch attached in front to the base of the coracoid had all but torn off backwards with it a strip of bone from the superior border of the supra-spinous fossa. As the base of the coracoid in its epiphysiary condition forms a part of the glenoid cavity just at its summit and along the concave part of its upper and inner border, we find these parts detached and displaced with the coracoid; the upper and inner end of the cotyloid ligament is torn through, and with the base of the coracoid the attachment of the outer limb of the cotyloid ligament is displaced unbroken, and the tendon of the biceps along with it. There is no lesion of the clavicle or any other part of the scapula, but it is of interest to note that the acromial epiphysis is joined to the spine by a diarthrodial joint.'

Before the Anatomical Society in November 1887 Prof. Curnow exhibited specimens of ununited coracoid epiphyses.

The author has no doubt that many specimens of fractures in adults —which are situated at the base, in the vicinity of the glenoid cavity — are in reality instances of traumatic separation ununited, or possibly of non-ossification from the time of birth.

In May 1887 the author showed before the Pathological Society (*Pathological Society's Transactions*, vol. xxxviii. 1887, p. 261) a specimen of separation of the coracoid epiphysis following a fall upon the shoulder.

George L., aged twelve years, was admitted into Guy's Hospital on October 11, 1886, under the care of Mr. Durham. Nine days previously he was said to have been thrown down by a dog, and to have fallen on his right shoulder, his right thumb also being bitten. Three days after, vomiting set in with feverishness and great pain in the shoulder. On admission the temperature was 103°·6; P. 124. There was a fluctuating area over the scapula, and some redness and puffiness over the back of the right hand. Incisions were made into the swelling on the dorsum of the scapula, and the infra-spinous fossa was found to be bare. Death took place early the next morning from pyæmia. At the autopsy it was found that the right scapula was almost entirely denuded of its periosteum, the subscapular, supra- and infra-spinous fossæ being bare, with the exception of the upper and lower angles, and full of bloody pus. The abscess cavity on the dorsal surface communicated freely with that in front by means of the shoulder-joint, and also over the neck of the bone. The joint was acutely inflamed and full of pus, the capsule partly destroyed, and the articular cartilages were beginning to be eroded. The scapula itself was of a greenish yellow colour, and, on section, infiltrated with pus. The coracoid epiphysis was completely detached, and only a small flake of the cartilaginous epiphysial line remained. The muscles were still attached to its apex, and around this process were the remains of what had apparently been a cavity full of blood, suggesting that this was the original seat of the disease—viz. that this process had been detached by the injury at its epiphysial line of cartilage, and that the injured tissue at the epiphysial line furnished a congenial soil for micro-organisms to flourish, acute osteomyelitis of the scapula taking place in a similar manner to that of the shaft of a long bone, and with it other signs of general infection.   There were pyæmic abscesses in the lungs, heart, brain, abdominal viscera, and fourth metacarpal bone.

This specimen is in the Royal College of Surgeons' Museum, No. 1218 E.   The catalogue gives the following brief description : ' A portion of a ·right scapula, the coracoid epiphysis óf which is completely detached.   The root of the epiphysis is denuded of its periosteum, and the *intervening cartilage is in great part destroyed*. In the recent condition the periosteum was stripped from the dorsal and ventral surfaces of the scapula by the formation of pus beneath it, and these abscess-cavities communicated freely above the neck of the bone.   On section the medullary tissue of the bone was infiltrated with pus.   From a boy, aged twelve, who died of pyæmia ten days after a fall upon his right shoulder.'

SYMPTOMS.—*Pain* over coracoid.

Inability to raise or adduct the arm, on account of the attachment of its biceps and coraco-brachialis muscles.

Mobility.—Preternatural mobility of the process may be felt on grasping this small fragment between the fingers and thumb, or on rotating or abducting the arm, or pressing on the tip of the process, whilst the scapula is fixed.   It may be grasped readily enough between the clavicular fibres of the pectoralis major and deltoid muscle if no displacement and swelling have occurred; but should these be present its depth from the surface will completely prevent its being grasped by the fingers.

Crepitus of the usual soft character, if there is but little displacement of the process.   If this cannot be detected on moving the process, it may be elicited by moving the. humerus at the shoulder-joint whilst the finger is placed in the depression between the deltoid and pectoral muscles in front.

Great swelling from direct violence.

If the coracoid process is *displaced* at all, it will be in the downward and inward direction, by the combined action of the pectoralis minor, biceps, and coraco-brachialis muscles.

A case has been reported by Dr. E. C. Huse, of U.S.A. (*Chicago Medical Journal and Examiner*, vol. xxix. August 1879, p. 175), but has not been confirmed by an autopsy.

M. Chauvel alludes (*Diction. encycl. des Sciences Médicales*, 1881, tom. quinzième, p. 294) to this form of injury when he says, in speaking of fractures of the base of the coracoid process, that fracture is sometimes met with in children at the line of junction of this epiphysis with the body of the scapula.

SEPARATION OF THE APICAL EPIPHYSIS of the coracoid might be brought about by the combined muscular action of the coraco-

M

brachialis, biceps, and pectoralis minor, and might give rise to great displacement of the tip of this process in a downward direction. The process of union in this case will probably only be by ligamentous tissue.

COMPLICATIONS. — Like the corresponding fractures in the adult, separation of the coracoid may be accompanied by either:

(a) Dislocation or fracture of the humerus, or (b) dislocation of the outer end of the clavicle.

TREATMENT.—If the separation has taken place at the base of the coracoid process, there will be but little difficulty in maintaining the fragments in good position, on account of the small amount of tendency to displacement through the attachment of the strong coraco-clavicular (conoid and rhomboid) and coraco-acromial ligaments.

Should, however, the separation occur at the apical epiphysis beyond these ligaments, nothing can be done to keep the separated fragment in its proper position through the combined action of the pectoralis minor, coraco-brachialis, and biceps muscles, but a small pad may be placed below the process, which will tend to support it in position.

The arm and forearm should always be flexed acutely, so as to relax the biceps and other muscles, and the elbow should be supported and the whole limb bound to the body. This may be effected by the hand of the injured side being fixed upon the opposite shoulder with the arm and elbow in the sling across the chest, while the scapula is supported behind by means of a soft broad pad.

CHAPTER III

SEPARATION OF THE UPPER EPIPHYSIS OF THE HUMERUS

ANATOMY.—In the first year of life the diaphysis of the humerus already attains the osseous shape which it keeps during the rest of life. Its upper end, which is in the first instance concave, and then a plane surface, is even now slightly convex, and fits into the cartilaginous epiphysis. The upward and inward extension of the diaphysis, the part which supports the head, is morphologically the same as the neck of the femur at this period.

During the first year, usually towards the middle of the year, osseous granules appear scattered in this cartilaginous end. Dr. Herbert R. Spencer (*Journal of Anatomy and Physiology*, vol. xxv. July 1891, p. 554) has found that a centre of ossification is not rarely met with in the head of the humerus at the time of birth. About the end of the first year these granules begin to group themselves into three centres, that for the head appearing first at the beginning of the second year, and that for the greater tuberosity during the third. The centre for the lesser tuberosity is not well marked until the end of the fourth year, at times as late as the end of the fifth. At this period these three centres are pretty accurately divided from each other by the anatomical neck and the bicipital groove; they begin to blend with each other about the sixth year (some anatomists state from the third to the fifth year), the lesser tuberosity joining first by its upper part with the head and greater tuberosity, and the latter being still separated from the head by a layer of cartilage. It is therefore possible to have a separation of the epiphysis of the head alone.

Somewhat later the greater tuberosity blends with the upper part of the head, and the large upper epiphysis is fully formed. It is entirely osseous at the age of puberty. This cup-like epiphysis includes the two tuberosities, the upper fourth of the bicipital groove, and the whole of the head and anatomical neck, as well as a very small portion of the bone external to the lesser tuberosity, between it and the anatomical neck, which constitutes part of the shaft in the adult. The limit of the epiphysial line on the inner side is situated directly below the cartilaginous articular surface of the head at its axillary margin and runs horizontally outwards, rising considerably in a point at the centre and terminating on the outer side directly below the tuberosities.

The cup-like epiphysis rests with its concavity upon the pointed concave end of the diaphysis. The cone-shaped end of the diaphysis only develops as age increases ; in infancy it is almost flat, and afterwards becomes slightly convex.

Each osseous nucleus of the head and tuberosities thus appears about the fourth or fifth year to be surrounded by cartilage—viz. that covering the articular surface and tuberosities, and that between the parts of the epiphysis.

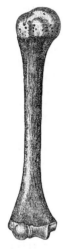

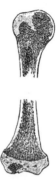

FIG. 25.—HUMERUS AT THE THIRD YEAR. (AFTER RAMBAUD AND RENAULT.) ABOUT HALF NATURAL SIZE

FIG. 26.—VERTICAL SECTION OF UPPER AND LOWER ENDS OF HUMERUS AT THE THIRD YEAR. (AFTER RAMBAUD AND RENAULT.) ABOUT HALF NATURAL SIZE

The three pieces of which the epiphysis is originally composed form by their union a kind of recess about the centre, which accurately fits the pointed pyramidal projection on the upper end of the diaphysis—a cone-like shape which has gradually developed as age advanced. Numerous small elevations and depressions are well marked over the surface.

Buttress-like ledges on the outer aspect of the upper end of the diaphysis support the greater and lesser tuberosities. As the bone grows the conjugal cartilage diminishes in thickness until it becomes a thin layer, and constitutes a weak point up to the time of final union of the epiphysis.

The younger the child the farther this line will be found from the head of the bone.

The epiphysis, when complete, is eleven millimetres thick in the centre opposite the depression for the central point of the diaphysis, twenty-two millimetres on the outer side at the tuberosities, and on the inner side, about the middle of the head, fifteen millimetres.

De Paoli gives the following table of measurements of the height and breadth of the upper epiphysis of the humerus in different individuals according to age.

The height is taken proportionally from the front half of a vertical coronal section dividing the head of the humerus into two halves, one anterior and the other posterior; the breadth is taken from the same section at the base of the epiphysis. He also measured the apparent height—that is, the distance from the middle of the upper surface and the base of the epiphysis.

Age	Height	Apparent height	Breadth
	mm.	mm.	mm.
Before birth	...... 11	...... 15	...... 18 ......
First year	...... 12	...... 19	...... 26 ......
Second	...... 12	...... 20	...... 28 ......
Fourth	...... 12	...... 19	...... 29 ......
Fifth	...... 12	...... 21	...... 37 ......
Sixth	...... 13	...... 20	...... 35 ......
Seventh	...... 15	...... 23	...... 38 ......
Eighth	...... 16	...... 24	... . 34 ......
Ninth	... { 16 ...... { 16	...... 24 .... —	...... 41 .... 39 ......
Twelfth	...... 14	...... —	...... 48 ......
Sixteenth	{ 18 .... { 16 ...... { 16	...... 29 ....,.... 24 .... 26	...... 41 .... 41 .... 40 ......
Seventeenth	... { 16 ...... { 18	...... — 24	...... 55 .... 40 ......
Eighteenth......................	...... 13	...... 26	...... 45 ......

This epiphysis does not begin to unite with the shaft until the twentieth year, or even a little later, and its central portion is the first to ossify on to the prominent point of the diaphysis, union being effected in the male somewhat later than in the case of the female. Some authors have stated that the union may not take place till the twenty-fourth year, or even later.

The epiphysial line marks the upper limit of the surgical neck of the bone in the adult.

In proportion as the spongy bone of the diaphysis at the level of the epiphysial line becomes rarefied and the medullary canal formed, the external compact layer of bone becomes thicker and more dense.

A trace of the line of union sometimes persists for a considerable time.

Posteriorly the line passes below the greater tuberosity, through the muscular fibres of the lowest thin part of the attachment of the teres minor into the shaft of the humerus. It is half to three-quarters of an inch below the level of the tip of the coracoid when the arm is hanging by the side of the body, but if the arm be abducted from the side, the outer margin of the line is almost precisely. on a level with this process. At fourteen years of age the outer margin is twenty millimetres below the acromial

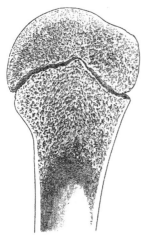

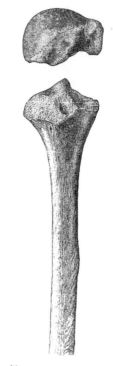

FIG. 27 —VERTICAL SECTION OF THE UPPER END OF HUMERUS AT THE AGE OF SEVENTEEN YEARS. ANTERIOR HALF OF SECTION, SHOWING THE CENTRAL CONICAL PROJECTION OF THE DIAPHYSIAL END AND CANCELLOUS STRUCTURE. ACTUAL SIZE

arch ; at eighteen years of age twenty-five to thirty millimetres below.

In the fully formed epiphysis the synovial membrane on the inner or under aspect, both towards the front and back, overlaps the epiphysial line for

FIG. 28.—UPPER END OF HUMERUS AT THE EIGHTEENTH YEAR

The epiphysis has been detached to show the pyramidal end of the diaphysis with its apex projecting upwards.

several millimetres, and the attachment of the capsular ligament corresponds here exactly to the epiphysial line. But separation of the epiphysis will not necessarily, except in cases of great violence, lead to opening of the articular cavity, inasmuch as the capsule is firmly attached to the epiphysis, and the synovial membrane passing off from the articular cartilage is but loosely attached to the diaphysis.

On the outer or upper surface the synovial membrane is far from the limit of the epiphysial line, the whole thickness of the tuberosities, with the capsular ligament, and many tendinous and muscular attachments to these processes intervening. The membrane approaches closer the line the nearer the inner aspect of the humerus is reached. In infancy, the synovial membrane is seen

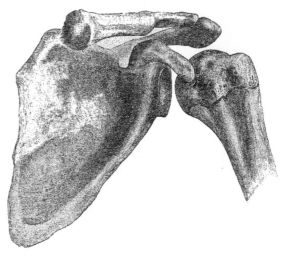

Fig. 29.—Bones forming the shoulder-joint at the twentieth year. Relationship of epiphysial junction of upper end of humerus

to pass over the upper surface of the cartilaginous epiphysis as far as the point where later on the osseous centres of the head and great tuberosities join together.

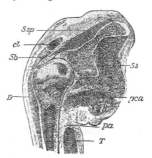

Fig. 30. Frontal section of the right shoulder-joint of a female infant æt. 1¾ years. Posterior half of section, the arm hanging vertically downwards

cl, acromial end of clavicle cut obliquely; *D*, deltoid muscle; *Sb*, synovial bursa beneath its origin; *Ssp*, supraspinatus; *T*, triceps; *pa*, profunda artery; *pca*, posterior circumflex artery; *Ss*, scapula. (A. v. Brunn.)

The synovial membrane appears to overlap the inner aspect of the diaphysis as age advances; at three years of age it overlaps it for two millimetres, at thirteen years for five or six millimetres (Sésary).

We see, therefore, that in infancy up to about the fifth year all the bony nucleus of the head is entirely within the capsule of

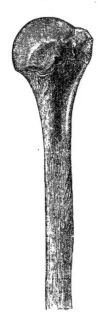

the shoulder-joint, while after this period, the ossific centres becoming blended with that of the head, part of this epiphysis is internal and part external to the synovial membrane.

The growth in length of the diaphysis principally proceeds from the upper epiphysis.

The muscles attached to this epiphysis are the subscapularis—to its lesser tuberosity—the supraspinatus, infraspinatus, and teres minor—to its three facets on the great tuberosity; the long tendon of the biceps occupying the groove between these two processes surrounded by the process of the synovial membrane of the shoulder-joint.

The capsular ligament is attached on the inner side at the level of the epiphysial line for rather more than the inner third of its extent, and then follows the rest of the line of the anatomical neck, between the head and the tuberosities.

FIG. 31.—UPPER EPIPHYSIS OF THE HUMERUS AT THE NINETEENTH YEAR. HALF NATURAL SIZE

E. M. Moore says: 'Taking the head of a bone from a subject ten years of age, parted by maceration, we find that the angle made by the junction of the plane,

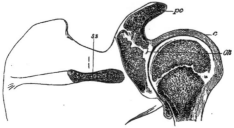

FIG. 32.—RIGHT SHOULDER-JOINT IN A SUBJECT ÆT. SIXTEEN.   THE ARM BEING PARALLEL TO THE MIDDLE LINE OF THE BODY, THE SECTION PASSES THROUGH THE CORACOID PROCESS OF THE SCAPULA AND THROUGH THE HEAD OF HUMERUS, ABOUT A QUARTER WAY DISTANT FROM ITS ANTERIOR ASPECT.   THE SYNOVIAL CAPSULE AND PERIOSTEUM APPEAR THICK ON ACCOUNT OF THEIR OBLIQUE DIVISION .

ss, spine of scapula; *pc*, coracoid process separated from the body of scapula by an epiphysial plate of cartilage, which increases considerably in thickness towards the articular surface; *on*, osseous nucleus appearing in the thickest portion of the cartilage (Uffelmann's osteo-epiphysis bicipitalis); *c*, capsular ligament. (Brunn.)

projected through the anatomical neck (which forms two-fifths of the whole surface), with the plane passing below the tuberosities, measures about 100 degrees.'

The periosteum passing from the epiphysis to the diaphysis is thick and strong.

AGE.—Instances have been recorded from the time of birth up to twenty-five years of age.

Dr. H. R. Wharton says ('Separation or Disjunction of the Upper Epiphysis of the Humerus,' *University Medical Magazine,* Philadelphia, January 1889, vol. i. No. 4, p. 212) that this accident is not a very unusual one in children from five to fifteen years of age as the result of falls upon the arm.

D'Arcy Power says (*Surgical Diseases of Children,* 1895, p. 171) : 'It is generally met with about puberty, and the separation results from direct violence to the shoulder. Separation of the whole epiphysis takes place after the sixth year, for it is only then that the nuclei of the head unite with that of the greater tuberosity to form a single mass.' As will be seen presently, separation does very frequently take place in infancy. The whole upper end of the bone is formed of one cartilaginous mass, in which the osseous centres for head and tuberosities appear. Therefore separation of any one of these component parts can only be effected by accompanying fracture of the cartilage uniting the centres, which must be an accident of extremely rare occurrence.

The author's own statistics are as follows :

Out of a total of *twenty-one pathological specimens* we must omit seven doubtful at the time of birth ; and seven in which the age is not stated (one of the latter being in a young person and one in a young adult) ; and in the remaining seven museum specimens, in which the age is given, two are at thirteen, one at seventeen, one at fifteen, one at eleven, one between four and five years of age, and one between three and four years.

In *seven compound cases,* in all of which the age is stated, two were at nineteen, two at fifteen, two at sixteen, and one at fourteen years.

Taking the whole *fourteen cases verified by dissection*; nine were from thirteen to nineteen years of age, six of these being from thirteen to sixteen—an average of thirteen years for those cases in which the age is stated.

Analysing the *twelve cases of arrest of growth,* the ages at which the separation is said to have taken place are : one at fourteen, one at eleven, one at ten, one at nine, one at eight, one at four, one at three, two at two, one at one and a half years, one at six months, and one in early infancy.

Among the *eighteen cases operated upon* for recent separation, or later for deformity, we find that : in one the age is not stated, two were at twenty-three, one at nineteen, one at eighteen, three at seventeen, three at sixteen, one at fifteen, one at fourteen, three at ten, one at nine, and one at seven years.

Taking the *sixty-one cases of simple separation*, the age is not stated in five (one of these, however, in a *child*) ; in thirty the age is stated to have been from thirteen to nineteen years of age—viz. four at nineteen, one at eighteen, one at seventeen, seven at sixteen, six at fifteen, six at fourteen, five at thirteen (amongst these thirty are recorded eleven cases from Guy's Hospital not hitherto published, and eight of these were from thirteen to seventeen years of age) ; twenty-four between four and twelve years of age—viz. six at twelve, three at eleven, two at ten, four at nine, three at eight, three at seven, and one each at six, five, and four years ; of the remainder, two in infancy, one at six months and the other at about thirteen months.

Analysing the *total* 119 *cases* recorded, in ninety-eight the age is accurately given, and amongst these the greatest number, sixty-six, occurred between the ages of nine and seventeen.

Hutchinson thinks that this injury occurs most often in boys from ten to fifteen years of age.

Dr. Jetter's seventeen cases from the Tübingen Clinic also give the maximum frequency of this separation from the tenth to the fifteenth year :

5 to 10 years	10 to 15 years	15 to 20 years	20 to 25 years
Five cases	Seven cases	Three cases	Two cases

He thinks, like many other surgeons, that the pure form of separation is most frequent during the earlier years of life.

SEX.—Out of forty-six cases, the sex is stated in thirty-seven, thirty-one being in males and six in females ; and out of a total of 119 cases, the sex being stated in 104, eighty-five were males and nineteen females.

ETIOLOGY.—Separation most frequently results from forcible traction of the arm outwards and upwards. According to Gurlt, it is produced by violence much greater than that which is the usual cause of fracture at the corresponding periods of life. He produced it by violent abduction while the epiphysis was fixed, and Colignon did so by violent abduction and rotation outwards of the limb.

Rognetta, by means of experiments, especially studied detachments of this epiphysis in the newly born. Salmon, however, in his experiments could not effect separation on the bodies of infants of less than a month old. According to Küstner's experiments on newly born children, separation is most easily effected by rotation of the upper extremity. Pajot separated this epiphysis by traction of a weight of nineteen kilogrammes after the soft parts had been removed from the articulation, but he found that, if these were preserved intact, it required a weight of thirty-five kilogrammes to effect its separation.

The injury may be occasioned by *direct* as well as *indirect violence*.

Separations the result of **severe direct violence** applied to the shoulder—such as the kick of a horse, a fall of a heavy box (1 cwt.) on the shoulder, a fall upon the shoulder (a projecting body striking it below the acromion), or some severe crushing accident (as being run over by a tramcar, waggon, or cart—are sometimes simple injuries, although out of seven cases known to have been produced in this way four were rendered compound.

Indirect violence.—We find in analysing forty cases that in the large majority (twenty-seven) the separation was produced by a blow or a fall on to the front or outer side of the shoulder, such as a fall from a waggon or from a tree sixteen feet high or less, or simply by a fall on the pavement from slipping on orange peel or whilst running. In one case the patient fell a distance of sixty feet from a warehouse.

Rollet says (*loc. cit. infra*) : ' As an element in the diagnosis let us also add the nature of the injury ; in the two cases which we mention, and in the four others observed by M. Poncet, the direct cause was a fall upon the prominence of the shoulder.'

In sixteen cases described by Dr. Jetter, twelve were caused by a fall upon the shoulder from a greater or less height—viz. varying from a man's height to seven metres high—on to the level ground or on to an object lying upon the ground ; once by a fall upon the shoulder, from slipping upon ice ; and twice by a fall on the out-stretched arm, causing forcible abduction. In three of the cases the mode of production was uncertain.

Bruns observed a case of separation of the upper epiphysis of the humerus in a boy aged fourteen who had fallen from a tree, a height of five feet.

Sir Charles Bell (*Institutes of Surgery*, vol. i. p. 3) says that he has known epiphysial separation of the upper end of the humerus occur from a boy firing a musket.

In two instances the violence was apparently even more *indirect*. It is stated in one instance that the separation was caused by a fall the height of a few feet on to the elbow ; while in another it was produced by the patient suddenly throwing, with great violence, his arms upwards and somewhat laterally ; in a third by the child being suddenly seized and raised by its arms ; and in a fourth case by the arms being caught between the spokes of a wheel.

Professor Kocher believes that violence applied from below, as in a fall on the outer side of the elbow, is often clinically the mode of production. He thinks that the abrasions and contusions frequently seen on the outer side of the elbow prove this.

On the dead subject the author has found that forcible abduction of the arm with rotation, especially outwards, is the most easy way to produce a separation of this epiphysis.

From this forcible abduction or elevation of the arm arise some of the frequent causes of dislocation in the adult.

Edmund Owen (*Surgical Diseases of Children*, 1885, p. 382) alludes to the case of a girl, aged eight, who had recently been under his care; the fracture occurred from the nurse twisting the child's arm behind her back, but with no great violence. Thus the humerus was converted into a lever of the first order, the fulcrum being found at the spot where the bone was brought into firm contact with the chest wall. On examining the joint under chloroform, crepitus of a peculiar 'mortary' feel was easily obtained. The end of the diaphysis projected somewhat outwards, and could be easily felt through the thin deltoid.

An interesting case is described by M. Ricard (S. Duplay and P. Reclus, *Traité de Chirurgie*, tom. ii. 1890), in which this epiphysis was clearly separated by a violent twist of the arm without any direct blow.

A youth, aged nineteen years, was seized by the middle of the arm during a quarrel, and violently twisted and pushed. Although no direct injury was received, the patient immediately experienced acute pain at the shoulder, with inability to move the arm. The next day there was found a fairly considerable swelling occupying the whole region of the shoulder and upper half of the arm, and extending upwards to the infra-clavicular region (rendering exploration of the latter very difficult), and also to the outer wall of the axilla. No abnormal projection, however, was detected. Active movements were impossible, and passive movements were only effected with much pain. The elbow was a little away from the trunk, but could be brought nearer with some pain. The sub-deltoid bursa and shoulder-joint appeared to contain abundant serous effusion. Direct pressure on the humerus and pressure on the elbow from below upwards gave rise to acute pain, which was limited to a spot two fingers' breadth below the acromion. Slight mobility was felt on seizing the arm by its lower extremity and rotating the humerus round its axis, while on placing the other hand on the shoulder very characteristic, but indistinct and muffled, crepitus could be plainly felt at the same spot as the pain. There was no appreciable shortening. Consolidation was effected with a certain amount of displacement of the humerus forwards, so that the head formed a marked angle with the axis of the humerus, being situated at its posterior and inner aspect. Movements, however, could be freely carried out.

In the following interesting case of incomplete displacement inwards of the end of the diaphysis recorded by A. Demoulin (*Archives générales de Médecine*, November 1893, p. 611) the separation was caused by a fall upon the elbow, the shoulder not touching the ground.

A pale thin girl (C. A.), aged fourteen years, came under the care of M. Duplay at the Hôpital de la Charité on February 4, 1893. About an hour previously she had fallen on to the right elbow whilst sliding on the pavement; this was followed by acute pain in the corresponding shoulder. On examination there was great pain on the slightest movement. The elbow was carried backwards and the arm somewhat abducted, the forearm being flexed at a right angle. Over the olecranon there was slight redness only; but no flattening of shoulder or projection of the acromion. In front of the deltoid region, two good fingers' breadth below the acromio-coracoid interspace, there was a slight projection forwards, with pain on pressure, but an absence of blood extravasation. The osseous border of this projection was about two centimetres broad, could be felt below the greater and lesser tuberosities, and had a prominent edge. Between this directly forward (and slightly inward) displacement of the upper end of the diaphysis and the head (which preserved its normal relations) a depression could be felt by the finger, but on the posterior aspect of the shoulder no depression could be made out under the epiphysis, although the thin condition of the patient rendered palpation very easy. No mobility, shortening of the arm, or crepitus was felt. The diaphysis was clearly not completely displaced off the epiphysis; however, the effect of rotation of the shaft upon the epiphysis could not be determined on account of the reflex contraction of the muscles about the shoulder. The least active movement of the arm was accompanied by great pain. The arm was put up in a sling. On the fourth day an unsuccessful attempt was made to reduce the displacement by traction on the lower end of the humerus, and again on the sixth day a third attempt under chloroform also failed; the limb was then put up in a plaster splint. From this time the patient experienced no further pain. The splint was removed on March 3, the twenty-seventh day. Although there was some wasting of the deltoid, consolidation was perfect, and rotation and all other movements of the shoulder-joint were completely restored. When the patient was seen a month later, after the use of massage, &c., the deltoid was normal, and the persisting deformity did not give rise to any inconvenience whatever.

Allusion is made below to separation during extraction of the child in delivery by dragging on the presenting arm, or by bringing this down when the legs and body were already delivered, or by the finger hooked into the axilla.

The following case has recently been recorded by Dr. J. Gurney Taylor (*University Medical Magazine*, Philadelphia, vol. ix. No. 2, November 1896, p. 118) as one of separation of the upper epiphysis of the humerus in a male infant, aged five months, due to simply lifting the child up by the arms. But it is a matter of some doubt if so slight an injury to a healthy bone could have produced such acute suppuration with pyæmia; it appears more probable that the affection was rather of the nature of infective arthritis of infants. Four days previous to admission into St. Christopher's Hospital for Children, the child at its christening ·had been picked up by the arms several times. From. that time he had cried continually, and the following day the left shoulder was noticed to be swollen. On admission the swelling had greatly increased, reaching from the insertion of the deltoid to the middle of the clavicle ; the axilla also was very much swollen. The skin was tense and red, and there was 'pitting' on pressure. Over the tendon of the biceps there was fluctuation. The head of the humerus was felt in its normal position, yet there was decided crepitus and great pain upon motion. A diagnosis was made of fracture of the humerus. The temperature was 104·5° F. and the pulse 180. Dr. H. C. Deaver opened the abscess, which contained about 2 oz. of pus. The humerus was intact, but the upper epiphysis was found to have separated. Pyæmia developed, and the infant died about two weeks from the date of the accident.

Muscular action.—The only recorded case of displacement by muscular action is that referred to by Colignon and quoted in Ashhurst's *Encyclopædia of Surgery*, vol. iv. p. 121. This remarkable case is also mentioned by Bouchut, as seen by Foucher (*Mémoire sur les disjonctions épiphysaires*) in the practice of M. Velpeau in 1855. A girl, previously in good health, aged thirteen years, is said to have produced this injury by muscular action in taking an embroidery frame down from a wall above her head. A sudden crackling, followed by acute pain, was experienced in the left shoulder. Considerable swelling and redness of the shoulder, with fever, appeared. An abscess formed, which was incised on the fourth day, letting out a great quantity of pus. It was noted at the time that the upper end of the humerus was broken. Suppuration continued, with diarrhœa and hectic, and death took place at the end of six weeks. The diagnosis was verified by the autopsy. The extremity of the diaphysis was in a state of necrosis at its upper third, and commencing already to be exfoliated. The epiphysial cartilage remained with the epiphysis, which was still in contact with the glenoid cavity, being held there by the muscles inserted into it and by the capsule of the joint. It had been separated from the diaphysis exactly at the conjugal cartilage. The periosteum, though still remaining attached to the epiphysis, was extensively separated. A vast purulent cavity occupied the axilla, being limited by the deltoid and great pectoral muscles.

It is questionable whether this was a true case of traumatic separation, or one rather of acute purulent epiphysial osteomyelitis followed by detachment of the epiphysis at the juxta-epiphysial region.

Other predisposing causes.—Mr. Cooper Forster had the case of Thos. H., aged four, under his care in Guy's Hospital in October 1878. Five weeks previously he had fallen on to his right shoulder, causing a separation of the epiphysis. Eight months before he had been trephined for a compound comminuted depressed fracture of the left parietal bone, and partial hemiplegia of the right side had since been present. A pad was placed in the axilla, and the arm secured to the body, and on his discharge twenty-six days afterwards there was good mobility of the arm.

PATHOLOGICAL ANATOMY. Separation of the cartilaginous upper end in the newly born infant or during delivery.—Such cases have been frequently recorded as having occurred from violent traction upon the arm or in the axilla during delivery, but in many of them there is every reason to believe that some disease or altered condition of nutrition was present in the bones.

Thus Bitot describes (*Journal de Bordeaux*, 1859, and *Gazette Médicale de Paris*, 1860) a very interesting case of separation of the upper epiphysis of the humerus which had been brought about by violent traction at the arm, combined with a see-saw movement. The shoulder was not deformed, but there was pain when the arm was moved. Death ensued at the end of twelve days, and at the autopsy the epiphysial separation was discovered and the humerus found to be notably diminished in size, being one centimetre shorter than that of the sound side.

From the shortening of the humerus (which was supposed to have taken place in the brief space of twelve days), from the altered condition of the bicipital groove and upper end of the bone found on comparison with the sound side, it is evident that the separation in this case cannot be considered as one due entirely to injury to a healthy bone.

The cases recorded by Bertrandi of Turin (*Opere anatomiche e cerusiche*, tom. v. Torino, 1787–8, p. 163), De la Motte, and Dubroca (*Bull. Médical de Bordeaux*, 1835) come under the same category. They are so open to doubt that the propriety of accepting them as true separations unaccompanied by disease or maceration must be carefully considered.

In some cases, however, union took place in eight to twelve days. In Dubroca's case the callus was very excessive, so that the shoulder was three times its proper circumference.

Examples in still-born and other new-born infants are doubtless of the same description, often caused by traction on the arm in shoulder presentation. No account has been taken in the present work of several other separations of the upper cartilaginous end of the humerus occurring in new-born infants, and produced by violent traction during birth, such as those related by Bruns, Durocher, Volkmann, Hamilton, Reichel, and others.

These epiphysial fractures of the humerus in the new-born are treated by Professor O. Küstner (*Annals of Surgery*, vol. i. No. 5, May 1885, p. 492; ' Ueber épiphysaire Diaphysen-Fractur am Humerus der Neugeborenen, *Archiv f. klin. Chir.* Berl. 1884,

xxxi. 310; 'Verletzungen des Kindes bei der Geburt,' *Handbuch der Geburtshülfe*, Bd. iii. Stuttgart, 1889). In their situation, from the fact that the junction of the cartilaginous upper end lies nearer the diaphysis, they approach more nearly fractures of the surgical neck in adults.

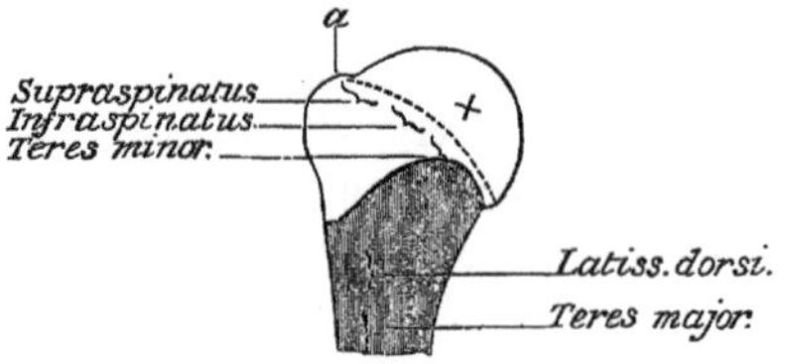

FIG. 33.—FRONTAL SECTION OF THE UPPER END OF THE HUMERUS AT BIRTH

×, head of the bone; *a*, greater tuberosity. It is seen that the junction of the cartilaginous upper end encroaches more on the diaphysis at this period than later. The attachments of the rotator muscles are indicated. (After Küstner.)

Pajot (*Thèse d' Agrég.* 1853, Paris) found that a weight of thirty-five kilograms (77 lb.) was sufficient to detach this epiphysis in the new-born, and only nineteen kilograms (41 lb.) were needed when the soft parts had been removed.

In Durocher's case (Chapelain Durocher, Thèse inaugurale, 8vo. Paris, 8 frimaire an xii.) the child died fourteen months after an injury of this kind.

In Volkmann's (*Beiträge zur Chirurgie*, 1875, S. 72) case of separation of the upper cartilaginous end of the right humerus in a newly born infant from traction during delivery, death took place on the fifth day. The separation was found to have taken place cleanly between the cartilage and the bone, except on the inner side, where the fracture ran somewhat through the bone. There was also an oblique fracture of the left clavicle and subluxation of the sterno-clavicular joint.

Separation of the upper epiphysis of the humerus after infancy.— Palletta, in his *Exercitationes Pathologicæ*, 1820, alludes (cap. vi. p. 59) to the possibility of separation of the upper epiphysis of the humerus; and Malgaigne, in his work *Anatomie chirurgicale*, considered this injury to be excessively rare. He says: 'It is only from the eighteenth to the twentieth year that the union of the epiphysis with the diaphysis is concluded, and up to that time separation of the epiphysis may take place. These separations are, however, very rare, and are more difficult of production as the child increases in age. I know of only four examples altogether; two brought about during labour, a third in a child whose age was not given, and the fourth observed by Champion in a child of eleven.'

Boyer, writing in the *Dictionnaire des Sciences médicales*, tom. xxii. p. 1, referred to separation of this epiphysis as a very rare accident, possible only in the very earliest years of life.

It is somewhat remarkable that so few specimens of this lesion are preserved in museums, since we recognise the injury during life as being of common occurrence. The author has been able to collect only eight.

Many compound separations, and cases operated upon for deformity, or for irreducibility soon after the accident, prove, however, that it is not so rare as is generally supposed.

Gurlt collected three cases in which the injury was caused during delivery (mentioned above), one each in children aged four, eleven, and fifteen years, and a specimen obtained three years after the injury.

Bruns collected only eleven cases confirmed by anatomical inspection ; all these are fully related below.

But, as Bruns says, this epiphysial separation occurs much more frequently than is generally supposed, and is one of the most common forms of the injury.

In all these specimens, and in compound separations, the whole of the upper extremity of the bone is detached—the head, with the tuberosities attached, being still in contact with the glenoid cavity of the scapula ; and the synovial membrane is often uninjured.

Separation of either of the tuberosities is possible before their union with the head—that is, up to the end of the fifth year. Such a lesion would probably be extracapsular, unless the violence were so severe ·as to lacerate the bicipital extension from the synovial membrane. The author cannot find any specimen of such a lesion or of simple separation of the osseous head. The latter is very improbable as the result of injury, and would be entirely within the capsule of the joint.

PURE SEPARATIONS.—*Pure separation through the cartilage* is extremely rare.

The separation took place, in Esmarch's case, through the substance of the conjugal cartilage, one layer of which remained attached to the epiphysis and another to the diaphysis.

In Foucher's case the whole of the epiphysial cartilage, as usually happens, remained with the epiphysis.

In one of two cases operated upon by Professor De Paoli of Perugia, the diaphysial end was said to be covered here and there with small areas of the conjugal cartilage.

According to Michniowsky, separation never occurs through the cartilage. Although this statement cannot be accepted, in a very large proportion of cases the conjugal cartilage becomes detached from the diaphysis through its ossifying line and remains attached to the epiphysis ; and often small granules of bone of the diaphysis still adhere to the conjugal cartilage, though they are not large enough to constitute a fracture of the diaphysis.

Out of Dr. Jetter's seven cases in which the diagnosis was confirmed by operation three were pure separations and three connected with an oblique fracture through the diaphysis ; in one the condition could not be made out with accuracy on account of the formation of two sequestra of bone. From these cases, Dr. Jetter believes that pure separations are more frequent in the earlier

N

years of life; but he records one in a woman aged twenty-three years.

PURE SEPARATIONS WITH DISPLACEMENT. **Complete displacement forwards and inwards of the diaphysis.**—Esmarch (*Archiv für klin. Chirurg.* 1863, Bd. iv. S. 585; also Caspar Nissen, *De resectionibus*, Diss. Inaug. Kiliæ, 1859, iv. S. 8) describes the case of a boy aged fifteen, whose left arm was seriously injured by a threshing machine. There was a lacerated wound at the inner margin of the deltoid muscle, through which the upper end of the diaphysis protruded five centimetres in length, with a thin layer of bluish cartilage covering it. The separation had taken place through the epiphysial cartilage, and the muscles were found to be much lacerated. The diaphysis could only be reduced after resection of two centimetres of its end and division of some muscular fibres. The wound rapidly healed, with free movement of the joint and two centimetres shortening. The separation had probably taken place in the midst of the conjugal cartilage.

In three of Dr. Jetter's cases which were operated upon for deformity the displacement was complete; the epiphysis had entirely left the diaphysial end, and had united to the side of the diaphysis, with which it was in contact. In two of the cases the displacement was extreme. In Dr. C. McBurney's case, treated by open operation for irreducibility of complete displacement of the diaphysis from the epiphysis, the separation was found to be exactly at the junction of the epiphysis and the shaft.

R. W. Smith thought that complete displacement of the diaphysis off the epiphysis was of very rare occurrence, and could not occur without being compound.

Incomplete displacement forwards of diaphysis.—The diaphysis is more frequently displaced only half the width of its diameter off the epiphysis, but the distance may be more or less than this.

There are two museum specimens and several others verified during life in which this form of displacement occurred.

Packard alludes to a notable example of epiphysial disjunction in the Mütter Museum (Ashhurst's *Encyclopædia of Surgery*, vol. iv. p. 122), in which the lower fragment overlapped the upper inwardly and in close contact with it, while the latter was tilted by the action of the scapular muscles, so that a space was left—filled up, however, by callus—between the two fragments at the outer part of the fracture.

Another specimen in the Musée Dupuytren, No. 91, is figured by Malgaigne in his treatise on fractures (*Traité des Fractures et des Luxations*, 1855, vol. i. p. 72; Atlas, plate i. fig. 4; Champion, *Journ. Complément du Diction. des Sc. Méd.* Paris, 1818, vol. i. p. 318; *Bulletin de la Faculté de Médecine de Paris*, 1812, No. vi. p. 117). There was a complete separation of the epiphysial line, but at the outer side of the diaphysis there was a small splinter torn off which remained attached to the epiphysis. The diaphysis was displaced inwards, passing beyond the epiphysis for several millimetres, and the epiphysis was connected with the diaphysis only on the outer side. The periosteum in many places was torn from the diaphysis, especially on the inner side, and was hang-ing to the epiphysis. The synovial capsule was lacerated towards the front and inner side. It was taken from a boy aged eleven, who was injured by his arm being caught in the spokes of a wheel and his body thrown violently backwards. The end of the humerus could be felt through a deep and contused wound at the outer part of the axilla, and there was extensive lacera-tion of the skin of arm and forearm. Death occurred on the seventh day from exhaus-tion. A portion of the skin of the arm had become gangrenous. The separation had not been detected before death. The artery, nerves, and muscles were intact.

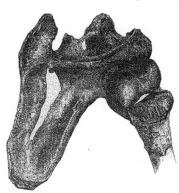

FIG. 34. CHAMPION'S SPECIMEN OF SEPARATION OF THE UPPER EPIPHYSIS OF THE HUMERUS (MALGAIGNE). ON THE OUTER SIDE A TAG OF PERIOSTEUM COVERS A SMALL SCALE, WHICH HAS BEEN DETACHED FROM THE DIAPHYSIS

In many cases which have now been operated upon for deformity, the epiphysis has been found placed upon and united to the outer aspect of the upper end of the diaphysis, which has not completely left the epiphysis.

The same displacement, although complete, occurred in H. E. Clark's case (*vide infra*).

Incomplete displacement backwards of the diaphysis is rarely met with. St. Bartholomew's Hospital Museum contains a specimen, No. 909 (*Catalogue of the Anato-mical and Pathological Museum of St. Bartholomew's Hospital*, vol. i. p. 132), in which the dia-physis is displaced backwards halfway off the epiphysis, the epiphysis retaining its normal position. The periosteum and part of the capsular ligament remain attached to the epiphysis on the inner and outer aspects. There is a rent in the periosteum on the posterior aspect through which the diaphysial end pro-jects. The diaphysis is not frac-tured, but a fracture extends through the body of the scapula

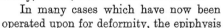

FIG. 35. INCOMPLETE DISPLACEMENT BACK-WARDS OF HUMERAL DIAPHYSIS (ST. BAR-THOLOMEW'S HOSPITAL MUSEUM)

and through the base of the coracoid process, indicating severe violence ; but unfortunately there is no history of this interesting specimen, excepting the statement that it was taken from a young person.

Thudichum, in his account of fractures occurring in the upper end of the humerus (*Ueber die am oberen Ende des Humerus vollkommenden Knochenbrüche*, Giessen, 1851) provides a description analogous to Malgaigne's preparation in a child four years old.

But in this case, from the figure given by Thudichum, it appears that the displacement is backwards. The preparation is in the Pathological Museum at Giessen, No. 35, 125 *a*. The capsule was torn in two places—at the inner side from the lesser tuberosity, and on the posterior aspect from the edge of the glenoid cavity of the scapula up to the greater tuberosity. The diaphysis projected backwards, and the periosteum was separated from it for a short distance. The capsular ligament was stretched and lengthened on the inner side.

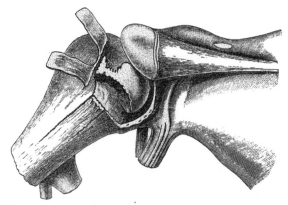

Fig. 36.—TRAUMATIC SEPARATION OF THE UPPER EPIPHYSIS OF THE HUMERUS. INCOMPLETE DISPLACEMENT BACKWARDS. (AFTER THUDICHUM, COPIED BY BRUNS, *Deutsche Chirurgie*, 1886, Cap. xi. S. 122)

The child from whom the specimen was taken had its left arm thrown violently and quickly upwards and in a lateral direction. It died from inflammation of the brain a few days later.

Dr. J. Ludw. Thudichum gives the following description ('Die Absprengung de Epiphysen,' *Illustr. med. Zeitschr.* 1855, Bd. iii. S. 188) and figures the same case. The child was three or four years of age. The separation was said to be complete through the epiphysial line, and was caused by the patient suddenly throwing its arm upwards and somewhat laterally. There was no displacement, on account of the ligamentous tissues about the tuberosities being intact; the periosteum, however, was partly separated from the diaphysis, and the capsular ligament torn in two places. Death resulted in a few days from other causes.

Complete displacement backwards.—A specimen of compound separation in which this form of displacement occurred has recently

(*St. Thomas's Hospital Reports*, N.S., vol. xxiv., 1895, p. 375) been placed in the museum of St. Thomas's Hospital. A boy aged 13 was run over by a van across the chest and sustained an anterior dislocation of the sternal end of the clavicle and a compound separation of the upper epiphysis of the left humerus, the bone protruding on the posterior aspect of the arm. The wound was cleaned, and through it the shaft and epiphysis were manipulated into position.

The periosteum was then stitched over the shaft to retain it in its normal axis. The joint apparently was not opened. Pneumothorax was present on the right side, and surgical emphysema appeared at the root of the neck in front and spread into the arms, neck, and abdomen. The wound in the arm suppurated, and although pus was evacuated from the chest, death took place on the sixteenth day. At the autopsy the pyo-pneumothorax on the right side was found to be due to a longitudinal rupture of the right bronchus. There were no fractured ribs.

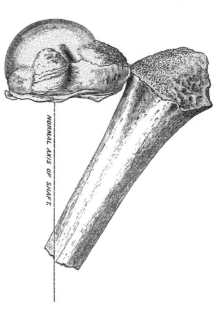

Fig. 37.—Pure separation of the upper epiphysis of the humerus with complete displacement backwards of the diaphysis (St. Thomas's Hospital Museum)

Complete displacement outwards of diaphysis.—Charles Williams describes (*Lancet*, July 15, 1865, vol. ii. p. 66) a case of compound separation in which the diaphysis was driven through the deltoid muscle. A farm boy, aged nineteen, was thrown from a cart-horse and fell with great force on to the right elbow, producing on the outer aspect of the right shoulder a transverse wound, through which the diaphysis protruded for one inch, penetrating the deltoid muscle. It was directed upwards, through the muscle above the level of the head of the bone; its upper surface was rough, and corresponded with the under surface of the epiphysial cartilage. Reduction was effected with ease after the removal of the prominent portion of the diaphysis. The diaphysis was drawn into the wound and placed under the epiphysis, which was still in contact with the glenoid cavity. The wound remained unhealed for a long time. Two years afterwards some necrosed bone was removed. Half a year later all the necrosed bone had come away. The shape and the rotundity of the shoulder were perfect and the union firm, so that the youth could move his arm in any direction, and had followed his occupation for some months. The case was under care for three years and seven months.

Malgaigne alludes to another compound case.

'Bichat says he has seen the lower fragment carried upwards with so much violence as to pierce the integuments and pass up much above the level of the head of the bone; and M. Guéretin has reported an instance in which the wound was caused by the lower fragment piercing through the deltoid and integuments. The patient was injured by the caving in of a gravel bank. The purulent discharge from this wound was enormous. Amputation was performed on the forty-ninth day, and death ensued on the sixty-third. It is remarkable that the amputation was intended to be and was supposed to have been done through the joint, but at the autopsy the head of the bone was found in place; its end was hollowed out to the depth of about one-third of an inch, and this concave surface had been mistaken for the glenoid cavity.'

In the case of compound epiphysial diastasis related by R. W. Knox (*Medical News*, Philadelphia, 1885, xlvii. p. 622) a lad, D. C., aged sixteen, received an injury whilst racing, his horse falling upon him. The shaft of the humerus protruded through the skin for one inch over the outer, or rather inferior, aspect of the deltoid muscle; and the end of the bone presented a transverse surface without spicules, comparatively smooth and devoid of cartilage. The head of the humerus could not be reached with the finger in the wound, but externally was felt to be *in situ*. Reduction was easily effected under chloroform, and an inside angular splint of zinc and shoulder-cap of felt moulded from the hand to the shoulder was applied. Rapid and complete recovery took place, and six months afterwards there was perfect movement and no appreciable difference in the size of the two arms.

A specimen of compound separation of the superior epiphysis of the humerus, with comminution of the diaphysis close to the line of the epiphysiary cartilage, was shown to the Pathological Society of Dublin by Dr. E. H. Bennett (*Proceedings of the Pathological Society of Dublin*, N.S. vol. vii. 1877, p. 220; *Dublin Journal of Med. Science*, 1877, vol. lxiii. p. 491). A powerfully built boy, aged about fifteen or sixteen years, was struck by the pole of a tramcar and knocked down, receiving, besides the injury to the humerus, an extensive fracture of the base of the skull and an impacted fracture of the shaft of the femur, from which he died in four or five hours' time. When the boy was admitted into Sir P. Dun's Hospital, the diaphysis was seen protruding for two inches through the skin on the outer side of the limb above the groove of insertion of the deltoid muscle, and the bone was entirely stripped of periosteum. On dividing the skin and deltoid muscle vertically the lower fragment could with some difficulty be replaced. On dissection a small part of the mammillated surface was present on the diaphysis, and the projecting points of the diaphysis in the centre and on the inside had been broken off, and were seen lying detached alike from the cartilage and diaphysis, except that a few shreds of periosteum still connected them to the cartilage. The periosteum, torn completely through on the outside, was stripped off the diaphysis down to the insertion of the deltoid, and even beyond this. It lay in shreds on the inner limit of the wound, and still retained its connections with the epiphysis undisturbed, the epiphysiary cartilage, as it were, preventing any detachment of it from the upper fragment.

The London Hospital Museum contains two specimens of this separation, No. 376 from a young adult, and No. 377 probably from a child four or five years old.

Juxta-epiphysial separation.—The separation, though a pure and complete one, may traverse the osseous material of the diaphysis, which directly adjoins the conjugal cartilage. A thin layer of the diaphysis in this manner remains adherent to the epiphysis. This is termed juxta-epiphysial separation by Ollier, and is probably a very frequent form of lesion, but it requires further confirmation by more specimens than those now recorded.

COMPLICATIONS.—*Separation with fracture of the epiphysis* can only result from severe direct violence.

In the London Hospital Museum, No. 372 (*Descriptive Catalogue of the Pathological Museum of the London Hospital*, 1890, p. 89), there is a specimen showing the epiphysis of the head torn off, and a vertical line of fracture separating the great tuberosity, the bicipital groove, and a portion of the lesser tuberosity from the head of the bone. The shaft of the bone has clearly been crushed, its upper end is wanting, and there are the marks of spikes on its surface. It is about two inches long, and the lower extremity is irregular, as if fractured.

Separation with fracture of the greater tuberosity.—Gurlt (*Lehre von den Knochenbrüchen*, II. Theil, S. 698, fig. 92) figures a specimen of fracture in the epiphysial line with fracture of the great tuberosity, which was separated from the head and shaft. The upper fragment was placed beneath the coracoid process, and was slightly hollowed out on the under side for the humeral shaft. It was taken from the body of a sailor aged seventeen, who had been thrown against the side of a ship and taken into Langenbeck's Klinik eight weeks after the injury. There was some projection of the acromion, and below the acromion there existed an arched projection, which could also be felt from the axilla, and was connected with the articulation. This projection became more prominent during abduction and movement of the arm backwards. The arm was slightly drawn backwards and abducted. The movements were very restricted, especially forwards. Ten days later an attempt at reduction was made by Schneider-Mennel's apparatus, and was followed by death from septicæmia (*Senftleben*, 1855).

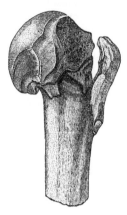

Fracture of diaphysis is a very frequent form of injury. The line of separation commonly deviates to some extent from the epiphysiary junction, and traverses somewhat obliquely the soft and friable osseous tissue of the diaphysis, so that the injury is partly a separation and partly a true fracture.

From the age of two or three years upwards a few osseous granules generally adhere to the epiphysial cartilage which has been detached, but these are not sufficiently large to constitute a fracture of the diaphysis.

The fragments detached from the diaphysis clinging to the epiphysis are often found to be small, but, on the other hand, large wedge-shaped splinters may be split off, as in P. Bruns's, Bennett's, Knox's, Champion's, and London Hospital cases.

Jetter thinks this combination of fracture and epiphysial fracture to be most frequent about the twentieth year.

The diaphysial fragments may be from the *outer side* as in Champion's case, or from the *inner side*. In one of Mr. Johnson Smith's cases (*loc. cit. infra*) the shaft of the humerus on the inner side was involved by a fracture of $2\frac{1}{2}$ inches in length ; in one of Bruns's cases by a fracture of the shaft on the outer side.

There was comminution of a portion of the diaphysis close to the epiphysial line on the inner side in Bennett's case.

Lange's case was accompanied by an oblique fracture of the diaphysis on the inner and posterior aspect, reaching for two inches below the epiphysial line.

Detachment of periosteum is one of the most important lesions. The periosteum, being loosely attached to the diaphysis and more strongly to the epiphysis, is always stripped off the diaphysial end to a greater or less extent, and has the appearance of a deep cup attached to the lower edge of the epiphysis, so that probably other muscles than those directly attached to the epiphysis—e.g. the lower fibres of the teres minor—will be detached with the periosteum and act upon this fragment. The periosteum is never stripped off from the epiphysis. In Foucher's specimen and many others it is clearly noted that the periosteum remained attached to the epiphysis, while it was extensively separated from the diaphysis. The extent of the detachment of the periosteum will vary, as a rule, with the intensity of the violence, and consequently with the amount of displacement of the diaphysis; as age advances and the periosteum becomes more adherent, the detachment will be less extensive.

The periosteal sleeve detached from the diaphysis may be five to ten centimetres in length.

Laceration and penetration of the deltoid at its anterior margin by the upper end of the diaphysis is of frequent occurrence where the displacement is considerable, but it will be found to a less extent in cases of incomplete displacement.

M. Rollet noted this lesion in three cases which had been operated upon. The author saw it also in one of Mr. Johnson Smith's cases.

The deltoid was lacerated in Pery's case.

This lesion will contribute very materially to the difficulty in reduction as well as, later on, to impaired functional activity of the limb; and, taken along with locking of the lower into the upper fragment, it forms one of the most urgent reasons for immediate operation.

Wounds.—Compound separation of the upper epiphysis of the humerus is a rare injury. P. Bruns, of Tübingen, collected four cases of compound separation.

In two out of seven cases of compound diaphysial separation of the upper end of the humerus, the wound was on the inner or front aspect of the shoulder to the inner side of the deltoid muscle; the other five were on the outer side penetrating this muscle. Two of the latter ended fatally. In the St. Thomas's Hospital specimen the end of the diaphysis projected on the posterior aspect of the arm.

Wound of axillary artery.—It is remarkable that the brachial plexus and other important nerves and vessels in the neighbourhood of the upper end of the humerus are not often injured.

One unique case is related by H. E. Clark (*Glasgow Medical Journal*, N.S. vol. xxvi. 1886, p. 206, plate, p. 210) of compound separation complicated with wound of the axillary artery. The wound of the soft parts was not very large, and there was very little laceration.

A boy, aged thirteen, had his arm caught in machinery, and was suddenly raised by the hand and arm with a jerk, the arm being drawn upwards and outwards. The injury was supposed to be a compound fracture of the humerus close to the head, the fragment protruding through the skin at the lower part of the axillary space. Although there was free hæmorrhage from the wound and the arm and hand were a little cold, with absence of pulsation in the radial artery, yet the colour of the skin was good and the fragment easily reduced under ether. Gangrene of the hand and wrist, however, set in on the fourth day, necessitating amputation at the shoulder-joint by Dupuytren's method and removal of the upper epiphysis, the operation being followed by good recovery. On dissection, the capsule of the shoulder-joint was found not torn at any part, and the tendon of the biceps still traversed the articular cavity; but that part of the capsule which extends below the anatomical neck was separated from the diaphysis along with the periosteum. The axillary artery was plugged above the line of amputation. The specimen is in the museum of the Glasgow Royal Infirmary.

Injury to shoulder-joint.—It is but seldom that this separation is complicated with any direct lesion of the shoulder-joint.

From the records of six cases Gurlt believed that laceration of the articular capsule was frequent.

The part of the capsular ligaments which extends below the line of the anatomical neck on the inner side is usually separated from the diaphysis with the periosteum, and so in the majority of cases escapes laceration.

Its proximity to the epiphysial junction should, however, make us guard against subsequent articular inflammation, and attempts at reduction of a supposed dislocation may soon be followed by symptoms indicative of articular lesion.

In Champion's case the synovial capsule was lacerated at the front and inner aspect.

Separation with displacement or dislocation of the epiphysial head. Although no specimen has been recorded of such a rare injury, the analogous accident in the adult has been frequently verified and its pathology studied. In most of those cases the lower fragment has been found lying on the outer side of the upper fragment, and more or less drawn upwards and outwards towards the glenoid cavity. For an excellent treatment of this subject Dr. Charles McBurney, and Dr. C. N. Dowd's article 'On Dislocation of the Humerus complicated by Fracture at or near the Surgical Neck, with a New Method of Reduction' (*Annals of Surgery*, 1894, April, p. 399), should be consulted. References will be found here to Oger's *Paris Thesis*, 1884, together with a list of published cases; and a very complete paper on this subject is given by Poirier and Mauclaire (*Revue de Chirurgie*, October 10, 1892). A satisfactory discussion of the subject is to be found in L. A. Stimson's *Treatise on Dislocation*.

At times the concomitant lesions are so extensive that death results in a few hours, as in Champion's case, where the child succumbed twenty-two hours after the accident.

Periostitis and necrosis of the suppurative kind are uncommon except in compound cases. They occurred in Foucher's case; an enormous abscess formed in the axilla, with commencing necrosis of the diaphysis, and terminated in death at the end of the sixth week from pyæmia.

In a case reported in 1878 by Esmarch (*Archiv für klin. Chirurg:* vol. xxi. 1878) a large abscess formed, and led to the removal of the epiphysis and a portion of the upper end of the shaft of the humerus; the injury had been mistaken for a dislocation of the shoulder, and two attempts had been made to reduce it. A useful limb was the result, for there was but little shortening and a free shoulder-joint.

Dr. Jetter relates a similar instance of secondary suppuration and necrosis of part of the epiphysis, as well as of the diaphysis, after separation. A boy (F. P.) aged seven years had fallen seven weeks previously from a tree about two metres high. There was great pain and swelling, but no wound. A sprain was diagnosed by a doctor, and leeches and ointment ordered. After eight days the father observed something projecting beneath the skin and took the child again to the doctor, who 'set' the arm and applied a stiff bandage. But three weeks later the father, perceiving pus soaking through the bandage, took it off and brought the child to the hospital on October 15, 1886. The boy was pale and thin, with diffuse swelling about the left shoulder, and a small granulating surface discharging thick pus situate between the acromion and coracoid process. The arm was shortened two centimetres ; the movements of the joint were free but painful. On October 19 a large sequestrum (one centimetre), showing the characteristic formation of the upper epiphysis of the humerus, was removed by means of forceps. The following day, under an anæsthetic, the movements of the joint were free, showing that consolidation had taken place. Suppuration was found to have extended down the inner side of the humerus. The abscess cavity was therefore scraped out, and a sequestrum of the upper part of the humerus removed about the size of a bean. By November 11 the functions of the arm were good, and the patient was discharged, the wound being nearly healed.

Compound separations not infrequently have been followed by septic wound infection, giving rise to profuse suppuration of the arm, secondary ostitis and periostitis from the stripping up of the periosteum and injury to the osseous tissue, and leading to more or less necrosis of the end of the diaphysis.

P. Bruns mentions (Langenbeck's *Archiv für klin. Chirurg.* Bd. xxvii. S. 240) the case of a boy aged nineteen who was thrown against a waggon-wheel by a falling weight. There was found a complete separation of the epiphysis, with only a few fragments of the diaphysis adhering to it, and the diaphysial end penetrated the skin and soft parts. Firm union took place, but with necrosis of the end of the diaphysis, which required, after the lapse of ten months, the removal of a sequestrum two centimetres in length involving the whole circumference of the bone.

Charing Cross Hospital Museum affords a similar example (specimen No. 37), and displays the epiphysis and upper part of the shaft of the humerus removed by Mr. Hancock from a lad who suffered separation of the upper epiphysis from accident, necrosis subsequently attacking the bone. The separation appears to have taken place completely through the epiphysial junction, although several necrosed plates of the inner and posterior aspects of the diaphysial end have been removed.

Necrosis also occurred in Charles Williams's case (*vide supra*).

Dr. G. Pery, of the Bordeaux Faculty of Medicine, has kindly furnished the author with an account of an interesting case published by him in 1861 ('Désépiphysation de l'extrémité supérieure de l'humérus,' *Union Méd. de la Gironde*, Bordeaux, 1861, tom. vi. pp. 49–51).

The separation was a compound one with displacement forwards of the diaphysial end of the humerus. Suppuration and sloughing of the wound ensued, and death took place on the sixth day. Paraplegia also complicated the case, being due to hæmorrhage into the spinal meninges.

Jean M., aged sixteen years, was admitted into the hospital November 3, 1860, under the care of M. Dupuy, having fallen from nearly the height of a second story. A doctor who saw him at the time replaced the end of the humerus, which protruded through the skin, but reduction was not completely effected. A temporary dressing was applied. The following day M. Dupuy noticed that the patient lay upon his back in a semi-unconscious condition. Paraplegia was present, with loss of power over the bladder and rectum. On the outer side of the shoulder, almost at the middle of the deltoid, there was an oblique wound four centimetres across, through which the index finger could feel the upper extremity of the lower fragment quite disconnected from the upper fragment. This extremity was unlike an ordinary fracture with its sharp projection, but, on the contrary, was rough in a uniform kind of way and somewhat rounded off. Separation of the upper epiphysis was diagnosed by M. Dupuy, and attempts were made to complete the reduction of the fragments, but without success.

Water dressings and a retentive apparatus were applied. Delirium followed, and on November 6 sloughing of the edges of the wound commenced with suppuration. On November 7 a counter opening was made at a dependent spot, letting out some fœtid pus, and a drain was inserted from one opening to the other. On November 9 the patient died in a comatose condition.

At the necropsy the thoracic organs and abdomen were found to be healthy, and there was no external lesion of the vertebral column. On opening the spinal canal small extravasations of blood were found on the inner aspect of the laminæ, and on the posterior aspect of the bodies of the vertebræ at the end of the dorsal and in the lumbar regions; but there was no appreciable alteration in the spinal cord. Beneath the skin of the right shoulder there was a collection of thick pus, and the deltoid was found to have been lacerated by the humeral diaphysis. The end of the diaphysis or lower fragment was rounded and but little roughened on the outer side, while on the inner side it was a little more so. The upper fragment, composed of the head and two tuberosities, was hollowed out corresponding to the end of the lower fragment. On the outer third of its surface the remains of the epiphysial cartilage were clearly to be seen. On the inner side, on the other hand, the thin compact layer which completes the diaphysial end above remained adherent to the epiphysial fragment. At the periphery there was some tearing away of the compact tissue, which dragged with it some small splinters of the diaphysis.

Gangrene of arm, from pressure on the axillary artery, occurred on the fourth day in Clark's case of compound separation, and in Hamilton's case.

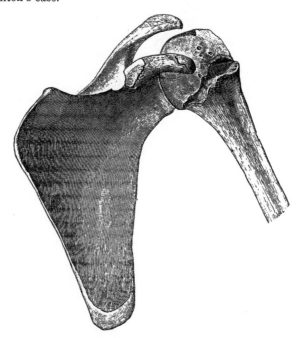

Fig. 39.—DIAGRAM OF SEPARATION OF THE UPPER EPIPHYSIS OF THE HUMERUS, WITH VERY LITTLE SPACE BETWEEN THE FRAGMENTS AND NO DISPLACEMENT

Ankylosis (osseous) is likely to occur in compound cases attended with suppuration, but no specimen has been recorded.

Separation without displacement may certainly occur, if we are to regard the numerous clinical examples recorded, but as yet it has not been anatomically verified.

SYMPTOMS.—Separation of the upper epiphysis of the humerus is not unfrequently met with, the mild form often occurring in private practice, whilst the more severe forms of displacement frequently come under the hospital surgeon's treatment.

Separation without displacement.—It is probable that the majority of the separations of the upper cartilaginous end of the humerus in early infancy are of this nature, while in older children detachment is undoubtedly common without any displacement of the diaphysis.

Pain and swelling are less marked than in separations accompanied by displacement. The pain is not severe on passive movement, yet the great loss of function of the shoulder is always a suspicious feature. The swelling about the shoulder comes on rapidly after the injury.

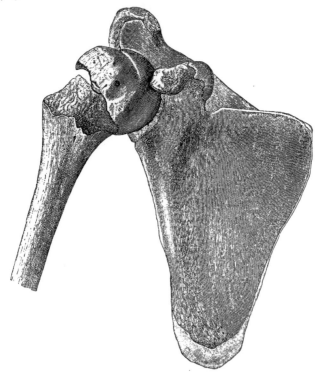

Fig. 40.—DIAGRAM OF SEPARATION OF THE UPPER EPIPHYSIS OF THE HUMERUS AT THE EIGHTEENTH YEAR. THERE IS A CONSIDERABLE GAP BETWEEN THE EPIPHYSIS AND THE DIAPHYSIS, WITHOUT ANY DISPLACEMENT FORWARDS OF THE LATTER. THE EPIPHYSIS HAS UNDERGONE SOME ROTATION IN THE GLENOID CAVITY

Deformity is absent; it will, in fact, often be thought that only a severe bruising or sprain at the shoulder-joint has occurred.

If traction, however, be made in the axis of the limb, and the swelling be not very great, a *slight depression* may be felt at the level of the junction cartilage, between the separated fragments.

Crepitus is of the usual peculiar soft or muffled character, for in these very simple cases in infancy displacement and fracture of the diaphysis are both absent. When present it is almost pathognomonic, and is produced by the rubbing of the two fragments one over the other.

Unnatural mobility will be very limited where no displacement exists. It may be produced in trying to obtain crepitus, and will be detected at the normal diaphysio-epiphysial line.

In effecting these movements, especially abduction, *a slight angle* is formed at the seat of separation.

In the following case there appeared to be little or no appreciable deformity at the time of injury. William McC., aged fourteen, came under the care of Mr. Durham at Guy's Hospital on March 28, 1885 (*Mr. Durham's Surgical Reports*, 1885, No. 312), having fallen 8½ feet off a gangway on to his left shoulder. There was much swelling and pain in the shoulder, but no deformity, the head occupying the glenoid cavity. Some antero-posterior movement of the humerus was permitted, with soft crepitus. Separation of the epiphysis with partial dislocation of the head was diagnosed later under chloroform. The treatment adopted was extension by weight on the arm and counter-extension by a jack-towel beneath the arms. After eighteen days there was good movement of the arm, and the boy was able to abduct it to a right angle from the trunk; there was, however, about one inch shortening.

Displacement of subsequent occurrence.—Should the nature of injury under these circumstances be overlooked at the time and the humerus be insufficiently supported, it is possible for the diaphysis to be subsequently displaced, the characteristic signs subsequently developing — viz. formation of slight hollow beneath acromion, projection forwards of diaphysial end, &c.

In the following case under the care of M. Davaine, recorded by Berges (*loc. cit. supra*), displacement occurred on the sixth day. In July 1889 a child, aged eight years, fell from a horse and complained of difficulty in moving its right shoulder. When examined almost immediately afterwards by a doctor, no sign of fracture or dislocation of the shoulder could be detected, and a diagnosis of simple contusion was made. The following day, as the patient still complained of pain on moving the arm, M. Davaine, after a careful examination, being unable to detect any sign of fracture or dislocation, and considering it to be a sprain, ordered the arm to be fixed in a sling. The patient was seen again by him on the following day without any new sign being noticed. The child, however, in spite of the sling, made frequent use of its arm, and on the sixth day M. Davaine found a projection (size of walnut) situated at the inner lip of the bicipital groove, about 2½ centimetres below the acromion; this, with its rounded upper border, might have been mistaken for the head of the humerus had not the latter been felt in the glenoid cavity. No ecchymosis, abnormal mobility, crepitus, or shortening on measurement was detected. M. Lannelongue then saw the case, and, making the diagnosis of traumatic separation of the upper epiphysis of the humerus, placed the arm in a plaster splint with continuous extension. On removing the splint on the twentieth day, the projection had totally disappeared, and the movements of the arm were normal. Only a slight wasting of the muscles due to the prolonged fixation was noticed, but this was soon remedied by the use of massage and electricity, and a month later the patient had completely recovered.

This displacement of the diaphysis occurring later when the patient is under treatment has also been noted by Jetter in three cases which had been under careful observation.

In none of them was there any displacement detected at the time of the accident. These three are recorded in another part of this chapter. The following is a fourth case.

M. N., eleven years old, fell from a first story four metres high on to the ground. Two days after (July 7, 1890) he came to the hospital. There was diffuse swelling and extensive contusion of the left shoulder. The humeral head was still in the glenoid cavity, and in the neighbourhood of the epiphysial line of the humerus abnormal mobility and marked crepitus were detected. Velpeau's bandage was applied. Ten days afterwards, on July 17, on changing the bandage, the diaphysis was found to project forwards and inwards. An anæsthetic was therefore given, and the fragments were replaced in their normal position by extending the arm and by pressure backwards on the lower fragment, but the deformity was reproduced as soon as the limb was let go. After reduction a second time, a plaster-of-Paris splint was applied to the trunk and arm, but even this allowed displacement two days later. The patient was finally treated for ten days by extension, lying upon his back with his arm elevated perpendicularly. After this, Velpeau's bandage was again applied, and on removing this eight days later the fragments were well united without much deformity, but the movements of the shoulder were restricted. After two years (March 20, 1892) there was to be seen on examination slight increase in the antero-posterior width of the shoulder, with slight displacement forward of the lower fragment. No measurable shortening or wasting of the arm supervened. All movements, especially elevation and rotation, were perfectly normal and painless.

Separation of the cartilaginous upper end of the humerus.—In infants separation will usually occur without any noticeable displacement of the fragments, and can only be recognised by abnormal mobility, soft crepitus, and swelling about the shoulder ; while loss of function and pain at the shoulder-joint are suggestive signs. The solution of continuity is somewhat further away from the head than when it occurs after the first few years of life, yet the dimensions of the epiphysis are now so small that the diagnosis is extremely difficult, especially when the displacement is not a marked feature.

The cases hitherto reported are too untrustworthy to throw any light upon the subject; yet fracture and dislocation are both so rare at this age that an epiphysial separation should always suggest itself.

Simple separation with displacement.—This is undoubtedly one of the commonest accidents of early life, and one frequently met with in the accident department of any large hospital; comparatively few cases, however, have been put on record. Sir Astley Cooper and other older writers speak of it as of common occurrence. It was also recognised by Sir Charles Bell, who says (*Institutes of Surgery*, 1838, vol. i. p. 110): 'I have known it occur from a boy firing a musket.'

Professor R. W. Smith, of Dublin, was the first to accurately describe it in 1847.

P. Bruns considers the injury as far from rare: out of fifteen cases of traumatic epiphysial separation which he had observed in the living subject, up to 1884, eight cases belonged to the upper epiphysis of the humerus.

Out of 105 cases verified by anatomical examination by Professor De Paoli, fourteen were of the upper end of the humerus.

The signs of simple divulsion of this epiphysis, owing to its anatomical relations, are comparable to those of fractures of the surgical neck of the humerus in so far as the displacements of the diaphysis are concerned, although they partake somewhat of the nature of a dislocation.

Sir Astley Cooper says: 'The signs of this accident are as follows:—the head of the bone remains in the glenoid cavity of the scapula, so that the shoulder is not sunken, as in dislocation; a projection of bone is perceived upon the point of the coracoid process, and when the elbow is raised and brought forwards this projection is rendered particularly conspicuous. By drawing down the arm the projection is removed, but it immediately re-appears upon giving up the extension, and the natural contour of the shoulder is lost. The diagnosis of this injury is not difficult, yet I have known the accident mistaken for dislocation. The point of the broken bone is felt at the coracoid process, and this is supposed to be the head of the os humeri; but with care the head of the bone can be felt still filling the glenoid cavity. When the elbow is rolled, the head of the bone does not obey its motion. Upon dissection of these cases in the young, the head of the humerus is found broken off at the tubercles, but it remains in the glenoid cavity.'

Incomplete displacement forwards of diaphysis. *Deformity.*—Considering that the solution of continuity always takes place in the same situation, it is not difficult to understand that the appearance of the shoulder should be so characteristic.

With so large a surface involved in epiphysial separation, and seeing that the upper end of the diaphysis is not a perfectly plane or transverse surface, but more or less pointed and fitting the concavity of the epiphysis as a kind of socket, it cannot be wondered that displacement is usually incomplete. In fact between separation without any appreciable displacement of the diaphysis, and separation where the latter almost penetrates the skin, many degrees of displacement are met with in practice. Moreover, the long heads of the biceps and triceps muscles will tend to keep the fragments in position.

The displacement forwards, or inwards and upwards, is no doubt kept up, if not caused in some degree, by the action of the coraco-

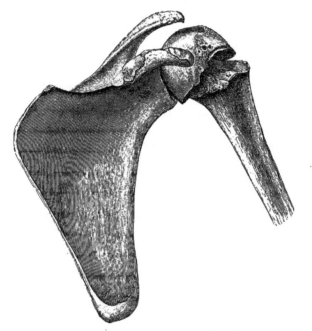

Fig. 41.—DIAGRAM OF SEPARATION, WITH LOCKING OF LOWER INTO UPPER FRAGMENT. THE HEAD OF THE BONE HAS UNDERGONE SOME ROTATION IN THE GLENOID CAVITY

brachialis, pectoralis major, teres major, and latissimus dorsi muscles which are attached to it.

The epiphysis will be directed a little outwards by the action of the subscapularis, supraspinatus, infraspinatus, and teres minor, which make the head of the bone perform a rotatory motion in the glenoid cavity, and tilt the lower end of the upper fragment upwards, so that its separated surface looks more or less outwards.

In fractures Boyer thought that these articular muscles, the supraspinatus, infraspinatus, and teres minor, elevated the fractured portion, because, the bone being thick, separation of the end must take place before displacement can occur.

If there is *great swelling* of the shoulder, axilla, or infraclavicular region, and much extravasation of blood into the subcutaneous tissue, it may be extremely difficult to determine with any exactness the nature of the injury.

Serous effusion into the articulation and into the subdeltoid bursa will also render the swelling more marked.

Mr. Hancock, describing separation of the upper epiphysis of the humerus in the *Provincial Medical Journal (Medical Times*, December 21, 1844, p. 249, and Braithwaite's *Retrospect of Med. and Surgery*, vol. xi. 1845, p. 247), and attempting to account for the signs of reproduction of the deformity, believed that in these accidents the long tendon of the biceps is either ruptured, or that by the fracture of the head of the humerus it is deprived of the fulcrum which it acquires in passing over that process, and is thus unable to antagonise the capsular muscles. The upper end of the bone is consequently drawn upwards and forwards by the supraspinatus and subscapularis muscles.

It is now certain that the diaphysis is mostly acted upon by the pectoral and other muscles described above, and that the scapular muscles, although powerfully acting upon the epiphysis, can have but little effect upon the lower portion of the bone. The tendon, moreover, of the biceps has never been found ruptured in this injury.

Professor E. M. Moore, of Rochester, U.S.A., in a paper read before the American Medical Association in 1874, and published in the *Transactions* for that year, has called attention to what he considers the true condition of the separated fragments in most of these cases, and to the proper remedy. He observes that the displacement is not usually complete, but that the upper end of the lower fragment is carried inwards to the distance of about onefourth of its diameter, when it is arrested by a convexity of the lower fragment becoming lodged in a natural concavity in the upper fragment. The smaller posterior facet of the superior diaphysial surface is locked with the larger corresponding anterior surface of the head. The upper fragment now becomes tilted by the action of the muscles attached to the tubercles, its internal margin ascending into the glenoid cavity, and its outer margin descending until it is arrested by the capsule.

If under these circumstances, as in reducing the fragments, the arm is carried forwards and upwards to the perpendicular line without extension, the upper fragment or epiphysis will remain fixed, being held fast by the capsule inserted into the posterior and under margin of the head, while the lower fragment or diaphysis, aided by the natural action of the muscles, will move outwards and resume its original position. The epiphysis will not participate in this movement, being fixed by the posterior part of the capsule, which is attached to it. The diaphysis slides back, producing a coaptation of the corresponding facet. See the figure in Agnew's

Surgery (1878, vol. i. p. 882, fig. 684), taken from Dr. Moore's paper.

Packard ('Artic. Fractures and Dislocations,' *Cyclopædia of Diseases of Children*, Keating, 1890, vol. iii. p. 1064) says: 'An important fact, pointed out by Mr. Jonathan Hutchinson and myself (*New York Medical Journal*, October 1866), is the rotation inward of the upper fragment by the action of the supraspinatus, infraspinatus, and subscapularis muscles, and this idea was again brought forward by Dr. Moore.'

The author is of opinion that the muscles lying parallel with the axis of the arm play an important *rôle* in carrying the lower fragment upwards until it is arrested by becoming fixed in the upper epiphysis, although the violence at the time of the accident is certainly the principal factor.

P. Bruns noted displacement upwards and inwards of the diaphysis in five out of eight cases which he observed in the living subject.

Jetter states that this displacement occurred in all of his seventeen cases, including recent and old cases. In four of the cases it was not present at the time of the accident, but it appeared later on.

The *prominence* which usually appears below the acromial end of the clavicle, to the outer side of and below the coracoid process, consisting of the upper end of the diaphysis, is not sharp, pointed, and irregular as in fracture through the surgical neck, but is smooth, more or less horizontal, transverse, or flat. Moving with every motion of the arm, when covered only by the skin and muscle, and feeling smooth or even slightly convex, it might be mistaken for the rounded head of the humerus; but it is less rounded than this, and in thin subjects the irregularities on the flattened surface may even be felt. It is quite unlike the end of a fractured bone. Frequently it is only the antero-internal edge of the diaphysial end that can be felt, but at other times a greater or smaller portion of the convexity of its upper surface may, as just stated, be perceived.

The situation of this projection has been noted by various writers as being beneath the deltoid, in front and below the acromion process, in front of the head of the bone beneath the joint, below the coracoid process, or forwards and upwards under the coracoid process.

It will vary according to the degree of displacement of the diaphysis, and in a small degree according to the age of the patient, or according to the presence or absence of the locked condition of the fragments which Professor Moore has so ably described from the cases seen by him. In some instances, therefore, it may be made to disappear by manipulating the arm in the manner he has indicated.

Moore says that the prominence is usually found about an inch and a half below the acromion and near the coracoid process. 'The curved line,' he says, 'from the acromion down to this projection has a long sweep, instead of the small sphere of the natural head. The appearance is pathognomonic, and may be safely trusted in diagnosis without insisting upon crepitus.'

Other observers give two' fingers' breadth below the clavicle in the neighbourhood of the coracoid process as the site of the projection, and others, again, one inch below the acromion in front of the shoulder.

Demoulin describes it in his case as a good two fingers' breadth below the acromio-coracoid interspace.

In Professor R. W. Smith's case it was found to be three-quarters of an inch below the coracoid process, and Hamilton states that in three of the cases reported by him the symptoms were present which are described by Professor Moore as characteristic of this form of injury. The projection was less marked and on a level with the coracoid process, or a little below it.

Packard says that in the few cases which he had seen the ridge has been less prominent than it is represented by Professor R. W. Smith in his work.

The truth of these observations is borne out if we look at the relationship of the epiphysial line to the coracoid process. It is almost on a level with it, and but little displacement of the shaft, with little rotation or descent of the epiphysis in the glenoid cavity, will be required to render it entirely so (see fig. 29).

Where the displacement inwards is greater, the diaphysial end will be felt below the coracoid process.

This projection of the diaphysial end follows all the movements imparted to the arm, which are effected with ease.

Professor R. W. Smith, in his work on *Fractures and Dislocations* (p. 199), clearly describes, and gives a figure of, this form of separation of the upper epiphysis of the humerus. He says, in his concise language: 'It is attended by a considerable degree of deformity, but of so striking a nature that there is no great difficulty in recognising the true nature of the injury. The axis of the arm is directed from above, within, and before, downwards, outwards, and backwards. The elbow, however, projects but little from the side, and can be brought into contact with it with facility. The head of the bone can be distinctly felt in the glenoid cavity; a slight depression is seen beneath it, and it remains motionless when the shaft of the humerus is rotated. The most remarkable feature, however, of this injury is a striking and abrupt projection, situated beneath the coracoid process, and caused by the upper extremity of the lower fragment or shaft of the bone, drawn inwards by the muscles which constitute the folds of the axilla. There is but little displacement as regards the length of the bone, for the extremity of the inferior fragment is seldom drawn so far inwards as to enable it to clear completely the surface of the superior.

'Were this to occur, the humerus would, of course, be drawn upwards by the muscles passing from the shoulder to the arm, in a direction parallel, or nearly so, to the axis of the humerus,.and a corresponding diminution in the length of the limb would result. This remarkable and abrupt projection does not present the sharp, irregular margin of an ordinary fracture; on the contrary, it feels rounded, and its superior surface is smooth and slightly convex. The latter can be felt as plainly as the cup-like cavity of the head of the radius in cases of luxation of that bone backwards at the elbow-joint. By pressing the upper end of the lower fragment outwards, and directing the elbow inwards, during extension and counter-extension, crepitus can be perceived and the deformity removed without much difficulty; but the moment the parts are abandoned to the uncontrolled action of the muscles the deformity recurs.'

The same author records (*Fractures and Dislocations*, p. 201) a characteristic and often-quoted case, of which he gives many details.

A boy, aged eight, was admitted into the Richmond Hospital under the care of Dr. MacDonnell. About a week previously he had fallen upon the shoulder, and at once lost the power of using the arm. There was no diminution of the natural rotundity of the shoulder, nor any unusual prominence of the acromion process. The head of the bone could be distinctly felt in the glenoid cavity, and it remained motionless when the arm was rotated; there was very little separation of the elbow from the side, but it was .directed slightly backwards. About three-quarters of an inch below the coracoid process there existed a remarkable and abrupt projection, manifestly formed by the upper extremity of the shaft, the upper surface of which was smooth and slightly convex, its margin having nothing of the sharpness which the edge of a recently broken bone presents in ordinary fractures. A crepitus was produced on replacing the fragments and rotating the shaft, the head of the humerus being fixed as far as it was possible to do so. The crepitus did not resemble the ordinary crepitus of fracture. All attempts to maintain the fragments in their proper relative position were in-effectual, although various mechanical contrivances were employed.

Mr. T. Holmes (*Surgical Treatment of Children's Diseases*, 1886, p. 249, fig. 39) figures a case in which all the features corresponded most accurately with those of Dr. Smith's, but he did not see it till eight weeks after the accident. The boy, aged fifteen, was then rapidly recovering useful motion in the joint.

In the museum of the Middlesex Hospital, No. 93, series xliii. (*Descriptive Catalogue of the Pathological Museum of the Middlesex Hospital*, 1884, p. 293), there is a cast of a shoulder showing this separation in a child; and Mr. Bryant also gives a representation of this injury (*Practice of Surgery*, vol. ii. 1884, 4th edition, p. 420, fig. 483) in a boy aged sixteen, who was under his care in Guy's Hospital in 1872. The end of the diaphysis of the right humerus was displaced forwards and inwards, and projected beneath the skin in front of the acromion as a rounded, slightly convex, prominence. The lad was carrying a box of fish (1 cwt.) on his head when he slipped and fell with the load on his shoulder. The head of the bone was in position, and on reducing the diaphysis backwards soft crepitus was both heard and felt.

On July 17, 1884, the author saw in consultation a boy (C.), aged fourteen years, with almost precisely the same symptoms. About $1\frac{3}{4}$ hours previously he had fallen from a tree a distance of fourteen feet to the ground; a branch, however, was said to have 'broken his fall.' The doctor said when he first saw the boy that the end of the bone was almost through the skin in front, but he was able to readily reduce it by pushing the shaft backwards. It went back with a 'jump,' so as to suggest to his mind a dislocation, yet the deformity had at once recurred to a slight extent. When the patient arrived the arm projected a little backwards and outwards, the elbow being only a short distance from the side. Three-quarters of an inch below the coracoid process there was considerable bruising and the characteristic angular projection of the diaphysis. This was accompanied by slight depression on the outer aspect of the shoulder about the middle of the deltoid. There was no shortening of the limb, which hung powerless. The head of the bone was felt in the glenoid cavity, and did not follow the movements of the shaft when this was rotated. The deformity was again readily reduced, being accompanied by a 'dummy' crepitus and a peculiar sensation as of the gliding of two more or less flattened surfaces one upon the other. The depression on the outer side immediately disappeared. The arm was kept to the side and wooden splints applied. In spite of the greatest care in endeavouring to keep the bone in its place, slight deformity remained in front at the end of a month. All the movements of the arm were very good, and there was firm union without shortening.

The depression here mentioned on the outer or postero-lateral aspect of the shoulder is situate below the head and tuberosities at the level of the epiphysial line. This, between the ages of sixteen and eighteen, is from one inch to an inch and a quarter below the acromion process, not quite down to the middle of the deltoid muscle. The distance will of course vary with the size of the patient.

The depression is often to be noticed still higher up, about half an inch below the acromion in cases of greater displacement; its presence may be accounted for by the rotation of the epiphysis in the joint, so that it takes an oblique or even perpendicular position, its separated surface looking more or less outwards, and its outer end being raised.

In other instances, the diaphysis being displaced forwards and inwards for less than half the extent of its upper end, the epiphysis with its cup-shaped hollow fits upon the outer part of the diaphysial end. The epiphysis is often rotated so that its inner edge passes upwards and its other end downwards.

Bergés quotes a case from M. Nimier's Thesis (Bergés, *De la disjonction traumatique de l'extrémité supérieure de l'humérus*, Thèse de Paris, 1890, p. 33 ; Nimier, Thèse, 1879), in which there was only a slight projection (of half a centimetre) of the anterior border of the lower fragment, and accompanied behind with a slight depression, indicating very little displacement of the diaphysis. The case was that of a child, aged nine years, which had fallen on to its left shoulder, fracturing the humerus above the insertion of the pectoralis major muscle. Reduction of the diaphysis was readily effected by manipulation and maintained by a simple bandage fixed against the trunk. Gentle movements by elevating the arm could be carried out on the fifteenth day.

H. E. Clark (*Glasgow Medical Journal*, N.S. vol. xxvi. 1886, p. 247) relates a case of separation with very little displacement inwards of the diaphysis. A boy aged fifteen slipped on a piece of orange-peel and fell on the pavement. On examination there was found extensive bruising of the shoulder, and when the head of the bone was fixed and the shaft moved in an angular direction the epiphysis was stationary, but if the shaft was rotated on its own axis *the epiphysis moved with the diaphysis*. A poroplastic splint was applied, and the patient did well.

Moscati diagnosed (*Mémoires de l'Académie Royale de Chirurgie*, tom. iv. 1768, p. 618 ; obs. 1, 1739) a case of separation of the upper epiphysis of the humerus in a girl aged nine years, who had fallen a short distance on to the upper part of her right arm, and had immediately lost all power of using it. The pain was very slight, but above the middle of the deltoid muscle there was an appreciable depression, and the head of the humerus had not left the glenoid cavity. Although there was but little abnormal mobility in all directions and no crepitus, a gliding movement was detected on moving the shaft. Perfect recovery ensued in a month and a half. The patient had been rachitic up to seven years of age.

A case of disjunction of this epiphysis is related by Dr. H. R. Wharton (*Med. and Surg. Reporter*, Phila. 1886, liv. p. 385), with slight projection in front and below the acromion process. The boy, who was aged twelve, fell off a waggon on to his left shoulder. There was slight flattening of the shoulder, and the arm rested against the side of the body. The head of the bone appeared to be slightly behind and below its normal position with reference to the shaft. Fergusson's dressing—roller bandage from tip of fingers to shoulder, and moulded pasteboard splint padded with cotton—was applied.

Bardenheuer has observed (*Deutsche Chirurgie*, 'Die Krank-heiten der oberen Extremitäten,' 1886, 1 Theil, S. 175) five cases of undoubted epiphysial separation of the upper end of the humerus, in all of which there existed a certain amount of angular displacement, and which could only be recognised by strongly abducting the elbow. In each there was the characteristic angular projection of the fragment forwards and inwards. Bardenheuer gives a figure of one such case.

The general aspect of the shoulder, apart from the deformity of the displaced diaphysis, is not materially altered. There is, in most cases, no loss of its natural roundness and smooth contour, but in others a slight flattening, or rather depression, may be seen on the affected side, never so distinct as in a dislocation. But its antero-posterior diameter is increased.

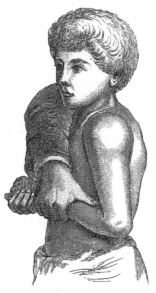

FIG. 42.—INCOMPLETE DISPLACEMENT FORWARDS OF DIAPHYSIS OF HUMERUS (AFTER BARDENHEUER)

Prof. Helferich depicts (*Atlas der traumatischen Fracturen und Luxationen*, 1895, tab. 28, fig. 2) the postero-lateral aspect of the shoulder of a boy aged fourteen years, in which the displaced diaphysis is well portrayed in this position. The displacement and characteristic angular projection of the diaphysis could, however, be best seen when the shoulder was viewed from above.

As we have seen in the preceding examples, the *arm hangs against the side of the body* in a helpless manner—all voluntary movements being nearly impossible, although there may be little or no displacement of the fragments. But it is more or less away from the side, the elbow being drawn slightly away therefrom in the abducted position, or at times projecting backwards and outwards when, as in many of the above cases, displacement is present in any degree.

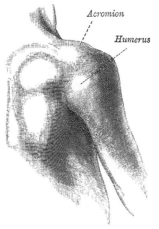

Acromion

Humerus

FIG. 43.—DISPLACEMENT OF THE DIAPHYSIAL END OF HUMERUS SEEN FROM THE POSTERO-LATERAL ASPECT (AFTER HELFERICH)

(The prominence of the humerus behind has been exaggerated by the artist)

The arm can be brought close to the side with ease, and other passive movements are tolerably free, although painful.

Moore says: ' The ability to convey the arm upwards and forwards, as well as upwards and outwards, is impossible much beyond a right angle with the body.'

Pain and swelling are often great. The swelling often extends over the whole of the shoulder and upper third of the arm, and takes place with great rapidity after the injury; it is always greater than in separation without displacement, and is due to the effusion into and swelling of the periosteum, as well as to the direct injury to the soft structures.

The presence of painful areas below the tuberosities is oftentimes very noticeable on pressure, and forms an essentially distinguishing sign from dislocation. Pain at the conjugal line is also experienced when pressure or a gentle blow is made from beneath the elbow upwards towards the acromial arch.

Increase of breadth of shoulder. Antero-posterior increase is seen when the shoulder is viewed laterally.

Mobility at about the epiphysial level may usually be recognised by grasping the epiphysial head and rotating the diaphysis; it is not great in amount and is absent when the fragments are locked together. Mr. H. E. Clark says in his case (*loc. cit. supra*): 'The head of the bone being grasped with the fingers of one hand, and the elbow with those of the other, and the shaft being made to move, it was found that if the movements were angular in their character, the epiphysis was quite stationary, showing how complete was the solution of continuity. If, however, the movement consisted in rotation of the humerus on its own axis, *the epiphysis moved with the diaphysis.*'

The *head of the bone* is always to be felt occupying its proper socket, even although, with the tuberosities, it may have undergone some rotation. We have also seen that it may or may not (*e.g.* without or with impaction of the shaft) rotate with the movements imparted to it. If the arm is gently moved without the head being grasped, it will rotate where there is the slightest degree of locking of the fragments. When, however, the displacement is more complete, the head of the bone will not obey the movements of the diaphysis when the arm is rotated.

The former fact, taken with the circumstance that dislocations are among the rarest of accidents in young subjects, renders it certain that the case recorded by Sir Astley Cooper (*Treatise on Fractures and Dislocations*, London, edited by Bransby Cooper, 1842, p. 431, and *Guy's Hospital Reports* No. ix.) belongs to this class of injury. A child, aged ten, was admitted into Guy's Hospital, having fallen upon the shoulder a distance of eight feet into a sawpit. There was inability to move the arm from the side and to support it without great pain. When the head of the bone, which still occupied the glenoid cavity, was fixed, the fractured end of the bone could be tilted and felt, and even seen, under the deltoid, by raising the arm at the elbow, but on rotation of the arm the head did not move. Crepitus was felt in raising the humerus and pushing it laterally outwards.

Crepitus.—The modified crepitus—which is usually described as 'muffled,' 'mortary,' 'feeble,' 'soft'—at any rate is much softer and less distinct than that which is met with in ordinary fractures, and must not be sought for too strictly without the use of an anæsthetic.

In many cases of incomplete displacement definite crepitus has been found difficult to obtain, for in certain cases on rotating the humerus the epiphysis will rotate with the shaft, the rounded diaphysis being locked in its concavity in the manner described above. The arm may even be bent somewhat towards the back of the trunk without crepitus being felt in these cases of impaction. In non-impacted instances, the head of the bone remaining without any movement during the manipulation of the shaft (especially if this is more of an angular than a rotatory character), crepitus will be elicited.

Crepitus may be absent also in the less frequent instances of complete displacement of the diaphysis from the epiphysis.

In Dr. C. McBurney's case, crepitus, it is especially noticed, did not exist on account of the displacement upwards and forwards of the diaphysis in front of the epiphysis—its rough end being felt just beneath the skin.

It can usually be felt in the different manipulations, such as pressing the upper end of the shaft backwards, drawing the arm inwards across the chest and at the same time extending it, which are necessary to effect reduction, thereby causing the two separated surfaces to pass in contact one over the other, or by fixing the head, rotating the humerus, and carrying the elbow inwards.

Crepitus was present in eight out of the eleven cases recorded by Bruns.

Dull crepitus was a notable sign in Wharton's, Moscati's, R. W. Smith's, Paletta's, Middeldorpf's (two cases), Hamilton's, and many other examples.

Mr. Le Gros Clark gives (*St. Thomas's Hospital Reports*, new series, vol. xvii. 1887, p. 2) the following note of a case in which crepitus was well marked :

'A lad, aged sixteen, was admitted into the hospital in consequence of a fall down a flight of steps, whereby his head, shoulder, and side were contused. The shoulder was swollen, and the deformity was thereby masked. Crepitus of a muffled character was elicited most readily by moving the arm backwards and forwards, especially when the hand was pressed up into the axilla ; the pain was referred to the front of the joint. When the swelling had subsided a large pad was placed in the axilla, and the shoulder was covered with a pasteboard cap. The boy soon recovered the use of the arm, and was dismissed at the end of the month.'

Jetter attributes the imperfectly marked crepitus as well as the small extent of the abnormal mobility to a partial preservation of the periosteum, and quotes the two following cases as instances.

CASE I. B. S., aged six years, on February 5, 1891, fell down ten steps of a stair. The following day she was brought to the hospital. The shoulder and upper half of right arm were greatly swollen, with tenderness on pressure. The arm appeared to be shortened. Under an anæsthetic there was abnormal mobility and soft-friction-crepitus at the epiphysial line during flexion, while the tuberosities of the humerus were fixed. During rotation the head in some degree accompanied the movements of the humerus, which was probably accounted for by a partial preservation of the periosteum. Velpeau's bandage was applied. By February 24 there was no swelling of the arm, but a slight angular projection of fragments could be felt at the epiphysial line; the arm was shortened by about one centimetre, and the head of the humerus rotated with the shaft. On March 4 electricity showed a partial degeneration of the deltoid muscle, the result presumably of contusion of the circumflex nerve at the time of the accident. The patient gradually regained the power in the deltoid, and could make active use of the arm for playing, eating, &c.

CASE II. H. K., sixteen years old, on August 16, 1891, was struck on the left shoulder by a falling empty cask, and came immediately to the hospital. Passive but not active movements were possible at the shoulder joint. At the epiphysial line there was some abnormal mobility without distinct crepitus; from this it was concluded that the periosteum, at all events on the outer side, was still intact. Velpeau's bandage was applied. On August 26 there was no effusion into the joint, and movement was good. Fragments united in very good position. On March 31, 1892, there was no wasting of the arm or appreciable shortening, and no deformity could be seen or felt. All movements, especially elevation and rotation of the arm, were normal, so that the patient was again perfectly fit for work.

Shortening.—Shortening, or loss of length of the arm, is generally absent in any marked degree in incomplete displacements, being not more than one to two centimetres. This means that there is but little tilting or overlapping of the fragments, that the periosteum is untorn, and the biceps tendon intact.

R. Dale (*Epitome of Surgery*, 1889, p. 65) and others say that there is neither shortening nor lengthening of the limb, but at the same time state that displacement readily recurs; but this cannot be very great in the cases to which they allude, in which there is this absence of shortening.

The following case of separation is reported by Hamilton (*Treatise on Fractures and Dislocations*, 7th edition, 1884, p. 260), which he had seen two weeks after the accident. There was then ½ inch shortening, the lower fragment projecting in front still ununited. The patient (Samuel R.), aged thirteen, fell through a hatchway, striking his shoulder. At the time the injury was diagnosed as a dislocation, and an attempt had been made to reduce it under chloroform. The result of this case was not known to Hamilton.

C. Puzey reported (*Liverpool Medico-Chirurgical Journal*, vol. v. 1885, p. 45) a case of separation with impaction, or rather locking, of the shaft into the concave under-surface of the epiphysis. Anthony B., aged twelve, was admitted into the Northern Hospital October 30, 1882, having some hours before fallen on his left elbow. The shoulder was swollen, especially anteriorly, with well-marked bony prominence 1½ inches below the acromio-clavicular joint, and at one point the skin was caught by a small spiculum of bone. Great pain resulted on movement. Under an anæsthetic the arm could be brought to the side and over the chest. The head of the humerus was in the glenoid cavity, and followed the movements of rotation made at the elbow, but these were accompanied by a rough sensation or click. The bony prominence, which appeared quite smooth, followed the movements of rotation, and the finger could be placed on its upper surface as on a ledge. There was ¾ inch shortening of the arm. The deformity failed to be reduced, so the arm was fixed to the side, and at the end of four weeks movements were commenced. At the end of two months there was perfect movement of the arm, the osseous projection rounding off, but with the same amount of shortening, viz. ¾ inch.

Moore describes the shortening of the humerus in these cases as 'from half to three-fourths of an inch.'

Professor Kocher (*Beiträge zur Kenntniss einiger practisch-wichtiger Fracturformen*, Basel und Leipzig, 1896) describes in detail and gives representations of seven cases of fracture about or through the epiphysial line (pertubercular fracture). In some the diaphysis had completely cleared the upper fragment, but in most it was incompletely displaced forwards and inwards, in one only forwards. The ages were in the case of the boys 18, 17 (two), 16, 10 years, in two girls 14½ and 12 years. Operation was subsequently performed in two of the cases for loss of function of the arms—a partial resection in one and a complete resection of the diaphysis in the other.

Effusion into shoulder-joint.—Effusion into the articular cavity has been noted in a few instances, coming on a few hours after the injury, but it is a noteworthy fact that in a large number of cases no evidence of synovial lesion has been present.

Although the synovial membrane extends below the upper end of the diaphysis on the inner aspect, immunity from injury of the articulation may be explained by the displacement forwards of the diaphysis (the most common form of injury), leaving the synovial membrane intact on the inner side, while lacerating the periosteum in front.

The following case of marked effusion into the joint is noted by Dr. Jetter.

F. B., aged fifteen, on May 24, 1882, fell upon the left shoulder in a gymnasium, and suffered immediate loss of power and movement of the arm. When seen the next day there was diffuse swelling of the whole shoulder and marked effusion into the joint. The head of the humerus remained in the articular cavity. Active movements were impossible, and passive movements painful, and these, when forcible, produced smooth crepitus. The end of the diaphysis was displaced forwards and inwards. After reduction, Leiter's coils were applied to the shoulder, then Velpeau's bandage. By June 3 the swelling had considerably diminished, and by June 7 the effusion into the shoulder-joint was very much less. The slight displacement forwards of the upper end of the bone was now very distinctly seen, and the epiphysis moved with it. On July 10 the patient left the hospital, and there was no subsequent shortening or loss of power in the arm, the patient being declared fit for military service.

Incomplete displacement, outwards.—Edmund Owen's case, already mentioned, was caused by indirect violence.

Incomplete displacement, backwards.—Although such displacement is probably not uncommon, the author is only able to record two instances. The specimen in the St. Bartholomew's Hospital Museum, and that figured by Thudichum, have both been referred to above; according to Küstner, the diaphysis in newly born children may be displaced backwards, as in a post-glenoid dislocation.

Complete displacement of diaphysis, forwards and inwards.—Several cases of complete displacement forwards of the diaphysis have been placed on record, but these are less frequent than the incomplete cases we have just discussed. Complete displacement was present in seven of the eight cases of compound separation described above, but it must be noted that in several instances the displacement was more forwards and outwards; in one only was it forwards and inwards. In these rare instances the epiphysis, being perfectly free from the diaphysis, will be very powerfully acted upon by the muscles attached to it, so that its separated surface will look more or less directly outwards. The diaphysis acted upon by the pectoralis major, latissimus dorsi, and teres major muscles is drawn upwards and inwards towards the coracoid process. Sometimes the smooth end of the diaphysis may be felt in the axilla.

Hamilton inclined to the belief that complete displacement was the more common form of separation, while R. W. Smith says : ' So great a degree of displacement as to enable the lower fragment to clear the under surface of the superior fragment must indeed necessarily be of very rare occurrence, and could scarcely happen without rendering the fracture compound.'

On abducting the arm, the convex end of the diaphysis can be felt in the axilla. The anterior diameter of the shoulder is increased, and the elbow can be brought to the side.

Numbness of the fingers may occasionally occur, as in the two instances recorded by Middeldorpf.

The characteristic displacement forwards and inwards of the diaphysis is also well shown in a case figured by Bruns (*Deutsche Chirurgie*, 1886, S. 126) in a girl aged fifteen years.

Complete displacement forwards above coracoid process.—The lower fragment, of an irregular transverse shape, will be situated immediately beneath the skin, and might be mistaken for the head of the bone.

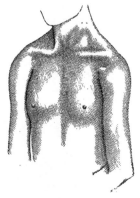

Hamilton gives (*Treatise on Fractures and Dislocations*, 7th edition, 1884, p. 261) the three following cases, which were probably examples of complete displacement, in which the upper end of the lower fragment was above the level of the coracoid process, and seemed to be directly beneath the skin.

FIG. 44.—SEPARATION OF UPPER EPIPHYSIS OF THE HUMERUS. COMPLETE DISPLACEMENT INWARDS OF DIAPHYSIS. (AFTER BRUNS)

CASE I. C. H., aged nineteen, in the delirium caused by fever, fell from a third-story window. Two physicians who were called in thought there was a fracture of the acromion process, accompanied by a dislocation of the head of the humerus, and they attempted to reduce it, but without success. Three weeks afterwards, Hamilton found a separation of the upper epiphysis of the humerus, and the upper end of the shaft projecting in front of the acromion process, a little above the level of the process and covered only by the skin. No union had occurred between the two fragments.

CASE II. John D., aged eighteen, fell about eight feet. The injury at first was believed to be a dislocation or fracture, and, the patient being placed under the influence of ether, attempts were made to reduce the deformity. The end of the bone seemed just under the skin, and almost ready to be thrust through, but the extension made it retire somewhat. Hamilton diagnosed a separation, although the shoulder was a good deal swollen. The upper end of the lower fragment could be felt distinctly—rough and serrated in front of the acromion process. On extension he was able to detect a slight crepitus or click, and on employing Dugas's test the elbow rested upon the front of the chest. One long splint was applied with a

sling under the wrist, but not under the elbow.   The fragments
united with very little deformity.   The diagnosis was confirmed by
Dr. Moore.

CASE III.   William H., aged nineteen, fell on a side-walk and
fractured the humerus at its upper epiphysis.   On the third day the
fragments were thought to have been reduced, and the limb was
secured in splints.   Subsequent attempts at reduction by Moore's
method under ether were unsuccessful.   The displacement was
complete, and the entire upper end of the lower fragment could be
distinctly felt.

Agnew (*Surgery*, Philadelphia, vol. i. p. 882) speaks of the
presence of a prominence immediately *above* the coracoid process

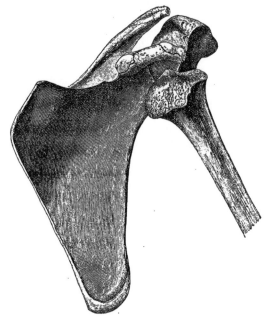

FIG. 45.—DIAGRAM OF COMPLETE DISPLACEMENT INWARDS OF DIAPHYSIS BENEATH
CORACOID PROCESS

of the scapula, with loss of power in the limb (the arm hanging
helpless by the side) as the signs which indicate the existence of this
fracture.   In Dr. C. McBurney's case the displacement was probably
of this description, the shaft being displaced upwards and forwards
in front of the epiphysis.

Complete displacement forwards below coracoid process is a more
common form of injury.

The upper end of the diaphysis is drawn upwards and inwards
just beneath the coracoid process.   In fact, this infra-coracoid projection is almost pathognomonic of the injury.   In this case, the

diaphysis having completely cleared the epiphysis, and lying on its inner side, the latter will be powerfully acted upon and rotated by the three muscles attached to it, so that its separated surface will look directly outwards instead of downwards. The rounded or slightly convex end of the bone can be readily felt with the fingers— in fact, in lean subjects nearly the whole of the epiphysial aspect of the diaphysis may be recognised by the characteristic cone-shaped projection at its middle—the sharp rim of bone, with the central elevated portion sloping off to the sides. The axis of the upper extremity is directed downwards, outwards, and backwards. Abduction of the arm will increase the deformity, while adduction with extension will render it less marked.

It is quite possible in thin subjects in which complete displacement has taken place, that on the lower aspect of the epiphysis a cavity may be felt in which the finger may be placed for nearly 1½ inches through the deltoid.

Mr. Bryant figures a case of complete displacement forwards of the diaphysis, projecting below the coracoid process, in a male patient aged sixteen years.

The slight hollow below the acromial arch is at times less marked than in incomplete displacement, on account of the rotation of the epiphysis in an opposite direction to that just alluded to. Its separated surface under these circumstances looks obliquely or perpendicularly inwards, and is in contact with the outer aspect of the diaphysis, as in Bruns's case.

The epiphysis, being fixed by the rotators of the arm, will not readily follow the movements of the diaphysis, unless it be held to it by the tough periosteum ; but even then it will only be movable to a small extent.

The diaphysis is held in its displaced position by the periosteum, as well as by the powerful muscles attached to its upper end.

Sir Astley Cooper, in alluding to the symptoms of this injury, says that the head of the bone remains in its place, but that the body of the humerus sinks into the axilla (where its extremity can be felt), and draws down the deltoid muscle, so as to lessen the roundness of the shoulder.

C. Puzey's case (*Liverpool Medico-Chirurgical Journal*, vol. v. 1885, p. 46) was probably an example of this form of displacement.

Thos. S., aged five, a delicate, unhealthy-looking child with eczema of the scalp and inflamed eyelids, had been run over by a light spring cart. Under chloroform the right shoulder was found to be much swollen, and the elbow away from the side, the smooth and rounded upper end of the humerus lying in the axilla. There was one inch shortening of the arm. Beneath the acromion the head and tuberosities of the humerus could be felt and moved. On fixing this fragment and rotating and drawing forwards the shaft, soft crepitus was noticed. When the arm was let go, the upper end of

P

the shaft rolled back into the axilla, and projected under the coracoid process. Suitable bandages were applied with a pad in the axilla. At the end of four weeks there was considerable osseous thickening but a good position of the fragments; and by the end of four months there was perfect use of the shoulder-joint and a good arm, with but little bowing forwards and inwards of the bone at the epiphysial junction, and no shortening.

One of the most marked cases of complete displacement of the diaphysis forwards seen by the present writer was the case of E. B., whom he had the opportunity of carefully examining when he was Surgical Registrar at Guy's Hospital. The girl, aged sixteen, was admitted under the care of Mr. Davies-Colley (Mr. Davies-Colley's *Surgical Reports*, 1884, No. 319), having been thrown out of a waggonette, one of the other people in the carriage falling on the top of her shoulder and the feet of a third person coming into direct contact with her shoulder. It was thought to be a dislocation of the shoulder; the following measurements, however, were obtained, notwithstanding the considerable swelling of the right shoulder, which measured $2\frac{1}{2}$ inches more in circumference than the left. The angular projection of the end of the diaphysis could be seen in front, and it was possible to place the tips of the fingers upon this transverse mass of bone, which was situated $1\frac{3}{8}$ inch below the coracoid process, and more than two inches below the acromial end of the clavicle. There was one inch and a quarter shortening from the external epicondyle of the humerus to the acromion process. The head was felt to be occupying the glenoid cavity, and the elbow was away from the trunk and pointed backwards and outwards. The diagnosis was fully confirmed under ether, and the diaphysis was easily replaced in its normal position by means of extension and manipulation. A guttapercha splint was afterwards moulded to the shoulder, but six days later the diaphysis was found to be again displaced. This was again reduced, and extension applied to the arm by weights with counter-extension. After twenty-one days the patient was discharged from the hospital with the limb in good position and the upper epiphysis firmly attach+d to the shaft.

Bergés quotes a like case from Nimier's Thesis (Bergés, ' *De la disjonction traumatique de l'extrémité supérieure de l'humérus*,' Thèse de Paris, 1890, p. 33; Nimier, Thèse, 1879), in which a child fell from a cart over four feet high. The upper end of the lower fragment, with its rounded outline, and its forward, inward, and slightly upward displacement, very like the displaced head of the humerus, pushed up the anterior wall of the axilla, below the coracoid process. However, the humeral head remained in position, for it could be felt below the coraco-acromial arch. The examining fingers could in the axilla easily feel the projection of the displaced end of the lower fragment and another behind belonging to the head in its proper position. Extension was employed, but the displacement was reproduced through the restlessness of the patient. Ultimately, firm union took place, with free and painless performance of motion.

Kirmisson relates (*Leçons cliniques sur les maladies de l'appareil locomoteur*, Paris, 1890) a good case of separation of the upper epiphysis of the humerus, with complete displacement of the diaphysial end to the inner side of the coracoid. Reduction was very easily effected, and perfect recovery took place, both in the natural contour and function of the arm and shoulder. Mayor's sling was the only apparatus employed.

Complete displacement, outwards and upwards.—The incomplete form of displacement furnishes the most frequent examples, but it has been met with in more complete form, especially in compound separations.

Shortening in both these forms is considerably greater than in the incomplete displacements; Moore says from half to three-quarters of an inch.

COMPLICATIONS.—*Injury to axillary artery* is of infrequent occurrence.

In H. E. Clark's case of compound separation, as well as in Hamilton's, the injury to the axillary vessels resulted in gangrene of the hand, &c.

Mr. Le Gros Clark records (*Lancet*, 1865, May 20, vol. i. p. 535) a case of separation of the head from the shaft of the humerus, the result of a fall from a height, complicated with singular chest symptoms.

J. H., aged twelve, hodman's boy, was admitted, December 2, into St. Thomas's Hospital, having fallen, half an hour previously, from a height of forty or fifty feet. Although there was considerable swelling of the shoulder, obscuring the nature of the injury at first, it afterwards became apparent that the epiphysis was separated from the shaft of the humerus, the length on the injured side being nearly an inch shorter than on the sound side, measuring from the acromion to the external condyle. There was no very marked falling in of the deltoid, but the upper extremity of the shaft of the bone penetrated between its fibres, and threatened to pierce the superjacent bruised skin. It was found impracticable to restore it to its direct and accurate relations with the head of the bone, and this state of affairs must have been due to the interposition of some tendinous fibres or to the impaction of the shaft in the head. The thin covering of skin over the upper extremity of the diaphysis ulcerated, but subsequently healed well. Good union and free mobility were ultimately regained. The interest of this case is, however, especially associated with the following condition, which supervened on the afternoon of the day after the patient was admitted. On visiting him Mr. Le Gros Clark found his face flushed, his respiration hurried and oppressed; but, though the dyspnœa was urgent, there was no lividity or coldness of the lips or extremities. The heart's action was forcible and frequent, but the sounds were normal. ·Over the left side of the chest there was *complete* dulness on percussion, and also absence of respiratory murmur, and, indeed, of any sound but the heart's action, except, perhaps, a scarcely perceptible murmur under the clavicle. Vocal thrill was equally audible on both sides. On the right side there was normal resonance on percussion, and the respiratory murmur was very distinctly audible—indeed, puerile. There was no cough nor expectoration. Four leeches were applied to the upper part of the chest, and relief almost immediately followed. On the following day the boy was breathing quietly, and in less than forty-eight hours all the above symptoms had disappeared, and the respiratory sounds on percussion and auscultation, as well as the heart's action, were perfectly normal. Mr. Le Gros Clark asks what was the cause of suspended respiration in the entire left lung. The extremely excited action of the heart seemed to indicate serious obstruction in the pulmonary circulation, and the result of treatment seemed to point in the same direction. If not engorgement of the lung from the violence done to the chest by the fall, what could it be, consistently with the rapid disappearance of the·symptoms?

Pressure upon brachial plexus.—The diaphysial end, if it be displaced far into the axillary space, may cause pressure upon the brachial plexus. This was probably the cause of the numbness of the fingers in two cases observed by Middeldorpf.

In one case (Middeldorpf, *Knochenbrüche*, S. 86, 1851) a boy, aged fifteen, after a fall from a stair, experienced very acute pain with complete loss of power of the arm, and any attempt at movement caused great distress. There was some falling in of the deltoid muscle, and the arm was abducted from the thorax at an angle of about thirty degrees, and shortened one centimetre. Numbness of the fingers was also present. High up in the axilla, beneath the vessels and nerves, the sharp edge of the bone could be clearly felt. Reduction was effected by powerful extension and pressure upon the edge in the axilla, and was accompanied by mild crepitus. There was no reproduction of the displacement on slight elevation of the arm. Union took place after fourteen days, without any deformity or loss of utility of the arm.

In the second case (Middeldorpf, *Knochenbrüche*, 1852) a boy, aged thirteen years, had fallen downstairs the previous day on to his left shoulder. Acute pain, numbness of the fingers, and loss of power of movement were experienced, with great swelling, especially of the deltoid, and abduction of the elbow. The lower fragment projected inwards and forwards into the axillary space. Crepitus and shortening were absent. Reduction was effected as in the preceding case, but recurred the next day, when a starch bandage was applied. Consolidation took place in seventeen days, without any trace of callus to be felt externally ; thirteen days later complete use of the arm was regained.

Separation with dislocation of the head of the bone.—It is possible in separations caused by very severe violence that the capsule of the joint may be more or less lacerated and the head of the bone displaced from its socket.

In March 1873 Mr. Durham had the following case under his care at Guy's Hospital. Robert. E., aged seventeen, fell from a warehouse a distance of sixty feet on to the pavement. On examination there was found considerable contusion and swelling in front of the left shoulder, a subspinous dislocation of the left humerus, with separation of its upper epiphysis, Colles's fracture (? separation of lower epiphysis) of left forearm, fracture of the upper third of shaft of right femur, and fracture of the clavicle. There was some numbness of the shoulder, but this was the only evidence of any nerve lesion. The head of the humerus could not be replaced ; the other fractures were treated with the usual splints. Two months later the patient was discharged with very fair movement of his shoulder.

The diagnosis of this complication must always be a matter of considerable difficulty, greatly increased by the swelling of soft parts about the shoulder. The presence of the epiphysial head of the bone in an unnatural position, the glenoid cavity not being occupied by it, and its failure to move when rotation of the arm is made, are the most characteristic signs. McBurney and Dowd (*loc. cit. supra*) point out that (in the adult) shortening of the limb and crepitus may or may not be capable of definition. A careful examination under an anæsthetic is imperative.

McBurney says : ' Usually the mobility of the shaft of the humerus, and the readiness with which it falls close to the side of the thorax, would prove the presence of fracture, the existence of dislocation of the head having been determined, but, as has been pointed out by Stimson (*Treatise on Dislocations*, p. 255), the same mobility may exist in a case of dislocation without fracture, provided the capsule of the joint has been sufficiently lacerated.'

DIFFERENTIAL DIAGNOSIS. **Sub-coracoid, sub-clavicular, and intra-coracoid dislocations** of the humerus forwards are the most common forms of injury likely to be mistaken for epiphysial separations.

Giraldès and R. W. Smith and others have drawn especial attention to the frequency of confusing these fractures with dislocations in children. The former surgeon says that in his wards he had a certain number of cases of separation of the diaphysis or epiphysis, all of which had been mistaken by practitioners for dislocations of the shoulder.

It should always be borne in mind that epiphysial separations can only occur at a period of life when dislocations are exceedingly rare ; and dislocation of the shoulder-joint in children is extremely so.

Mr. Henry Morris records (Holmes, *System of Surgery*, 1883, vol. i.

p. 972) a case of dislocation forwards in an infant fourteen days old, and Mr. Mayo Robson, of Leeds, describes (*Lancet*, July 26, 1890, p. 172) a case of supra-coracoid dislocation of the right humerus in a youth aged sixteen. At the time of operation by exploratory incision, there was, in addition, a split fracture separating the great tuberosity from the bone and extending down the shaft, and the glenoid cavity was filled with callus. Fraser (*American Journal of the Medical Sciences*, 1869) replaced the dislocated head of the bone in a boy aged fifteen years, and obtained a good result. These rare cases may almost be disregarded in practice : separations of the upper end of the humerus replace dislocations before the twentieth year.

The end of the diaphysis situated in front of the shoulder, being slightly convex and rather smooth, may be easily mistaken for the head of the bone, displaced below or above the coracoid process— especially as the central conical projection is the first part to ossify on to the epiphysis, so that it may readily be broken off and cause this surface to appear flatter than it otherwise would do. But it is never so smooth, rounded, or situated so high in the axilla as in dislocation. On the other hand, it has an abrupt anterior ledge situated lower down and smaller than the normal head of the bone. The skin often presents over the displaced lower fragment a peculiar depressed appearance ; it is held firmly over the projection and cannot be moved over it, while occasionally a distinct pit is seen in the integument on attempting to replace the diaphysis in its natural position. This condition of the skin is the result of the penetration of the muscular fibres of the deltoid, deltoid aponeurosis, and even the superficial fascia by the diaphysial end. It is not met with in dislocation.

In a large proportion of the cases described above a diagnosis of dislocation was at first made.

Jetter says that out of seven cases operated upon for deformity and loss of function of the arm after union had taken place the displacement had, on five occasions, been diagnosed as a dislocation, and attempts at reduction had been made by the medical attendant.

As late as June 1893 we find (according to Lejars) a case being mistaken at one of the French hospitals and vain attempts made at reduction by Kocher's method.

Dr. J. F. Erdmann, of New York, mentions (*New York Medical Record*, October 26, 1895, p. 586) the case of a boy (M. McG.), aged sixteen, who had fallen upon his shoulder six weeks before. He had been an inmate of one of the large New York hospitals, and was being treated for a sub-coracoid dislocation of the humerus. There was no swelling, but marked flattening of the shoulder, broadening from before backwards, and $1\frac{1}{4}$ inch shortening. A slightly convex deformity, continuous with the shaft, with the bicipital groove well marked upon it, was found beneath the acromion, and downwards and in front, practically sub-coracoid, a round, fairly movable mass was felt. A diagnosis of epiphysial separation was then made and operative treatment recommended, but refused.

The author has seen the same mistake made at the hospitals in London.

There are many other signs, as well as the prominence referred to above, in which epiphysial separation and dislocation somewhat resemble one another. Great bruising and swelling render the diagnosis still more difficult.

Unnatural mobility of the upper end of the bone is mostly, but not invariably, present in separation, and consequently cannot be considered as diagnostic from dislocation; it is nearer to the joint as infancy is approached. For the head of the bone remaining in the glenoid cavity is usually motionless when the shaft is moved, except in the cases of incomplete displacement with impaction described above.

In this connection H. E. Clark observes (*vide supra*): ' One noteworthy sign which may be found useful in the diagnosis of such cases is this: the head of the bone being fixed with the fingers of one hand, while the elbow was held with those of the other, the shaft was made to move with the result that if the movements were angular in their character the epiphysis was quite stationary, a fact which showed how complete was the separation of the bone. If, however, the movement consisted in the rotation of the humerus on its own axis, the epiphysis moved with the diaphysis. This may be explained by the convexity of the upper end of the lower fragment fitting into the cup-like surface on the under surface of the upper fragment; this arrangement of the parts, while allowing angular movement to take place at the line of separation, will not permit rotatory movement of the one upon the other.'

The shoulder still *retains its general rotundity.* Although there may be some depression (one inch or more) below the acromion, it is not immediately below the acromion process, nor does it extend at all backwards behind this process, as in dislocations. There is, therefore, no projection of the acromion, nor any deep excavation immediately below it, inasmuch as the epiphysis still retains its normal position, and, in thin subjects, may be felt below the acromion process when there is an absence of great extravasation of blood.

The *head* of the bone, often distinctly felt *in its socket,* is one of the best distinguishing signs. It is often placed obliquely in the glenoid cavity—being retained there by the muscles attached to the epiphysis and by the capsule of the joint—and may rotate with the diaphysis if the locking of the fragments is very firm; in complete displacements it does not move with the diaphysis.

The fragments are not easily maintained in position after reduction, the deformity immediately recurring on letting the parts go free, except where the two fragments can be made to fit accurately one in the other. On the contrary, in dislocation after reduction the parts usually maintain their normal position, and the movements are again very free.

Professor R. W. Smith says, in reference to diagnosis : ' The chief diagnostic signs are an abrupt projection beneath the coracoid process, caused by the upper end of the lower fragment, and the immediate recurrence of the deformity when the means employed for its reduction cease to be in operation.' In another paragraph he says : ' There is no fracture incidental to the upper end of the humerus in which it is more difficult to maintain the fragments in their proper relative position.'

Modified crepitus may be felt during reduction, and, if present, is characteristic.

Shortening is not usually marked, except in complete displacement.

There is *no fixation* of the limb in its abnormal position, as in dislocation.

The elbow *does not project to such a very marked degree* from the side of the body as it does in dislocation, nor is there any difficulty in bringing it into contact with the side of the trunk.

Dugas's test (L. A. Dugas, *Trans. Amer. Med. Association*, vol. x. p. 175) is most useful. The hand of the affected side can *easily be placed* by the surgeon upon the *opposite shoulder*, while at the same time the elbow may be brought against the front of the chest. If this can be done readily there is no dislocation.

Acute *pain* is also felt *at the epiphysial line* on pressure and during manipulation.

Chloroform should be given in all cases where there is the slightest doubt about the diagnosis or where difficulty is subsequently experienced in reduction.

In one of the cases of complete displacement seen by Hamilton *a fracture of the acromion process with a dislocation* of the head of the humerus was believed to have taken place. Such an error could not have occurred if the above means of diagnosis had been carefully applied.

When, however, a true *dislocation is associated with a fracture* of some part of the neighbouring bone, as of either of the tuberosities (not uncommon with forward dislocation), the anatomical neck, &c., the signs are usually so obscure as to render the diagnosis well nigh impossible. They have been mostly recognised after death.

An exploratory incision under strict antiseptic precautions, as advocated by Mayo Robson, should be undertaken in all such cases, at any rate when ordinary means of reduction have failed. The same operation must be carried out in *all epiphysial separations accompanied by dislocation*, whether partial or complete ; or even excision of the head may be required.

Fracture of the surgical neck.—So many signs of this transverse fracture in the adult are obviously the same as in separation in children—namely, the general character of the deformity, direction of the displacement, unnatural mobility, shortening of arm, causation &c.—that we have to rely upon the *age of the patient* and upon the fact that the fracture takes place in the immediate vicinity of the conjugal cartilage. In youths, during the period of growth, a direct injury to the shoulder is more likely to be followed by epiphysial separation than fracture of the surgical neck, therefore in them every solution of continuity in this situation should suggest the former lesion, especially if accompanied by deformity. M. Coulon describes (*Fractures chez les enfants*, Paris, 1861, p. 127) two or three cases of supposed fracture of the surgical neck in children.

M. de Saint-Germain (*Chirurgie des enfants*, Paris, 1884, p. 178) says that he has seen several cases of fracture of the upper extremity of the humerus in children, but believes they are rare.

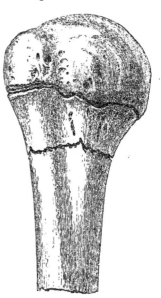

The angular, convex, or smooth *end of the diaphysis*, upon which, in complete displacements, the examining finger may be placed as upon a ledge, is unlike the sharp pointed projection of a fracture, which is situated somewhat lower than in separation. Even in incomplete displacements the exact seat and character of the diaphysial end or edge are most important for diagnosis.

D. W. Cheever, of Harvard University, puts the matter as follows (*Boston M. and S. Journal*, 1893, cxxviii. p. 585): 'Separation of the epiphysis is practically about the same thing as fracture of the surgical neck; it takes place within a

FIG. 46.—DIAGRAM OF SITUATION OF SEPARATION AND FRACTURE OF THE UPPER END OF THE HUMERUS IN CHILDREN
(Actual size)

fraction of an inch of the same locality, and whether the epiphysis or the surgical neck will give way depends on the age of the patient. Then these two are combined usually under the ordinary name of fracture of the surgical neck.'

It is very improbable, however, that the line of fracture in the adult, which is generally very irregular, will be transverse—in fact, it is never so tranverse as in separation of the epiphysis. Transverse fractures, again, are often impacted, and so do not permit any movements between the fragments; in epiphysial separation some lateral movement may commonly be obtained of the diaphysis on the epiphysis on moving the arm, whereas in the impacted fracture no such movement can be effected, the upper fragment rotating at the shoulder-joint. According to Poncet, the chief points in the diagnosis of this injury are the age of the patient, the high position of the lesion in the immediate neighbourhood of the shoulder-joint, and the displacement forwards and inwards of the lower fragment.

The *muffled crepitus*, when present, is characteristic. Seeing that the separation may be only partial, being accompanied by a fracture of the shaft as in Mr. Johnson Smith's case, the crepitus more distinctive of an ordinary fracture will be met with. The soft crepitus will then be obscured by the fine dry crepitus of the fracture.

The signs of **separation of either tuberosity** in the child will for the most part be negative and obscure, and indistinguishable from *fracture of the tuberosities in the adult*.

Both will be extrascapular, and caused by direct violence to the shoulder. Some increase in breadth of shoulder, localised, pain at the epiphysial line, and the possibility of seizing the separated process between the fingers and replacing it in its natural position when the arm is abducted, will be present both in separation and fracture.

Both those limited injuries are distinguishable from separation of the whole epiphysis by displacement forwards in the case of the lesser tuberosity and by displacement backwards in that of the greater tuberosity, giving rise to a projection which is movable, and a gap or depression between it and the rest of the upper part of the bone. Crepitus will be absent, or with difficulty obtained in these fractures by grasping the process and rotating the arm.

The head of the bone will not as a rule rotate in the glenoid cavity if the remaining portion of the upper end of the humerus be broken through at the epiphysial junction.

Sprains and contusions of the shoulder in childhood offer some of the most difficult cases for diagnosis from epiphysial separation with little or no displacement. In this connection the author would refer the reader to Ollier's description of juxta-epiphysial sprains.

TREATMENT.—The treatment of this separation will vary with the particular character of the lesion presented—with or without displacement, or accompanied by some complication.

Where displacement is absent, or has been reduced, the treatment will not differ from that of fracture of the upper end of the humerus, care being taken to prevent any subsequent displacement or movement of the fractured surfaces, and thereby to guard against the possibility of arrest of growth of the bone, whilst the arm is fixed to the side by a simple bandage, with or without a cap of felt or other material over the shoulder.

Mr. Thomas Callaway (*Dislocations and Fractures of the Clavicle and Shoulder-joint*, 1849), in describing the ease with which several cases of fracture of the surgical neck of the humerus, occurring at Guy's Hospital in children at puberty, were reduced and maintained in position, does not even allude to the frequent occurrence of epiphysial separation at almost the same point.

They certainly present much greater difficulties in treatment than fractures of the surgical neck, on account of the lesion of the bone being placed higher in position, especially on the inner side, thus rendering the upper fragment very short and difficult to be fixed by a retentive apparatus.

INCOMPLETE DISPLACEMENT.—In certain cases of *incomplete* displacements of the epiphysis, the deformity is so slight that but

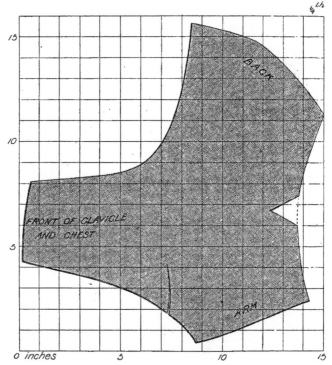

FIG. 47.—PATTERN IN HOUSE-FLANNEL OF PLASTER-OF-PARIS SHOULDER CAP FOR A CHILD OF EIGHT YEARS

Reduced to one-quarter size on scale of inches.

little manipulation of the upper end of the epiphysis is required to replace the fragment, and therefore but simple measures are required to retain the same in proper position. In these the reduction of the fragments is usually maintained. Simple fixation of the arm to the side and flexion of the elbow are often sufficient for this purpose, the chest affording a very good support for the diaphysis; or a plaster-of-Paris splint, taking in the shoulder and arm, in the form of a cap with the arm bandaged to the side and a wedge-shaped axillary pad, may be necessary.

Reduction in the more simple cases is effected under an anæsthetic by pressing with the greatest gentleness the upper end of the lower fragment backwards and outwards with one hand, and by making extension or traction at the elbow with the other hand and at the same time drawing the elbow forwards and upwards. In these incomplete cases reduction by this or Moore's method can only be successful if the deltoid has not been transfixed by the diaphysial end, a complication which so often happens in the more complete displacements.

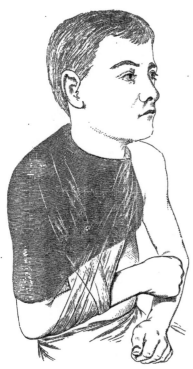

FIG. 48.—METHOD OF APPLYING PLASTER-OF-PARIS SPLINT TO TRUNK AND UPPER EXTREMITY

The following cases have been treated at Guy's Hospital upon this simple plan with favourable results.

No. 1. W. H., aged thirteen, was admitted under the care of Mr. Durham, November 20, 1874, having fallen off a van on to his right shoulder. There was diagnosed a separation of the upper epiphysis of the humerus with considerable contusion around the joint; arm was bandaged to side, and some days later a felt cap was applied. Discharged December 15, 1874.

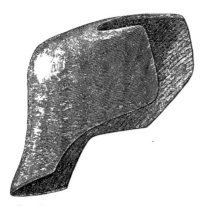

FIG. 49.—PLASTER-OF-PARIS SPLINT REMOVED

No. 2. H. L., aged sixteen, admitted under the care of Mr. Bryant, October 16, 1876. He fell off a swing on to his right shoulder, causing separation of the upper epiphysis with much bruising; arm was fixed to chest by bandage. Discharged November 7, 1876.

No. 3. Eliza B., aged seven, under the care of Mr. Howse, was admitted on July 5, 1877. She had been run over by a cart, the wheel passing over her right shoulder. There was found to be a fractured clavicle, and separation of the upper epiphysis of the humerus. The arm was fixed to the side, and ten days later a gutta-percha splint moulded to shoulder. Discharged August 8, 1877.

An accurate diagnosis should in all cases be made under an anæsthetic before swelling, which rapidly ensues, takes place. The fragments should then be gently replaced in position. The author would add that the medical attendant should not undertake the entire responsibility. However skilfully the injury may have been treated, he is sure to be blamed for any deformity, or any arrest of growth of the limb, that may result.

COMPLETE DISPLACEMENT.—Separation with *more or less complete displacement forwards* may be one of the most difficult injuries to treat at the upper end of the humerus. It should be reduced by means of extension and abduction of the arm, assisted by direct pressure upon the displaced diaphysis.

Prompt reduction is absolutely essential if the functions of the shoulder are to be rapidly restored.

Moore does not believe that extension alone will produce complete reduction. He says : ' Traction does not produce reduction, for the reason that it does not remain in place after it appears to be reduced ; the symptoms recur as soon as the extension ceases.'

E. F. Lonsdale relates (*A Practical Treatise on Fractures*, 1838, p. 179) a case of locking together of the fragments in a boy about twelve years old, which shows the difficulty of complete reduction. The fracture was situated apparently through the lower limit of the epiphysis of the bone, about an inch below the tubercles ; the fractured end of the shaft of the bone was projecting anteriorly under the acromion, being almost through the integument. The portion of bone was so jammed in this position that long continued extension, very violently applied, could not reduce it ; the joint was not injured, and the bone united, with no other deformity than this small prominence that was felt beneath the skin. Mr. Lonsdale continues : ' It was difficult in this case to say upon what the opposition to the reduction depended, for the muscular power of the boy was small, and acted but very slightly.'

The elbow and forearm should not be raised, otherwise the upper end of the diaphysis will tend to be displaced forwards again.

Even when the fragments have been reduced, it has been found extremely difficult to retain the bones in their proper position.

After the lapse of three or four weeks, on taking off the splints, there will at times be found, in spite of every attention, some displacement forwards, or irregularity or unevenness at the line of union. The union is quickly effected, probably from the great vascularity of the epiphysis, and the number of muscles attached to it.

The functions of the joint are very seldom permanently impaired, and the projecting mass of bone will mould down and become rounded off in the course of time with the subsequent growth of the bone, so that after two years the angular deformity becomes scarcely perceptible.

Jetter alludes in three instances to this continual displacement of the lower fragment forwards and inwards, in spite of careful treatment by Velpeau's bandage. Two of these have been related above, the third is as follows :

M. T., nine years old, fell on March 25, 1891, from a loaded waggon upon her left arm. On admission to hospital the next day there was great swelling of the left shoulder and upper third of arm,

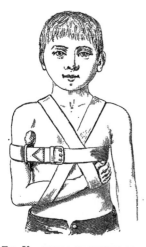

FIG. 50.—METHOD OF APPLYING BAN-
DAGE AFTER THE DIAPHYSIS HAS BEEN
RESTORED TO ITS NORMAL POSITION
The moulded shoulder cap is not
shown

deviation of the axis of the humerus, the head of which still occupied the articular cavity, with typical displacement upwards and inwards of the lower fragment. Abnormal mobility and soft crepitus were also present. The fragments were easily reduced by extension, and Velpeau's bandage was applied; but, in spite of this, displacement occurred again the next day. The arm was therefore elevated and extension employed. This kept the fragments in good position, but the extension had to be removed after five days on account of some excoriation at the bend of the elbow. Velpeau's bandage was again applied for nine days, when the displacement had reappeared, which necessitated a resort to the former method of treatment till April 16, when it was removed, and there was no further displacement.

On April 19 the patient was discharged with all the movements tolerably free.

In all cases it is advisable to insert a flat soft pad into the axilla, and the arm must be bandaged to the chest as in a fracture of the clavicle, assistance being supplied by a moulded poroplastic splint or other material for the sake of compression and rest to the deltoid and other muscles.

At Guy's Hospital, in 1874, Mr. Birkett treated, with an excellent result, a case of separation of the upper epiphysis of the right humerus by means of a gutta-percha cap to shoulder. Michel K., aged seven, had been run over by a van, the wheel passing over his shoulder. Twenty-eight days later there was good union and no appreciable deformity.

Or the arm may be placed on a pyramidal pillow, inserted after Dupuytren's method into the axilla, and the arm bandaged to the body. The hand of the injured arm may be placed upon the opposite shoulder, as in fractured clavicle; occasionally this is the only position in which reduction of the fragments can be maintained.

Mr. Durham treated a case at Guy's Hospital in this manner. Sam S., aged fifteen, fell off a cart, pitching on to his left shoulder, and causing separation of the upper epiphysis of the humerus. A pad was placed in the axilla, and the elbow bound to the side. He was discharged from the hospital after a month. There was then firm union, and all movements of the arm were good, but the shaft still projected somewhat forwards. In this case an inside splint was applied in addition, but this could not be of great service, inasmuch as the separation is close to the head of the bone.

Some surgeons prefer to abduct the limb from the trunk to a right angle or less, with or without a posterior splint passing over the scapula. This method entails great incon-

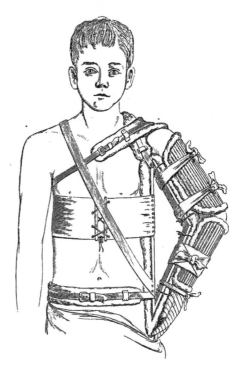

Fig. 51.—MIDDELDORPF'S TRIANGLE, CONSISTING OF A DOUBLE INCLINED PLANE FRAMED OUT OF THREE BOARDS

The longest side is fixed to the trunk by straps. whilst the arm, bent to an obtuse angle, is placed upon the two shorter sides, and fixed there by bandages or Gooch's splinting. (After Esmarch)

venience, as the patient will be confined to his bed. In other respects it will be found to be very efficient in remedying the displacement, and bringing the upper end of the lower fragment into complete apposition with the epiphysis, which has undergone rotation.

A laminated plaster-of-Paris splint may be applied with the arm in the abducted position, the patient lying upon his back.

Unfortunately, the reduction is often by no means easy, great difficulty being experienced from the locking of the fragments and the small size of the upper fragment. The head of the humerus, by a firm grasp of the thumb and fingers on either side, may be restrained enough to produce crepitus, but not enough to answer the necessities of reduction.

Mr. E. M. Moore's method ('Epiphysial Fracture of the Superior Extremity of the Humerus,' *Trans. American Med. Association*, 1874, p. 296) of reduction of incomplete displacement forwards of the diaphysis by completely drawing the arm at right angles to the trunk without extension has already been mentioned. The reduction is effected by carrying the humerus forwards and upwards to the perpendicular line. When once reduced the displacement has shown no tendency to recur, any simple apparatus being sufficient to complete the cure. The arm is then carefully lowered and fixed in this position. Mr. Moore has verified the correctness of his opinion by having in this manner effected the reduction with great ease in three cases which came under his observation. The patients were respectively six, fourteen, and sixteen years of age.

In the first case reduction was effected on the fourteenth day, in the second case on the second day, and in the third on the seventeenth day. In both of the latter ineffectual attempts had been already made to reduce what was supposed to be a dislocation. In order to maintain the reduction all that was found necessary was to bring the arm down beside the body while in a state of moderate extension, and to secure it with a Swinburne extension splint. In all three cases there was a perfect result. The restoration to full use was accomplished in less than thirty days.

Others have employed Moore's method with equally good results.

Packard, in this connection, says (*Cyclopædia of Diseases of Children*, Keating, 1890, vol. iii. p. 1064) : 'I would venture to express my belief that a better plan is to follow the upper fragment with the lower, first by extension, overcoming any impaction that may exist, and then carrying the elbow upwards and outwards, so that the arm shall be at an angle of perhaps forty-five degrees with the body, in which position it can be readily supported by means of a splint, one branch of which should be applied to the side of the chest, the other to the inner side of the arm. After a week or two the splint may be changed so as to lessen the angle, and again two or three days later, and so on until the arm is brought down close to the body.'

Dr. Chas. H. Richmond (*New York Medical Journal*, November 1877, No. 26, p. 504) diagnosed this separation in a boy aged nineteen, who had fallen backwards a distance of six feet to the ground, and successfully reduced the displacement by Moore's method, the arm being carried upwards and forwards while extended. There was slight depression existing beneath the acromion, with the characteristic forward and outward projection a little below, together with ' muffled ' crepitus. A splint was applied, and at the end of four to five weeks the result was perfect.

When this form of displacement has been followed by successful reduction by this method, it appears to be less liable to become again displaced, owing to the irregularities and the cup-like manner in which the separated surfaces fit together when once reduced.

Continuous extension may be employed after complete reduction, and for cases of constantly recurring displacement. It has principally been found useful in older children, and is effected by means of a weight attached to the extremity, a wedge-shaped cushion in the axilla being of assistance in preventing the displacement of the lower fragment.

A simple method of continuous extension is that employed by Lannelongue. The shoulder, trunk, and arm, as far as its lower part, are surrounded by a plaster trough made with a bandage, in which a wooden splint is firmly fixed, descending a short distance below the elbow. To the lower end of this some india-rubber tubing is attached and fastened above to the lower end of the arm. The forearm is fixed to the trunk by a sling.

In spite of all perseverance, skill, attention, and the use of extension, counter-extension, and other mechanical means, it has in exceptional instances been found impossible to effect reduction.

Hamilton describes the following case (*Treatise on Fractures and Dislocations*, 7th edit. 1884, p. 261) of Joseph S., aged sixteen, who fell backwards down a flight of steps, striking his back and arm near the shoulder, and causing a separation of the upper epiphysis of the left humerus. It was supposed that there was a dislocation of the humerus, and an attempt had been made to effect reduction with the heel in the axilla and without an anæsthetic. He was seen by Hamilton the following day, when, all efforts at replacement proving ineffectual, splints were applied. The patient left the hospital nine weeks afterwards with the fragments united, but overlapping at the point of fracture, the upper end of the lower fragment being in front of the upper fragment. The limb was shortened one inch, but its motions were free and its utility unimpaired.

Demoulin, Hutchinson, and others have described many similar cases (see under PROGNOSIS, SEQUELÆ, &c.). Some go so far as to believe that irreducibility is the rule after separation of the upper epiphysis of the humerus. But we need only point to Kirmisson's and other cases in which perfect reposition of complete displacement was most easy, and followed by absolute recovery of the shape and use of the arm.

R. W. Smith says (*loc. cit. supra*, p. 202) : ' I am sure that, however experienced the practitioner may be, he will find the treatment of the case embarrassing, and that it will require the exercise of all his ingenuity and skill to prevent a certain amount of displacement from being permanent, and to counteract the influence of the muscles, which unceasingly act upon the lower fragment. The consolation, however, remains that, notwithstanding the deformity, the patient will ultimately regain the almost unimpaired use of the limb.'

One of the chief difficulties of reduction occurs, however, from the *insertion between the epiphysial fragments* of bands of periosteum, fascia, or muscle, or from the penetration of the periosteal sheath by the diaphysial end.

Union of fragments by operation, resection of diaphysial end, &c.—In *recent cases*, in which it is found to be impossible to reduce the deformity on account of the displacement of the diaphysis, and in which it is probable that the utility of the arm will suffer in consequence, the propriety of cutting down upon the fragments, resecting the end of the diaphysis, directly placing the fragments in position, and wiring the fragments together will at once suggest itself to the surgeon.

This especially applies to cases of complete displacement, and others where the difficulty of retaining the fragments in position is great. The presence of the diaphysial end beneath the skin in front of the shoulder indicates that it has passed through the deltoid, transfixing and lacerating the front portion of the muscle.

At a meeting of the Society of German Surgeons in 1888 (Sajous, *Annual of the Medical Sciences*, vol. iii. G. 3; *Annals of Surgery*, February 1889, vol. ix. No. 2, p. 153) Professor Helferich (Greifswald) narrated the history of a case in which he had cut down upon the separated epiphysis of a humerus. At the same meeting Bruns reported two cases, and Woelfler one, of separation of the epiphysis, with dislocation of the head, successfully treated by excision of the upper fragment.

In Professor Helferich's case (*München med. Woch.* No. 40, 1887) a lad of sixteen, while wrestling, fell violently to the ground, striking the left shoulder. The head of the humerus was found in its normal position under the acromion, while the rounded upper end of the shaft was displaced forwards and inwards, under the coracoid process, from which position it could be slipped up and down, and, when strong downward traction was made, soft crepitus was developed. An apparent shortening of the arm of $1\frac{1}{2}$ centimetres was observed. All attempts at reposition proved unsuccessful owing to the interposition of soft parts between the fragments, and an incision was made in front of the shoulder. The upper end of the humerus had penetrated into the axilla through a buttonhole slit in the periosteum and capsule, which latter it was found needful to incise before reduction could be accomplished. The fragments were then fastened together with a long awl-shaped steel pin, which projected beyond the surface at the line of sutures. This was removed at the first change of dressings at the end of eight days. The shoulder-joint regained its function in a short time.

In the case of a boy aged ten years, recorded by Dr. Jetter, resection of the diaphysial end for complete displacement only left 1·7 centimetres shortening after the lapse of nine years.

Dr. Fred. Lange, of New York, has published (New York Surgical Society, November 22, 1886, *Annals of Surgery*, vol. v. 1887, p. 448) another case in which operative measures were resorted to as an immediate method of treatment. He describes this as a fracture of the humerus with interposition of soft parts treated by operative replacement.

A boy, aged ten, fell about eight feet, striking his right shoulder, and sustaining a fracture of the humerus immediately below the head; the lower fragment had apparently perforated the deltoid muscle, and, with a sharp edge, was fixed in the deep layers of the skin without penetrating it. A distinct protrusion was formed on the anterior aspect of the shoulder, the elbow being thrown backwards so that the axis of the bone was directed abnormally to the front. The lower fragment could not be released from its abnormal attachment, even after the swelling and tension had markedly subsided. On the seventh day, the patient being placed under ether, an incision was made over the displaced fragment, and the slit in the deltoid enlarged. A separation was then found in the epiphysial line as far as the middle of the bone, whence a line of fracture went in an oblique direction downwards and backwards, its lowest point being about two inches below the epiphysial line. In order to bring the fragments into proper apposition, it was necessary to elevate the arm above the horizontal line and to give it a decided outward rotation, at the same time bringing it slightly forwards. The periosteum and fibrous attachments on the edge of the upper fragment were not torn exactly in the line of the fracture, but at a short distance below, so that they overlapped the edge of the upper fragment and had to be turned up, a condition similar to that found in fractures of the patella. The periosteum had to be slightly indented, and then coaptation could be effected. The long head of the biceps was not torn, but lifted out of its groove and dislocated to the inner side; with the lower fragment, it returned to its normal relations. Union without necrosis and complete cicatrisation ensued. The upper fragment, by the action of the muscles inserted into the greater tuberosity, was abducted and rotated outwards; consequently, during the after-treatment the corresponding position of the arm was maintained with slight extension by means of a splint passing from the posterior aspect of the arm over the back to the opposite scapula.

Dr. F. W. Murray described (*Annual of the Universal Med. Sciences*, 1891, vol. iii. I. 3) a case of separation in a patient seventeen years old with displacement of the end of the shaft inwards, in which he found it necessary to excise ¾ inch of the shaft. Kirmisson (*Leçons sur les maladies de l'appareil locomoteur*, Paris, 1890) has also adopted the same procedure. M. Rollet states that a patient of M. Poncet was readily admitted into the military service five years after a similar operation.

M. Rollet (*vide supra*) expresses himself thus : ' In cases in which this displacement cannot be reduced, and where the upper end of the lower fragment has either perforated the skin, or, after having torn through the fibres of the deltoid, forms a very prominent subcutaneous projection, it is necessary to resect the extremity of the displaced lower fragment of bone. By such operation alone— which, being an extra-articular one, presents very little if any danger—can deformity be removed, and the functions of the injured limb completely restored.'

Professor Erasmo de Paoli, of Perugia, recommends (*Communicazioni della Clinica Chirurgica Propedeutica dell' Università di Perugia*, Perugia, 1891) the method of fixing the fragments by means of one or two sutures of sterilised silk. These buried silk sutures appeared to him to be preferable to the steel pin used by Helferich, because they permitted an immediate and perfect closure of the wound. The permanent presence of this extraneous material in connection with the epiphysial cartilage appeared to him to have also the advantage of exciting formative activity in it, and correcting the slight shortening produced by the resection.

The two following cases operated upon by De Paoli were not quite recent, being ten days and seventeen days respectively after the accident. The displacement of the lower fragment was absolutely irreducible by external means. The difficulty of reduction was caused by the powerful resistance of the periosteal sleeve attached to the epiphysis, as well as by the rapid formation of adhesions with the surrounding structures, and by the displacement of the epiphysis upwards and backwards. Consolidation in the abnormal position had already commenced in so short a time. With regard to this it is interesting to note in the second case that after seventeen days there was no longer any trace of mobility of the fragments. In both cases it was necessary to remove a small portion of the diaphysial end.

Case 1. B. R., aged fourteen, fell, on May 4, 1891, from a height of three metres, striking his shoulder. He was at once seen by a doctor, who suspected fracture of the upper end of the humerus with great displacement, and attempted the reduction of it under an anæsthetic ; a bandage was applied to retain the parts in position. On May 14 he was admitted to the hospital. Beneath the coracoid process there was to be seen and felt a dome-shaped prominence one inch in width, the head of the humerus occupying its normal position ; this, as well as the diaphysial end, followed the movements of the arm, but when the former was firmly fixed with the fingers, only the projecting diaphysis moved. The boy could move his arm backwards and a little forwards and inwards, but incompletely elevate it. The right humerus was shortened 2½ centimetres as compared with the left.

The diagnosis was made of traumatic separation of the upper epiphysis of the humerus with marked displacement and commencing consolidation. On June 20, 1891, a vertical incision was made from the apex of the acromion downwards over the projecting end of the diaphysis, which was readily recognised, and covered here and there with small areas of epiphysial cartilage. The union already established between the two fragments was broken across by means of a raspatory and by forcible adduction. To effect reduction it was necessary to pare away a small amount of the end of the diaphysis, and after the lower aspect of the epiphysis had been freshened by scraping, the two fragments were united together with a stout sterilised silk suture. Catgut suture was used for the periosteum and deltoid, and silk for the skin. A small drain was inserted in the lowest part of the wound, and the wound dressed antiseptically, the shoulder being fixed immovably in the abducted position.

On June 23rd the patient was sent home, there having been no rise of temperature. On July 21 the boy had never had any pain of any kind, the dressings were removed, and perfect union was found, with all deformity corrected. Active and passive movements of the shoulder were perfectly free.

Case 2. T. B., aged seventeen, fell from a tree, seventeen days before his admission into the hospital, on to some stony ground, striking his left shoulder. Pain and swelling of the shoulder were felt at the time, but of this he took no notice and attempted to continue his work. Becoming worse, he was sent to the hospital by the local doctor. On examination an abnormal projection was noticed two inches from the apex of the acromion process continuous with the humeral diaphysis; it had a sharp anterior edge, and a somewhat convex upper surface. The shoulder retained its normal convex shape.

The upper epiphysis of the humerus appeared somewhat bulky, but was in its normal position. Active movements were very restricted in every direction. Passive motion, with the exception of abduction, was altogether free, and the epiphysis moved freely with the projecting diaphysis. The left humerus was shortened three centimetres. Separation with great displacement of the humeral diaphysis was diagnosed.

On June 4, 1891, an incision was made over the projecting lower fragment through the antero-internal aspect of the deltoid, which was adherent to it. The adhesion between the fragments was broken down by forcible movements. A portion of the bone, 1½

centimetres in length, had to be removed by a saw. · It was then
seen that the separation did not wholly follow the epiphysial line,
but that a splinter of the diaphysis had been broken off from its
postero-internal aspect. The two fragments, after being replaced
in perfect apposition, were united by two sutures of sterilised silk
passed through the bone. The periosteum was next sutured, then the
muscle, and finally the skin. Antiseptic dressings were employed,
and an immovable. bandage applied. On July 9 the patient was
discharged. There had been no pain and no rise of temperature.
On July 13 the patient was seen again ; there was then perfect union
of the fragments, and normal freedom of movement of the shoulder-
joint.

M. C. Walther (*Revue d'Orthopédie*, Jan. 1897, No. 1, p. 40) operated successfully for irreducible displacement on a lad aged seventeen,
three days after the accident. Whilst at play the lad had fallen
heavily from his comrade's back to the ground on to his left shoulder.
There were the characteristic signs of displacement forwards and inwards of the diaphysis, the end of which presented the usual ' plateau '-
like surface. Under an anæsthetic reduction of the displacement
was found impossible, although several attempts by extension of the
upper limb were made ; a vertical incision was therefore made over
the front of the shoulder, and the irreducibility was found to be due
to the projection through the deltoid of the lower fragment, which
was made fast in a narrow buttonhole of muscle substance. Even
after a wide incision of the muscle, and having the fragments under
direct observation, it was still impossible to make the proper coaptation of the fragments. A second cause of irreducibility appeared to
be the preservation of a wide band of intact periosteum, which held
the fragments so firmly that their replacement was impossible. After
having resected from the diaphysial fragment the length necessary
to obtain reduction, M. Walther simply reunited the soft parts
without employing any suture to the bone, since there now remained
between the fragments no obstacle to their proper coaptation,
reduction being complete. The separation was not perfectly pure,
inasmuch as a vertical splinter of the diaphysis was detached from
its posterior and inner aspect and remained attached to the epiphysis.
Consolidation took place readily and uniformly, the arm being secured
in Hennequin's apparatus. The result at the end of the second
month was perfect ; there was no deformity and. no restriction of
movements, which could be carried out fully and with their natural
force.

Helferich (*Fracturen und Luxationen*, 3 Auflage, München,
1897, S. 133) gives two figures of another case before operation seen
from the outer aspect and from above. The girl (L. V.), aged
fifteen, had fallen from a high heap of straw upon her left shoulder.
Fourteen days later (October 1894) she came under treatment,
and the displaced diaphysis was replaced by means of an anterior

incision and fixed in position by a steel pin. Consolidation took place, with good mobility of the joint.

Finally, the author would insist that in separations with considerable deformity which are irreducible, and in others where the impaction of the fragments is an important and possibly the only factor in the causation of the subsequent loss of functional activity of the limb, operative measures should not be delayed. They should also be undertaken in the rare examples of complete displacement of the diaphysis from the epiphysis, where the epiphysis has undergone considerable rotation. Operation should also be practised in cases where there is evidence of pressure upon the axillary vessels or brachial plexus of nerves. In these instances the diaphysial fragment must be replaced, for by no other surgical method can this satisfactorily or effectually be accomplished.

In the larger proportion of cases the operation is extra-articular, and at the present day it cannot be considered so grave as before the introduction of aseptic and antiseptic methods, wound infection being absent.

The new skiagraphy will, in the near future, undoubtedly furnish some exact data upon which the surgeon may rely in deciding upon the advisability of an operation.

Replacement and union of fragments by operation without resection of the diaphysis will sometimes be found sufficient in recent cases.

It should be recommended in the cases of great and irreducible displacements of the diaphysis, especially if associated with any of the complications already enumerated, and in the younger periods of childhood, when many years of growth still remain to the humerus. Laceration of the periosteum and muscles, folding of their torn fibres over the diaphysial end, or their intervention between the fragments, being the most frequent causes of irreducibility, simple aseptic incision over the protruding diaphysis, division of the soft structures, and enlargement of the rent in the periosteal sheath will be enough to enable the bone to be gently replaced in position.

After pegging the fragments together by means of pins to prevent displacement, the divided edges of the periosteum and capsule should be carefully sutured with carbolised catgut or silk, then the edges of the muscles, and finally the skin.

Antiseptic dressings should then be carefully applied, and a drain inserted if considered necessary.

Passive motion should be commenced in from two to three weeks, and the other subsequent treatment carried out as in a recent fracture.

At the New York Surgical Society, November 13, 1895, Dr. Chas. McBurney (*Annals of Surgery*, February 1896, p. 177) presented a boy in whom separation of the upper epiphysis of the humerus had been treated by open operation. The patient was

fifteen years of age, and was first seen in the previous June,
five days after he had fallen in a gymnasium upon his left
shoulder. The shoulder was then uniformly swollen and the skin
red, the temperature was 101° F., and the pulse rapid. The head
of the bone was in the glenoid cavity and separated from the shaft
at the epiphysial junction. Crepitus did not exist, for the shaft was
displaced upwards and forwards in front of the epiphysis, and its
rough end could be felt but a short distance beneath the skin.
Ether was administered, but reduction could not be accomplished
by traction and manipulation. McBurney therefore made a vertical
incision about three inches long over the prominent upper extremity
of the shaft. The fracture was found to be exactly at the junction
of the epiphysis and shaft, and the latter projected through nearly
the entire thickness of the deltoid muscle. The periosteum had
been split vertically, and it and the muscular fibres were so folded
under the upper end of the shaft that reduction could not be made
without incision. These soft parts being held aside with retractors,
reduction was easily effected, and accurate apposition of the bone ends
obtained. The slit in the periosteum was then closed with catgut,
and the more superficial wound closed in the same way with
drainage. The wound healed cleanly and rapidly. The movement
at the joint was now entirely restored, and one arm could be
used quite as well as the other. No difference in the length of the
two humeri exists, although the boy has grown much since the
injury.

In another instance reported by Dr. Jetter (*Beiträge zur
klinischen Chirurgie*, 1892, S. 373) resection of the diaphysis was
found to be unnecessary.

Maria R., aged twenty-three, on May 19, 1890, was pushed
into a ditch and fell upon the right shoulder. She was unable to
move the arm, and cold fomentations were applied on account of the
great swelling. The arm was then 'set' by a doctor, and a plaster-
of-Paris bandage applied for four weeks. Five weeks after the
accident the patient was admitted into the hospital. There was
about one centimetre shortening, and the usual displacement forwards of the diaphysis, its end being directly below the coracoid
process. Abduction, flexion, extension, and rotation were very
limited.

After division of the soft structures, and breaking down of the
uniting callus by rotating the arm, the fragments could be separated
from one another. The fracture followed the epiphysial line, and
the lower fragment, after it had been freed of adhesions and part of
its periosteum, could be readily replaced in position without resection of its end. As the lower fragment had some tendency to become displaced subsequently, the arm and hand were placed in the
elevated position. When seen nearly two years later (1892) the
movements of the humerus were normal, with the exception of slight

limitation of outward rotation. There was no deformity, and the woman could again do any sort of work.

Resection and replacement of the diaphysial end in old cases of separation were first recommended and carried out by Bruns in 1884 for correction of the deformity and restoration of the function of the limb, elevation and rotation of the limb being especially impaired. Arrest of growth, which may result from great displacement, must also be taken into consideration. In two instances which had not been recognised at the time of accident as epiphysial separations, and had united with so much displacement that the utility of the arm was greatly impaired, Bruns (*Centralbl. f. Chirurgie*, 1884, S. 277; *Mittheilungen aus der chirurgischen Klinik zu Tübingen*, i. 1884, S. 243; *Beiträge z. klin. Chirurg.* Bd. i. 1885, S. 241) cut down by a longitudinal incision along the outer edge of the diaphysis under strict antiseptic precautions, separated the united fragments with a chisel and raspatory, removed a portion (one centimetre in one case and two centimetres in the other) of the end of the diaphysis, and successfully replaced them in their natural position. In one case the fragments fitted so firmly against one another after this procedure that the epiphysis moved freely when the diaphysis was manipulated, and there was no tendency to displacement. In the other case, the fragments were retained in position by placing the elbow in front of the chest and the hand on the opposite clavicle. No osseous suture was used.

The first case was that of a young man (B. S.), aged twenty-four (a very exceptional age for this injury), who four weeks previously had fallen (1882) from the eighth step of a staircase to the ground, striking his shoulder.

The second was that of a boy (A. H.), aged ten years, who had fallen, five weeks previously, on to his shoulder from about the sixth step of a ladder.

Both were diagnosed as dislocations, and attempts made to reduce them, in the first without any success, and in the second the deformity, though reduced for a time, was soon reproduced.

The characteristic deformity was well marked in both, the diaphysis, with its rounded end, being displaced upwards and inwards against the coracoid process, and the epiphysis firmly united to it, although the fragments were probably only in contact at their edges. All movements of the arm in both cases were greatly interfered with, but more especially rotation and abduction. In the first case the shortening measured two centimetres, in the second one and a half centimetres.

At the operation the separation of the epiphysis in the boy's case was found to be a pure one, whilst in the other it only took place through the inner half of the epiphysial line, and then ran obliquely outwards through the diaphysial end. In both the epiphysis had rotated on its antero posterior axis very considerably, so that its separated surface looked inwards, and was in contact with the outer side of the displaced diaphysis.

In both consolidation took place in three or four weeks, the free mobility of the arm being completely restored, and the deformity obliterated. In the boy's case nine years after the operation (1892) all movements of the shoulder were complete, and he could work perfectly with this arm. Only a slight wasting of the deltoid and three centimetres shortening of the humerus could be detected.

Dr. Jetter (a former assistant of Bruns) adds two other examples from the Tübingen Clinic. After resection of the diaphysial end and reduction, the fragments were kept in position by means of steel pins, which were removed between the second and third weeks.

Case I. A lad (J. B.), aged nineteen years, on July 28, 1890, fell from a height of seven metres in a barn, and the handle of a pitchfork which he was carrying was thrust into the right axilla. Great pain and inability to move the arm were immediately experienced. No diagnosis was made by the doctor, who applied an ice-bag, and later on, electricity. On September 1, 1890, the patient was admitted to the hospital on account of the impaired use of the arm. The diaphysis of the humerus was detached at the epiphysial line and displaced forwards and inwards. The fragments had united, as the head moved with the shaft. Elevation of the arm could not be effected, and rotation was limited.

After division of the soft structures, the uniting callus was divided by a chisel. On the inner side the separation was accompanied by a fracture of the diaphysis. Reduction could only be effected after resection of one centimetre of the end of the diaphysis. The fragments were held in position by means of two steel pins. By September 8 the wounds had healed without drainage. On September 26 the patient was discharged; shoulder-joint normal. Three weeks later, pins were removed. Movements of joint quite free.

Case II. A boy (A. M.), aged nine, fourteen days before admission, 1891, fell from a tree on to his face with his left arm outstretched. The end of the diaphysis was displaced forwards and inwards, near the coracoid process, two fingers' breadth below the acromio-clavicular joint. The head of the bone occupied the glenoid cavity, and moved with the diaphysis. The humerus was shortened about one centimetre, and the movements of the joint were greatly hampered, rotation being almost impossible.

On October 17, the usual incision over the end of the bone was made, the fragments divided through their uniting material, and one centimetre of the diaphysial end resected. The diaphysis was then replaced and fixed with two pins. On November 4 the patient was discharged with a starch bandage, and on November 13 the pins were removed, the fragments having consolidated in good position. When seen on April 1, 1892, the shoulder-joint was free in every way, and the power in both arms appeared to be almost equal.

Where there appears to be no tendency to displacement or separation of the fragments after they have been placed in contact, simple suture of the periosteal covering of the fragments, combined with deep sutures to the fascial structures round the joint, will suffice, instead of making use of the osseous suture.

Lejars successfully adopted this plan (*Revue de Chirurgie*, August 1894, p. 636) in the following operation for the relief of deformity of the shoulder and impaired function of the upper limb.

A boy aged sixteen years came under his care at the Necker Hospital in June 1893. On May 12 he had fallen and struck his right shoulder against the ground. On getting up he experienced great pain and was unable to use his right arm, so that he had to hold it up with the other hand. He went to a hospital, where subcoracoid dislocation was diagnosed and an attempt made (of course unsuccessfully) to reduce it by Kocher's method. The swelling, which was considerable, and the pain prevented a complete examination, but by the first few days in June, when he was admitted, the effusion of blood had diminished, so that there could be made out below the coracoid process a rounded osseous projection which elevated the skin and looked somewhat like the dislocated head of the humerus, although smaller and having a less regular outline. It rolled to and fro during rotation of the arm, showing that it was clearly in direct continuity with the shaft of the bone. Beneath the acromion the humeral head could be felt in position. It moved slightly with the arm. The diaphysis of the humerus was displaced upwards, forwards, and inwards, and a distinct gap left on the outer side of the epiphysial line. Consolidation was almost complete. The diagnosis of old separation of the upper epiphysis of the humerus was very clear. There existed also extreme loss of functional power—so much so that, as regards flexion and abduction, these were scarcely represented. The deltoid was already markedly atrophied. Operative interference appearing to be the only thing capable of rectifying matters, on June 15, the patient being placed under chloroform, a long incision was made in front of the shoulder along the pectoro-deltoid furrow and the inter-muscular space widely opened out, after ligature and division of the cephalic vein. This gave sufficient access to the seat of the old injury. The pointed and cone-shaped end of the diaphysis was found to be almost in contact with the coracoid process, the line of consolidation ran very obliquely outwards, and the uniting callus was already solid. After the use of the rugine for clearly displaying the ends of the bones, M. Lejars with chisel and mallet removed the callus, resected about two centimetres of the sharp end of the diaphysial fragment, and made the two surfaces which he wished to bring in contact quite regular. The lower fragment could now be made to glide fairly easily under the epiphysial fragment, so that the continuity was re-established and the direction of the bone made perfectly straight. As the surfaces of the two fragments then corresponded tolerably well, it was considered sufficient to use four simple periosteal ligatures of silk applied to the antero-internal aspect of the humerus, to insure the fragments keeping their proper position. Some catgut was used to unite the peri-articular planes of fibrous tissue and the separated borders of the pectoralis major and deltoid. The skin was united without any drainage, iodoform dressings were applied, and careful fixation made by means of plaster.

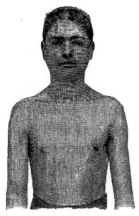

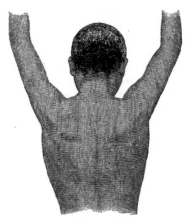

FIG. 52.—OUTLINE OF SHOULDER PERFECT, WITHOUT ANY OF THE DEFORMITY WHICH WAS PRESENT BEFORE OPERATION. (LEJARS)

FIG. 53.—THE ARMS COMPLETELY ELEVATED. (LEJARS)

There were no important after results. At the end of three weeks the apparatus and dressings were removed, and union was complete ; the humerus was not only firmly united, but in a perfectly straight line, and without the existence of any trace of the deformity in front. Massage and electricity were now commenced, and continued regularly every day.

When the patient left the hospital, on July 28, the movements of the upper extremity were already very free ; he could place his hand to his head and abduct his arm almost to a right angle (the scapula being fixed). Extension was the only very limited and difficult movement. Electricity and massage were continued every second day. Improvement rapidly took place after the end of July, so that the patient went to work again. When seen quite recently (1894) the functions of the shoulder were almost complete ; there was the normal range of movement, without any trace of deformity, of atrophy, or rigidity of the joint (see figures).

M. A. Ley (*La Presse Médicale Belge*, No. 33, 16 Août 1896, p. 257) records a similar example of resection and replacement of the diaphysial end of the humerus in simple separation of the upper epiphysis in a boy aged 16½ years. The operation was undertaken three weeks after the injury (April 3, 1896) by M. Lambotte, for repeated recurrence of displacement after reduction and after the application of a plaster bandage. An exact diagnosis was not made previous to the operation, beyond that a fracture of the upper end of the humerus was discovered. The usual symptoms of displacement forwards of the humerus with soft crepitus were present. The deltoid muscle was found to be almost transfixed by the end of the diaphysis, which still had a little of the conjugal cartilage adherent to it. Reduction of the diaphysis was effected, but on the slightest movement the displacement was reproduced; three to four centimetres of the end of the bone were therefore removed. The periosteum was found to be torn and separated from the shaft for a considerable extent. Iodoform gauze dressings and Desault's apparatus were then applied, and the after results were excellent. Seventeen days after the operation the wound was almost completely healed and union perfect. About a fortnight later the patient could freely elevate his arms, and there was scarcely any deformity; two months afterwards, through the employment of active and mechanical movement, the functions of the shoulder-joint were quite restored, with only half a centimetre shortening. M. Ley believed that a tuberculous family history in this case predisposed to the epiphysial separation. It was the result of direct violence; the patient, whilst at play, having been thrown to the ground, with a comrade falling upon him and striking him on the right shoulder.

The results of the operation being so successful, we ought to carefully consider the question of resection and suturing when the active movements of the arm are merely limited, and not confine our operative interference to cases in which all or nearly all movement is lost.

Mr. W. Johnson Smith, of the Seamen's Hospital, Greenwich, showed before the West Kent Medico-Chirurgical Society (*British Medical Journal*, February 28, 1892; and *Lancet*, March 5, 1892, p. 526) a patient in whom compound separation of the incomplete variety, with displacement forwards and inwards, and an extensive fracture of the diaphysis, had occurred two and a half months previously. The lesion resulted in distortion and uselessness of the arm. The subject of this injury, W. L., aged eighteen, a Danish seaman, was admitted into the Seamen's Hospital on January 28, 1891. On November 16, 1890, he had fallen from the topsail yard on to the deck, injuring his head and left shoulder. He stated that there was a large wound in front of the joint, through which immediately after the accident a long piece of bone protruded. This, in the course of the voyage, which lasted till January 26, gradually fell back into the wound, and was covered over by scar tissue. There was no medical man on board the ship, and the patient was treated simply by rest and the application of ointments to the wound. At the time of the patient's admission, the left upper limb as compared with the right was wasted and cold. He could move the limb freely at the elbow and wrist, but the movements of the shoulder were much retarded. He could move the elbow away from the side of the chest to the extent of about 1½ inches only. The length of the left arm, measured from the acromion to the external condyle, was 11¼ inches; that of the right arm 12¾ inches. In front of the shoulder, beginning about 2 inches below it, was a broad irregularly-shaped cicatrix measuring 3 inches in the vertical direction. Immediately beneath this, projecting under the skin, near the coracoid process, was a prominent hard projection, formed by the upper end of the shaft of the humerus displaced inwards and forwards. The upper end of this portion of the bone, which had evidently been detached from the head, was smooth, even, and slightly rounded. The head of the humerus seemed to be in its normal position, and could be rotated. After attempts had been made without success to restore the free action of the shoulder-joint by passive movements, ether was administered on February 17, and the prominent portion of bone exposed by a vertical incision about 4 inches in length. The anterior two-thirds of the upper end of the shaft presented a free surface, which was quite flat and smooth. The posterior third, on the other hand, was united to the anterior and inner portions of the upper segment of the humerus, and the posterior and outer surfaces of the shaft near its upper end had contracted firm osseous union with a long piece of bone 2½ inches in length continuous with the head, or rather with the anatomical neck. The union between the two segments of the humerus having been severed by bone forceps, and a portion of the posterior spine of bone removed, the upper end of the shaft was applied to the under surface of the head and fixed in its normal position by a loop of thick wire, and also by an ivory peg driven through the anterior surface of the shaft into the cancellous tissue of the upper segment. The wound, having been drained and closed by superficial sutures, was covered by cyanide gauze and a large pad of wood-wool. The patient did well after the operation, and was discharged on May 17, quite free from any deformity in front of the shoulder, which joint the patient could move very freely, and, according to his own report, as well as that on the right side. In a letter written in August he stated that he had been at work for some time as a seaman.

One of the cases recorded by Jetter and one by Bruns revealed a less extensive fracture of the diaphysis.

Resection of the projecting diaphysis in old separations.—After the lapse of some weeks, or even months, for severe deformity and impairment of utility of the arm, removal of the displaced diaphysial end may be had recourse to.

In these instances it is only necessary to remove the rarefied anterior projecting portion of the diaphysis, after separating it from the lacerated fibres of the deltoid. The posterior part, about two-thirds of the thickness of the bone, will be found firmly consolidated with the epiphysis. The epiphysis should not under these circumstances be separated from the shaft.

M. E. Rollet (*Lyon Médical*, March 29, 1891) reports two cases of détachment of the head of the humerus that came at the same time under the care of Professor Poncet, of Lyons. One patient was aged fifteen and the other seventeen years. In each the deformity at the seat of injury and the impairment of the function of the limb were relieved by resection of the upper extremity of the lower fragment at five and a half and seven weeks respectively after the injury. In the first case the girl, while running, had fallen upon the antero-external aspect of the left shoulder and experienced acute pain in the shoulder ; ecchymosis and some swelling appeared, with inability to use the arm. Eight days after the accident she noticed a projection at the upper part of the arm. On her admission on the twenty-fifth day there was a marked projection in front of the shoulder, five centimetres below the middle of the space between the coracoid and acromial processes. It was visible beneath the skin, which appeared to be almost penetrated.

Where the epiphysial separation is associated with a fracture of the diaphysis and the loss of function is not very marked, this simple process of removal of the small portion of the diaphysis which projects too much will not interfere with the connection of the head with the rest of the diaphysis.

Dr. Jetter records a case of this kind of a boy (K. E.), aged sixteen years, who had fallen upon his left arm while sliding on the ice on New Year's Day 1891. The arm was 'set' under chloroform by a doctor, and a dressing applied for fourteen days, when passive motion was commenced. An osseous projection being noticed at the end of four weeks, another attempt was made to 'reset' the arm, and a plaster-of-Paris bandage applied for another four weeks. The patient was then admitted into hospital for the very marked loss of use of the arm. The arm was shortened one and a half centimetres. An incision was made (March 19) over the bony protuberance, which was two fingers' breadth below the coracoid process, the soft parts divided, and the periosteum detached from the bone. The inner half only of the diaphysis was found to be separated at the epiphysial line, and to project away from the epiphysis, while the outer half was broken off by a longitudinal fracture of the diaphysis. This outer portion, to which the head was still attached, was displaced backwards and downwards, and

had united in this position.   The projecting end of the diaphysis presenting the epiphysial surface was merely chiselled off, and the soft
parts reunited, with drainage.   The patient was discharged on
March 28 perfectly cured.

Dr. Chas. L. Leonard (*The American Journal of the Medical
Sciences*, August 1896, p. 143) records an example of diastasis of
the proximal epiphysis of the humerus, with overlapping of the
fragments and union in a faulty position.   The state of the parts
was revealed by means of the Röntgen rays.   S. B., aged sixteen
years, fell heavily on the left shoulder while playing football in
December 1895.   He passed through the hands of two doctors,
and was subsequently sent to the University Hospital of Pennsylvania for operation.   A longitudinal incision through the deltoid
towards its anterior border showed the proximal end of the
lower fragment overlapping the upper fragment by about two inches,
with firm bony union between the two fragments.   The upper end
of the lower fragment lay beneath the coracoid process and interfered
materially with the function of the joint.   The upper portion of the
lower fragment was resected. giving the joint free motion.   The
patient made a good recovery.   The skiagraph showed the position
of the fragments after the operation and their lateral union in a
faulty position.

M. C. Walther (*Revue d'Orthopédie*, Jan. 1897, No. 1, p. 43)
operated upon a similar case for irreducible displacement of the
diaphysis forwards, inwards, and upwards in front of the epiphysis.
The 'plateau'-like surface of the end of the diaphysis was well
marked.   Fixed in this position it led to decided functional impairment of the injured limb, the range of elevation and forward
projection of the arm being restricted by contact of the displaced
diaphysial fragment with the coracoid process.   (A front and a
profile drawing of the deformity are given by this author.)   The
patient was a lad aged eighteen years, who had fallen from a
scaffold about four metres high.   At the beginning of the sixth week
after the accident a vertical incision was made over the projecting
bone on the outer side of the pectoro-deltoid groove.   As a mass of
callus had already formed between the posterior aspect of the displaced epiphysis and the front of the epiphysis, M. Walther had to
determine between two procedures ; either to completely resect the
callus in order to place the fragments absolutely in apposition, or to
freely remove the projecting end of the diaphysial fragment without
interfering with the callus, now so very solid.   He decided to resect
only the end of the fragment, to carve away the callus, and to model
it in order to efface the projecting angle.   This he performed for
two reasons : the desire to profit by the consolidation already
established, and also the difficulty which apparently would be present
in resecting the callus from a very robust and muscular subject, in
a very deep operation wound.   The result was very good.   Although

elevation of the arm forwards was not perfectly complete, on account of the slight projection forwards which the callus still made, this slight limitation of movement did not entail any loss of function of the limb.

Professor Kocher (*Beiträge zur Kenntniss einiger praktisch-wichtiger Fracturformen*, 1896, Basel und Leipzig) has performed resection of a portion or the whole of the diaphysial end eight times.

Excision of head of the bone, leaving the epiphysial cartilage *in situ,* has been suggested for angular deformity and impairment of movements of the shoulder-joint. The severity of the operation precludes its performance under these conditions, while there is nothing to recommend it.

COMPOUND SEPARATIONS.—The majority of compound separations will require *resection of the end of the protruding diaphysis* before reduction can be accomplished, notwithstanding the laceration of the soft parts.

After the fragments have been placed in position and the wound irrigated, they must be retained in proper apposition by means of ivory or steel pins, or by means of wire sutures.

This has been done by Esmarch and others, and a plaster splint applied. Antiseptic methods and dressings should be carefully applied to the wound. Many of the untoward complications so frequently recorded have probably been due to failure in, or want of, antisepsis.

The first authentic case on record of resection of the diaphysial end in compound separation of the upper epiphysis of the humerus by gunshot wound was M. Roux's in 1837 (*La Presse Médicale*, 1837, July 12). A youth (R.), aged fifteen, received (March 20, 1837) a gunshot wound, with the muzzle held close to him, the bullet penetrating the right shoulder-joint and fracturing the head of the humerus. · A month after the accident, M. Roux performed resection of the upper end of the bone below the surgical neck. The operation was most successful, the arm recovering all its movements. The examination of the part removed showed a complete separation of the epiphysis by the bullet, which had shattered the epiphysis and penetrated the diaphysis.

In the case of a boy aged fifteen years, operated upon by Esmarch (Casper Nissen, *De resectionibus*; Dissert. inaugur. Kiliæ, 1859; *Archiv für klin. Chirurg.* Bd. xxi. S. 835), reduction of the diaphysis could not be effected, even after division of the lacerated muscles in the wound, and resection of two centimetres of the diaphysial end. At the end of three months all movements of the shoulder-joint were completely restored, and the arm—shortened only 2 centimetres—was still useful for all kinds of work.

The following instance of compound separation, recorded by Mr. Johnson Smith, of the Seamen's Hospital, Greenwich (*Lancet*, March 5, 1892, p. 526), shows the good results which may be

R

obtained by this procedure. It is especially worthy of note, for it appears that although nearly 2½ inches of the shaft were excised, sufficient new bone was formed from the periosteum which remained, and from the separated ends, to compensate for about 1½ inch of this, and to form a bone apparently perfect.

John F., an Irish boy, aged fourteen, was admitted on August 18, 1891, with an injury to the right shoulder, complicated by protrusion of bone through a wound in the axilla. All that could be learnt as to the cause of this injury, which had occurred about half an hour before admission, was that the right sleeve of the patient's coat had been caught in some machinery, and that the arm had been violently wrenched. The boy, when first seen in the ward, was pale and collapsed. The injured arm was abducted and rotated outwards, and there was much swelling over the outer side of the shoulder. In the outer boundary of the lower third of the axilla there was a transverse wound about 2½ inches in length, through which protruded the upper end of the shaft of the humerus detached from the head. This protruded portion of bone, which was 2 inches in length, was completely denuded of periosteum. The upper surface, which was also quite bare, was even over its anterior third, then rose into a small rounded elevation, and shelved off obliquely to the posterior surface of the bone. The anterior half of the surface was smooth, and presented a continuous layer of compact bone tissue, whilst in the posterior half the spongy tissue was exposed, as if a small portion of the upper end of the shaft had been broken away. There was no bleeding from the wound at the time of admission, and the patient's clothes were but slightly stained by blood. On examination of the seat of injury, whilst the patient was under the influence of ether, it was found that the protruded end of the humerus had passed between the median and ulnar nerves, and that one surface of the bone rested upon and firmly compressed the main artery. The denuded portion of the shaft of the humerus was thrust through the wound in the axilla and sawn off. The detached portion from which the periosteum had been stripped away measured 2½ inches in length. The shortened end of the shaft then fell back into the axillary space, and rested very near to the head of the bone. The capsule seemed to be intact, and no orifice could be found leading into the joint. As there was much swelling in front of the shoulder, it was found impossible to ascertain whether or not the long tendon of the biceps had been ruptured. A drainage tube had been thrust to the bottom of the wound; this was closed by sutures, and the seat of injury covered by a large wood-wool pad. A firm pad was placed in the axilla, and the upper limb bandaged to the side of the chest.

The patient progressed favourably after the operation. During the first three weeks the recorded temperature was usually normal, and never higher than 99·5°. The wound healed slowly, but without any discharge of pus. The movements of the arm were much restricted for some weeks, but when the boy was discharged, on October 13, they were quite free. He could then lift the limb a little above the level of the shoulder, and move it to the full extent in the forward and backward directions. The movements of rotation were much restricted.

On January 12, 1892, the movements of the right arm were quite free in every direction, and this limb, the boy asserted, was as strong and useful as the left one. There were no signs of muscular atrophy, and no appreciable difference could be observed in the thickness of the two limbs. Repeated measurements were made of both arms from the tip of the acromion to the external condyle, but shortening of not more than 1 inch could be discovered on the right side. The right shoulder was rounded, and did not differ in external appearance from that on the opposite side. There was clearly firm union between the head and the shaft of the bone. The boy had since the middle of November been employed in manual labour, consisting mainly in moving heavily laden wheel-barrows.

If the *large axillary vessels or nerves* are irremediably damaged, *primary amputation* is usually indicated.

Much, however, may be done to save the limb in young subjects, even under these unfavourable circumstances.

Separation with dislocation of the epiphysial head.—Treating the separation until firm union has occurred, and then using the repaired shaft for extension, rotation, or leverage in attempts at reduction, cannot be too strongly condemned at this early age. The dislocation should always be reduced first by operative measures, the difficulty of reduction by other means being due to the small size of the epiphysial fragment destroying the power which the shaft has to control its movements.

Seeing that it is almost impossible to reduce the head of the bone in these extremely rare cases, an incision should be made with antiseptic precautions through the skin and deltoid muscle from the acromial end of the clavicle down to the seat of separation, and the epiphysis replaced in position. It will be found necessary to open the capsule of the shoulder-joint before the epiphysis can be reduced. This should be accomplished by direct manipulation of the head into its place by pressure of the thumb and fingers, or by means of traction made upon it by a traction hook inserted into a hole drilled in it after the method advocated by McBurney (*Annals of Surgery*, April 1894, p. 408). The fragments should then be fastened together in their normal position by means of pegs or other sutures.

Riberi's method (made use of in adults) of treatment by passive motion employed from the commencement, so as to establish a false joint at the point of fracture, the dislocated head of the bone being left unreduced, is quite out of the question in the case of children.

Massage, electricity, &c. — Much may be effected, often very rapidly, by active and passive movements carried out day by day, supplemented by massage and by electricity where there is great loss of power and usefulness of the limb or rigidity, the result of too long fixation, with atrophy of the muscles.

The following case described by Curtillet (*Du décollement traumatique des épiphyses*, Lyon, 1891, p. 100) under the care of M. Levrat, was one in which great loss of functional power of the limb and want of any improvement of the fixed position of the arm against the trunk was rapidly and very successfully treated after the lapse of six months by massage and by repeated daily movements of the limb.

A boy (E. L.), aged nine years, entered the hospital on November 28, 1890. Six weeks previously the child's shoulder had been jammed between a wall and the edge of a cart, causing very acute pain, with great swelling and complete loss of power over the arm.

A doctor applied two leeches but no apparatus, and, at the end of four or five weeks, first a doctor, and then a bone-setter, attempted to reduce the supposed dislocation. When examined, the arm was found to be carefully fixed by the patient to the side of the body with the forearm forcibly flexed against the front of the chest. The scapula moved when attempts were made to move the shoulder-joint.

There was no flattening of the shoulder, but below the coraco-acromial arch the rounded head of the humerus could be felt in its normal position, and moved with the shaft of the bone. The edge of the diaphysial end displaced forwards from the epiphysis could be seen and felt 5 centimetres below and a little external to the apex of the acromion, and above it a very clear depression. The circumference of the arm was here 2 centimetres greater compared with the opposite side, and its length from the acromion to the epitrochlea 2 centimetres less. Each day massage was employed with systematic movements while the scapula was fixed; and an excellent result was obtained, so that at the end of a month the child left the hospital with almost complete recovery of all movements and usefulness of the limb.

PROGNOSIS, SEQUELÆ, &c.—The progress of these separations will naturally depend upon the character of the injury.

In simple separation, without displacement of the diaphysis, laceration, or any extensive stripping of the periosteum, union of the fragments by callus is rapid and the prognosis as a rule very good; though occasionally, as will be pointed out presently, arrest of growth takes place.

It is an important fact that *firm union* by osseous material is the usual termination. Notwithstanding that so large an osseous surface is involved, consolidation will be complete in two or three weeks. Even if displacement or deformity remains, the movements of the shoulder are ultimately entirely restored. Indeed, the author has not been able to find any authentic example of non-union of this epiphysis which was permanent.

Professor R. W. Smith, writing in 1867 (Address in Surgery, British Med. Association, *Brit. Med. Journal*, Aug. 17, 1867, p. 122 ; see also *Fractures and Dislocations*, 1847, p. 202), says : 'I have already mentioned the anatomical error into which some have fallen, of supposing that the tubercles of the humerus formed a portion of the shaft of the bone, and it has been to them a matter of surprise that in cases of separation of the epiphysis, osseous union should occur, the head of the bone being, according to their statement, detached from all connection with living structures.

' Vidal (de Cassis) has observed (*Traité de pathologie externe*, tom. ii. p. 114) that the occurrence of osseous union would be easy to conceive if the head of the bone formed one body with the tuberosities. Had M. Vidal examined in the young subject the situation of the line of the epiphysis, he would have learned the simple anatomical fact that, in the injury under consideration, the tubercles formed a portion of the superior fragment ; and that the epiphysis comprised not only the head of the bone, but likewise the entire of both tubercles, with that portion of the bicipital groove which is situated between these processes ; and he would not have stated, as he has done, that in cases of separation of the epiphysis the lower fragment was acted upon by the supraspinatus and infraspinatus, for he would have seen that these muscles were attached to the superior fragment.'

There can therefore be no difficulty in the matter of the blood supply to the head, which is so intimately connected with the tuberosities, nor any difficulty in understanding the occurrence of the osseous union of the fragments.

Hamilton reports a case of delayed union in a child thirteen months old, which is often quoted as a case of non-union. However, it is not conclusive, as the ultimate result is not stated nor the possibly diseased condition of the bone from some constitutional affection excluded.

In 1855 M. B., aged thirteen months, fell sideways from his cradle, causing some injury to the arm near the shoulder. He was taken to an empiric, who called it a sprain and applied liniments. Three weeks after the accident he was brought to Hamilton, who found the arm hanging beside the body, with little or no power on the part of the child to move it. There was a slight depression below the acromion process, and considerable tenderness about the joint ; but the shoulder was not swollen, nor had it been at any time. The line of the axis of the bone, as it hung by the side, was directed a little in front of the socket. On moving the elbow backwards and forwards, the upper end of the shaft moved in the opposite direction with great freedom, and could be distinctly felt under the skin and muscles. This motion was accompanied by a slight sound or sensation, not unlike the grating of broken bone, but much less rough. There was no shortening of the limb. When the elbow was carried a little forwards upon the chest, the fragments seemed to be restored to complete coaptation ; and of this Hamilton judged by the restoration of the line of the axis of the shaft to the centre of the socket, and by the complete disappearance of the depression under the point of the acromion process. Suitable dressings were applied to retain the arm in this position ; but five months after the injury was received the fragments had not united, and the child was still unable to lift the arm, although the forearm and hand retained their usual strength and freedom of motion. The same crepitus could occasionally be felt in the shoulder, and the same preternatural mobility. The shoulder was at this time neither swollen nor tender.

Altered shape of the shoulder and limb.—In incomplete displacements terminating favourably we find the deformity that remains is slight, without any shortening or disturbance in the function of the limb. But hitherto, from the difficulty of complete reduction of the diaphysis, there has not uncommonly been found some projection of this portion of bone, so that after repair has taken place many of the initial signs of this lesion are still present. This prominence of the bone, however, will rapidly become rounded off in its subsequent growth, and the deltoid and other muscles as they increase in bulk will hide even considerable deformity. The utility of the arm as regards movements, especially at the shoulder-joint, is surprisingly little impaired. Although the injury may have been overlooked, and the deformity be extreme, the amount of movement is often considerable.

Deformity is often great after complete displacements, and considerably interferes with the function of the limb ; while in many others the deformity, though present in some slight degree, does not give rise to any great interference with its utility. Indeed, when these patients are seen some years after the injury, no disturbance in the function of the limb is present, and the deformity is then hardly appreciable.

Dr. Jetter relates four cases to show the completeness of the return of function of the extremity associated with slight deformity, and sometimes shortening.

CASE I. B. W., aged eleven years, was hurled from a machine, striking his left arm against a cart-wheel. He was immediately admitted into hospital (October 23, 1885). The whole of the shoulder was very much swollen. At the level of the epiphysial line, on the outer side, a slight depression was felt, and the axis of the arm deviated a little. The epiphysis was in its normal position, and did not rotate with the humerus during passive motion, which was painful. No crepitus. Leiter's coils were applied. On October 30 Velpeau's bandage was employed, with plaster of Paris, as in fracture of the clavicle. On November 5 the patient was discharged, and by December 14 the fracture was perfectly united and the movements free, but the lower fragment projected somewhat forwards and inwards. When seen seven years afterwards (March 18, 1892), the patient was a big strong fellow, with the muscles of both arms equally well developed, and the function of the left arm quite as good as that of the right, so that without experiencing any pain he could work well as a bricklayer. On the inner side of the humeral neck, however, there was a slight convexity forwards of the bone, and a shortening of about 1 centimetre.

CASE II. A. W., aged thirteen, on October 3, 1887, fell from a tree to the ground, about a man's height, alighting upon her back and right shoulder. The humerus was found to be broken, and was attended to by a doctor, who kept the patient in bed for eight days, putting the bone into position and applying a bandage. The patient then came to the hospital (October 9), complaining of great pain in the shoulder, which was somewhat depressed, though its rotundity remained unaltered. The arm was slightly abducted, with a bending forwards of its axis at the upper third. This became more marked on elevating the limb. Slight crepitus at the epiphysial line was felt during passive movement, and, on fixing the head of the humerus, there was only slight abnormal mobility but no shortening. The shoulder was put up in plaster of Paris, and a Velpeau's bandage applied. On its removal (October 24) there was no deformity or swelling, and the head of the bone moved with the shaft. Patient was discharged on October 28. When seen five years later (March 20, 1892) the muscles of both arms were equally well developed, no displacement was to be seen or felt, and there was no shortening. All the movements of the joint were free, and the patient was perfectly fit for work.

CASE III. F. E., aged fourteen years, two days previously fell from a height of about two metres upon her left shoulder. On her admission to the hospital (June 28, 1889), the upper half of the arm and the shoulder were greatly swollen and painful. The head of the bone was still in position, and the tuberosities moved with the humerus as long as they were not held firmly, but directly the head was held fast it did not rotate with the bone. There was no crepitus. Velpeau's bandage and Leiter's coils were applied. The bandage was removed on July 6, and on July 20 the swelling had much diminished. A projection forwards of the upper end of the diaphysis could now be felt at the epiphysial limit; rotation and all movements were good, with the exception of abduction, which was imperfect. Three years later (March 20, 1892) the shoulder, on examination, had somewhat increased in its antero-posterior diameter. Consolidation had taken place, with slight displacement forwards of the lower fragment. Measurement showed no shortening. The muscles were equally developed in both arms; elevation of the arm was possible, and the patient was again perfectly able to do her work.

CASE IV. F. S., twelve years old, on June 30, 1889, fell down stairs upon her left shoulder. On examination there were the usual appearances of epiphysial separation with contusion. A Velpeau's bandage was applied, and removed six days later. On July 20 the deltoid was found to be somewhat wasted, the end of the humeral diaphysis projecting forwards. On July 31 the patient was able to elevate the arm horizontally, and the shoulder was no longer painful. Three years later (March 22, 1892) the muscles of the arms were found to be equally well developed. No measurable shortening was observed, but there was still slight displacement forwards of the lower fragment. Abduction, rotation, and all other movements were normal, and the girl was fully able to perform her duties.

Malgaigne states that he had seen a separation of the head of the humerus, sustained at an early age, and united with great displacement; the arm had lost its power, hanging atrophied and nearly useless beside the trunk, but the union, though unsatisfactory, was very solid.

Mr. William Lynn, Senior Surgeon to the Westminster Hospital, as long ago as 1833, commented (*Lancet*, December 28, 1833, p. 517) on the case of a girl (L. C.), aged eleven years, under the care of Mr. Guthrie at the same hospital, which formed the subject of a lecture by Mr. Guthrie on 'A Peculiar Kind of Injury of the Shoulder-joint.' On October 8 the child had fallen out of a second-story window upon her shoulder. There was a considerable prominence visible in front beneath the coracoid process, which might have been mistaken for a dislocation of the head had it not been for the irregular projection of the bone, and the fact that the head could be felt and moved in the glenoid cavity. The projection of the end of the humerus followed the movements imparted to the elbow. The arm could be elevated and the hand placed on the top of the head, the elbow also could be brought close to the side with ease, although it tended a little backwards. The forefinger could be made to sink into a hollow between the projecting end of the bone and the head of the humerus. The arm was shortened half an inch, and there was great swelling of the shoulder. Mr. Lynn found the joint broader and flatter than normal, and the limb shortened about 1 inch. Under the anterior part of the deltoid there was a broad and flat projection—manifestly the upper end of the humeral diaphysis. The head of the bone was felt to move (with the shaft) in the glenoid cavity. All the movements of the joint were performed somewhat imperfectly, from the angular union that had taken place, although the integrity of the joint had probably not been invaded. Mr. Lynn also felt another projection beneath the deltoid, which he took to be the epiphysis of the acromion, and this, being supported by the head of bone, had speedily united.

Mr. Guthrie alluded to a similar case in a boy, who also had good use of the arm.

R. W. Smith gives (*Fractures and Dislocations*, 1847, p. 204) a representation of an example of fracture through the line of the epiphysis, united by bone, and states that it exhibits very well the displacement which the upper end of the lower fragment usually suffers under the influence of the action of the muscles constituting the folds of the axilla. It has been drawn inwards, but not so far as to enable it to clear the under surface of the superior fragment.

So great a degree of displacement as this would imply is of very rare occurrence, and could scarcely happen without rendering the fracture compound.

Dr. Wharton ('Separation or Disjunction of the Upper Epiphysis of the Humerus,' *University Medical Magazine*, Philadelphia, January 1889, vol. i. No. 4, p. 212) relates the case of a girl, aged seven years, who, in going down stairs, tripped and fell upon her right arm. Upon examination a few hours after, the right arm

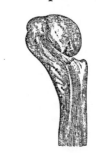

FIG. 54.—OLD FRACTURE OF THE HUMERUS THROUGH THE LINE OF THE EPIPHYSIS UNITED BY BONE. DISPLACEMENT OF THE LOWER FRAGMENT INWARDS.
(R. W. SMITH)

was found to be helpless, and any attempt to move the arm was followed by pain; there was no rigidity in the neighbourhood of the shoulder-joint, and the arm could without difficulty be brought in contact with the side of the body. There was no flattening of the shoulder, but a marked prominence in front and to the inner side of the acromion process of the scapula. On grasping the arm at the elbow and gently rotating it, and placing one hand over the prominence in front of the acromion, the smooth upper-end of the humerus could be felt moving under the hand, the head of the bone still remaining in the glenoid cavity. Reduction was effected by extension upon the arm from the elbow and by pressure backwards upon the projecting end of the humerus. Dull crepitus was elicited by rotating the arm during the same movements. A moulded splint was applied to the shoulder and arm, and the arm fixed against the side of the body, the hand and forearm being supported in a sling. This apparatus was renewed every second or third day, and finally removed at the end of the fourth week, the union at this time being quite firm. The patient had a good range of motion at the shoulder-joint, and subsequently regained the full use of her arm, although a very perceptible projection of the upper end of the humerus could be plainly felt in front of the shoulder-joint immediately above the coracoid process.

In Durocher's case the separation of the epiphysis occurred during birth, and was found on the death of the child at fourteen months to have been followed by shortening of the diaphysis of the humerus for a quarter of its length. The muscles of the shoulder were also considerably atrophied.

Hutchinson once examined (*Med. Times and Gazette*, March 10, 1866 ; *London Hospital Reports*, vol. i. 1864, p. 89) a lad, aged thirteen years, in whom it seemed probable that both upper and lower epiphyses of the right humerus had been detached. There had been separation of the lower epiphysis in the left arm and a fracture of one clavicle. These complicated injuries had been sustained in a fall from a ship's mast eight months previously. The right humerus was much shortened, partly by arrest of growth and partly by union with displacement.

Dr. Charles T. Parkes, Professor of Surgery in the Rush Medical College, Chicago (*International Clinics*, vol. i. 1891, p. 128), describes the following case in a clinical lecture. A boy, ten years of age, fell from a fence five weeks previously, producing an epiphysial fracture, as was shown by the unusually well marked projection about two inches below the acromion process on the anterior surface of the arm. This prominence was just beneath the shoulder-joint, and directly continuous with the shaft below. The lower end of the humerus projected too far backwards as compared with the uninjured bone. The upper end of the lower fragment had been displaced so far forward that it stood entirely away from the direction of the short fragment still attached to the head of the bone ; the broken surfaces were absolutely separated from each other. On moving the shoulder-joint there was some limitation to the full degree of motion on the injured side ; still, it moved freely and easily in all directions within this limited range of motion.

Dr. Parkes continues : ' This case also gives an excellent illustration of angular deformity, forward in this instance and extreme in degree. It also demonstrates that firm and solid union will take place between broken bones, even if the broken ends are not anywhere in contact with each other, provided one of the broken ends is held in contact with some portion of the shaft of the other fragment. Notice again that, notwithstanding the presence of this deformity, the boy has a very useful and movable joint. The extent of range of motion is limited somewhat, but with use will increase from day to day until it is restored quite to the normal condition. Is any operation advisable in this case to overcome the deformity ? I think not, unless it be the rather simple one of exposing the upper end of the lower fragment and chiselling away this projection, mainly to prevent ulceration of the skin covering it, which seems imminent.'

. In the following case, described by Dr. J. H. Pooley (*New York Medical Journal*, 1875, xxi. p. 139) the projection of the shaft in front of the shoulder was after treatment nearly as marked as at the time of the accident.

A girl (Alice F.), aged twelve years, fell from a tree on to her left shoulder, separating the upper epiphysis of the humerus. The arm was quite useless, and painful on movement. There was some slight depression of the shoulder, but no globular swelling, like the head of the humerus in the axilla; but in front, one inch or more below the joint, a peculiar pointed but not sharp projection. Under chloroform there was found unnatural mobility near the shoulder, with obscure crepitus. A pasteboard splint was moulded to the shoulder and outer side of the arm, and the arm was brought close to the side and the elbow raised. Three weeks later the splint was removed and passive motion commenced. Union had taken place, but there was still some projection in front. At the end of several months the arm was practically as good and useful as the other, the movements being all but perfect, although the prominence in front was still quite noticeable, though less marked, with half an inch shortening.

In Charles H. Richmond's case (*New York Medical Journal*, 1877, No. xxvi., p. 504) the deformity was the same as at the time of fracture.

A girl, aged ten, fell backwards from a height of three or four feet, causing a separation of the superior epiphysis of the humerus. The forward and outward projection of the lower fragment, with its rounded margin, produced marked deformity. There was but little shortening, and only 'muffled' crepitus was present. Reduction was effected and a leather splint applied to the outside of the shoulder, with extension. On removing this subsequently the deformity was found to be the same as at the time of the fracture. Five or six years later the deformity still existed, although much smoothed down.

Ricard, in Duplay and Reclus' *Traité de chirurgie*, tom. ii. 1890, p. 456, figures a specimen of separation of the upper humeral epiphysis united apparently by osseous material, but with considerable angular deformity (see figs. 55 and 56).

Hutchinson alludes (*Med. Times and Gazette*, March 10, 1866, p. 248) to a lad, aged fourteen, who was brought to him on account of deformity, some time after the accident, when the swelling had disappeared. The lower fragment was displaced forwards, and the finger could be laid on a flat ledge of bone a third of an inch wide, looking directly upwards and presenting the irregularities characteristic of an epiphysial surface.

In all the examples just quoted there must have been great detachment of the periosteum accompanying the displacement, while the difficulty experienced in reducing these epiphysial separations, leading either to total failure or incomplete coaptation of the fractures, no doubt accounts for the prevalence of deformity after this form of injury. Bruns has noted deformity in five out of eight cases under his observation.

To sum up the signs remaining a few months after the accident, we may find the following very characteristic appearances, seen also in certain fractures of the surgical neck of the humerus, and described since 1645 by Boyer, Debrou, Hennequin, Decamps, and many others. Slight flattening of the shoulder, with some atrophy of the deltoid, biceps, and muscles of the arm. Half to one inch shortening. Long axis of the arm directed backwards and outwards, and the forearm semiflexed. Marked impediment to the movements of the arm, although the hand can be placed on the opposite shoulder. Slight depression below the acromial arch from stretching of the deltoid. The head of the humerus is in position, and follows the movements of the arm, showing that the fragments are well united. In front of the shoulder, 1½ to 2 inches or more below the acromion process, there exists a very considerable and characteristic projection,

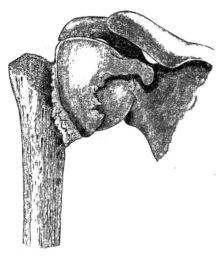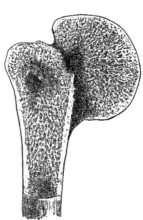

FIG. 55.—DISJUNCTION OF THE UPPER EPIPHYSIS OF THE HUMERUS, UNITED WITH LOCKING OF THE UPPER END OF THE DIAPHYSIS IN THE EPIPHYSIS. RICARD'S SPECIMEN. (AFTER DUPLAY AND RECLUS)

FIG. 56.—SECTION OF RICARD'S SPECIMEN. (AFTER DUPLAY AND RECLUS)

somewhat rounded in front but flattened above. (This projection of the diaphysial end forwards and inwards towards the coracoid process may be so great as to be in contact with this process, or there may be only some irregularity and thickening about the epiphysial line.) Considerable loss of function. Loss of active power in the hand and whole extremity, while passive movements, although free, are limited.

Deformity is so very much like dislocation that attempts have frequently been made to reduce the supposed displaced head of the bone.

Mr. Hutchinson says (*Medical Times and Gazette*, March 10, 1866, p. 247) that a few months after a separation of the epiphysis it is very likely that all the appearances of a dislocation will be assumed. Owing to the altered form of the neck of the bone, the head is gradually displaced downwards, until a hollow is caused under the acromion, the aspect being exactly like that of a dislocation. The head of the bone may even be felt in the axilla, though not so low down, nor so distinctly as in a true dislocation. It may be thought that a dislocation has been overlooked. The appearance is usually produced when the patient begins to use his arm, and if present at first it always increases. The neck of the humerus would come to resemble in form the neck of the femur of a young subject, and subsequently the elevation of the arm by the deltoid would push the head of the bone lower and lower in the glenoid cavity.

Hutchinson has seen reduction attempted not unfrequently. He relates the following case. A boy, aged fourteen, was brought to him in the belief that a dislocation had been overlooked. The deformity was very considerable—a hollow under the acromion, the head of the bone felt in the axilla, and the fibres of the deltoid stretched. The symptoms then present (two months after the injury) were said not to have been there at first. Irregularity and thickening were felt about the line of the epiphysis, and by pressing the arm straight upwards the subacromial hollow was almost filled up.

Non-union of the epiphysis is often alluded to by writers, but, as has been already stated, the instances of false joint recorded up to the present time cannot be relied on.

Reichel, in his work, figures and minutely describes a specimen in the possession of Ludwig (Leipzig) which is open to much doubt. The head of the left humerus he describes as separated as a cap from the diaphysis, more than an inch below the great tuberosity, so that this limb was shorter than the other. It was said that the separation had taken place in infancy, and that there was an entire absence of osseous union, and a false joint produced. It was said also that this was probably the result of too early movement of the limb.

Those cases related by Durocher, Bertrandi, and Hamilton as occurring in newly born infants are in like manner open to considerable doubt. They were all probably due to disease.

Loss of power and utility of the arm, apart from the causes just mentioned, may be the result of too long fixation of the limb, and consequent muscular atrophy, even though the displacement may not have been very great.

From the close relationship of the synovial cavity to the inner part of the epiphysial line it might be supposed that subsequent articular rigidity is a frequent consequence of separation, but this is not usually the case.

Reichel's case, and another, described by Palletta (*Exercitationes pathologicæ*, Mediolani, 1820, iv. p. 59) in a youth, aged fifteen, are quoted by Rognetta as examples of deformity and shortening in cases where the injury was not diagnosed or was badly treated. Palletta saw his case one month after the injury, which was from a fall from a high roof on to the shoulder. The end of the diaphysis was two fingers' breadth below the acromion, and the arm was shortened a thumb's breadth. The motions, at first very limited, were ultimately completely restored.

Ankylosis, the result of neglect of proper treatment, is well shown in Hoffa's case.

Bony ankylosis of the shoulder-joint, from some cause difficult to explain, followed in four of J. Hutchinson junior's cases. However, in one suppuration had occurred.

Shortening of the arm as the result of imperfect reduction or of the impossibility of keeping the fragments in position is very frequent. It is well exemplified by Hamilton's and Puzey's cases.

In Jetter's cases which were treated at the time of the accident no appreciable shortening could be found on examination.

TABLE OF SHORTENING IN INCOMPLETE DISPLACEMENTS AFTER TREATMENT

Surgeon	Sex of patient	Age	Amount of shortening	Date of measurement	Shortening at time of accident
Hamilton	Male	13 years	½ inch	14 days	Not stated
Hamilton	Male	16 years	1 inch	9 weeks	Not stated
Pooley	Female	12 years	½ inch	several months	Displacement 1 inch or more below joint
Durham	Male	14 years	1 inch	18 days	Not stated. Partial dislocation of head
Richmond	Female	10 years	A little, same as at time of accident	5 or 6 years	A little shortening
Puzey Johnson	Male	12 years	¾ inch	4 weeks	¾ inch shortening
Smith	Male	18 years	1½ inches	2½ months	Not stated. Complicated with fracture of diaphysis

Arrest of growth of the humerus.—The upper epiphysis of the humerus is mainly concerned in the growth in length of the bone, the average increase in length of the humerus through the upper end during life being about 18 centimetres—more than double, according to Vogt's calculations, that of the lower end.

The upper epiphysis from the tenth year will add 7 to 10 centimetres to the length of the humerus, whilst the lower epiphysis adds only 1·5 to 2 centimetres.

The accounts of conical stump published by Mr. Owen (*Lancet*, October 3, 1892), by Dr. Lediard (*Lancet*, January 9, 1892, p. 88), by Dr. Félix Lejars (*Leçons de chirurgie*, 1893–94), and others, show how active the upper epiphysis of the humerus is, and bear out the fact that conical stump is very apt to result in the arm after amputation.

Injuries to the cartilaginous junction of the epiphysis with the diaphysis, which are of almost daily occurrence, have been comparatively seldom followed by arrest of growth of the shaft. Yet its occasional occurrence should place the surgeon on his guard, so that the nature of the injury may be thoroughly explained at the time to the patient or friends so far as the future condition of the limb is concerned.

This serious interference with the proper development of the bone has taken place after the most simple injuries to the upper end of the humerus. In several cases the injury has been entirely overlooked; in others the injury was obscure and left unrelieved, while in others it was recognised as an epiphysial separation. The author is unable, therefore, to agree with those who believe that arrest of growth of the bone never need be feared in simple separation.

At the age when this separation is most common—viz. ten to seventeen years—arrest of growth will not occur to any important extent.

It has been thought by some writers that epiphysial separations which are not simple, but accompanied by fracture of the diaphysis of the humerus, may lead to premature ossification of the cartilage produced during the formation of the callus, and bring about an arrest of growth.

Others, again, believe that arrest of growth is dependent upon the displacement of the diaphysis. However, in Knox's, Hamilton's, the author's, and many other cases, there was no shortening, although displacement was a notable feature.

In several separations of the upper epiphysis of the humerus which Dr. Wharton had under his observation (loc. cit. supra) he could detect no difference in the growth, development, or usefulness of the arm, although the injury had occurred several years previously.

No arrest of growth followed any of the compound injuries.

There is usually no loss in the proper thickness of the shaft, the bone continuing to grow by means of the periosteum. This is especially noticed in Bruns's, Vogt's, Dittmayer's, and Hoffa's cases.

Albert Hoffa describes (Berliner klinische Wochenschrift, No. 4, S. 49, January 28, 1884, and Revue des Sciences Médicales, No. 48, October 15, 1884, vol. xxiv. fasc. 2, p. 637) a case of arrest of growth in the length of the arm, with ankylosis of the shoulder-joint, following traumatic separation.

A man, aged twenty-nine, received a blow at the age of nine years from the butt end of a gun on the right shoulder. Although there was great pain, the injury was not treated at the time, as the boy concealed it from his father. A subsequent attempt to restore the mobility of the arm was unsuccessful. There was no further injury, inflammatory process, or disease to account for the deformity, viz. considerable flattening of the shoulder, projection of the acromial arch, and atrophy of the trapezius and deltoid, which reacted, however, to electricity. All the other muscles, as well as those of the forearm and hand, the clavicle and scapula, presented no difference from those of the left side. The right arm was as thick as its fellow, but shortened 6½ centimetres (2·559 inches). The humeral head was displaced forwards, upwards, and inwards, and at the level of the epiphysiary line an angular bend in the bone could be felt. The shoulder-joint was completely ankylosed, rendering abduction impossible, all the other movements of the arm being carried out through the scapula.

At the Congress of the German Surgical Association of Berlin in 1877, Vogt (Langenbeck, *Archiv für klinische Chirurgie*, 1878, Bd. xxii .S. 341) exhibited a patient, aged twenty, who since his tenth year had suffered from complete cessation of growth in the length of the left humerus, following an injury which at the time was thought to be a sprain, but which was doubtless, he said, a traumatic epiphysial separation of the humerus with displacement. From that time the arm entirely ceased to grow in length, while the functions of the limb were unimpaired, excepting that a slight difficulty was experienced in abduction. All the muscles of the arm and forearm were well developed, with the exception of the deltoid and trapezius, which were much atrophied. The shortening of the humerus amounted to 13 centimetres (5·121 inches), while the growth in thickness was the same as on the opposite side.

Dr. J. F. Erdmann, of New York, mentions (*New York Medical Record*, ·October 26, 1895, p. 587) the case of a boy (J. D.), thirteen years of age, who was knocked down by a mail waggon and thrown forward on to his right shoulder. When seen within half an hour after the injury swelling was very slight and pain considerable, but no deformity; unnatural mobility was felt high up, and by grasping the shoulder with the left hand, and moving the arm with the right, grating of a peculiar soft character was obtained. He was discharged at the end of the third week, and the family reported ' that you would not know the arm had been broken.' Measurements, four years after the injury, revealed a shortening of three-quarters of an inch.

Bruns relates (Langenbeck, *Archiv für klinische Chirurgie*, 1882, Bd. xxvii.) two cases which came under his own observation. In one, almost identical with that of Vogt, a healthy, powerfully built man, aged forty-nine, had fallen when two years old from the arms of the nurse on to his right shoulder. The injury was treated, ·and no signs of inflammation followed, but the longitudinal growth of the arm. did not progress from this time, whilst the growth in thickness of the bone was not arrested. The shortening of the right humerus was enormous, amounting to 14 centimetres (nearly 6 inches); the neighbouring bones, clavicle, scapula, radius, and ulna and muscles were normal. All movements of the shoulder-joint were free except abduction, so that the patient could not elevate the arm above the horizontal position. There was some deformity or irregular projection, probably caused by displacement of the diaphysial end.

In the other case, a boy, aged twelve, had in his fourth year sustained an injury to his left arm by being lifted violently up by his arms. A sudden 'crack' was felt, and he found he could not use the arm.

Epiphysial separation was diagnosed, and a plaster of Paris splint was applied for some weeks. Bruns found a shortening of about four centimetres of the humerus, whilst the growth of the forearm was perfect. The shoulder-joint was completely ankylosed, so that all movements of the arms were carried out through the mobility of the scapula. Slight atrophy of the muscles of the arm and an indistinct projection of the diaphysis close to the epiphysis were found.

Helferich figures (*Atlas der traumatischen Fracturen und Luxationen*, München, 1897, Tab. 34, Fig. 2) the case of a man (Bertram, 1878) who had considerable shortening of the right humerus from arrest of growth, the result of an injury in very early youth to the epiphysial cartilage of the upper end of the humerus.

In common with many other observers, this surgeon believes

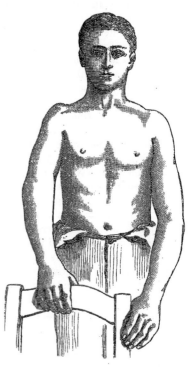

FIG. 57.—ARREST OF GROWTH OF HUMERUS AFTER INJURY TO ITS UPPER EPIPHYSIS. (AFTER HELFERICH)

that the amount of shortening is greatest when union has taken place with considerable displacement. It will, of course, vary according to the time which has elapsed since the accident.

The two following cases, mentioned by M. Curtillet as described by Dittmayer (Dittmayer, *Th. de Würzbourg*, 1887 ; Curtillet, *Du Décollement traumatique des Épiphyses*, Lyon, 1891), illustrate this very well.

In the first case a boy, aged thirteen years, had fallen on to his right shoulder at the age of eleven. Very acute pain in the shoulder and inability to move the arm were experienced at the time. Soft crepitus and abnormal mobility were detected on examination by a doctor, who fixed the arm in the adducted position with a pad in the axilla. At the end of three weeks the

S

arm was placed in a simple sling, and eight days later this was removed, and no further treatment adopted, as the patient appeared to be completely cured. No inflammatory condition was subsequently observed. On admission into hospital the right shoulder was found to be flattened, a depression was to be seen below the acromion, and at the same spot the humeral head could be felt still occupying its normal position. The deltoid muscle was wasted, but yet reacted to electricity. The osseous projection of the end of the diaphysis could be seen and felt displaced forwards and inwards in Morenheim's fossa. The shoulder-joint was completely ankylosed, and only slight abduction could be effected through movement of the scapula.

The clavicle, scapula, other bones, muscles, and joints of the forearm were normal, and the thickness of the arms on the two sides was the same. The shortening of the right arm, amounting to 2½ centimetres, was considered by Dittmayer to be due to arrest of growth following the disjunction, for the overlapping of the fragments could not have produced the same amount of shortening.

The second case was that of a boy, aged fourteen years, who had fallen, at the beginning of April (1887), from a ladder on to his right arm. Acute pain was felt, with loss of power over the limb. A disjunction of the upper humeral epiphysis was diagnosed, with displacement inwards and upwards of the diaphysis. Middeldorpf's triangular apparatus was applied, and the bone rapidly united by osseous material. Active and passive movements of the limb were obtained ; massage and electricity were employed successfully in restoring the function of the limb. However, on the patient's admission to the hospital, he could not carry out the movements of the arm completely nor elevate it above the horizontal position. There was some deformity due to the incomplete reduction of the displacement, and as a consequence of the ossification of the epiphysial line there was an arrest of development which gave rise to a shortening of 3 centimetres, but there was no diminution in the thickness of the limb, nor any other abnormality of the bones or soft parts.

Bryant mentions (*Guy's Hospital Reports*, third series, vol. viii. 1862, plate) having seen a woman, aged thirty, whose humerus was shortened five inches from a fall on the right shoulder in early infancy. There was atrophy of the deltoid and complete ankylosis of the shoulder-joint, but with the forearm well developed. Although the accident had not been followed by any suppuration, the case was a somewhat uncertain one, as due to traumatic causes alone.

A similar instance of three inches shortening of the humerus with impaired movements is recorded by Humphry in the *Royal Medico-Chirurgical Transactions*, vol. xlv. 1862, p. 285. The woman, aged seventy, had been told that the arm was natural at birth, but had been injured at the shoulder when she was six months old.

Mr. A. H. Tubby mentions (*Lancet*, June 6, 1891) a similar case of 3½ inches shortening of the humerus in a young lady, aged twenty-five years, who was injured at the age of three years by being lifted up by the right hand. The injury was diagnosed at the time as diastasis of the upper end of the humerus.

TABLE OF CASES IN WHICH ARREST OF GROWTH FOLLOWED SEPARATION OF THE UPPER EPIPHYSIS OF THE HUMERUS

Surgeon	Sex of patient	Age	Amount of shortening	Age when injured	Nature of injury, &c.
Hoffa	Male	29 years	6½ centimetres	9 years	Blow on shoulder from gun. No treatment
Vogt	Male	20 years	13 centimetres	10 years	Thought to be a sprain
Bruns	Male	49 years	14 centimetres	2 years	Fall from nurse on to shoulder
Bruns	Male	12 years	4 centimetres	4 years	Violently lifted by arms
Bryant	Female	30 years	5 inches	a few months	Injury to shoulder from a fall
Shearer	Male	53 years	4 inches	Not stated	Not stated
Tubby	Female	25 years	3½ inches	3 years	Diagnosed as epiphysial separation
Helferich	Male	?	?	very early youth	" "

Arrest of growth from inflammation due to traumatic causes.—In the *Guy's Hospital Reports*, 1862, 3rd series, vol. viii., Mr. Birkett reports an example of shortening by six inches, which was clearly due to extensive inflammation and suppuration about the upper epiphysis. A cicatrix was present.

Bidder and Langenbeck mention like cases. In Bidder's case the humerus was shortened six to seven centimetres, which was attributed by the patient to vaccination improperly performed.

Mr. Jonathan Hutchinson reported (*British Medical Journal*, July 25, 1885, p. 152) a remarkable case of arrest of growth of the left humerus in a young lad aged sixteen. The shortening amounted to four inches, and resulted from an injury followed by inflammation and ankylosis at the age of a year and a half. The injury was believed to have been slight, but it was followed by inflammation, and the arm was said to have been kept at rest for six months. There was bony ankylosis at the shoulder-joint, but there was no proof that the epiphysis had been detached. The clavicle and scapula were thin and atrophied, which might have been attributed to the absence of motion at the joint.

Dr. F. Shearer (*Brit. Med. Journal*, October 10, 1885, p. 700) also records an instance of four inches shortening of the arm in a man aged fifty-three, following a fracture of the humerus near the right shoulder-joint sustained at two years of age, which was doubtless a case of separation of the epiphysis, and, as in the cases just alluded to, was followed by inflammation and the formation of an abscess. There was no ankylosis of the shoulder, and therefore no atrophy of the shoulder girdle as in Hutchinson's case.

The same observer mentions a more authentic case which he had seen of a man aged fifty-three, whose arm was shortened by four inches, measuring from the tip of the acromion to the olecranon process. In other respects the right arm was well developed, and likewise the forearm. The shoulder-joint was not ankylosed, and there was no wasting of the muscles of the shoulder.

Arrest of growth may follow fractures other than epiphysiary separation.

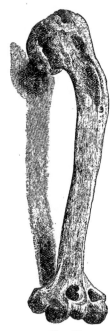

Fig. 59.
(Guy's Hospital Museum, ½ size)

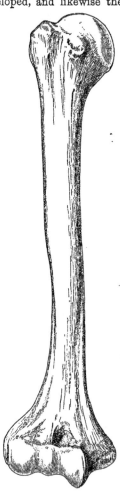

Fig. 58.—UNINJURED HUMERUS
(Guy's Hospital Museum, ½ size)

In the museum of Guy's Hospital there is a specimen of arrest of growth of the left humerus for three and a half inches after what was probably a fracture of the shaft at eight years old. The author removed it, as well as the opposite humerus, while acting as dresser to Mr. Bryant. Figured in Bryant's *Practice of Surgery*, 4th ed. vol. ii. 1884, p. 425.

Necrosis of the diaphysis and suppuration have been a common result of compound separations.

Necrosis occurred in Williams's and Bruns's cases and is seen in the specimen in the Charing Cross Hospital Museum. Extensive osteomyelitis and suppuration of the joint occurred in Esmarch's case in a child of five years. The head of the bone and the upper end of the diaphysis were excised with a good result—viz. a useful arm, with but little shortening, and a free shoulder-joint. Suppuration occurred in one of Hutchinson's cases, in a boy aged fourteen.

Gangrene, &c.—Although *gangrene* occurred in two instances, *permanent paralysis* from pressure and injury to the brachial plexus had not followed in any.

CHAPTER IV

SEPARATION OF THE LOWER END OF THE HUMERUS BEFORE PUBERTY

ANATOMY.—The lower end of the humerus, comprising the external and internal epicondyles, and the lower quarter of the coronoid and olecranon fossæ (Krause), remains cartilaginous from birth up to

the third year, with the exception of some scattered osseous granules in the capitellar portion.

Henle says this centre in the capitellum is distinguishable towards the second year. The author has often observed a distinct nucleus about the middle of the second year. Humphry notes its appearance at a few months after the centre of the head of the bone—viz. during the first year.

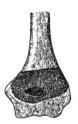

At the end of the third year the nucleus of the *capitellum*, which is therefore the first of the four centres to appear, attains a considerable size, and is situated at the beginning towards the inner side of this process, but rapidly spreads, so that at the termination of the sixth year the whole of this is in-

FIG. 60. — VERTICAL SECTION OF THE UPPER AND LOWER ENDS OF THE HUMERUS IN A CHILD AGED TWO YEARS AND NINE MONTHS

vaded. It also extends inwards so as to form the outer half of the trochlear surface, ending by becoming much thinner at the bottom of the trochlear groove, and it remains disconnected with the rest of the articular end of the humerus for more than ten years—i.e. till the fifteenth or sixteenth year. By the sixteenth year the whole of this portion of the articular surface is entirely osseous, and forms a hemispherical mass, with its convex surface below and in front towards the cup of the radius, whilst its upper slightly excavated surface is presented towards the end of the diaphysis.

The next centre to appear is that for the *inner epicondyle* (epitrochlea), which does so about the fifth year (Henle), or the fourth or fifth according to Sappey, though it may be delayed in its appearance until the tenth or eleventh year.

In the cartilage of the *trochlea* an osseous centre next becomes visible towards the projecting part or inner lip of this surface. Sometimes there are two, the second smaller one being more external and soon blending with the larger. This appears between the eleventh and twelfth years, at times a little later.

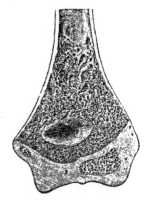

FIG. 61.—FRONTAL SECTION OF LOWER END OF HUMERUS AT THE AGE OF SIX AND A HALF YEARS. ANTERIOR HALF OF SECTION. CENTRES OF CAPITELLUM AND INTERNAL EPICONDYLE WELL DEVELOPED. ACTUAL SIZE

The last to appear is the nucleus for the *outer epicondyle*, which does so at the thirteenth or fourteenth year (Henle), sometimes a little later, in the middle of the cartilage forming this process; the latter is soon ossified throughout its small extent, and unites a year or two later—about the sixteenth year—with the two portions forming the articular surface.

The lower end of the humerus varies much in the times of complete ossification of its different component parts. They may all be entirely ossified as early as the fourteenth year, often as late as at the sixteenth year.

A most careful study of the exact shape and extent of this epiphysis, and of the articular connections and muscular attachments, is very essential to the proper understanding of the numerous and complicated lesions of the elbow-joint which occur in young subjects.

It is certain that separations of a portion (not the whole) of this wide epiphysis are much more frequent than they have hitherto been generally supposed to be.

Formation of the lower epiphysis.—Great confusion has existed amongst British and other writers with regard to the nomenclature of

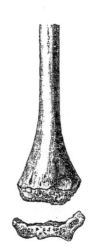

FIG. 62.—LOWER END OF THE HUMERUS, ABOUT THE ELEVENTH YEAR, SHOWING THE CARTILAGINOUS EPIPHYSIS DETACHED (AFTER RAMBAUD AND RENAULT)

At this age the centres of capitellum and internal epicondyle are fairly large, while some osseous granules indicate the centre for the trochlea. The epiphysis rises some millimetres above the lateral portions of the diaphysis. The fully formed coronoid and olecranon fossæ are limited below by the epiphysis.

the different parts of this epiphysis. The French terms introduced by Chaussier of condyle and epicondyle for the usual ones of capitellum and external epicondyle, and trochlea and epitrochlea for the trochlea and internal epicondyle, might well be adopted. In the older text-books of anatomy the terms inner and outer condyles, which are still adopted by most surgeons, have been applied to the internal epicondyle and external epicondyle. Not infrequently the condyles have vaguely been alluded to as including parts of the trochlea or capitellum respectively ; these names are still employed in this way by many American surgeons.

We still find in most anatomical works that the fully formed epiphysis is composed of four centres—internal condyle, external condyle, trochlea, and capitellum—and that these form the lower end of the humerus. They do so in the infant, and for the first few years of life ; after this time the end of the bone is very differently constituted.

Alex. Manquat (*Essai sur les décollements épiphysaires traumatiques*, 1877), in common with a few anatomists, makes a grave error when he says : ' The epicondyle (external epicondyle) unites with the condyle (capitellum) towards the fifteenth or sixteenth year, and the *epitrochlea (internal epicondyle) to the trochlea a little later, at the sixteenth or seventeenth year.*'

About the fifteenth or sixteenth year, the two portions of the articular surface formed by the capitellum and trochlea blend together (commencing at the groove of the trochlear surface) and produce one articular surface ; the external epicondyle is then joined on. These three portions form by their junction the lower epiphysis of the humerus, which does not include the internal epicondyle. This is relatively to the developing shaft much thinner than the cartilaginous lower end of the humerus of infancy, consequently the epiphysial line of junction is much nearer to the articular cavity than in the earlier period of life.

The internal epicondyle forms a distinct epiphysis by the downward growth of the diaphysis separating it from the rest of the end of the bone, which usually unites with the diaphysis without blending with the trochlea. This junction is effected from the eighteenth to the twentieth year, but as late as the twenty-fifth year traces of the line of junction may still be seen.

The lower end of the bone decreases relatively in size as childhood advances. The transverse measurement from the apex of the internal epicondyle to that of the external epicondyle is exactly six centimetres at the age of seventeen years, and its vertical depth is only eleven millimetres at the middle of the trochlear surface, while the width from epicondyle to epicondyle during the third year is about three centimetres, and the vertical depth seven millimetres. At fourteen and a half years the width is rather more than four and a half centimetres, and the depth eight millimetres.

It will thus be seen that as age advances the increase in size of the lower end of the bone is rather in width than in vertical depth. The point of junction of the trochlear and capitellar portions of the lower epiphysis at the middle of the trochlear groove at the sixteenth year is the narrowest portion of the bone, and much more likely to be broken across, detaching one or other portion of bone rather than the whole epiphysis separating at this age.

De Paoli gives the following table of measurements of the height and breadth of the lower epiphysis of the humerus in individuals of various ages taken in frontal section (dividing the epiphysis in two parts, one anterior and the other posterior).

Age	Height at the middle of the trochlea	Height at the middle of the condyle	Breadth at the upper part
Before birth. . .	.. ...6 mm.......	.... .. 8 mm.......	.........22 mm.
One year . . .	......6 ,, ...	......10 ,, ...	.........29 ,,
Two years . . .	......6 ,, ...	......— ,, ...	... .35 ,,
Four years . . .	......7 ,, ...	...... 8 ,, ...	.........36 ,,
Five years . . .	......6 ,, ...	......11 ,, ...	.........36 ,,
Six years . . .	......6 ,, ...	......11 ,, ...	.........37 ,,
Eight years . . .	......6 ,, ...	......12 ,, ...	.........41 ,,
Nine years . . .	......6 ,, ...	......12 ,, ...	.........40 ,,
Ten years . . .	......7 ,, ...	......11 ,, ...	.........41 ,,
Eleven years . . .	......4 ,, ...	......10 ,, ...	.........42 ,,
Thirteen years . .	......5 ,, ...	......10 ,, ...	.........42 ,,
Fifteen years . . .	......5 ,, ...	......10 ,, ...	.........52 ,,

It is common to find an error in surgical works as to the fully formed epiphysis. Thus Erichsen, alluding to separation of the lower epiphysis of the humerus as a frequent accident in children, makes the statement that in this accident the trochlea, the capitellum, and the condyles are broken off from the shaft, which remains *in situ.*

The anatomical difference of the lower epiphysis of the humerus at puberty and the lower end of the same bone in infancy led R. W. Smith to suppose that this epiphysis was only composed of the trochlea and capitellum, so that the epiphysial line ran below the epicondyles at all ages.

The upper surface of the lower end of the bone in childhood, when removed from the shaft, presents a number of projections which fit on to corresponding depressions on the end of the diaphysis. It is somewhat cup-shaped, or lipped, at the sides, rising about a quarter of an inch above the diaphysis. In infancy it is almost flat.

The olecranon and coronoid fossæ, as seen at the twelfth year, are formed almost entirely in the diaphysis, and are limited below by the osseous margin which corresponds to the epiphysis. While in infancy the cartilaginous epiphysial end completes the lower part of the olecranon fossa, in the fully formed bone the fossa is formed in no way by the epiphysis.

It is an error to suppose that the epiphysial line is transverse in the youth. It is almost so at birth, when the whole of the lower extremity of the humerus is cartilaginous, and remains like this for a few years, completely above the epicondyles. The diaphysis in its growth enlarges, thickens at each side to form the lateral projections, and extends downwards, forming the whole of the olecranon fossa; but it is especially on the inner side, towards the internal epicondyle, that the increase takes place, apparently at the expense of the epiphysis. The humeral diaphysis penetrates, as it were, the trochlea, and gives great support to this part of the epiphysis, the separation of which will become more difficult after the age of four years. However, on the outer side the epiphysis remains much thicker—nearly double the size of the trochlea—is not invaded by the diaphysis, and consists of more than half an inch of bone as seen from behind, above the articular surface of the capitellum.

So that at about thirteen years of age the epiphysial line will be seen to be placed very obliquely downwards and inwards, the epiphysis on the inner side being thin, and limited precisely by the cartilage-clad area in front and behind. On the inner side it rises slightly towards the internal epicondyle, which at this age is almost separated from the rest of the lower extremity of the growing diaphysis. The external epicondyle is very rarely isolated in the same manner from the epiphysis.

The epiphysial line at this age is relatively much nearer to the articular surface than in infancy, from the increasing growth of the diaphysis. It is still, as in infancy, above the external, but below the internal epicondyle, which is now excluded from its formation. The epiphysial line of epiphysis proper, comprising the external epicondyle, capitellum, and trochlea, is therefore very obliquely placed if we draw a transverse line uniting the apex of the two epicondyles. The plane of the articular surface likewise makes an acute angle inwards with the same transverse line. On the outer side the epiphysial line terminates above the external epicondyle, and on the inner side below the internal epicondyle. The distance from the latter increases slightly as the diaphysis grows downwards, and the internal epicondyle is further removed from the epiphysis until the time of complete union.

This epiphysis after its complete formation rapidly unites to the diaphysis, being firmly welded on by the seventeenth year. After this year the growth in length of the humerus is therefore arrested as far as the lower extremity is concerned, but it is carried on by the epiphysis of the upper extremity till adolescence.

Some anatomists have stated that the external, but more frequently the internal epicondyle, after being quite developed and osseous, often remains isolated for a considerable number of years, sometimes for life.

Relations of the synovial membrane to the epiphysial lines.—The lower extremity of the humeral diaphysis has very extensive relations with the synovial membrane.

The synovial membrane, as seen at fifteen years of age, passes for some distance upwards over the epiphysial line of cartilage, both in front and behind the lower end of the humerus. In front it is thick, and but loosely connected with the diaphysis, and springs from the articular surface. It is readily detached from the coronoid and radial fossæ in front, whereas behind it is much thinner and extends upwards from the articular surface, being firmly attached to the lower part of the olecranon fossa beneath the lobe of fat fitting the upper part of this cavity.

Hence it is obvious that the synovial membrane may be easily torn through, and the articulation liable to be opened at the olecranon fossa in separations of the lower epiphyses. On a vertical median section we see that at the olecranon fossa the synovial membrane overlaps the diaphysis for 0·008 millimetres at three years of age, and for fifteen millimetres at thirteen years of age (Sésary). Behind the capitellar portion of the epiphysis, the synovial membrane does not quite reach up to the epiphysial line.

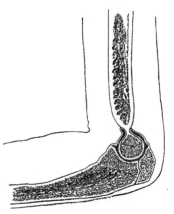

The synovial membrane on the *outer side* passes up on the outer aspect of the capitellum above the articular surface as far as the external epicondyle, rendering it possible for the synovial membrane to be opened here in separation of this process.

On the *inner side* the synovial membrane does not extend upwards

FIG. 63.—SAGITTAL SECTION OF THE ELBOW-JOINT ; HUMERO-ULNAR ARTICULATION IN A YOUTH AGED FIFTEEN AND A HALF YEARS, SHOWING THE RELATION OF THE SYNOVIAL MEMBRANE TO THE EPIPHYSIAL LINES

over the inner aspect of the trochlea, much above the epiphysial line ; about three-sixteenths of an inch below the internal epicondyle. Therefore, detachment of this process is not necessarily accompanied by opening of the articular cavity.

The epiphysial line lies more deeply in the joint during childhood than it does in infancy.

Detachment of the capitellar or trochlear portions of the epiphysis must necessarily be associated with opening of the articular cavity, through the fracture of the articular cartilage uniting these two portions about the middle of the trochlear surface. This opening of the cavity will happen whether these portions of the epiphysis are connected with the corresponding external and internal epicon-

dyles or the contrary. The external epicondyle will most likely
accompany such a separation of the capitellum from the fifteenth
to the seventeenth year of age.

The *capsule* of the joint is attached to the humerus immediately
above the coronoid and radial fossæ in front, and is continuous at the

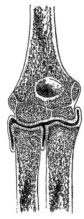

sides with the lateral ligaments, which
are merely thickened portions of the
capsule. It is attached here to the
lower aspects of the external and internal epicondyles. Behind, it is attached
to the humerus in a line passing
through the upper part of the olecranon
fossa; below, to the edges of the olecranon and coronoid processes of the
ulna, to the edge of the greater sigmoid
cavity, and to the orbicular ligament
surrounding the head of the radius.

The precise relationship of the articular structures is important not only
from the occurrence of the separation
being attended by a fracture into the
joint, but from the facility with which
the extensive synovial membrane in-
flames in the case of separations in
its neighbourhood. The effusion into
its cavity renders both the diagnosis

FIG. 64.—FRONTAL SECTION OF BONES
FORMING THE LEFT ELBOW-JOINT
OF A CHILD FOURTEEN YEARS NINE
MONTHS OLD. FRONT HALF OF
SECTION. ᴇRELATION OF SYNOVIAL
MEMBRAN TO THE EPIPHYSES

and treatment more difficult.

The close proximity of the median and musculo-spiral nerves,
and brachial vessels in front, and the ulnar nerve behind, to the
end of the diaphysis must always be remembered.

AGE.—Composing the thirteen *pathological specimens* here collected there were four at the age of two years, one at four, one at
ten, one at thirteen, two 'in children,' and two in which the age was
not given. In two old separations the age was between four and six.

Out of the seventeen *compound* cases the age is given in
thirteen—two at thirteen, one at eleven, two at ten, one at eight
and a half, one at eight, one at seven, three at six, and one at three
years of age. In three the age is not stated. In one the separation
occurred in a girl, and in another the age is given as fifteen
(Bryant's); the latter is a dubious one, inasmuch as the condition of
the parts at the time of operation is insufficiently stated. It may
have been a very unusual case of delayed ossification of the epiphysis.

In the author's own records of forty-two *simple* cases, one in a
recently born child is very questionable. Apart from this—there
are six in which the age is not stated; three occurred in young
children, and one in a boy. The youngest patient was one year and
eight months, and the two oldest thirteen years old; two cases occurred

at twelve, one at eleven, two at ten, two at nine and a half, two at nine, nine at eight, three at seven, three at five, three at four, and one at two years of age.

Out of the total of *seventy-two cases*, the age was given in fifty-five, while seven were in children or young boys, and forty-four occurred from about the second up to the tenth year.

Although some surgeons consider this injury to be very rare after the age of four years, certainly it is only possible as a complete separation of the whole lower end before thirteen years of age.

D'Arcy Power says (*Surgical Diseases of Children*, 1895, p. 174) : ' The lower epiphysis may be separated at any time up to the thirteenth or fourteenth year, though the separation is somewhat more frequent under four years of age.'

Out of fifty-two cases collected by Mr. Hutchinson junior (*Brit. Med. Journal*, December 31, 1893) twenty-four were simple separations (fifteen under his own care), twenty-three complicated, mostly compound ; and five cases of old separation of the epiphysis. He thought that clean separation was present probably only in the minority. The youngest patient was eighteen months old, the oldest fourteen years.

Out of fifty cases of fracture of the lower end of the humerus which came under the care of Dr. C. A. Powers of New York, nine were over twenty years of age and forty-one were under. Of the forty-one, thirteen were under five, twelve between five and ten, thirteen between ten and fifteen, and three between fifteen and twenty years of age.

SEX.—In only two of the author's cases is it stated that the accident occurred in girls, but it should be noted that in a very great number of instances mention is merely made that the accident occurred to children.

ETIOLOGY.—Separation of the entire epiphysis is usually produced by *direct violence* applied to the elbow, such as a fall upon the elbow while bent, or the passage of a cartwheel over it, or a kick from a horse.

In other cases the violence is more *indirect*, the force being transmitted through the bones of the forearm, as by a fall upon the outstretched hand, the forearm being semiflexed.

In one case the patient had fallen upon the hand, and in another a boy fell across the back of the extended limb.

Separation has been known to occur from a fall upon the palm of the hand, the forearm and elbow being at the time in the extended position ; also from falling on the forearm.

On the dead body, it is remarkably easy to separate the lower epiphysis of the humerus in infancy by forcible hyper-extension or flexion of the forearm ; more especially the author has found it detachable from the third to the eighth year. Schüller and others have made the same observation.

In 1876 Berthomier found in his experiments that less violence was required to effect epiphysial separation than to fracture the lower end of the humerus. He observed that direct traction on the forearm led usually to an epiphysial fracture of the humerus; that it was perfect and pure up to ten years of age, and accompanied by small scales of bone beyond that age; and he believed that falls upon the hand which produced an injury of the elbow always produced a more or less perfect separation of the lower epiphysis of the humerus.

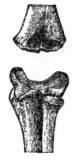

FIG. 65.—DIAGRAM OF SEPARATION OF THE LOWER END OF THE HUMERUS BEFORE PUBERTY

Separation produced in the body of a girl aged six and a half. The whole cartilaginous mass of the lower end of the humerus, consisting of both epicondyles, the trochlea, and capitellum, is cleanly detached.

Bardenheuer thought that separation was most frequently brought about by adduction or abduction of the forearm while in the extended or flexed position.

The narrow lower end of the humerus escapes detachment in many falls upon the elbow on account of the protection afforded by the bones of the forearm, as well as by its own elasticity. It is at this early period—i.e. up to the eleventh or twelfth year—almost entirely composed of cartilage; a much greater amount of force will consequently be required to separate it than if it were osseous, so that Gurlt and others are right in believing that on the living subject this lesion always requires a great degree of violence for its production.

PATHOLOGICAL ANATOMY.—Of all injuries to the elbow-joint, those to the epiphyses of the humerus are the most important and complicated.

Writing in 1886 (*Bulletins et Mémoires de la Société de Chirurgie,* Paris, 1886, N. s. xii.) M. Farabeuf says, very erroneously, that separation of the whole lower end of the humerus cannot occur after about the fourth year; but his experiments and remarks upon the osseous epiphysis of early puberty, formed by the capitellum, trochlea, and external epicondyle, which he calls the lower epiphysis, are interesting, and will be alluded to in Chapter V.

Other surgeons have, on the contrary, declared separation of the lower epiphysis of the humerus to be the most frequent of all epiphysial separations. From the published records it appears to be not uncommon, but not so much so as some other epiphysial separations; yet cases examined anatomically have been seldom met with. Up to the time of Bruns's paper four cases only had been recorded as verified in this way.

Gurlt considered it a very rare injury.

Bardenheuer agrees (*Deutsche Chirurgie*) with Schüller's opinion that it is far more frequent than is generally supposed, and says that three times he has resected cases of old injury in which the whole epiphysis in children of four to six years of age had been broken off the diaphysis and displaced backwards. The function of the limb was considerably impaired, flexion being quite impossible In two cases the capitellum, together with the external epicondyle, was separated and accompanied on the inner side with a fracture above the trochlea.

Malgaigne very rightly classes disjunction of this epiphysis with supracondyloid fractures of the humerus.

The lower epiphysis of the humerus is often found to be detached in severe direct injury or crushing of the elbow and arm. Polaillon mentions (*Affections chirurgicales des membres*, 1885, p. 687) the case of a little boy, aged seven and a half years, whose right arm was crushed under the wheel of a carriage. Through an extensive wound the elbow-joint was seen to be opened, and the lower epiphysis of the humerus separated. The humeral diaphysis was broken into several fragments and the muscles pulped. Death took place from shock six hours after disarticulation of the shoulder.

The separation takes place in the usual position in the ossifying layer immediately adjoining the epiphysial cartilage.

It is possible for it to occur in the cartilaginous layer itself, but no specimens exist. Yet a portion of the cartilage has remained attached to the diaphysis in several of the compound separations of part of the epiphysis recorded in advancing childhood.

St. Thomas's Hospital Museum, No. 115 (*Descriptive Catalogue of the Pathological Museum, St. Thomas's Hospital*, Part I. 1890, p. 22, 2nd edition), contains the best specimen of a complete and pure separation of this epiphysis, presented by Sir William MacCormac. It consists of the lower part of a child's humerus, showing a complete separation of the lower epiphysis along the normal line of junction (see fig. 66).

The epicondyles remain with the trochlea and capitellum as a whole. The internal epicondyle has an osseous centre of $\frac{2}{3}$ of an inch in diameter, and the external has dragged away a few granules of the diaphysis along its base. The diaphysis is otherwise uninjured.

Stimson says (*Treatise on Fractures*, 1883, p. 411) : 'There is also a specimen in the museum of Bellevue Hospital, U.S.A., of the bones of the forearm of a child with a shrunken cartilage attached, which seems to be the lower epiphysis of the humerus.'

In St. Mary's Hospital (*St. Mary's Hospital Museum Pathological Catalogue*, 1891, p. 10) is a specimen, No. 94, of a pure separation of the lower epiphysis of the humerus, the separation passing exactly through the epiphysial junction without any fracture of the diaphysis, but the olecranon is fractured into three pieces. No cartilage remained on the humeral diaphysis, the separation being in the juxta-epiphysial layer of new bone. It was taken from a child aged about four years, whose arm was 'jammed' in a gate.

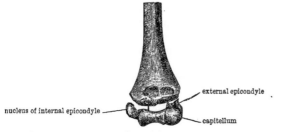

FIG. 66.—PURE SEPARATION OF LOWER END OF HUMERUS BEFORE PUBERTY.
(ST. THOMAS'S HOSPITAL MUSEUM)

In this specimen most of the articular end is cartilage ; that in connection with the external epicondyle forms a cap to the bone of the shaft. For this drawing the author is indebted to Mr. S. G. Shattock, who kindly sketched it for him.

The brachial artery was bruised and subsequently thrombosed, but the separation was a simple one. The limb was amputated by Mr. Page at the shoulder-joint, traumatic gangrene threatening to spread upwards (see fig. 67).

St. George's Hospital Museum contains a specimen of united fracture a quarter of an inch above the epiphysial line which was only distinguishable from epiphysial separation during life by the rough loud crepitus. The diaphysis was displaced forwards, and the gap behind filled up with new bone. The specimen is described by Mr. Holmes in the *Path. Soc. Trans.* vol. xiii. p. 186.

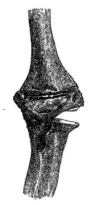

FIG. 67.—COMPLETE SEPARATION OF THE LOWER END OF THE HUMERUS AT ABOUT FOUR YEARS OF AGE. (ST. MARY'S HOSPITAL MUSEUM)

In the London Hospital Museum is a specimen, No. 389 (*London Hospital Museum Catalogue*, 1890, p. 92), of compound fracture near to the line of the lower epiphysis. The lower end of the upper fragment projected into the wound, and was accordingly sawn off. The line of junction of the epiphysis was pretty nearly followed. The patient recovered with a stiff elbow.

Separation with vertical fracture of epiphysis into elbow-joint. It is quite possible for simple separation to be complicated with a vertical fracture into the elbow-joint, either between the trochlea and capitellum, or through the trochlea at the junction of the two epiphysial portions.

There is, however, no specimen in existence showing this form of lesion.

Separation, with slight fracture of the diaphysis.—As the period of childhood advances, in all probability the greater will be the likelihood of separation being accompanied by a detachment of some small portion of the diaphysis. This is, indeed, a not uncommon form of injury Even in infants, a portion of the bone may be torn away.

In 1818 Champion (*Journal Complément. du Diction. des Sci. Méd.*, Paris, 1818, tom. 1, p. 323) described the case of a boy, aged thirteen, whose arm had been caught (1816) by the sleeve and rolled round seven times by some machinery.

The separation was without difficulty made out on account of the absence of swelling of the arm—the easily recognised lower end of the humerus being twisted from before backwards, and from within outwards. The displacement was readily reduced by twisting the forearm in an opposite direction.

On dissection there was revealed a complete separation of the lower epiphysis of the humerus, together with a thin flake from the posterior and outer part of the diaphysis the size of a finger-nail, half an inch in width and a quarter of an inch in thickness. The periosteum was stripped from the outer side of the diaphysis up to the insertion of the deltoid, and the anterior and posterior capsular ligaments of the joint were lacerated in front and behind, as well as the portion of the synovial membrane which corresponded to the separation of the epiphysis. Compound fracture of the bones of the forearm rendered primary amputation of the arm necessary, and the patient recovered. The epiphysis preserved its relations with the bones of the forearm by means of the lateral and capsular ligaments.

In the London Hospital Museum, No. 550A (*loc. cit. supra*, p. 121), is a specimen of separation of the lower epiphysis of the humerus, accompanied by fracture of the femur a short distance above the inferior epiphysial line, and other injuries. They were caused by the parents, who, whilst drunk, dragged the child about by its limbs. The child's age is not stated, but it was probably about two years.

Partial separation, with fracture of diaphysis.—A very common condition, as seen by the number recorded below under compound separations.

The outer portion of the epiphysis, consisting of the capitellum and external epicondyle, appears to be most often detached, the fracture then passing through a portion of the diaphysis above the epiphysial line of the internal epicondyle and trochlea.

Mr. Jonathan Hutchinson junior's specimen at the Royal College of Surgeons Museum, 1888, No. 940A, is a good example.

It consists of the right elbow-joint, from a child aged two, showing incomplete detachment of the lower epiphysis of the humerus, the periosteum being torn from the back of the diaphysis.

The line of separation has followed almost exactly the epiphysial disk, except at the inner side, where a small piece has been wrenched off the diaphysis for ¾ inch in height and ½ inch in width. The injury was due to the child being violently dragged about by the arm.

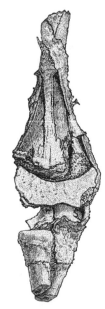

Schüller found the same condition in his experiments, and Bardenheuer alludes to the frequency of this form of injury.

Mr. Jonathan Hutchinson junior's specimen, Royal College of Surgeons Museum, No. 940ʙ, 1889, comprises the lower end of the left humerus from a child aged two years, who fell out of bed sixteen days before death (which was due to croup). The lower epiphysis has been separated, taking with it a small part of the adjacent diaphysial end on the inner side, while on the outer half it is through the epiphysial line. The displacement was backwards and inwards. Under treatment with an angular splint, bony union had already occurred to a great extent, chiefly through cartilaginous formation. But some lateral displacement, with forward projection of the diaphysis, may still be seen in the preparation.

Fig. 68.—Partial separation, with fracture of the diaphysis. (Royal College of Surgeons Museum)

Hamilton showed, before the New York Pathological Society (*New York Medical Journal*, September 1865, p. 461), a partial separation of the lower epiphysis of the humerus. A girl, aged ten, had fallen on her elbow. Three weeks afterwards the upper fragment was thrust through the skin. Resection was refused by the parents, so amputation was performed. The line of separation passed partly through the epiphysial line and partly through the diaphysis.

Dr. Little, at the same society, May 1865 (*New York Medical Journal*, vol. ii. 1866, p. 133), presented the lower end of a humerus, with a portion of the epiphysis, which he had removed. The injury which occasioned its removal was a fracture which extended half across the epiphysial line and then across the lower extremity of the bone higher up. The patient recovered with a stiff arm.

Bardenheuer alludes (*loc. cit. supra*) to two cases of old separation of the capitellum and external epicondyle, together with fracture above the trochlea on the inner side, in which he performed resection for loss of function, flexion being entirely lost. The ages were from four to six years of age.

A partial separation of the inner and middle portion of the lower humeral epiphysis is portrayed by Helferich (*Atlas der trauma-tischen Fracturen und Luxationen*, 1895, Tab. 30, Fig. 1*a* and 1*b*). There existed also a transverse fracture and fissure of the humeral shaft, and a longitudinal fracture of the ulna associated with a separation of the olecranon epiphysis. The radius was uninjured. The injury to the child's arm was caused by a severe machinery accident which necessitated amputation.

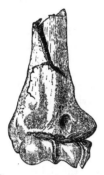
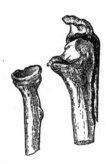

FIG. 69.—PARTIAL SEPARATION OF EPI-PHYSIS, WITH FISSURE AND TRANSVERSE FRACTURE OF THE SHAFT (AFTER HELFERICH)

FIG. 70.—SEPARATION OF THE OLE-CRANON EPIPHYSIS, WITH LONGITUDINAL FRACTURE OF SHAFT (AFTER HELFERICH, SAME CASE)

COMPOUND SEPARATIONS. **Pure separations.**—Many compound separations have revealed the precise condition of the separated fragments. Mr. Hutchinson says a compound fracture at the line of the epiphysis is necessarily a compound fracture into the joint, since it was barely possible the joint should not be opened. The author cannot agree with this unless it be a complicated case, and associated with a vertical fracture into the articular surface, or with a fracture between the internal epicondyloid portion and trochlea surface, opening the synovial membrane at that spot.

In the following instance part, at any rate, of the epiphysial cartilage adhered to the diaphysis.

Mr. Jonathan Hutchinson related, from the London Hospital, the case (*Medical Times and Gazette*, April 7, 1866, p. 360) of a lad, aged thirteen,. in whom the lower end of the diaphysis projected through a large laceration in front of the left elbow. From the character of the exposed surface it was clear that the line of epiphysial junction had been almost accurately observed.

Although there was no difficulty in reduction, the end was resected, as it was thought that sufficient extension could not be effected through the injury to the soft parts ; the lower end of the upper fragment would certainly have rested in front of the lower fragment and elbow-joint, and deformity would have resulted. The lower margin of the fragment removed was capped with the epiphysial cartilage. The lad subsequently had his elbow bent at a right angle and quite stiff, but he could use his arm well. Mr. Hutchinson says the ankylosis at the elbow was unavoidable, and must have occurred whatever the treatment had been. It is probable that this was an unusually complicated case of separation, suggesting also a fracture between the internal epicondyle and trochlea, opening the synovial membrane on this side, and a fissure extending between the trochlear and capitellar portions.

Spillman (*Bull. de la Soc. de Chirurg.*, Paris, 1875, November 10, p. 771) records the following case of compound separation in the epiphysial line directly above the epicondyle and epitrochlea.

The boy, aged eleven years, fell off a mule at full gallop, causing a transverse wound four centimetres long on the outer side of the biceps tendon, one centimetre above the bend of the left elbow, through which the end of the diaphysis protruded. The diaphysis was separated directly above the epicondyle (external epicondyle) and the epitrochlea (internal epicondyle), and comprised a small portion of the olecranon fossa. It was only after resection of forty-three millimetres of its end under chloroform that reduction was effected, the periosteum being carefully preserved. There was no fracture of the epiphysis penetrating the joint. The elbow was placed in splints in a semiflexed position, and the patient recovered the complete use of his arm, although he fell about the ninth week and refractured the humerus a little above the site of resection, which caused a small sequestrum to separate in the eighteenth week.

Spillman also mentions a second case (*Bull. de la Soc. de Chirurgie*, Paris, 1875, p. 772) which presented a precisely similar lesion to the last, with detachment of the periosteum and a small flake of the diaphysis. The child (O. A.), aged six years, had fallen from a wall one metre high. The same difficulty was experienced in reduction of the displaced diaphysis, and it was necessary to remove twenty-eight millimetres of the diaphysial end before it could be effected. With the exception of the formation of a small abscess on the inner side of the arm, which was opened, the wound healed, and consolidation took place in about five weeks' time, the humerus of each side being equal in length; and the child had completely recovered when it left the hospital a month later.

Dr. Lange, of New York, had a similar case (Hamilton, *Fractures and Dislocations*, 1884, p. 291, fig. 80) of compound separation of this epiphysis, the separation following the conjugal cartilage. The epiphysis was removed through the wound, with a portion of the diaphysis, and the patient recovered with a useful arm.

Maisonneuve (*Clinique Chirurgicale*, 1863, tome i. p. 533) met with a compound separation of the lower epiphysis, the shaft projecting a considerable distance through a large lacerated wound at the lower and antero-external part of the arm, whilst the lower epiphysis remained in its normal position. The periosteum was completely stripped off the protruding bone for about four centimetres, but remained adherent to the epiphysial cartilage below, and was torn longitudinally for the passage of the shaft. The diaphysial end was regular and perfectly free from any fracture, and was an exact counterpart of the supra-epiphysial portion of the bone. The patient, a boy (A.) aged seven, had fallen about three metres with his left hand stretched forwards. Reduction was effected with some difficulty, and Maisonneuve replaced the bone within its periosteal sheath. The limb was kept semiflexed with a plaster splint. In two months the wound healed, and a complete recovery ensued after the lapse of eighteen months, all the movements of the limb having recovered to their fullest extent by the regular active use of the arm combined with massage and sulphur baths.

In his address in Surgery (*British Medical Journal*, 1867, vol. ii. Aug. 17, p. 123) at Dublin, 1867, R. W. Smith alluded to a case under the care of Dr. Hutton in the Richmond Hospital, Dublin. The injury was compound, the extremities of the radius and ulna, surmounted by the epiphysis of the humerus, projecting through a large transverse wound, which was placed at the back of the elbow; and an opportunity was thus afforded of observing the anatomical characters of this injury and the relative position of the bones which is not presented when the wound is situated in front of the articulation. Two projections were visible posteriorly, both placed above and behind the plane of the condyles, the inner formed by the olecranon, the outer by the capitellum of the humerus surmounting the head of the radius.

The *Indian Medical Record* (Calcutta), April 1, 1892, vol. iii. p. 119, contains the following case of separation of the lower epiphysis of the humerus and protrusion of the upper fragment through the skin, reported by Surgeon Captain Geo. S. Thomson, M.B., Indian Medical Service (Deesa). It occurred in a little boy three years of age. Whilst playing he fell from a bridge on February 27, 1892, alighting on his right elbow, which was then in a bent position; he was a very heavy child for his age, and a *compound* fracture of the humerus just above the condyles was produced. The upper fragment—consisting of the shaft of the bone down to the coronoid and olecranon fossæ and including a small portion of the thin lamella of bone between those hollows—projected externally for fully one inch through a large wound at the outer side of the arm above the elbow-joint. The lower fragment and elbow-joint were carried upwards and backwards behind the shaft of the bone to its inner side. The forearm was slightly flexed upon the arm, at an angle of about thirty degrees at the elbow; and the hand and forearm were held pronated. The child complained of very little pain, and there was but trifling hæmorrhage.

An attempt was made to reduce the displaced fragments by gentle manipulation, but this resulted in failure, owing to the contraction and rigidity of the muscles surrounding the elbow. Under anæsthesia the fracture was readily adjusted.   The wound was cleansed with perchloride of mercury lotion; and iodoform, sal alembroth wool, and angular splints were applied. Next day the dressings were re-applied and the limb was put up in a plaster-of-Paris bandage in a semiflexed position; a window was then cut in the bandage when it had set, and through this *dry* antiseptic dressings were applied to the wound. *Eight* days after the accident the plaster-of-Paris bandage was slit up, and the amount of union present warranted passive motion being employed in a very steady and gentle manner in order, as far as possible, to prevent ankylosis.   The moulded plaster-of-Paris splint was re-applied, but was dispensed with the third day following, and passive motion was persevered with daily. The wound healed without suppuration, and was completely healed on March 12, or fifteen days after the accident. The child regained the perfect use of his arm, and could place it on his head, on the opposite shoulder, and up to his mouth; in fact, all the motions of the elbow-joint were unimpaired at the date of the report—twenty-one days after the accident.

Dr. John Ashhurst published in the *University Medical Magazine*, Philadelphia, April 1892, p. 518, another example of compound separation of the lower epiphysis of the humerus, in which resection was performed.

Wm. F., aged eight years, was admitted to the University hospital, when the upper fragment, consisting of the diaphysis of the humerus, projected nearly three inches from a large triangular-shaped wound on the anterior surface of the arm a short distance above the elbow.   The brachial artery could be seen stretched across the wound, pulseless, but apparently uninjured, while the arm below the seat of injury was cold. The question of amputation arose, but the youth of the patient, combined with the fact that the wound was produced by the protrusion of the bone itself from within outwards, and that the main vessels were probably uninjured, impelled Dr. Ashhurst to make an attempt at saving the arm.   In order to effect reduction an inch of bone was removed, after which the protruding part was easily replaced. A counter-opening was made, a drainage-tube passed through, and the wound closed, after having been thoroughly washed out with a warm solution of bichloride of mercury, 1 in 2,000. It was then dressed antiseptically, and the arm placed on an internal angular splint. The circulation returned to the hand in a few hours. At the first dressing, on the fifth day, the drainage tube was shortened, and at the second dressing, six days later, it was removed. Passive motion was practised as soon as the external wound was healed. The splint was removed in eight weeks, and the arm supported by soap plaster and a bandage. The union eight weeks after the injury was firm. There was then some movement at the elbow-joint, with very good motion in the direction of pronation and supination.

Dr. Harry Finley kindly sent the author the notes of the following case which came under his notice. Alex. A., æt. seven years, was admitted to Carlisle Infirmary, July 11, 1894, under Dr. H. A. Lediard. He had fallen whilst climbing some iron railings. On examination, the lower end of the diaphysis of the humerus was protruding through a vertical wound just large enough to admit its passage, about one and a quarter inches from the centre of the bend of·the elbow-joint. The bone was quite bare of periosteum and cartilage. The deformity was very well marked, the forearm being halfway between supination and pronation, movable without pain and displaced backwards; but for the appearance of the humerus it would have looked much like a dislocation of the forearm backwards. However, the lower epiphysis could be readily felt, there being no effusion. Reduction not being accomplished, even after some enlargement of the wound, a piece of the shaft about three quarters of an inch long was sawn off, within an hour, under chloroform, and the shaft was then easily replaced and found to have its proper relation to the periosteum. The epiphysis appeared to be entire, without fracture into the joint. After the usual douching, &c., a small drainage tube was inserted and the wound closed. The tube was removed on the fourth day. The arm was put up in an anterior splint, and an internal right-angled splint on alternate days till August 6, when the patient was discharged. In December all the movements of the joint were excellent, and there was no backward or other displacement, and very little if any thickening around the end of the diaphyses. The 'carrying angle' was increased about 20°. There was no more than $\frac{3}{4}$ inch difference in the length of the two arms.

Compound separation, with fracture of the diaphysis.—Fracture of the diaphysis to a greater or less extent is usually observed in compound separations.

In 1864 Dr. J. C. Reeve, of Ohio (*Hamilton's Fractures and Dislocations*, 7th edition, 1884, p. 291, fig. 79; *Cincinnati Lancet and Clinic*, November 23, 1878, p. 386), saw a girl, aged ten, who had fallen a few feet, striking, probably, her elbow. The separation being compound, the end of the humerus protruded in front. Union not having occurred at the end of three weeks, as the arm had been kept for about two weeks on a wooden splint without a particle of padding, and the olecranon was projecting from a large ulcerated wound behind, the condition of the arm rendered amputation necessary. A small fragment of the shaft came away with the epiphysis.

Dr. J. A. Macdougall (*Edinburgh Medical Journal*, March 1891, p. 827) mentions the following case of compound separation with a shaving of the shaft attached. B. G., a little lad of ten, fell from the railing of an outside staircase, and in landing pitched upon his right elbow. On examination it was found that the shaft of the humerus

protruded from a ragged and contused wound on the outer side of the
arm immediately above the elbow, the fracture having taken place a
little way below the expansion of the condyles. The separation had
occurred immediately above, and passed through the line of the
epiphysis from before backwards, and it was noted that the periosteum was entirely stripped from the posterior surface of the exposed
humerus for nearly an inch. Primary excision was performed, and
gave a very excellent result.

Bardenheuer also removed the diaphysial end of the humerus,
which projected directly forwards in a second case—figured by him
(*Deutsche Chirurgie*)—complicated with fracture of the posterior
part of this end, which remained attached to the epiphysis.

In a case alluded to by Mr. Hutchinson junior (*British Med.
Journal*, 1893, December 30, p. 1417), the detachment followed the
epiphysial line exactly, except at the extreme external part. The
patient was aged thirteen. Primary amputation was performed.

In the majority of the pathological specimens, and in the compound separations just mentioned, the epiphysis was displaced more
or less *backwards* from the diaphysis.

Displacement forwards of the epiphysis.—A unique case of transverse fracture of the lower end of the humerus immediately above
the epiphysial line, with displacement forwards, indistinguishable
from pure separation of the epiphysis, and associated with separation
of the olecranon epiphysis, came under the author's observation in
1893.

On May 17, 1893, a girl, H. B., aged six years, fell from a third-
story window, her head striking the pavement below. She was
admitted to the Miller Hospital a quarter of an hour after the accident, with fracture of the parietal bone and severe concussion of
the brain. There was severe contusion and swelling of the elbow,
with what was believed to be separation of the lower epiphysis of
the humerus, fractured olecranon process, and fracture of the shaft
of the ulna about the junction of the upper and middle third. She
recovered from the fractured skull, and the injured humerus and
ulna appeared to unite very well, although there was some deformity.
However, she was admitted again on July 25, with the history of
having fallen twice downstairs upon her elbow. The movement of
the elbow, which was pretty free when she left the hospital, was
now very restricted. Flexion was only possible to an angle of 125°,
and extension to an angle of 135°. The olecranon process was now
found to be separated about half an inch from the rest of the
bone, and firmly fixed at the back of the elbow. On August 10
(three months after the accident) she was placed under the author's
care for operation by Mr. Thomas Moore, who had been in charge of
the case. The movements of the elbow-joint were then very slight,
flexion being prevented by the impact of the head of the radius
against the front of the lower end of the humerus, and there was

much deformity. The condition of the elbow only permitted excision of the joint, which was performed.

Examination of the parts removed by this excision showed that the whole epiphysis and epicondyles of the humerus had been removed, together with a small portion of the lower end of the humeral diaphysis, the greater portion of the cup-like end of the radius, the olecranon process, and a portion of the upper end of the ulna. The humerus had been transversely fractured immediately above the epiphysis, so that the track on each side almost touched the cartilaginous epicondyles, whilst in the centre it was rather more than a quarter of an inch above the epiphysial line. The epiphysis, showing a considerable osseous

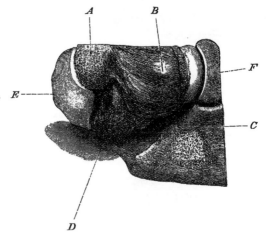

Fig. 71.—FRACTURE OF DIAPHYSIS DIRECTLY ABOVE EPIPHYSIS. DISPLACEMENT OF EPIPHYSIS FORWARDS. SEPARATION OF OLECRANON EPIPHYSIS. PARTS REMOVED BY EXCISION. (NATURAL SIZE)

A, Lower end of humerus. B, External epicondyle. C, Upper end of ulna. D, Space at olecranon fossa between the olecranon fragments filled with fibrous tissue. E, Olecranon epiphysis displaced and united to lower end of humerus. F, Portion of head of radius.

nucleus in the capitellar and commencing ossification in the internal epicondylar portion, was displaced forwards with the head of the radius and the ulna, and firmly united to the lower end of the humerus in this position. The capitellum of the humerus thus looked directly forwards, and the anterior margin of the radial cup in this displaced position had come in contact with the front of the humerus. The cartilaginous epiphysis of the olecranon was displaced rather more than half an inch backwards off the upper end of the ulna, and firmly fixed to the lower end of the diaphysis of the humerus posteriorly. The space between the olecranon, upper end of the ulna, and posterior aspect of the epiphysis of the humerus was occupied by dense fibrous tissue (see figures).

The child made an excellent recovery, and obtained a most useful and freely movable joint.

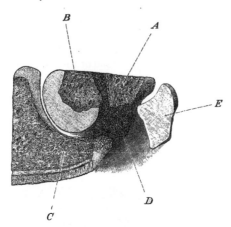

Fig. 72.—ANTERO-POSTERIOR VERTICAL SECTION OF SAME SPECIMEN
(NATURAL SIZE)

A, Diaphysis of humerus. B, Epiphysis with a small portion of the diaphysis. C, Ulna. D, Space between olecranon fragments. E, Olecranon.

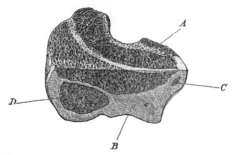

Fig. 73.—FRONTAL VERTICAL SECTION OF THE HUMERAL PART REMOVED

A, Lower end of diaphysis of humerus. B, Lower epiphysis. C, Commencing ossification of internal epicondylar portion. D, Osseous nucleus of capitellum.

Displacement outwards.—Mr. Bryant had a case of compound separation of the lower epiphysis of the humerus under his care at Guy's Hospital in October 1876, in which the epiphysis is said to have been displaced outwards. The patient (Eliza W.), aged fifteen, was injured by the passage of the wheel of a cart over her left arm. The wound was dressed with compound tincture of benzoin, and the arm placed on an outside angular splint. Seven weeks later the elbow could be flexed to some extent.

Displacement inwards and backwards.—Bardenheuer gives two figures of a case of incomplete displacement inwards of the epiphysis and forearm in a girl (C. S.) upon whom he operated. The diaphysial end of the humerus, displaced outwards and forwards, was removed, and is represented in one of the drawings (see *Deutsche Chirurgie*). The radial fossa was completely hollowed out, and before the operation its inner edge was mistaken for the anterior edge of the trochlea. The epiphysis was displaced backwards, carrying with it a portion ($\frac{1}{4}$ to $\frac{1}{3}$ centimetre) of the posterior part of the diaphysis, which formed a firm band of continuity between the displaced epiphysis and the diaphysis. At the operation the joint was opened, but this was followed by complete restoration of the function of the joint.

Displacement inwards.—In the case already mentioned under the care of Mr. Hutchinson junior, the line of separation followed only halfway the epiphysial disk, diverging for the other half into the diaphysis. Bony union occurred, with some lateral displacement inwards. (Royal College of Surgeons Museum.)

Detachment of periosteum.—In displacement of the epiphysis backwards, the periosteum is mostly detached from the posterior aspect of the lower end of the diaphysis.

In two of Bardenheuer's cases of old separation the periosteum had evidently been separated at this part, for a complete new shell of thin bone had formed which so exactly took the normal position of the bone that at first sight it looked like the bone itself, but was thinner and narrower. The humerus itself, with the olecranon fossa above the epiphysial line, projected in front in line with the axis of the shaft, whilst the thin, narrow new layer of bone behind made an angle with it.

OTHER COMPLICATIONS.—**Injury to the brachial artery.** Pressure upon the brachial artery leading to its occlusion has been met with in a few compound separations.

Professor R. W. Smith exhibited to the Pathological Society of Dublin (*Proceedings of the Pathological Society of Dublin*, N.S. vol. iv. 1870, p. 109) a cast of a recent example of separation of the lower and epitrochlear epiphyses of the humerus, the diaphysis having protruded through a large transverse rent in the integuments, just above the flexure of the elbow. A few moments before his admission, the boy, aged eight and a half, was thrown to the ground from a donkey, and on examination half an hour afterwards the following conditions were noted. Two inches of the diaphysis protruded through the wound ; the periosteum was detached along with the articular epiphysis and that of the epitrochlea ; the coronoid depression was distinctly seen ; the temperature of the limb, below the seat of the injury, was normal, but the pulsation of the radial and ulnar arteries could not be felt. The absence of pulsation was noted very shortly after the receipt of the injury. The pulsation ceased to be distinguishable at the point of bifurcation of the brachial artery, but the temperature of the limb continued normal. The patient being under the influence of chloroform, the forearm was semiflexed, and the epiphysis of the humerus (still resting upon the radius and ulna) was found to have passed backwards and upwards with these bones. Dr. Smith completely reduced the fragments, restored the parts to their normal relative position, and the limb was then secured in an angular splint in the semiflexed position. The patient left the hospital at the end of five weeks. The ultimate condition of the limb was as follows : the range of motion of the elbow-joint was extensive, though neither complete extension nor perfect flexion was possible. The lower end of the humerus formed a slight projection in front, while posteriorly two prominences were plainly visible, which were as nearly as possible on the same level ; the inner was formed by the olecranon, and the outer by the capitellum, surmounting the head of the radius. When the boy was last seen the pulsation had not re-appeared in either the radial or ulnar artery.

Laceration of elbow-joint.—In Champion's case of simple separation accompanied by other severe injuries, the anterior and posterior ligaments, as well as the part of the synovial membrane which corresponded to them, were lacerated.

Laceration of the brachialis anticus.—This muscle may be torn at its lower part, either in front or at the sides, by the displaced end of the diaphysis.

The *biceps tendon* may be *displaced* somewhat to either side.

Dislocation of elbow.—Mr. C. J. Bond, of Leicester, has recorded (*Provincial Medical Journal*, March 1, 1895, p. 133) a unique case of *separation of the lower epiphysis of the humerus*, together *with a dislocation of the elbow-joint*. A boy of twelve fell off a bicycle, and was thought ' to have a fractured elbow.' The arm was put up in the extended position in splints for some weeks. When Mr. Bond saw the boy, six weeks later, the appearance was that of a backward dislocation of the elbow, except that the shortening was in excess, and the prominence on the anterior aspect of the joint was larger than usual. As no reduction or alteration of the relation of the bones could be effected under chloroform, three months after the accident the joint was opened by a vertical posterior incision, and by sawing across the olecranon. The following condition was then found : the lower epiphysis of the humerus carrying the articular surfaces had been separated from the shaft, and had re-united at a right angle with it ; and, the radius and ulna having also been displaced somewhat backwards, the articular end of the epiphysis of the humerus lay on the ulna in front of the coronoid process. Mr. Bond first tried by chiselling through the line of union of the epiphysis to bend that straight, and bring it into a line with the shaft, and then to carry the ulna and radius forwards, and so reduce the dislocation. This was so far successful ; but the same difficulty occurred here which so frequently occurs in dealing with soft parts which have contracted up in any new position after injury—namely, the difficulty that, when the bones were in position and the dislocation reduced, the olecranon could not be brought down anywhere near the end of the ulna, so that the joint could not be closed posteriorly, nor the bones be kept in position. The loosened epiphysis was therefore removed, the forearm bones replaced, and the olecranon wired; the wide flattened end of the shaft of the humerus now lay in the articular concavity of the ulna, and formed the new elbow-joint.

Primary union of the wound occurred, and the recovery was soon complete. Mr. Bond saw the patient eighteen months after operation, and the limb was a very useful one; the patient could flex and extend through an angle of 45 degrees, and get his hand up to his mouth. The forearm was in the position midway between pronation and supination, but there was no further movement of that kind.

LATER COMPLICATIONS.—*Suppuration* has frequently occurred after compound separations. It may also take place after sloughing of the skin from pressure of the displaced diaphysis.

Gangrene has ensued, especially in compound cases that have been neglected.

SYMPTOMS. SEPARATION WITHOUT DISPLACEMENT.—Separation is not necessarily accompanied with displacement, the parts being held by the periosteum and other soft tissues; but from the comparative thinness of this epiphysis in the antero-posterior diameter it is not likely to be free from some degree of displacement, even though the violence may have been slight. The signs about to be mentioned will then be absent.

Besides the *age* and the *history* of the accident, we have only *unnatural mobility* at the level of the diaphysio-epiphysiary junction to guide us. This, on account of the lipping of the epiphysis on each side, will be more marked in the antero-posterior direction than in the lateral; but even lateral movement is often obtainable. The elbow should be grasped with one hand upon the epicondylar portion of the humerus, and the lower end of the shaft of the humerus with the other, and gentle pressure made.

' Muffled ' *crepitus* will usually be absent or difficult of detection.

Stripping up of the periosteum may be expected to have occurred, and to give rise to considerable subsequent thickening about the lower end of the bone in a short interval of time.

G. A. Wright (Ashby and Wright, *Diseases of Children*, 1889, p. 642) thinks it is possible that in some instances the violence may strip up muscles and the thick loose periosteum without any fracture or diastasis, and this injury of the periosteum may be the cause of that subsequent thickening.

SEPARATION WITH DISPLACEMENT.—Such great confusion has arisen with regard to these epiphysial separations of the lower end of the humerus amongst even modern writers that it is necessary to state clearly the nature of separation in each. In these, as in all other separations, the author has taken the anatomy of the epiphyses as the only true guide for a correct description of these lesions. It would only be confusing to discuss the correctness or incorrectness of the terms applied to the different portions of the bone in each case that has been recorded. All that can be done is to give as clear a description as possible, based on anatomical and experimental grounds, of the nature of the lesion likely to be met with in each case.

The injury under consideration—which should be more correctly described as separation of the lower end of the humerus—is more rare in its pure form than the similar separation at the upper end of the humerus. The lower osseous epiphysis proper is formed by the external epicondyle, the capitellum, and trochlea, the internal epicondyle constituting a distinct epiphysis attached to the humerus. But this arrangement only takes place after puberty, about the thirteenth year, by the growth of the diaphysis. Before this period the internal condyle is still part of the lower end of the humerus. Consequently it is impossible for complete traumatic separation of the entire epiphysial end of the humerus, including in this term both epicondyles and the whole of the articular surface, to occur after this period. The internal and external epicondyles are separated, together with the rest of the articular portion, as a complete mass, so that the line of separation slopes downwards from *above* each epicondyle, and then runs almost transversely above the articular surfaces.

Separation of the lower end is infrequent compared with separation of the part of the epiphysis or articular surface occurring after this period.

Writing in 1884 Hamilton said that he had never met with a case; and Agnew (*Agnew's Surgery*, vol. i. 1878, p. 889) says the injury is very rare.

Hutchinson says (*Medical Times and Gazette*, Jan. 5, 1884, p. 1) it is quite possible for the whole epiphysis to be clearly separated from the shaft by a transverse line of detachment, which permits the condyles and epicondyles to pass backwards together with the bones of the forearm. 'I have seen many examples of complete transverse detachment of the whole lower epiphysis. Most of them have come to me late on account of awkward union, but in a certain number I have had an opportunity of examining the state of things immediately after the accident.'

They are rightly placed by Malgaigne (*Traité des fractures et des luxations*, 1847, p. 542) among *supra-condyloid fractures* of the humerus ('fracture sus-condylienne'), thus: '*Fractures sus-condyliennes de l'Humérus.* Je désigne sous ce nom ce que Dupuytren appelait *fracture de l'extrémité inférieure de l'humérus*, afin d'établir plus de précision et d'exactitude dans le langage. C'est donc une solution de continuité qui sépare toute l'extrémité articulaire du corps de l'os, sans pénétrer dans la jointure ; et chez les enfants, qui y sont plus sujets que les adultes, il y a probablement, dans beaucoup de cas, une disjonction de l'épiphyse.'

Dupuytren, Vidal (De Cassis), and Adams (*Cyclopædia of Anatomy and Physiology*, vol. ii. p. 68) also correctly state that the deformity is not accompanied by any changes of the normal relations existing between the olecranon and the condyles (epicondyles). The symptoms of supra-condyloid fractures and separations of the whole lower epiphysis are so similar that it is often very difficult to distinguish the one from the other.

Dupuytren, moreover, remarks that whatever may be the prominence of the olecranon posteriorly, it is never further distant from the condyles of the humerus than in the normal condition of the parts in the case of fracture, but that in dislocation the separation is very considerable.

Dr. E. M. Moore is of opinion that supra-articular fracture of the humerus in a child is almost always epiphysial.

DISPLACEMENT BACKWARDS OF THE EPIPHYSIS. **Deformity.**—In the majority of cases the lower fragment comprising the epicondyles and the whole of the articular portion is displaced backwards to a greater or less extent by the force of the injury, carrying with it the radius and ulna, while the lower end of the diaphysis projects in front of the elbow, producing an appearance very similar to that of dislocation of both bones backwards.

The forearm is semiflexed at an angle of about 25 degrees by the action of the brachialis anticus and biceps muscles, the hand in a position midway between supination and pronation, and the arm powerless.

The olecranon projects posteriorly, being drawn upwards and backwards by the triceps, and is in normal relation with both the external and internal epicondyles. The external epicondyle is also in natural relation with the radial head below. The tip of the olecranon and the epicondyles are in the same line when the elbow is extended, and below the line between the two epicondyles when the elbow is flexed to a right angle. The antero-posterior diameter of the elbow is greatly increased just above the elbow.

The depression behind the elbow above the displaced epiphysis is somewhat wedge-shaped, due to the curving inwards of the triceps, which is prominent.

The deformity is very readily effaced by slight force.

Among the earliest cases recorded was one under the care of M. Dupuytren, 1832 (*Leçons orales de clinique chirurgicale*, 1832, tom. iii. p. 396), in which the displacement was backwards, the lower end of the humerus projecting in front. The injury had occurred a month previously, and was mistaken for a dislocation, attempts being made to reduce it. The fragments were united in a bad position, which caused considerable loss of extension of the elbow-joint. Unfortunately the age of the patient is not given; it is only stated that the case was that of a young child.

In separations of the whole lower epiphysis which Packard has seen, the lower fragment has always been carried backwards, the radius and ulna following it, and the lower end of the upper fragment projecting somewhat strongly in front of the elbow.

Sir Astley Cooper mentions a case which was most probably an epiphysial separation.

A boy, aged nine years, was admitted into Guy's Hospital with a fracture of the condyles of the humerus above the elbow-joint, which had been caused by his being thrown from a cart and having fallen upon his elbow. The following symptoms were present: forearm slightly bent, with considerable projection backwards of the radius and ulna; while just above the projection there was a hollow in the back of the arm, so that the appearances much resembled those of dislocation. On extending the forearm reduction was effected, but the deformity was immediately reproduced directly this was discontinued. Splints were employed for ten days, when they were occasionally removed, and passive motion commenced.

The displaced diaphysis differs very much in characteristics both from a dislocation and a fracture. Its anterior edge under the brachialis anticus is somewhat rounded and quite regular, unlike the sharpness and irregularity of a fracture; at the same time its lower surface is convex, even, and smooth, unlike the trochlear and capitellar surfaces of the joint. The breadth of this lower end of the upper fragment is greater than in the case of a fracture above the condyles of the humerus, but considerably less than in the case of dislocation, when it is equal to that of the opposite humerus.

The line of separation takes place nearer the end of the bone than in a true supra-condyloid fracture, as in the adult, and consequently the lower edge of the diaphysis is usually situated somewhat lower, almost *on a level* with the flexure of the elbow. In fracture the prominence is *above* the fold of the elbow and in dislocation much *below*, so that it is often very difficult to feel the articular surfaces.

Although the end of the diaphysis in the first few years of life will be found to be transverse, yet as puberty is reached the epiphysial line becomes oblique from without inwards, and from behind forwards, and will often allow some rotation or twisting of the epiphysis, so that the inner epicondyle is placed behind the corresponding outer condyle of the humerus, and the external epicondyle somewhat in front of the corresponding part of the humerus. Either epicondyle, in consequence, appears very prominent on the inner or outer side.

Mr. Hutchinson showed before the Pathological Society (*Pathological Society's Transactions*, vol. xv. 1864, p. 199) a photograph of this injury taken half an hour after the accident. A boy, aged ten, fell off a horse in front of the London Hospital, and was at once carried in, enabling the state of the parts to be examined before any swelling had obscured them. The olecranon projected prominently, and the tendon of the triceps stood out as in dislocation backwards of the radius and ulna. The sharp ends of the bone just above the condyles could be easily felt; the inner one, indeed, was almost through the skin, and the outlines of these parts made it clear that the shaft was completely detached from the epiphysis. The lowest parts of the condyles themselves could be felt to be still *in situ*—i.e. having passed backwards with the ulna and radius. It appeared to be a complete transverse detachment, of the whole of the three parts of which the lower epiphysis of this bone is composed. Even in the photograph the prominence forwards of the lower angles (condyles) of the shaft was easily recognised. In front of the joint, just over the tendon of the biceps, there was a very deep dimple, caused, no doubt, by the skin being tied down by attachment to the fascia. Swelling took place with great rapidity. No difficulty was experienced in effecting reduction, but the deformity was reproduced as soon as the restraining force was removed. A splint was applied to the back of the arm and elbow, and a pad placed over the lower end of the shaft kept it in place. A second rectangular splint was applied to the inner aspect of the arm.

The same surgeon saw another child who had fallen off a tree a short time previously, and under chloroform diagnosed a complete detachment of the lower epiphysis of the humerus.

It was easily reduced, but at once returned. A rectangular concave back splint was applied, and very little displacement resulted.

Mobility of the forearm and lower end of the humerus with the epicondyles, especially in the antero-posterior direction, is nearly always a prominent feature.

Another very important sign is the great tendency to **reproduction of the deformity.** Reduction is easily effected by the application of gentle extension, pressure of the diaphysis backwards and of the elbow forwards, and the limb regains its normal appearance, but when the extension is discontinued immediately shortens again, whilst the deformity recurs—the powerful action of the muscles passing from the arm to the forearm being the chief factor in producing this result. In dislocation the bones are not disposed to become again displaced after reduction.

This was well marked in Hutchinson's case just related, and also in another case alluded to by the same author (*Medical Times and Gazette*, January 5, 1884, p. 2) of a girl aged twelve, who fell from

U

an apple-tree. Ether being administered, he was enabled to make an examination of a most marked example of transverse separation. It was not difficult to get the bone into place, but almost impossible to keep it there. It was put up in a moulded back splint.

Muffled crepitus.—During extension and replacing of the fragments by grasping the arm in one hand and the forearm in the other, the fragments are made to move backwards upon each other. The characteristic ' muffled ' crepitus will usually be detected.

It will be found to be more characteristic and more easily obtainable in this than in any other form of epiphysial separation. However, on the contrary, crepitus may be absent, although a disjunction is present.

Writing in 1837 (*Presse Médicale*, No. 55, July 12, 1837, tom. i.) M. Roux drew special attention to this sign in lower humeral separation.

A child of ten or eleven years had a severe fall, in which the ground was struck by the palmar aspect of the right hand. When seen by M. Roux some hours afterwards the following signs were present, which led him to diagnose disjunction of the lower end of the humerus : pain in the humero-ulnar articulation, no noticeable swelling ; depression on either side of the olecranon, and the tendon of the biceps rendered prominent by a firm, hard, osseous mass. Replacement of the limb to its normal position was effected by moderate extension, and ' soft ' crepitus was produced by the rubbing together of the granular surfaces of the fragments, which were invested with a layer of ossifying cartilage. The crepitus was characteristic and somewhat feeble, but differed from that which is felt in the case of fracture. The arm was maintained in the flexed position, and the reduced epiphysis fixed by an apparatus. The parents made light of the injury, and took the apparatus off on the thirteenth or fourteenth day. The child used its arm, now free, in a very irregular manner—perhaps had a fresh fall ; at any rate, the same evening he was unable to move his arm. A doctor who was consulted thought there was some simple rigidity about the articular ligaments. However, when the child was seen by M. Roux three months afterwards, the arm was still about a quarter flexed. Extension was impossible and flexion very limited. The deformity of the joint was irreparable, and in the position described by Hippocrates as ' coude de belette.'

H. E. Clark, of Glasgow, relates (*Glasgow Medical Journal*, vol. xxvi. p. 248) a somewhat doubtful case in a recently born child, which he diagnosed as separation on account of the peculiar crepitus and mobility of the condyles with the forearm. The arm appeared to be paralysed from birth. The result of treatment was good, the elbow being flexed at a right angle.

If a fracture of the diaphysis accompanies the separation, the dry crepitus then obtained will obscure the more characteristic crepitus.

Shortening of arm.—On carefully measuring the arm from the prominence of the external and internal epicondyle to the acromion process, shortening of the humerus from $\frac{1}{2}$ inch to an inch will be found.

The active movements of the elbow in flexion and extension of the forearm are limited, mostly on account of the pain, never absolutely wanting, as in dislocation. Flexion is usually more painful than extension. Passive movements of pronation and supination are permitted to a great extent, and are more extensive than in intra-articular lesions, e.g. in the corresponding separation in youth, viz. separation of the trochlea, capitellum, and external epicondyle.

It must always be remembered that attempts at extensive movement cause great pain, and the above signs can only satisfactorily be detected while the young patient is under the anæsthetic. Without its use some damage is sure to be done to the soft structures—e.g. the periosteum may be still further stripped up, or the synovial membrane lacerated.

Shortening of forearm.—The forearm as seen from the front is shortened, as in dislocation.

The distance from the front of the displaced diaphysis to the styloid process of the radius will be found shortened as compared with the opposite side.

Swelling occurs with great rapidity after the accident, obscuring the various prominences of the displaced bones, and rendering the diagnosis very embarrassing.

In Hutchinson's case, just quoted, the quickness of the swelling was very noticeable, although no time was lost; yet before the photograph could be completed the contour of the parts had been to a large extent concealed.

The lapse of a few hours is quite sufficient to obscure the parts completely by such a swelling, which extends upwards and downwards beyond the seat of separation. It will then be absolutely necessary to place the patient under an anæsthetic and make a careful examination of the injured elbow. An anæsthetic would have to be given even for the proper reduction of the fragments and the application of splints; all violent attempts at reduction will only increase the gravity of the injury.

Where a surgeon sees the case before swelling has taken place an exact diagnosis can easily be made.

Dr. John Watson, of the New York Hospital, records (*New York Journal of Medicine*, N.S. vol. xi. November 1853, p. 430) the case of a girl, aged twenty months, who had her elbow injured by the mother suddenly wrenching the limb in attempting to lift her. The whole arm, when seen by Dr. Watson on the fourth day, was too much swollen to make out very clearly the exact nature of the accident. But eleven days later this had subsided, and it was apparent that the shaft of the humerus had been separated from

its cartilaginous expansion at the condyles. By the use of angular
pasteboard splints the reduction was maintained, and the disjoined
condyles united again to the shaft after about four or six weeks.
Hamilton also quotes Dr. Watson's case. It is exceedingly doubtful
whether this was a true case of traumatic separation in a healthy
subject, but it is quoted here on Hamilton's authority.

In four days' time the periosteum, which has been stripped
off from the displaced shaft, especially behind where an interval is
left between it and the diaphysis, although still adherent to the
epiphysis, pours out abundant inflammatory material. A day or
two later the outlines of the bones will have been quite obscured
by the new osseous material, and the diagnosis then becomes
absolutely impossible.

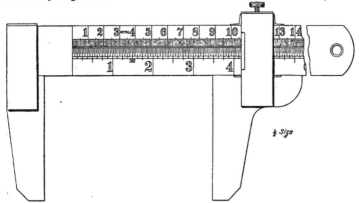

FIG. 74.—CHESTERMAN'S STEEL CALLIPER GAUGE FOR MEASURING HEIGHT AND
WIDTH OF THE EPIPHYSES AT THE VARIOUS AGES
Divided: inches into thirty-seconds, centimetres into millimetres and halves

This interval between the diaphysis and the epiphysis the author
has noticed in all the experiments made by him on the dead body.

Ecchymosis about the elbow is often very marked from extravasated blood.

The **breadth between epicondyles** is not altered, thereby distinguishing it from separation of the lower epiphysis during the
period of youth.

COMPLICATIONS.—**Injury to the brachial artery.**

The close relation of the brachial artery to the front of the
lower end of the diaphysis is a fertile source of danger. Yet it is
remarkable how often the vessels at the head of the elbow escape
injury. Probably their curved position and great mobility tend to
bring this about.

In Professor R. W. Smith's case of compound separation absence
of pulsation was present from the bifurcation of the brachial artery
downwards, due to pressure upon this vessel.

T. Bryant (*Practice of Surgery*, 4th edition, 1884, vol. ii. p. 369) alludes to the case of a boy aged nine years. The lower epiphysis of the humerus, with the bones of the forearm, was displaced backwards : the anterior border of the diaphysis injured the brachial artery and occluded it. Reduction was effected and splints applied. At the end of six weeks there was good movement of the joint, and pulsation had returned in the radial, but not in the brachial, artery. This appears to be the same case as that of a boy who had fallen downstairs and separated his epiphysis, with occlusion of the brachial artery, recorded by Chas. Wood in the *Guy's Hospital Gazette*, July 1878, p. 82. The age of the patient is, however, given here as five years.

Bryant also gives (*Brit. Med. Journal*, May 30, 1896, p. 1487) the following case of separation of the lower epiphysis of the humerus from the diaphysis, and displacement of the epiphysis with the bones of the forearm backwards, with occlusion of the brachial artery. A boy, aged five years, was admitted into Guy's Hospital on May 27, 1878, under his care, having injured his elbow one week previously in falling downstairs. The limb was cold, swollen, and pulseless below the elbow. The forearm, with the lower epiphysis of the humerus, was displaced backwards, and the anterior edge of the extremity of the diaphysis was pressing seriously upon the brachial artery, which was in front. When the deformity was reduced pulsation did not return in the vessel. The limb was put into a good position and fastened in a splint after having been raised and well wrapped up in cotton-wool ; everything went on well. Subsequently, on the seventeenth day after his admission, or the twenty-fourth day after the accident, pulsation returned in the radial artery, but when the child left the hospital in the sixth week no pulsation had returned in the brachial artery below the seat of injury. At that spot the vessel was clearly occluded.

G. A. Wright gives the following case (*Guy's Hospital Reports*, third series, vol. xxiv. 1879, p. 52) of occlusion of the artery for twenty-two days, caused by an ill-applied anterior angular splint ; fortunately no ill results followed. S. M., aged five. On May 11, 1878, the boy fell from some banisters upon his right elbow ; separation of the lower epiphysis of the humerus resulted from the injury, the lower fragment, as usual, being displaced backwards, while the end of the diaphysis projected forwards prominently upon the anterior surface of the arm. The arm was placed upon an anterior right-angled splint with the object of correcting the deformity produced by the contraction of the triceps. Eleven days later (May 22), great swelling of the limb having ensued, a fresh examination showed absence of pulsation in the radial artery at the wrist, the arm being cold. The patient was then admitted into the hospital. The splint having been removed, the swelling subsided, pulsation returned in the radial and ulnar arteries on June 2, and the boy was discharged with complete power of pronation and supination, but very limited flexion and extension, and much callus about the seat of injury.   In this case the occlusion of the artery probably depended upon direct compression between the lower end of the diaphysis and the splint; a result pointing to the advisability of avoiding the use of anterior splints in these cases, as also in the similar condition of dislocation backwards of the radius and ulna with fracture of the coronoid process, and consequent tendency to recurrence of dislocation, although anterior splints are the best adapted to remedy the deformity.

Dr. Bristow relates (*Brooklyn Medical Journal*, vol. ix. April 1895, No. 4, p. 250) a case of compression of the brachial artery by diastasis of humerus in backward dislocation of ulna that had occurred at Long Island College Hospital.   A diagnosis of dislocation of the ulna backwards had been made, but on a more careful examination there was found a diastasis of the humerus with projection of the upper fragment forwards into the bend of the arm. There was no pulsation of the radial and ulnar arteries, the forearm being quite cold.   The pressure of the upper fragment against the artery could not have lasted more than three-quarters of an hour, for the child had only been injured one half-hour before being examined, and in fifteen minutes the fragment had been reduced and the arm put into an angular splint.   A clot must have formed from the compression in a very short time indeed.   The collateral circulation was produced in the forearm, however, through the precaution which was adopted to practically omit all bandages on the forearm.   Pulsation returned in the vessels at the end of five days.

Dr. Bristow pointed out that a bandage properly applied may yet result in gangrene if the artery has been occluded by the pressure of the anterior fragment.   In this case it would not have been difficult for this occlusion to have escaped notice at the time, and a very slight pressure on the forearm might be just sufficient to overcome the force of the collateral circulation, and gangrene might result, although there was no undue pressure.

A case in which the pressure was such that no pulsation could be detected in the vessels at the wrist is alluded to by Mr. Jonathan Hutchinson (*Med. Press and Circular*, 1885, p. 461, November 18). It had been mentioned to him by his son, who has referred to another case (*Brit. Med. Journal*, November 3, 1894, p. 967), quoted below, in which the end of the diaphysis passed through the soft tissues in front of the elbow between the brachial artery and the biceps tendon.

In Page's case gangrene occurred as the result of the bruising and thrombosis of the brachial artery.

Injury to nerves.—It is remarkable that the large nerve trunks —such as the musculo-spiral, the median, or ulnar nerve—are not frequently affected. The ulnar nerve, being in close contact with the internal condyloid portion of the diaphysis of the humerus, would appear to be especially liable to injury; but fortunately, in the usual form of injury, the upper diaphysial fragment passes forwards and the nerve escapes injury. The ending of the musculo-spiral in front of the outer end of the humerus, and the median nerve, also in front, are, together with their branches, equally liable to be involved and produce loss of sensation, pain, or paralysis in the parts supplied by them, although examples have been rarely published.

All these complications are frequently met with in fractures of the lower end of the humerus.

G. A. Wright, however, says (loc. cit. supra, p. 645) that implication of the musculo-spiral nerve in the callus of a separated lower epiphysis of the humerus is not uncommon, and there may be paralysis of the nerve for a time; usually this disappears, and he thinks that no hasty operation for the release of the nerve is called for.

In one of Mr. Jonathan Hutchinson junior's cases (Brit. Med. Journal, Dec. 30, 1893), 'pulsation at the wrist was stopped by the forward projecting diaphysis, and there were marked signs of pressure on the median nerve. These symptoms disappeared on reduction, and recovery was perfect, excepting that flexion was limited to a right angle.'

Wounds.—In many instances this injury has been complicated by a wound rendering the lesion compound, vide cases of R. W. Smith, Champion, Spillman (2), Reeve, Lange, Bryant, Hutchinson, Thomson, Ashhurst, Lediard, MacDougall, and Maisonneuve. The wound is usually placed in front of the flexure of the elbow. In the second case of Spillman's it was a transverse one just above the elbow, in Lediard's it was vertical. In one case recorded by Professor Smith the wound was situated at the back of the elbow, through which the lower epiphysis protruded. Sturrock's case (vide infra) was followed by suppuration, and the range of movement limited to less than a right angle.

Fracture of the bones of the forearm.—Champion's case was complicated by compound fracture of the bones of the forearm, and Wight (Annals of the Anatomical and Surgical Society, Brooklyn, N.Y., October 1880, p. 433) met with a somewhat similar case in a boy aged eight, who fell from a cart and sustained a greenstick fracture of both bones of the forearm, less than an inch from the wrist-joint. There was displacement to an angle of about 45 degrees. Reduction was effected by forcible manipulation. No crepitus was elicited. Separation of the lower epiphysis of the humerus also existed, with extensive extravasation around the elbow-joint. The case was treated with a double-angled splint. Passive motion of both joints was begun on the third day, and good union was obtained, although at the time of the report the movements of the elbow were still somewhat hindered by excessive deposit of callus. The wrist motions were almost perfect.

Stripping up of the periosteum occurs in all cases, probably to some extent even in separation without displacement.

In the form of displacement which we are now considering—viz. backwards of the epiphysis—allusion need only again be made to the space left behind between the detached periosteum and the posterior aspect of the diaphysis.

In compound separations the detachment of the periosteum has been effected for nearly halfway up the shaft on one side. It is also noted in Spillman's case.

Synovitis of the elbow is a very common complication, especially in its milder forms. Suppuration of the joint is rarely met with except as the result of extension from a suppurating focus in its neighbourhood.

At the period in which this form of diastasis occurs, laceration of the synovial membrane will necessarily be less frequent than in later years, when the separations are frequently partial and complicated. Moreover, the earlier the age the less firm is the synovial membrane attached to the olecranon fossa and posterior aspect of the diaphysis. During the first few years of life this depression is so little developed, and the synovial membrane is so loosely attached to the bone in this situation, that it is likely to escape any serious injury.

In a case under the care of Mr. Durham at Guy's Hospital in July 1876, a boy (John G.) aged eight, had fallen off a donkey into the road and separated the lower epiphysis of his humerus. There was found a great amount of effusion into the elbow-joint. The patient did well, the arm being put up in lateral splints.

Suppuration of joint or limb has been noted in several of the compound cases.

In a few neglected examples the skin over the displaced diaphysis has sloughed from pressure, and given rise to suppuration.

Displacement outwards of epiphysis.—The few cases the author has been able to find recorded include one under the care of Mr. Howse, at Guy's Hospital, in June 1888. Joseph S., aged seven years, tumbled and fell, striking his right elbow on the ground. There was found a separation of the lower epiphysis of the humerus, with displacement outwards and somewhat backwards. The lower end of the diaphysis projected forwards above the bend of the elbow-joint, and the relation of the internal condyle to the olecranon process was not altered. Soft crepitus was felt, and the deformity could easily be reduced, but it re-appeared when the parts were relaxed. An anterior rectangular splint was applied, and the patient did well, so that he was able to leave the hospital on the sixteenth day, though the elbow was still considerably swollen.

The following case was seen by the author with Dr. Hearnden, of

Sutton, Surrey: L. E., aged eight years, on September 17, 1894, fell off a summer-house about ten feet high, detaching the lower epiphysis of her left humerus, which was displaced outwards and very slightly backwards, the inner side of the diaphysis being found, on examination, in its displaced position to the inner side above the internal epicondyle. There was considerable contusion over the inner side of the elbow, and the radial artery could not be felt to pulsate at the wrist. 'Dummy' crepitus was well marked, with mobility in the lateral direction. The fracture did not implicate the joint. There was also a fracture of the lower end of the radius, about three-quarters of an inch above the epiphysial line, the wrist with the hand being displaced backwards and the shaft of the bone forwards. There was

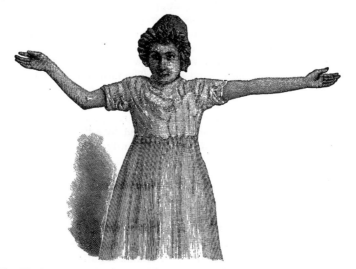

FIG. 75.—DISPLACEMENT OF LOWER EPIPHYSIS OF HUMERUS OUTWARDS, WITH INJURY TO MEDIAN NERVE. AMOUNT OF EXTENSION AT THE ELBOW-JOINT THREE MONTHS AFTER THE ACCIDENT.

loss of sensation of the whole index-finger and the outer side of the middle finger. Both fractures were easily reduced; an anterior rectangular splint, to include the separated epiphysis as well as the fractured radius, was applied, and an external rectangular splint with a short lateral splint on the inner side, to prevent the displacement of the shaft inwards. Four days later there was great swelling of the elbow, the forearm, and the whole of the hand, and numerous blebs had formed over the elbow. There was also effusion into the joint. The loss of sensation, coldness, and inability to flex the index-finger still persisted; the inner splint was therefore removed, although the injury to the median nerve was probably caused at the time of the accident and not by any undue pressure of the splint. Seven days after the accident the splints were removed, and displacement inwards of the diaphysis was found to still exist. The radial artery could now be felt pulsating, and there was some return of sensation in the middle finger. The anterior rectangular and outer splints were re-applied. On the thirteenth day a posterior rectangular splint was applied, with interruption at elbow, but at the end of a week this made no alteration in the condition of the median nerve, for the index-finger still could not be flexed, and there was the same area of loss of sensation. The humerus continued a little displaced inwards, but the elbow-joint could be freely moved and the fracture of the radius had firmly united in good position. In the second week in December, 1894, although pronation, supination, and flexion of the elbow were almost perfect, extension could not be effected beyond 135 degrees, on account of the pain, presumably from pressure upon the injured median nerve. The inner projecting angle of the dia- physis, after the swelling had cleared up, was now very prominent on the inner side ; it was therefore decided to remove the projecting portion of the bone, which was done with antiseptic and aseptic precautions, no drainage being used. The median nerve was found in front of the outer edge of the projection, and had to be drawn aside during the operation. A week or two afterwards the sensation and use of the index finger suddenly returned, and have remained ever since. Their restoration was preceded by a tingling sensation. The extension of the forearm was subsequently perfect, no deformity being noticeable.

Mobility of the epiphysis and elbow-joint is most marked in the lateral direction, distinguishing the injury from dislocation outwards of the elbow.

Displacement outwards, with fracture of the diaphysis, is not an un-common form of injury. The following is an example which the author had the opportunity of seeing some days after the injury. A girl, aged seven, came under the care of Dr. F. D. Atkins, of Sutton, on August 23, 1893. She had fallen from a tree five or six feet high on to the ground, striking her left elbow. When seen by Dr. Atkins within an hour after the accident there was already very great swelling, and the lower epiphysis of the humerus was displaced outwards. Chloroform was immediately administered, the displacement reduced, and the elbow put up on an anterior rectangular splint. When the author saw her there was still great swelling with ecchymosis about the joint, but mobility in the antero-posterior and lateral directions, crepitus, dis- placement of the epiphysial fragment outwards and slightly back- wards, and the normal relations of the epicondyles rendered the diagnosis clear. Chloroform was again given, and the fragments replaced in position ; but, notwithstanding all efforts, there was a great tendency for the displacement outwards to recur. A sharp- pointed process on the outer side, a small portion of the diaphysis, half an inch long, remained connected with the outer part of the epiphysis above the external epicondyle. The anterior rectangular

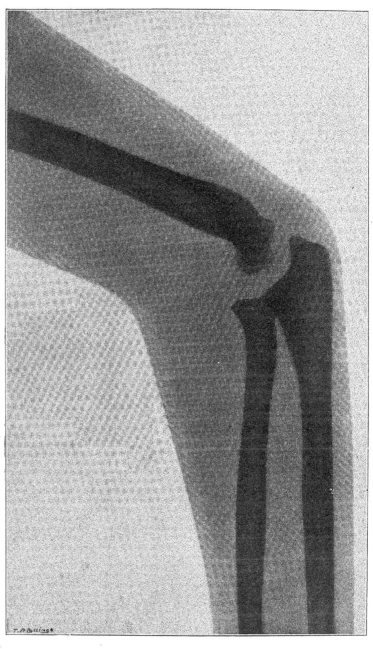

DISPLACEMENT FORWARDS OF LOWER EPIPHYSIS OF HUMERUS.

Dr. CAMPBELL POPE's case.   Taken by Dr. F. H. Low.

splint was again applied. The diaphysis became again displaced, in spite of the careful application of the splints. Slight sloughing of the skin occurred over the end of the diaphysis, a small portion of which was subsequently removed.

Displacement inwards of epiphysis.—This, like the preceding lateral displacement, is very rare and likely to be overlooked.

The case from the Children's Hospital, Pendlebury, quoted below is, however, a good example of this injury.

Displacement forwards of epiphysis.—Mr. Jonathan Hutchinson's case, alluded to below, was probably of this variety. His son also alludes to another case of forward displacement under his care (*British Medical Journal*, December 20, 1893, p. 1418). The author's case of fracture directly above the epiphysial line with displacement of the epiphysis forwards has already been described. The thin edge of the diaphysis may be felt behind in these instances.

Separation of part of the epiphysis, with fracture of the diaphysis.—This is a very frequent injury near the elbow-joint in children, and might with good reason be placed in a separate group. The author has seen many instances ; the following is one of them. A girl, Edith L., aged eight years, was under the care of Mr. Wm. F. Hearnden, of Sutton. She had fallen a distance of five feet on to her elbow. The fracture had traversed more than the inner half of the epiphysial line, and thence passed upwards obliquely through the diaphysis to above the external supracondyloid ridge. When the author saw the case in 1890, four months after the accident, there was still visible some projection forwards of the diaphysis in front, and great thickening about the lower end of the bone. All movements of the elbow were excellent, with the exception of complete extension, which was

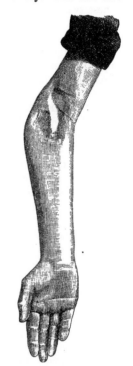

FIG. 76.—PARTIAL SEPARATION, WITH EXTENSIVE OBLIQUE FRACTURE OF THE DIAPHYSIS OF THE HUMERUS. (MR. W. F. HEARNDEN'S CASE)

prevented apparently by the callus in the olecranon fossa behind. Union was complete.

J. Hutchinson junior states that a clean separation at the epiphysial disc is probably uncommon after the age of five or six, but that it may occur some years later, and that in over fifty cases it was present probably only in the minority. The youngest patient was one and a half years old, and the eldest fourteen years.

The signs present are as follows : *Projection* of portion of the end of the diaphysis forwards. *Crepitus* characteristic of fracture. The *epicondyles* in normal relation with olecranon, while the *pointed end* of the lower fragment of the diaphysis may be felt about the external or internal supra-condyloid ridge, and perfect *movements of joint.*

Separation of the epiphysis, with vertical fracture into joint.—In addition to the signs already given of separation of the lower epiphysis of the humerus, there is that of unnatural mobility of the portions of the epiphysis. On grasping the inner and outer portions of the epiphysis, with the accompanying epicondyles, with each hand, these two portions will be found to move backwards and forwards, one upon the other. Such movement will probably be accompanied by crepitus.

If the upper fragment be driven downwards or the olecranon upwards between the portions of the epiphysis, the increase in the breadth of the elbow from one epicondyle to another will be a notable feature.

DIFFERENTIAL DIAGNOSIS.—Epiphysial separations are much more frequent at the elbow-joint than dislocations ; in fact, the latter are comparatively rare.

Many of the signs of traumatic separation are common to it and to fracture above the condyles and to dislocation of both bones of the forearm backwards, which is most frequent about the age of puberty ; but the diagnosis is generally easy, provided an anæsthetic be given. It should be arrived at as soon as possible before any swelling has occurred. Even should this have taken place, it is very undesirable that the injured arm be left for the inflammatory swelling to subside.

In all cases in which the signs are at all indefinite, an anæsthetic should be at once administered and a thorough examination made.

Dislocation of the elbow-joint (both bones of forearm backwards).— In dislocation as well as separation the arm is semiflexed, or nearly so.

The following points met with in dislocation are sufficient to prevent its being mistaken for diastasis :

1. Immobility of forearm.

2. Absence of crepitus.

3. No tendency for deformity to be reproduced after reduction, which is often difficult to be carried out.

4. End of humerus deeply placed in flexure of elbow, and often not to be felt. In separation the diaphysial end is felt on a level with it.

5. The relations of the olecranon process to the epicondyles very markedly changed, the distance between them being greatly increased.

6. No shortening of arm.

7. Seldom produced by a fall on the elbow, as in diastasis or fracture.

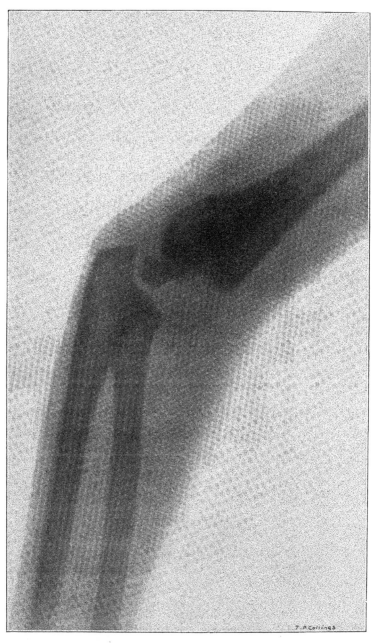

DISPLACEMENT BACKWARDS OF LOWER EPIPHYSIS OF HUMERUS,
WITH FRACTURE OF DIAPHYSIS.

Four months after injury. Child aged eight years. Dr. CAMPBELL POPE's case. Taken by Dr. F. H. Low.

8. The top of the olecranon is raised much above the normal horizontal line passing through the epicondyles of the humerus.

9. Elastic stiffness is a distinguishing sign mentioned by Dr. L. C. Lane, of San Francisco. It is a slight rebound of the forearm with an elastic jerk when it is flexed or extended. This rebound is much less or wholly absent in supra-condyloid fracture.

As R. W. Smith remarks, the observations of Dupuytren respecting the danger of confounding fracture immediately above the elbow with dislocation backwards apply with peculiar force to the injury we are considering.

'If,' says this distinguished surgeon, ' the opinion that the case is one of luxation be acted upon, extension and counter-extension are employed, the reduction is accomplished without much difficulty, and the surgeon congratulates himself upon the ease with which he has restored the bones to their places. But soon the displacement is reproduced, and at the end of a few days, in the midst of the swelling, something unnatural is felt. This accident is generally ascribed to the patient, who is charged with being intractable. The reduction is again effected, but the deformity soon recurs, and considerable swelling then supervenes. As long as this condition lasts the surgeon continues severe, but when the swelling has disappeared, after the lapse of a few weeks, he discovers the error which he has committed ; but the mischief cannot now be repaired, the motions of the joint are never perfectly regained, and the deformity is incurable.'

Dupuytren relates (*On the Injuries and Diseases of Bones*, Sydenham Society, 1846, p. 103) the case already alluded to above, in which such an error had been made, and deformity consequently resulted.

In the latter end of 1832 a young child was brought to him, who, a month previously, had fallen whilst in the act of getting on a donkey. Two doctors were successively called in, who pronounced the case to be one of dislocation, and treated it accordingly. When Dupuytren saw the child's arm there was an irregular tumour in front, which was evidently the lower extremity of the humerus ; the olecranon forming a prominence behind. From the tender age of the patient, he believed that there was a separation of the epiphysis ; the two fragments were united, but with deformity.

A rare case of compound dislocation of the elbow-joint without fracture is described by Chauncy Puzey (*Lancet*, 1893, July 8, p. 87). ' The boy, aged nine years, had sustained a compound dislocation of the right elbow-joint. The sharp trochlear portion of the lower end of the humerus had penetrated the soft parts in front of the joint, and, with the inner condyle, appeared on the front of the upper part of the forearm, tightly embraced by the skin, through which it had burst. The forearm was considerably shortened by the backward displacement of its bones, and the elbow was kept fixed at a point

about halfway between extension and a right angle.   The hand
and lower part of the forearm was dusky in hue, and the radial pulsation at the wrist was barely perceptible.   The dislocation, after some
difficulty, was reduced, the joint drained, and an aseptic dressing
applied.   The boy made a good recovery, and an examination of
the joint one year later showed recovery, with unimpaired movements of the joint.'

Simple contusion of elbow.—In instances where the displacement
of the epiphysis is not very great, great swelling and ecchymosis
may completely mask the slight deformity present, and cause its
being mistaken for a simple contusion.

Fracture above the condyles.—This form of fracture is common
enough in children.   Hamilton says that of eighteen fractures at
this point, twelve occurred in children under ten years of age, the
youngest being two years old.

There is a good specimen of this in St. George's Hospital
Museum described by Mr. Holmes.

The error of confounding a diastasis with a fracture is not so
disastrous as confounding it with a dislocation, since in the former
case the mistake is of comparatively slight importance, inasmuch as
the same treatment is applicable to both.   The latter must always
be considered as a serious error.

Out of sixty cases of injury to the elbow-joint in children, recorded
by Guedeney from M. Vincent's clinic during seven years, twenty-
seven were of the lower end of the humerus (excluding injuries to
the epicondyles and articular processes).   Of these, thirteen were
diagnosed as separations of the lower epiphysis of the humerus,
ten as fractures of the lower end of the humerus (two being
compound), three T-shaped fractures, and one Y-shaped fracture.

The following points in epiphysial separations will assist in
distinguishing them from fractures :

1. Muffled crepitus.
2. The lower end of the upper fragment. has greater breadth than
   in fracture.
3. The line of separation is nearer the end of the bone and the
   anterior projection of the diaphysis on a level with the fold
   of the elbow ; in fracture it is usually above it.
4. The anterior projection in diastasis has a rounded extremity
   unlike the projections of the sharp ends of a fracture.

Mr. Holmes showed, at the Pathological Society in 1862 (*Path.
Soc: Transactions*, vol. xiii. p. 187), a specimen of fracture, about
¼ inch above the epiphysial line, in which the injury was only
distinguishable during life from separation of the epiphysis by the
distinctness of the crepitus.   The child was aged nine years, and had
fallen three months before upon her elbow.   She died of chorea.
There was a large smooth mass of bone on the posterior aspect,
filling up the gap that would otherwise have been left by the pro-

jection of the upper fragment forwards, so that no irregularity was seen here. But in front the upper fragment projected beyond the lower by a large irregular prominence, half as thick as the humerus itself.

The London Hospital Museum contains two specimens of fracture of the lower end of the humerus a little above but close to the epiphysial line. They were both removed from boys the subjects of compound fracture. The author's specimen figured above (p. 281) also shows this form of fracture.

Berthomier pointed out that the usual seat of this form of fracture is lower than is generally supposed.

M. Hallé presented to La Société Anatomique de Paris, in November 1886 (*Bull. de la Soc. Anat.* 1886, p. 647), a specimen of an elbow of a child whose age was not given. During life, after the swelling had disappeared, the displacement of the head of the radius and of the olecranon suggested incomplete dislocation of the elbow inwards. On the death of the child shortly afterwards from broncho-pneumonia complicating measles, there was found a supra-condyloid fracture detaching the trochlea, the condyle (capitellum), and the epitrochlea (internal epicondyle). The course of the fracture was lower than the usual situation of fracture of the lower end of the humerus, but was, on the other hand, higher than the epiphysial line.

Comminuted fractures of the lower end of the humerus are of frequent occurrence, and have the characteristic feel of a 'bag of beans.'

It is very probable that several of the fragments traverse the epiphysial line, but will in no way allow of the injury being considered in any other light than that of a fracture. The separation of the epiphysial portion may .pass through the capitellar, trochlear, or epiphysial line, or through the line of the epicondylar epiphyses, the fissures between the fractures and epiphysial fragments communicating in numerous directions.

Although great swelling and extravasation of blood are present in a very marked degree, it is surprising to see how completely the function of the limb will be regained in these young subjects. Crepitus is very easily detected.

Guedeney gives details of *seven* cases diagnosed as fractures of the lower end of the humerus in children : female aged six years, male aged eleven years, male aged seven (complicated by fracture of the lower extremity of the bones of the forearm), male aged seven and a half years, male thirteen years, female two years, and male nine years (? pressure on brachial artery). *Three* were cases of fracture of the lower end of the humerus *complicated with wounds* in children : female aged three and a half, female aged six, and female aged eight and a half years. (In the last case numerous fragments of bone were removed from the lower end of the humerus by means of incision on the outer side and on the inner side through the seat of the wound.) *Three* were cases diagnosed as T-*shaped fractures* of the lower end of the humerus in children aged—male (?) six years, male six years, and male six and a half years. *One* case was diagnosed as Y-*shaped fracture* of the lower end of the humerus in a male (?) child aged twelve years. All were treated by fixation in the extended and supine position, and later on in the flexed position.

The most valuable aid in the treatment as well as in the diagnosis of epiphysial separations at the elbow-joint has been recently developed under the Röntgen rays and in the additional use of the fluoroscope. As Professor W. B. van Lennep, of Philadelphia, says : 'Not only is the diagnosis greatly facilitated, but, what is of more value, the position of the fragments can be inspected from day to day with the fluoroscope after the application of non-metallic splints. Subsequent taking down of the dressings, with its accompanying pain and disturbance, can thus be often avoided. So, too, the approximation of the fragments may be accurately accomplished under the guidance of the eye.' He gives (*The Hahnemannian Institute*, January 1897, vol. iv. No. 3, p. 15 ; *Hahnemannian Monthly*, February 1897) an illustrative skiagraph of separation of the lower epiphysis of the humerus in a child aged four years. There was the usual displacement of the epiphysis backwards, which had been presumably reduced. It is interesting to notice the splint faintly outlined in the skiagraph, while the nails holding its two pieces together are distinctly seen. The other dim shadows are the padding and bandages. The olecranon epiphysis gives the impression of a separation there.

Dr. Chas. L. Léonard (*American Journal of the Medical Sciences*, August 1896) also gives a skiagraph of diastasis of the distal epiphysis of the humerus. W. McL., aged eleven years, came to the University Hospital of Pennsylvania on March 31, 1896, with fracture of the humerus. The history was of a fall from a wall five feet high to the pavement, striking the left hand. The patient weighed about seventy-five pounds ; he sustained no other injury. The case was diagnosed and dressed before the skiagraph was developed, the latter demonstrating the correctness of the diagnosis and showing the position of the fragments resulting from this form of epiphysial separation.[1]

PROGNOSIS AND RESULTS. Union.—Good firm union always results, and takes place very rapidly, for in common with all epi-

---

[1] Dr. O. Büttner and Dr. K. Müller give the following practical remarks on the use of the screen and photographic plate in the Röntgen process (*Encyklopädie der Photographie*, Heft 28, 1897, S. 105 ; *Tecnik und Verwerthung der Röntgen'schen Strahlen*):

'In the case of fractures and luxations the use of the screen is to some extent precluded, as the pain caused by moving the patient would be too great. Pyknography (i.e. the representation of the shadows on a photographic plate) is therefore of special value in such cases. The plate may be wrapped in paper and placed under the limb, and the exposure may be made by a trustworthy attendant. With a spark of twenty centimetres the exposure should be from ten to thirty minutes, according to the thickness of the part.

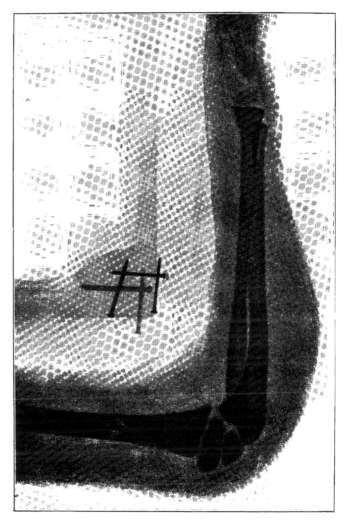

SEPARATION OF LOWER EPIPHYSIS OF HUMERUS.

Shadows of the splint and padding are seen.   Prof. W. B. Van Lennep's case.

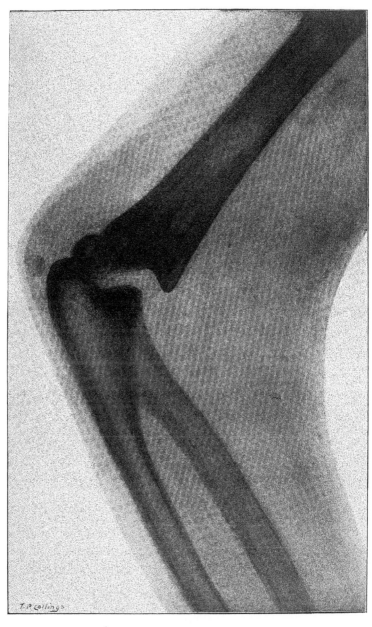

SEPARATION AND DISPLACEMENT BACKWARDS OF THE LOWER EPIPHYSIS OF THE HUMERUS.

Dr. CHAS. L. LEONARD's case.

physial separations these injuries unite with greater rapidity than fractures.

Although in even the simplest cases union takes place, some impairment of the functions of the joint may ensue from one or other cause (to be presently described), so that a perfect recovery cannot be said to be the invariable rule. It is therefore prudent in all cases to impress early upon the minds of the parents or friends the idea or suggestion of an unfavourable prognosis. It is always necessary to be most cautious in this matter.

In the following case recorded by C. A. Sturrock (*Edinburgh Hospital Reports*, vol. ii. 1894, p. 600), eight months after the injury (displacement backwards of the epiphysis), there was only

Fractures and displacements of the superficial bones are scarcely to be seen with the screen, but by proper direction of the latter the authors have been able to see good shadow outlines of the shoulder-joint. The details are completely rendered on the plate.

'In a plate given of the pyknogram of a fracture of the humerus through the "anatomical neck," taken four weeks after the accident, the contours of the bones, the acromion, the glenoid cavity, the scapula, the ribs, and the upper arm are quite distinct. It is clearly seen how the articular surface of the head is displaced laterally. A bridge of periosteum, which has separated from the diaphysis of the upper arm, has already produced bone and therefore appears as a shadow. In the humerus the medulla and compact tissue are distinctly differentiated. An important advantage of the pyknographic image is that the healing process may be watched from day to day. We can see the healing process in the living body, instead of having the difficulty of studying it in specimens obtained only casually.

'As plaster of Paris and splints do not obstruct the rays much, we can see if the re-adjustment of the broken bones or luxations is accurate, and if the callus is converted normally into bone. False union may be avoided more and more. Those who are accustomed to inspect all fractures in several directions with the screen, and also to photograph them, will be astonished to see how defectively fractures are healed even when they have been considered perfect examples. There can be no question that pyknoscopy will do good service in the effective treatment of injuries to the extremities, and that new and unsuspected improvements will be made in the direction of remedial treatment of traumatic lesions. According to our observations, defective "setting" is not infrequently brought about by the interposition of small splinters of bone between the fragments.

'With recent injuries, especially to the joints, the accumulation of blood renders the use of the screen more difficult, but it does not interfere with a photograph. Injuries to the vertebral column can always be recognised in children, but with greater difficulty in adults.

'Especially favourable objects for observation are articular fractures, and those rare fractures which have hitherto presented insurmountable difficulties to the methods of diagnosis, for which recourse could only be had to mere supposition—e.g. fractures of the hand and tarsal bones of the foot, &c., and more particularly those of the glenoid cavity of the shoulder and hip. We can see small splinters of bone in a joint and proceed to their removal, if necessary.

'We need not point out how much this knowledge means to surgical procedure, nor of what importance it is that we have other means than the sense of touch to guide us when operating upon badly united fractures. A large number of cases of injuries to joints will doubtless present themselves that have healed under conditions of movement, in which we are enabled by pyknoscopy to observe directly the impediments to motion, and thus to adopt proper operative treatment. Fractures and other injuries that were difficult to recognise formerly may now be distinctly seen and placed graphically before laymen. The pyknogram will therefore be of use to convince the patient himself, and those interested in him, of the necessity of a useful operation.'

For further practical details of this process the reader must be referred to Dr. D. Walsh's recent book, *The Röntgen Rays in Medical Work*, London 1897.

a slight degree of thickening traceable above the joint, no shortening, and perfect movement.

W. H., aged 12, admitted to Royal Infirmary, Edinburgh, on February 6, 1893, with a history of having fallen on his bent wrist when running, and of having felt something 'give way' in the region of the elbow. Under anæsthesia, it was found that the articular surface of the lower end of the humerus, along with the radius and ulna, was displaced backwards; the shaft of the humerus, to which were attached both the condyles (*sic*), formed a projection in front of the elbow. On manipulation, cartilaginous crepitus was readily obtained: when the arm was flexed to a right angle the deformity disappeared, and the relation of the bony prominences was apparently normal. The parts were accordingly placed in splints in this position for two weeks, when passive movements—at first very gentle, afterwards more forcible—were commenced, and continued for ten weeks. After the splints were removed the arm was retained on alternate nights, first in the flexed, then in the extended position. The earliest movements were exceedingly painful, and necessarily very limited in range. On one occasion, five weeks after the accident, the boy absented himself for some days, and when he returned for treatment the arm had become much stiffer. Eight months after the accident, except for a slight degree of thickening above the joint, no trace of the injury could be discovered; there was no shortening, and the range of movement was perfect. The case is of further interest in that some years previously the boy had sustained a compound diastasis of the lower end of the other humerus. Suppuration had occurred, and the range of movement was less than a right angle.

Deformity is found to be very great where the injury has been mistaken for a fracture.

One of the chief objects in the treatment is to prevent the projection forwards of the diaphysis, and this can be successfully accomplished by careful treatment. Unless this deformity be remedied early, there is sure to be some restriction of movement of the elbow-joint.

Mr. Hutchinson says that after union has occurred with a certain amount of deformity, the surgeon, unless well acquainted with the subject, is apt to suppose that he has overlooked a dislocation. Several such cases had come under his notice, and in some it had been proposed to attempt reduction. He mentions (*Medical Times and Gazette*, January 1884, p. 2) the case of a boy who was brought to him for stiffness of the elbow a month after the accident. Two years previously he had excised one of his knee-joints. He had now fallen downstairs, and, instead of breaking his ankylosed lower limb, had displaced the epiphysis of one elbow. Union had occurred, with much displacement backwards still remaining. The swelling had pretty well disappeared, and the outline of the lower end of the bone was easily distinguished. The elbow was at an obtuse angle, and its area of flexion was very limited. Free movements were instituted and were followed by much improvement at the end of a year, but the power of flexion was far from complete.

Mr. C. G. Wheelhouse, in a clinical lecture on the Surgery of the Epiphyses in 1885 (*British Medical Journal*, March 7, 1885, p. 475), mentions the case of a child who had been treated for a supposed simple dislocation backwards of the bones of the forearm under the care of the late Mr. Teale. There resulted a considerable amount of deformity, with tolerably free movements of the joint, accompanied, however, by some permanent stiffness and locking. After careful examination Mr. Wheelhouse came to the conclusion that the injury had been a dislocation accompanied by a fracture through the epiphysis, and that, though the joint had not been restored to its original condition of perfection, the result was, for such an injury, very excellent, and one with which the parents of the child should have had every reason to be content. But they were not, and taking legal advice upon the subject, they threatened an action at law against Mr. Teale. They were only dissuaded from it with difficulty.

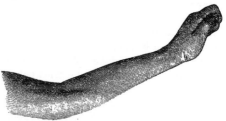

FIG. 77.—HYPER-EXTENSION OF ELBOW AFTER DISPLACEMENT FORWARDS
OF DIAPHYSIS OF HUMERUS

Great deformity, accompanied by hyper-extension at the elbow-joint, existed in the following example of old separation with displacement backwards which came under the author's care in May 1895. Eight and a half months previously the girl (Dorothy C.), aged six years, had fallen in the playground at school and injured her left elbow. The injury was said to have been treated as a sprain and lotions had been applied. Probably at this time there was little deformity, but on admission to the Miller Hospital there was a large projecting mass of bone discovered in front of the elbow, most marked towards the inner side. This was clearly the lower diaphysial end of the humerus, and over its edge the brachial artery could be seen and felt pulsating. The epicondyles and olecranon held their normal relations. While movements of pronation and supination were absolutely perfect, flexion at the elbow could be effected only to a right angle. Extension, both active and passive, was greatly beyond the normal limit, the forearm posteriorly being at an angle of 125 degrees with the arm (see fig. 77).

x 2

After incision of the skin the author removed the projecting inner angle of the diaphysis by means of a chisel. The brachial artery and median nerve lying over the bone had to be drawn aside at the time of operation. Primary union of the wound took place, and at the end of six months flexion was greatly increased, reaching even 50 degrees. The patient could touch the front of her shoulder, which she could not do before the operation. The whole limb had gained in muscular power, but hyper-extension at the elbow remained the same.

In a few rare instances, in spite of all care, some deformity will remain with considerable thickening; in the course of some months, however, the parts become so much remodelled that the final result is usually good.

Lannelongue lays it down that fractures of the elbow in children are serious lesions and difficult of cure, and that it is saying too much to assert that after one of these fractures all the proper movements will be preserved.

Besides the specimen of *displacement forwards of the epiphysis* described above from the patient whose elbow the author resected, there is another case, to which Mr. Hutchinson alludes, where a man had a very curiously shaped elbow, which looked altogether narrower than usual; the olecranon projected a little, but not so much as would have been expected; and he came to the conclusion that the reverse of the usual state of things had taken place, and that instead of the epiphysis with the ulna and radius being carried behind the humerus, the opposite condition of displacement forwards had occurred.

Limited movement.—Where the joint has been patiently and carefully treated, good movements of flexion and extension are to be ultimately expected in most cases; although the friends of the patient should always be made to clearly understand that the joint must be stiff for some time—probably for many months—subsequent to the injury.

The movements of pronation and supination are rarely affected.

Limitation of movement may be due to (1) *Stiffness and thickening of the joint* from (a) implication or laceration of the synovial membrane; (b) from extension to the joint of the inflammation at the seat of the separation; (c) from the limb being kept at rest too long. (2) *Excessive deposit of callus*, either in front or behind the articulation, which may hinder the movements of the elbow, as in Wight's case. (3) *Imperfect reduction of fragments.*

Exuberant callus, by its presence, may cause the greatest impediment to the functions of the limb, especially if the displacement has not been entirely corrected. It is produced by the periosteum, which may have been stripped up or otherwise injured, and the close proximity to the conjugal cartilage and growing end of the bone also conduces to its formation. In like manner at an earlier period after the injury, the newly formed callus may produce pressure upon the brachial artery or median, ulnar, or musculo-spiral nerves in the vicinity of the elbow-joint. The provisional callus filling up the olecranon and coronoid fossæ often hampers for some time the free movement of the elbow-joint.

Ankylosis of elbow.—At first sight it would appear that ankylosis after injury to the elbow-joint in children was more common than after injury in the neighbourhood of other joints. The multiple character of its functions in part accounts for this.

In rare instances the joint remains permanently affected and stiff.

Considering that the attachment of the capsule of the joint is above the epiphysis, especially in front, it is not surprising if articular inflammation and subsequent rigidity should ensue, unless the fragments be accurately placed in normal position. Yet M. Guersant, in reporting (*Bulletin de la Société de Chirurgie*, 1861, 2ème Série, tom. i. p. 679) a case of separation of the lower epiphysis of the humerus with displacement backwards, seemed astonished that at the end of a month there was still some impediment to free movement of the elbow. The patient was a boy aged eight who had fallen on to his elbow, and the usual signs were present.

M. Sée and some other surgeons believed that the subacute inflammation and plastic infiltrations of the articular and periarticular structures are brought about by effusion of blood and serum.

Jonathan Hutchinson's case of resection for compound diastasis resulted in an elbow bent at right angles, and quite stiff.

The advocates of the treatment by the extended position of the joint maintain that the liability to ankylosis after this method is much less than after treatment in the flexed position. However, most British surgeons maintain that the latter position is the one in which the ultimate results are better, at any rate in the form of the injury under consideration.

Implication of nerves.—The musculo-spiral, the median, and ulnar nerves are each of them liable to be implicated in the abundant callus which is often present, extending even up the humerus for some distance, and their injury may give rise to paralysis, loss of sensation, hyperæsthesia, vesication, &c.

Resection of the callus pressing upon the nerve may be required, that the nerve may be set free.

Hamilton relates (*Fractures and Dislocations*, 8th edition, 1891, p. 240) a case in which a fracture just above the condyles occurred at the age of four years. Appreciable deformity remained at the age of twenty-seven years. The patient could not then completely supinate the forearm. The whole arm was weak, and the ulnar nerve remarkably sensitive. The ulnar side of the forearm, and also the ring and little fingers, were numb, and had been in this condition ever since the accident. In another case of fracture, which occurred nine months previously in a lad aged nine years, he had operated by sawing off the projecting end of the upper fragment. This fragment was lying in front of the lower one, and the skin covering its sharp point was very thin and tender. There was no ankylosis at the elbow-joint, but the hand was flexed forcibly upon the wrist, the first phalanges of all the fingers being extended and the second and third phalanges flexed. Supination and pronation were lost. The forearm and hand were almost completely paralysed, and at times very painful. The ulnar nerve could be felt lying across the end of the bone. The projecting fragment was exposed and removed, and the nerve lifted and laid aside, but a year later the arm was found to be in the same condition.

Dr. Deanesley (*Lancet*, April 22, 1893) thinks, however, that in many cases of this kind the paralysis is present soon after the accident, but is often overlooked, and is due to the imperfectly reduced separation of the epiphysis ; also that, although the paralysis might be attributed to pressure of callus involving the nerve (for in his cases much callus was thrown out), yet it did not appear to him to be very well established that this is ever a real cause of nerve paralysis. He expresses his belief that, nerve lesions not being thought of, paralysis and contracture of muscles are confused with the general weakness and stiffness so often left for a considerable time after the fracture has united.

Paralysis, however, of the musculo-spiral nerve produces the characteristic and familiar wrist-drop, which is little likely to be overlooked. If any doubt as to the existence of nerve lesion remains after the examination of the voluntary power, sensation, and attitude of the limb, it can generally be set at rest by testing the electric excitability of the muscles and nerves to the faradaic and galvanic currents. Faradaic excitability is usually lost, while galvanic irritability, on the other hand, is retained, and in some cases is increased.

Dr. Deanesley recommends that as a rule no attempt should be made to deal with the nerve injury until the fracture is soundly united. The whole limb should be treated with systematic rubbing, and with faradaic or galvanic electric currents. No operation should be advised unless there is reason to believe that there still exists some pressure or traction on the nerve which can be relieved, 'or any marked displacement of the bony fragments.' He relates (*Lancet*, April 22, 1893, p. 928) the two following cases from the General Hospital, Wolverhampton :

(1) *Separation of lower epiphysis of left humerus ; paralysis of musculo-spiral nerve.*—A boy, aged eight years. The accident, caused by a fall on February 18, 1892, was recognised by the usual signs. After reduction the elbow was immobilised at a right angle by plaster of Paris. When this was removed at the end of four weeks there was much bony thickening about the lower end of the humerus, and the elbow was very stiff. There was also

complete paralysis of all the muscles supplied by the musculo-spiral nerve below the elbow. These muscles gave no response to faradaism, but responded to a smaller minimal galvanic stimulation than the corresponding muscles of the opposite side. No loss of sensation could be detected. Friction, passive movement, and the galvanic current were employed daily. Recovery of voluntary power began in the supinators on March 9, and was complete in all the affected muscles on May 2, although then, and for long after, there was no recovery of faradaic excitability. Redundant callus having been absorbed, it was found that the displaced fragments had not been perfectly reduced, the lower end of the shaft being in front of and overlapping the lower fragment, forming a prominence at the front of the elbow which stopped flexion at a right angle. Extension was also slightly limited. In other respects the limb was perfectly normal.

(2) *Separation of lower epiphysis of right humerus ; paralysis of musculo-spiral nerve.*—A boy, aged eight years. The accident was caused by a fall off a gate on September 6, 1892. The displacement was reduced and the limb put up on an internal angular splint. On September 10 he was found to have complete paralysis of the extensors of the wrist and fingers and of the supinator longus. No anæsthesia was detected. This resembled the previous case in almost every respect, both in the imperfect reduction of the fragments and in the result. The muscles, which had lost faradaic, but preserved galvanic, excitability, were treated daily with one or other form of electricity. Recovery began in the supinator on October 27, and was complete in all muscles on November 27, the patient having been under treatment nearly three months.

Numerous similar cases are recorded by Callender, Hamilton, and others.

Lange records (*New York Medical Journal*, April 28, 1883. p. 469) the case of a girl, aged eight, who, after a fracture close to the lower end (supra-condyloid fracture) of the humerus, experienced pain at the seat of injury, the wrist and fingers being flexed, with a very limited degree of motion. A sharp edge of bone could be felt. An incision was made, and the median nerve found flattened against the edge of bone ; above this point the nerve was thickened. The nerve was loosened and the edge of bone excised, with decided relief. The colour and temperature of the limb were also markedly improved. A curious point is that in this case the growth of the nails, as indicated by ridges on them, was interfered with previous to the operation.

In a case of Volkmann's, after resection and reduction of the protruding diaphysis for compound fracture, persistent paralysis of the musculo-spiral nerve resulted, although the elbow-joint was movable.

Gangrene.—The possibility of the occurrence of gangrene from interference with the circulation in the brachial artery should ever be present to the surgeon's mind. The vessel may be unavoidably pressed upon by the lower end of the upper fragment, or may have been injured at the time of the accident, but this serious mishap may be the result of a badly fitting splint or bandages applied too tightly; especially is this true of the plaster-of-Paris dressing.

Shortening of arm.—Unless very great difficulty has been experienced in keeping the fragments in position, and some over-lapping remain, there will be found to be little or no shortening of the arm in separation; yet it is usual to find half an inch or more shortening after fracture above the epicondyles.

Arrest of growth in length of the arm.—Although the increase in the length of the humerus takes place in a very small degree at the lower end of the bone, it is possible that the injury may be followed by a partial arrest of development or irregular growth in the lower end of the humerus.

Vogt reckons that the increase of the humerus through the lower epiphysis is only about 7 cm. for the whole period of life. After the tenth year the epiphysis only adds about 1 cm. to the increase in length of the bone, so that after the twelfth year of life the influence of this end of the humerus in causing any appreciable shortening of the arm can have but little value.

M. Goyrand (*Bulletin de la Soc. de Chirurgie*, 1861, p. 534) watched for eight years the development of the humerus in a case of epiphysial separation of its lower end, in which the injured limb was developed absolutely like the other. The patient was a girl, who had met with the injury to her arm from a fall at the age of three years.

Suppuration may result from periosteal inflammation; it is certainly less common after this form of separation than after many others. It is, however, more often met with after compound separation.

Mr. Hutchinson refers (*London Hospital Reports*, 1864, vol. i. p. 89) to a case of suppuration after epiphysial injury in a sailor lad, who fell from a ship's mast and received severe and complicated injuries. The patient had fracture of one clavicle and separation of three epiphyses. Of his right humerus both the upper and lower epiphyses were detached, and about the lower injury suppuration occurred. In his other arm there was separation of the lower epiphysis of the humerus, and here again suppuration occurred. Eight months after the accident union had taken place at all the injured parts, but with the characteristic deformity at each. The right humerus was already considerably shortened, partly by arrest of growth, but chiefly by union with displacement. The lad (who was aged fourteen, and was growing very rapidly) had not been treated at the hospital.

In over fifty cases J. Hutchinson junior found that suppuration never occurred unless the injury had been compound from the first, and had become so owing to sloughing of the over-stretched skin. The youngest patient was eighteen months, the oldest fourteen years old.

Suppuration of the elbow-joint may occur (1) by extension from periosteal inflammation ; (2) by wound of the synovial membrane.   It is frequent in compound separations.

Suppuration occurred in Sturrock's case, leaving the range of movement less than a right angle.

Necrosis of diaphysis is a not uncommon result in compound separations.

Marjolin, in a short article upon 'Fracture of the Humerus above the Condyles in Children' (*Journal de Méd. et Chir. Prat.*, Paris, 1863, xxiv. 397–399), remarks that M. Velpeau was wont to observe in his lectures that one of the worst things that could happen to a young surgeon beginning practice is to meet with a case of traumatic injury of the elbow in a child.   Marjolin believed this to be very true regarding complicated and obscure injuries, which so often occasion errors of diagnosis and of prognosis fatal to the practitioner's reputation.   Such cases require the utmost care in examination, for the whole subsequent progress and treatment depend upon an accurate diagnosis.

TREATMENT.   Simple cases.—The treatment is, for the most part, the same as in supra-condyloid fracture.   Reduction of the deformity is effected without any difficulty in most cases by extension and gentle manipulation of the diaphysial end.   For this purpose the humerus should be grasped with one hand and the forearm with the other or by an assistant.

To maintain the fragments in good position is often a question of extreme difficulty, so great is the tendency of the deformity to be reproduced.   This is to a large extent dependent upon the character of the disunited surfaces, the powerful action of the triceps and other muscles upon the ulna and lower epiphysis of the humerus, the small size of the lower fragment, and its proximity to the elbow-joint.

The elbow should be fixed at a right angle and a *plastic splint* (previously cut out and prepared by means of a paper pattern shaped to the sound limb) moulded to the elbow accurately, evenly, and firmly.   The elbow and fragments should be kept in the corrected position until the mould is quite hard.   The splint should extend well up the arm and down the forearm to the wrists, so that the whole length of the limb may be supported.

It matters but little of what material the splint is composed, provided that it will harden at once.   Flannel soaked in plaster of Paris, gutta-percha, Cocking's poro-plastic splinting, &c., are all good.

Croft's plaster-of-Paris lateral splints, with an interval on the anterior and posterior aspects of the elbow, the author has found to be one of the best forms of splint in injuries about the elbow-joint in children. These splints can be readjusted day by day as the

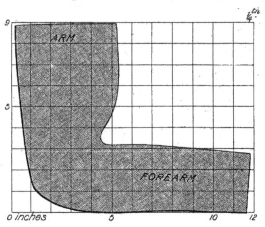

FIG. 78.—PATTERN FOR INNER PIECES OF LATERAL SPLINTS WITH ELBOW AT RIGHT ANGLES. FOR A BOY OF FIFTEEN YEARS

Reduced to one quarter size on scale of inches. Splints for all ag may be cut from this pattern

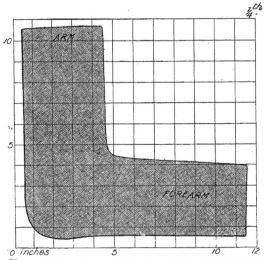

FIG. 79.—PATTERN FOR OUTER PIECES OF LATERAL SPLINTS WITH ELBOW AT RIGHT ANGLES. FOR A BOY OF FIFTEEN YEARS

Reduced to one quarter size on scale of inches

swelling subsides, and be evenly and carefully bandaged again to the limb.

Croft's splints consist of four pieces of common house flannel accurately cut to the shape of the joint and adjoining portions of the limb to which they are about to be applied. Two of the pieces are used on each side of the limb, leaving a gap or interval a half to three-quarters of an inch wide on either lateral aspect (or on the front and back when antero-posterior splints are required). The two external pieces

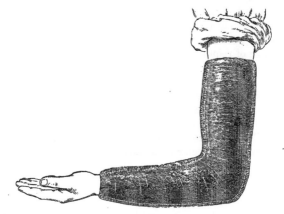

FIG. 80.—SEMIDIAGRAMMATIC VIEW OF CROFT'S LATERAL SPLINTS OF PLASTER OF PARIS APPLIED TO ARM AND FOREARM

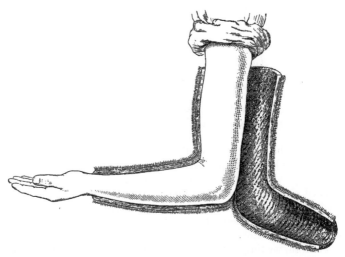

FIG. 81.—THE SAME WITH OUTER SPLINT LAID ASIDE BY THE MUSLIN BANDAGE ALONG THE WHOLE OF GAP IN FRONT AND OF GAP BEHIND IN THE FOREARM PORTION

are soaked in plaster of Paris of the consistency of cream, and placed on the outer surface of the two internal pieces. The whole is retained in position by means of bandages made of porous muslin, and rolled on evenly without tension, while the limb is held in the required position until the plaster sets (see fig. 80). The splint may be readily removed by cutting the muslin bandage through at the gaps left on either side between the edges of the flannel. One side only of the splint may be removed or laid aside in a hinge-like manner for the necessary examination of the joint by merely cutting through the bandage on one aspect of the limb (see fig. 81).

On account of their danger, plaster of-Paris-bandages should be scrupulously avoided.

Some surgeons use pasteboard, leather, &c.; but these have the disadvantage of requiring some time to harden. Others recommend the hand and forearm to be evenly bandaged before the splint is applied.

A simple rectangular posterior splint of wood, or other material, shaped in a concave manner, will often be found sufficient.

An interruption at the elbow is an advantage to the back splint. Sir Astley Cooper added a short splint in front of the arm to correct the tendency to displacement forwards.

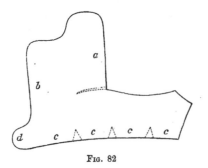

Fig. 82

Hamilton preferred a thick sheet of gutta-percha, moulded and applied accurately to the limb. It should be extended over the shoulder, the back of the arm and forearm to the wrist. The splint should first be lined with woollen cloth or some such material. A pretty large pledget of fine cotton-wool is laid in front of the elbow-joint to prevent the bandage from excoriating the delicate and inflamed skin, and great care taken to protect the bony eminences about the joint, or, rather, to relieve them from pressure, by increasing the thickness of the pads in a horseshoe shape above and below these eminences.

Packard, writing in Keating's *Cyclopædia of Diseases of Children*, describes the following splint, which meets the indications, and which, he says, has given him the best results. Measuring by the sound limb, a piece of binder's board is cut out—or, for a very young child, a piece of pasteboard—in the shape shown in the diagram (fig. 82). This is then again cut in the dotted lines, and it will be seen that *a* can be turned over so as to fit along the front of the arm, while *b* will be on its inner side, and *c* on that of the forearm.

The portions, *c, c, c, c,* turned up, will steady the forearm and hand, while *d* is turned up so as to push the olecranon forward and, along with it, the lower end of the lower humeral fragment. Properly padded, this splint is secured by means of a bandage accurately applied from the fingers to the shoulder, and the hand and forearm are supported by a sling.

Anterior rectangular splints to the elbow, made of wood or other material, are to be avoided for many reasons. First, as Packard remarks, the obliquity of the line of the articulation is not sufficiently recognised, and the application of splints which lie straight across the front of the joint pushes the trochlea upwards, and so presses the upper and inner angle of the lower fragment behind the opposing point of the upper fragment. Secondly, the epiphysial line of cartilage itself is not quite transverse, but extends obliquely downwards and inwards, so that however easy it may be to secure the diaphysis backwards, it will be found almost impossible by these measures to remedy the twisting which, as it were, the epiphysis undergoes.

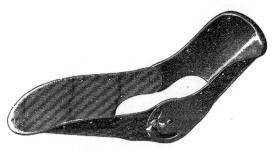

FIG. 83.—WINCHESTER'S TIN SPLINT. CAN BE PLACED AT ANY ANGLE BY MEANS OF JOINT AT ELBOW OR BENT TO THE REQUIRED WIDTH AT THE SIDES BY MEANS OF WRENCHES

Thirdly, the pressure of the splint at the bend of the elbow will tend to injure the brachial artery by compressing it against the projecting upper fragment.

Many observers have written upon the treatment of fracture of the elbow-joint in children, and these injuries have been the subject of many discussions before different societies. Some blame the flexed position with fixation as the cause of ankylosis; others blame the condition of the joint.

Hamilton says that Dr. Physick's simple angular side-splints, made of wood, without joints, are still used by some American surgeons in fractures about the elbow-joint.

Various forms of angular splints with a hinge at the elbow, some fitting the forearm and arm accurately, are all more or less cumbersome.

A combination is often useful, such as a gutta-percha, leather, or Gooch splint on one side, and on the other an angular splint reaching from the shoulder to the end of the fingers; or a leather or gutta-percha splint moulded behind the elbow, and a small wooden splint to the front of the arm, with a pad over its lower end, between it and the projecting part of the diaphysis.

The author is convinced that, as a rule, all injuries to the lower end of the humerus should be treated with moulded rather than manufactured splints.

The splint should be applied as soon as the diagnosis has been made, and, if possible, under the influence of an anæsthetic. By this means the formation of a projection in front may be avoided. No time should be lost in waiting for the swelling or inflammation to subside, for even after the lapse of a few days it will be found almost impossible to accurately re-adjust the fragments.

Fractures about the elbow-joint are treated by fixation in many positions, viz. complete flexion, semiflexion, complete extension, and incomplete extension, any of these being combined with pronation or supination of the forearm.

Hitherto, with the exception of fracture of the olecranon and some few others, each surgeon has had his own particular method for all fractures, irrespective of their nature.

In this country Mr. Jonathan Hutchinson is one of the chief advocates for treatment in the flexed position, but, at the same time, he states (*Medical Times and Gazette*, 1866, vol. i. p. 515) 'that it is difficult, if not impossible, to effect accurate coaptation of the fragments. There is almost certain to be some overlapping; but still, the bent position is the best one.' His son gives (*British Medical Journal*, December 30, 1893, August 11, 1894, and November 3, 1894) the results of fourteen cases treated with splints in the flexed position. 'In six the result, as regards absence of deformity and the elbow movement, was practically perfect. In the remaining eight a certain amount of limitation of extension and flexion—usually about 20 degrees in either direction—with thickening of the lower third of the humerus, remained when the patient was last seen. In only one was the power of rotation in the least affected, and it need hardly be said that a range of flexion amounting to 80 or 90 degrees is, whilst not ideal, of extreme value to the patient.'

Powers mentions two cases of separation of the lower epiphysis of the humerus in children aged two and six years respectively, and in each a perfect result was attained by simple confinement at a right angle, the lower fragment being drawn well forward.

Mr. Christopher Heath and many other British surgeons still employ this method.

Malgaigne, Marjolin, Coulon, Boyer, and Nélaton always employed the semiflexed position in fractures about the elbow.

König, Goyeneche (*Fract. du coude chez les enfants*, Thèse de Paris, 1872), Hamilton, and other more recent writers maintain the advantages of the same position, the forearm being flexed at 90 to

100 degrees. In this position the flexor and other muscles attached to the epicondyles are relaxed, and the tilting forwards of the lower fragment is prevented.

Others prefer to fix the elbow in the rectangular position for a week or ten days, and then change the angle day by day, without passive motion.

Dr. E. M. Moore employs a lateral angular splint, and every alternate day flexes the elbow more and more until the hand can touch the neck; the forearm is then carried downwards by degrees, and the process is reversed, but the arm is never brought out perfectly straight.

Others, again, prefer to treat these fractures with the forearm flexed to less than a right angle with the arm.

Bardenheuer recommends permanent extension, in the first instance, for this form of injury, and many French surgeons hope that the flexed position may be entirely given up; while Pitha and Billroth and other German surgeons go so far as to say that juxta-epiphysial separations can only be reduced by means of extension.

Ricard, however (in Duplay and Reclus's *Traité de chirurgie*, 1890), still advises treatment by fixation in the rectangular position, but advocates early movement (fifteen to eighteen days in children), rubbing, massage, &c., to guard against ankylosis.

In spite of all the advantages claimed for it even from the days of Hippocrates, this plan is one that cannot be recommended.

Liston, and a few other British surgeons, also treated supra-condyloid fracture in the straight position.

M. C. Guedeney, in his thesis upon the treatment of fractures of the elbow in children (Thèse de Lyon, Mars 1893), gives an account of sixty cases of fractures about the elbow, at ages varying from six to seven years, treated (with the exception of three) by a modification of the principle laid down by Laroyenne and advocated by his pupil, Berthomier, in 1875—viz. by fixation in complete and permanent extension. This modification, introduced by M. Vincent, of Lyons, consists of fixation in the extended position for a time, alternating with flexion in the supine position. The results, at the time of leaving the hospital or later on, in many cases were said to have been excellent, but some eight of them were very incomplete; in five the results were unknown. Immediately, or a few days after such an accident, under an anæsthetic, the fragments are reduced and the limb immovably fixed in complete extension and supination by applying a posterior trough splint of plaster, or silicate, extending from the shoulder to the fingers. A small tongue-piece over the palm of the hand passing between the thumb and fingers ensures perfect fixation in the supine position. This allows free access to the limb in front, and does not, as some have said, exercise too great constriction; neither is the position unbearable for children. The pain at first experienced passes off in two days. The dressing is usually changed on the day after its first application, and re-applied.   On acute pain, or other sign of compression, the splint must be removed at once. On the eighth to the tenth day, according to the swelling, the splint is removed and the forearm slightly flexed, the joint being now carefully examined.   Consolidation will have occurred to a great extent, and does not prevent the limb being put up in the flexed position for eight or ten days in a plaster trough.   At the end of this time (the twentieth day) the fracture is perfectly united, and passive motion is commenced ; or, if ununited, the splint is left on some days longer, or a third one is applied as the first in the completely extended and supine position.

M. Vincent himself adds : ' The position is alternately total extension and flexion, more or less at a right angle.   At each renewal of the immovable apparatus slight movements are carried out at the articulation.'

Of the following thirteen cases of separation of the lower end of the humerus published by M. Guedeney, in four the displacement of the epiphysis was more or less backwards, in four there was little or no displacement, and in five the displacement is not stated.

Displacement backwards.   I. *Juxta-epiphysial disjunction of the left humerus.*—Boy (J. L.), aged eleven years, was admitted May 31, 1890, having fallen on his left side with the forearm bent.   Juxta-epiphysial fracture of the lower end of the humerus was diagnosed. The arm was directed obliquely from below upwards, and from without inwards.   There was little bruising or swelling, but crepitus was distinct.   Under an anæsthetic the fragments were placed in position, and a plaster apparatus applied in complete extension. On June 22 consolidation was complete, but there was abundant callus ; arm and forearm in same axis, with a tendency to adduction.   There was no ankylosis, all movements being free.   The forearm was bent to a right angle and the elbow put up again. The following day the child left.   Results unknown.

II. *Juxta-epiphysial disjunction.*—Boy (P. C.), aged four, admitted May 6, 1891, having fallen from a height of one and a half metres on to the right arm.   The humerus was found displaced in front of the lower fragment.   Reduction was effected by extension and counter-extension, and a posterior plaster splint was applied in the extended and supine position.   When seen after some time there was no ankylosis.   The limb was sound, and displayed a perfect result.

III. *Epiphysial disjunction, with displacement backwards.*—A girl (M. B.), age not stated, admitted June 20, 1884 ; she had fallen upon a staircase on to her elbow, and was treated at first by a bone-setter in the country.   When seen there was swelling, traces of extravasated blood, projection of the humeral end forwards, of the olecranon backwards, with a depression above and two or three centimetres shortening.   Complete extension could be carried out, but flexion only halfway.   Under an anæsthetic a sharp ridge could be felt in the bend of the elbow. Reduction was effected, and the limb fixed in the extended position. On July 11, flexion was limited to a right angle, and there still existed marked swelling. On July 18, the extent of movements had increased. Passive movements were now commenced, and the elbow fixed in the flexed position. Left the hospital January 25, 1893. Parents stated that the child was quite cured, and that she does not recollect which was the injured arm.

IV. *Disjunction of the lower epiphysis of the humerus.*—A girl (A. J.), aged eight years, was admitted August 3, 1885, having fallen from a wall a height of about two metres on to her right elbow. Slight swelling without bruising was noticed; the movements of the joint were free, and there was abnormal mobility, but no crepitus. The lower part of the humerus projected forwards and inwards, the epiphysis being displaced backwards and outwards. The fragments were immediately reduced by extension and counter-extension, and a plaster splint was applied in the extended position. On August 30 the splint was removed; good consolidation took place, after which passive movements were carried out. On September 18 the child left the hospital; on February 5, 1893, she was seen again. The result was perfect; all movements of the elbow were normal, extension being even a little exaggerated. The child said that this arm was now stronger than the other, and could do needlework. No trace whatever of callus.

Little or no displacement. V. *Epiphysial disjunction of the humerus.*—Boy (P. M.), aged nine and a half years, admitted November 5, 1885, after a fall on the elbow. There was considerable swelling about the elbow, bruising of the lower part of the arm, and limitation of movements. At the lower end of the humerus there was a little abnormal mobility and distinct crepitus, but no displacement. Silicate splint applied in the extended position. *November 9.*—Slight swelling of fingers. *November 18.*—Swelling still remained; the arm put up in silicate splint flexed at a right angle. On December 17, all swelling gone, and complete union of the fragments. The result was perfect, the arm having recovered the use of all movements.

VI. *Disjunction of the lower epiphysis of the humerus.*—Boy (P. M.), aged nine and a half, fell on the elbow. There was some ecchymosis, but no displacement. Silicate splint applied in the completely extended position. Dressing removed at the end of fifteen days, and forearm placed in the flexed position. On removal of the last splint there was no more swelling, and all the movements of the elbow were good.

VII. *Disjunction of the lower epiphysis of the humerus.*—Boy (J. B.), age not stated, admitted July 21, 1885, after a fall from an apricot tree. There were swelling and abnormal mobility above the humeral epiphysis, and very little displacement. Reduction was effected, and a plaster splint applied in the extended position.

July 30, 1885.—Left the hospital with a new splint. Patient could not be traced again.

VIII. *Juxta-epiphysial disjunction of the humerus.*—A boy (P. D.), aged seven years, admitted January 8, 1892, after a fall from making a false step. Immediately there was loss of power, and the arm (especially a little above the elbow) and the forearm were swollen and painful. Movements of the joints were free, but extreme flexion dragged backwards the lower fragment of the humerus. Crepitus was present. Reduction and fixation with silicate splint in extension. *January* 18.—The result was good ; a plaster splint applied in the semiflexed position (135 degrees). *February* 16.—Flexion beyond a right angle difficult and painful. *February* 28.—The abundant callus hindered flexion, while the other movements were preserved.

Displacement not stated. IX. *Epiphysial disjunction of the lower end of the humerus, with fracture of the radius and ulna.*—A girl (Julia M.), age not stated, admitted April 1887, having fallen the previous day from a chair on to the ground. There was effusion of blood about the left elbow, olecranon uninjured. The radius and ulna were fractured at the lower end, with a small wound in front of forearm. *April* 22.—Under an anæsthetic, reduction and plaster splint applied in extended position. Seen in January 1893, six years after, the elbow had rapidly recovered, and preserved all its movements, including pronation and supination.

X. *Juxta-epiphysial disjunction of the lower end of the humerus.* A boy (Chas. M.), aged eight years. No details are given, but under chloroform a plaster splint was applied in extreme extension and supination. The child did not attend the hospital again, and the results were unknown.

XI. *Juxta-epiphysial disjunction of the right humerus.* — Boy (A. B.), aged five years, admitted December 23, 1890, after a fall upon a stone. The usual treatment was carried out. When seen on March 18, 1893, there was a perfect recovery ; the child could use his arm in every direction, the injured limb being as strong and sound as the uninjured one. An appreciable amount of callus still persisted. Although complete flexion could not be carried out, all the other movements of the limb were free.

XII. *Juxta-epiphysial disjunction of the humerus.*—Boy (L. S.), age not stated, admitted November 28, 1890, fell upon his elbow while carrying a load. No details are given except that he was treated by the usual method. Rigidity of the joint persisted for some time. On March 7, 1893, he could flex and extend his arm ' as he wished.' No pain or swelling ; complete recovery.

XIII. *Juxta-epiphysial fracture of the humerus.*—A boy (F. E.), aged thirteen, admitted October 14, 1891, after a fall upon the front of the left forearm. The arm seemed to have been subjected to a twisting movement, which detached the lower epiphysis. The line appeared to be oblique, and to involve the joint. Crepitus was distinct, notwithstanding the swelling; radius and ulna intact. Reduction was effected by means of strong extension, and the limb was fixed in a plaster apparatus in the extended position. *October* 25.—Fresh apparatus applied in the extended position. *November* 17.—Passive movements were carried out, and the arm put up in the flexed and supine position in a metal trough splint. When seen on January 25, 1893, the child had recovered all the movements of his limb.

By this method the advantages of the flexed position are said to be added to the complete reduction of the fragments gained by the extended position. Compound fractures are treated in the same way after the wound has been cleansed.

Older cases of ankylosis, &c., however, are treated by M. Vincent by forcible replacement of the fragments, and put up in the flexed position.

T. W. Nunn (*Clinical Society Transactions*, vol. xxv. p. 245), Allis, Illingworth (*Brit. Med. Journal*, February 1889), Berthomier, Bardenheuer, Warren (*Trans. American Med. Association*, vol. i. p. 174), Frere, Lauenstein of Hamburg (Langenbeck's *Archives*, vol. xxxvii.), Stimson, L. C. Lane, and others, including Billroth and Koenig, have of late years advocated putting up the limb in all injuries of the elbow in the straight position, with the forearm prone.

They claim that the deformity of cubitus valgus or cubitus varus, so frequently seen after treatment in the rectangular position, is to a great extent obviated, and a much earlier return of mobility of joint and usefulness is obtained.

Bardenheuer combines traction with extension in all these fractures. He has for five years (1888) treated all elbow fractures with permanent extension, both longitudinal and transverse, and with satisfactory results. Of course in this method of treatment the patient is confined to his bed for some weeks.

Dr. Lauenstein says, in support of this plan, that in the extended position the bones of the forearm afford a lever in adjusting the fracture of the lower end of the humerus; the anterior part of the capsular ligament is kept on the stretch, thereby lessening 'the danger of the bones of the forearm becoming entangled in the callus, and of the mobility of the joint being interfered with;' also that the surgeon can, in this position, 'readily detect any deviation from the normal direction of the axes of the humerus and bones of the forearm.' He advises (*Beitrag zum Centralblatt für Chirurg*. No. 24, 1888), for all fractures of the lower end of the humerus, treatment in the extended position, having for six years had good success in all his cases. He thinks that the surgeon should not be content with the preservation of the mobility of the joint, but that the deformity of cubitus valgus or varus, which is so prejudicial to the ulterior welfare of the patient, should also be seriously considered in treating such cases. An autopsy upon a

T-shaped fracture showed him that the flexed position produced bending, not at the joint, but at the seat of fracture. Previous to this he had employed this position for all fractures of the elbow.

Koenig in the same year, 1888, recommended the extended position for hospital practice, and the angular splint for private patients.

Nunn believed that in the extended position there was less danger of the anterior part of the capsular ligaments of the joint being involved in the callus, as it was held on the stretch, and that the risk of ankylosis was diminished, especially as the position permitted of effectual application of the ice-bags for the control of inflammatory action.

Wagner and Sonnenburg, while admitting the value of this method, claimed (1888) that some cases do better when treated in the right-angled position.

In 1875 Berthomier (*Mécanisme des fractures du coude chez les enfants ; leur traitement par l'extension*, Paris, 1875) following the views of Coulon, Marjolin, Pézerat, Laroyenne, and others already mentioned, recommended the extended position in transverse fractures of the lower end of the humerus. They believed that reduction was much more perfect in the extended than in the flexed position, and that it was not accompanied by the subsequent deformity met with under the latter mode of treatment. In a large number (eighty) of fractures and epiphysial separations of the lower end of the humerus, as a result of experiments on the bodies of children of all ages, but more especially from two to ten years, M. Berthomier came to the conclusion that the extended position was the best for maintaining the fragments in position. He quotes twelve cases of fracture of the elbow in the living subject, observed in the Lyons Hospital, in which good results had followed treatment by the extended position, and is of opinion that all fractures of the elbow—with the exception of that of the external epicondyle, in which he considers the flexed position the best—ought to be fixed in the extended position.

In a communication to the French Congress of Surgery in 1888 Berthomier adds 'that the flexed position is an obstacle to the reduction and coaptation of the fragments, and may give rise to ankylosis, whereas in extension and supination the coaptation is perfect,' the lower fragment being firmly held posteriorly by the olecranon, and in front by the detached periosteum and the anterior ligament, which form a very resisting splint. He thinks that ankylosis and stiffness following fractures of the elbow in children are always due to incomplete reduction of the fragments, and not to inflammation of the joint brought about by intra-articular fracture.

Dr. A. Hanbury Frere, speaking of the treatment of separation of this epiphysis, says : ' In these cases the fragment can be brought into good position, when the arm is straight, by traction on the forearm; and, therefore, the arm should be dressed in the straight position with plaster or starch bandage, keeping up gentle extension on the forearm till the dressing has set.'

To an admirable article on 'Fractures of the Bones of the Elbow-joint,' by Dr. L. C. Lane, of San Francisco (*Transactions of the American Surgical Association*, vol. ix. 1891, p. 393), the reader may be referred for the treatment of all such fractures by extension.

Many American surgeons believe that the 'carrying function' of the limb—viz. the normal angle outwards which the forearm makes with the arm in full extension—can only be preserved by adopting the extended position. Although in certain fractures (alluded to later on) involving the elbow-joint, the displaced fragments may be more completely reduced by the extended position, the author believes that

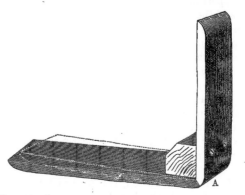

FIG. 84.—AUTHOR'S ANTERIOR RECTANGULAR SPLINT FOR THE LEFT ELBOW

The dotted lines are inserted to show the amount of outward deviation of the forearm piece. The angle at A is not transverse, but slopes obliquely to the inner side, according to the natural obliquity of the elbow-joint

separations of the lower end of the humerus are best treated in the flexed position, provided always that the natural obliquity of the elbow is fully maintained.

Mr. Jonathan Hutchinson says that the muscles retain the lower fragment in such a position that the joint itself is always flexed; and, therefore, if we straighten the arm there will be backward displacement.

The author's own experience agrees with this; the usual displacement backwards of the epiphysis is not nearly so well remedied in the fully extended position as when the forearm is flexed.

He is therefore of opinion that epiphysial separation of the lower end of the humerus is best treated by the flexed position, however strongly the position of full extension may be urged in the treatment of some of the other forms of injury to the elbow-joint in children.

For an excellent *résumé* of the various opinions as to the straight and rectangular positions in fractures of the elbow-joint, the reader should consult Dr. A. Hanbury Frere's valuable papers in the *Provincial Medical Journal* for January, March, and April, 1892, and Dr. J. B. Roberts's excellent contribution to the *Transactions of the American Surgical Association*, vol. x. 1892, p. 15.

No absolute rule can be laid down applicable to all separations or fractures. The mechanism and form of displacement are so totally different in each separation, whether of the lower end of the humerus or of one of the other epiphyses, that it is manifestly unscientific to treat them all by the same method.

Professor J. S. Wight, of Brooklyn, enumerates (*Annals of Surgery*, vol. xvii. August 1893) some cases of fracture of the lower end of the humerus, treated in the nearly extended (straight) position, in which ankylosis of the elbow-joint resulted. He argues from these in support of the bent position—that is, by treating all cases of fractures of the elbow-joint in the rectangular position.

In five cases recorded by him which had been treated in the extended position, midway between complete extension and right-angled flexion, the ankylosis and disability of the arm were very great, so that operative measures were resorted to, and with good result. In four other cases Dr. Wight used 'forcible joint infraction' to remedy the ankylosis. Two of these had been treated by the above method, one by a right-angled splint, and one (the only case) by a fully extended straight splint.

In one other case, treated by a nearly straight splint, the limb was very much disabled. Operation was in this case emphatically declined.

Dr. H. L. Smith, of Boston, U.S.A., has lately (*Boston Medical and Surgical Journal*, October 1894, p. 386) made a series of experiments with a view of determining the best position of the arm in the treatment of fracture involving the joint. He found, in fractures of the inner or outer side—internal or external condyle (*sic*)—T-shaped fractures, and transverse epiphysial separations, that the deformity was always reduced and the fragment firmly locked in position by flexing the forearm into the acute position (45°), with the forearm semi-pronated.

It is possible, in certain forms of this injury, that semi-pronation and extreme flexion may bring about a greater amount of movement of the elbow, but further experience is desirable upon this point.

Dr. W. Bruce, of Dingwall, suggests (*British Medical Journal*, October 24, 1896, p. 1201) simply reducing the fracture, bending the elbow to an acute angle, and laying the arm across the chest over a thick sheet of cotton-wool. A bandage enveloping the trunk and injured limb is then applied. The arm is undone daily and inspected.

Without any fixation.—The fear of ankylosis has led many surgeons, from the time of Hippocrates and Celsus, to treat fractures

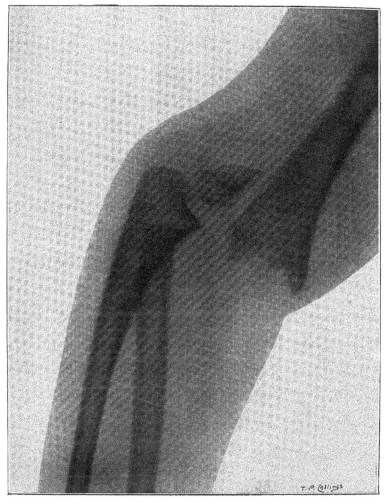

SIMPLE SEPARATION OF LOWER EPIPHYSIS OF HUMERUS WITH COMPLETE
DISPLACEMENT BACKWARDS.

From a girl aged five years.   Irreducibility of epiphysis.   Wiring to diaphysis after open incision and reduction.
Elbow joint uninjured.

Mr. THOMAS MOORE'S case.   Taken by Mr. THOMAS MOORE.

about the elbow without any fixation of the fragments by splints or apparatus. This method has of late years been revived, especially by French surgeons. The elbow is simply placed in a sling, and passive movement commenced from the time of the injury and increased at intervals. At the Société de Chirurgie, Paris, this subject was discussed in 1880, and again in 1886. Tripier, of Lyons, in 1888, thought that immediate passive movement and massage should be carried out in injuries to the elbow-joint in children, both intra- and extra-articular, provided there was no displacement.

The plan cannot be too strongly condemned.

Passive motion should be commenced very early. At the end of seven or eight days the splint should be removed, and, while the' limb is firmly grasped at the seat of fracture, gentle flexion and extension of the joint through a small arc should be made, without inflicting pain, and the splint re-adjusted.

This should be repeated every second or third day, a larger arc being made each time. At the end of three weeks the splint should be left off, and the arm placed in a sling. By this time the limb will have almost regained its usefulness.

Gentle passive motion should still be kept up and all violent attempts at movement avoided, the amount of movement being progressive at each time of application.

If great pain, with effusion into the joint, is produced, the elbow must be allowed rest for a few days. In fact, many of the older children will not submit to movement if it is in any way painful, and will not come back again for treatment; at least, this has been the author's experience in hospital practice.

Dr. L. C. Lane, in his extension treatment, commences passive motion on the second or third day, and repeats it daily for twenty-five days. The forearm should be flexed twice to a right angle slowly and deliberately, whilst the seat of fracture is grasped securely. The patient should offer no resistance. At the end of this time the arm is unbandaged, flexed to an angle of 60 degrees, and carried in a sling. The patient may then commence voluntary movements.

Later on flexion and extension should be repeated several times daily, in order to counteract the shortening of the peri-articular structures through cicatricial contraction.

Mr. Joseph Bell, of Edinburgh, teaches that fractures near the elbow in young people should be kept quiet for a period corresponding to the age of the child, a day for each year; e.g. a child of five years for five days, of ten years for ten days.

Other surgeons prefer to wait for three weeks before commencing passive motion, but there does not appear to be any advantage in allowing this lapse of time, at any rate in the case of children.

The thickening and stiffness of the joint will subside in time.

To attempt to hasten this by forcible flexion or manipulation would
be disastrous, and followed by disjunction of some neighbouring
epiphysis. Several months are often required in children to completely re-establish the mobility by gentle movement and massage.

Active motion.—The child should be taught to exercise its elbow
in different ways. These movements may alternate with the
more careful and methodical movements carried out by the surgeon
in the later stages of treatment. Active movements are more productive of serious results than passive motion. In the latter, if
properly carried out, there should not be any mobility whatever
at the seat of separation.

Electricity, massage, friction, are of great utility in the later
stages, when there is much atrophy of the muscles of the arm
and forearm, although the usual result is that when union is complete the mobility of the joint is generally perfect. But even when
deformity is present and the motions much restricted, great benefit
will be obtained in time. In the course of years the end of the
bone will become remodelled, until scarcely any trace of the lesion
remains.

Partial separation with oblique fracture of the shaft.—The treatment is the same as for complete separation, but greater difficulty
will be experienced in keeping the fragments in position on account
of the oblique direction of the fracture.

Separation of the epiphysis with vertical fracture into joint.—The
treatment will be the same as for simple separation, with the
exception that it will be found more difficult in this case to keep
the fragments in proper position. Some deformity is, therefore,
sure to result, and probably some permanent stiffness of the joint,
through the lesion being an intra-articular one.

Compound separations.—Reduction of the protruding diaphysis is
usually impossible without *resection* of a portion of its end. If
sufficient be removed, it will be found easier to keep the fragments
in position, and there will be less likelihood for displacement to
recur. Spillman removed rather more than an inch in one of his
cases, and one inch and three quarters in another, before reduction
could be effected. Both terminated in recovery.

The wound must be carefully cleansed, and all portions of the
bone removed that are seen to be soiled with mud or other foreign
matter. If the joint has been opened, it should be syringed out
with carbolic or perchloride lotion (1 in 2000), and any pieces of
bone which are wholly detached from the periosteum and other
tissue must be removed. Care should be taken to fix the elbow at
a right angle with the forearm in the prone or half-prone position, the
most useful position in the event of ankylosis supervening, which
is very likely to occur if the strictest cleanliness of modern surgery
be not adhered to.

Maisonneuve was able to successfully replace the bone, which protruded for four centimetres, and cause it to re-enter its periosteal sheath without resection of the diaphysial end.

Dr. R. W. Smith did the same in a case where there were signs of pressure upon the brachial artery.

In Hutchinson's case, after excision of the upper fragment which protruded, the patient recovered with a stiff elbow.

Erichsen removed the projecting end of the shaft of the humerus in a case of compound separation. An excellent result, without impairment of freedom of action of the joint, followed the operation.

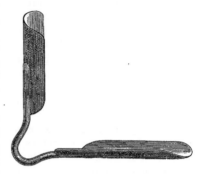

The author has collected seventeen compound cases, many of which recovered the function, and obtained a useful arm.

These cases, being so often septic before coming under treatment, take many weeks, or even months, to heal, and the suppuration present is often accompanied by necrosis of fragments of bone. But J. Hutchinson junior has mentioned (*Brit. Med. Journal*,

FIG. 85.—JONES'S POSTERIOR TROUGH SPLINT OF TIN, WITH INTERRUPTION FOR COMPOUND INJURIES AT THE ELBOW-JOINT. THE FOREARM PIECE CAN BE BENT INTO THE SEMI-PRONE POSITION OR BE DEFLECTED OUTWARDS

November 3, 1894, p. 967) a case under his care in which there was very little suppuration and no necrosis, although the periosteum had been completely stripped up to the deltoid insertion. The diaphysis had worked through the soft tissues in front of the elbow between the brachial artery and the biceps tendon. It was impossible to effect perfect reduction without cutting off one inch of the shaft. In this case a careful trial was given to extension, but it had to be abandoned after a day or two.

Lange (*loc. cit. supra*, fig. 80, p. 290) found it necessary in his case to remove *the epiphysis as well as a portion of the shaft*, the patient recovering with a useful arm. But this must be a very exceptional case in the present days of antiseptic surgery, even though the compound separation involve the elbow-joint.

The old plan of *excision* of the whole joint in all cases of compound injuries into the joint is no longer justifiable.

Beach reports (*Boston Medical and Surgical Journal*, January 4, 1877) a case of compound fracture and separation of the lower epiphysis of the humerus, with crushing of the ends of the radius and ulna, in a boy, aged eight, who had been run over by a horse-car. *Excision* of the joint was adopted, and the patient made a perfect recovery, the arm being as useful as the other, although three inches shorter.

Mr. Jonathan Hutchinson junior summarises (*British Medical Journal*, December 30, 1893) the records of fifteen compound cases where the diaphysis protruded through the skin.

'In six of these the diaphysis was reduced more or less perfectly; one recovered with an almost perfect arm, one with thrombosis of the brachial, and a third with paralysis of the musculospiral. The other three ended in amputation—one primary, two secondary, owing to gangrene from the artery being torn or obliterated by splint pressure. In three cases a more or less complete excision of the joint was performed; one recovered with very good movements, one with a stiff elbow, the third with a fairly movable one. In six cases the projecting diaphysial end was cut off in order to procure reduction; four of these ended with most satisfactory results, one recovered with an ankylosed elbow, and the sixth underwent amputation at the end of three weeks because no union had occurred. In two of the fifteen cases an action for malpractice was brought.'

Primary amputation.—Extensive lesions of the soft parts, or injury to important vessels or nerves, may render amputation necessary. But even in apparently hopeless cases much may be done to save the upper extremity in young subjects.

Extensive stripping-up of the periosteum, laceration of the ligaments of the elbow-joint, and compound fracture of the bones of the forearm, necessitated primary amputation in Champion's case. Recovery followed.

Secondary amputation.—In compound separations, should gangrene, or extensive suppuration, with its consequent dangers, threaten the life of the patient, secondary amputation must be performed.

In Reeves's case (*loc. cit. supra*) amputation was performed at the end of three weeks, on account of the condition of the arm, no union having occurred.

Deformity, if quite recent, may be treated by breaking up the soft uniting material under an anæsthetic, and replacing the bones in their natural position.

Dr. Robert Abbe brought before the New York Clinical Society, 1886 (*New York Medical Journal*, October 23, 1886, p. 469), three cases in which the epiphysial separation had been overlooked at the time, two of which he had successfully treated by breaking up the uniting callus by means of lateral flexions and over-extension, and reducing the displacement of the fragments.

CASE I.—Five weeks before coming under observation, a boy, five years old, had fallen headlong from a wagon, striking with his left elbow under him. An examination under anæsthesia showed marked deformity, with forward prominence of the shaft. The biceps tendon had slipped to the inner side of the shaft. The callus having been broken up by manual force, reduction was effected, and a plaster-of-Paris splint applied. At the end of three weeks and a half the splint was removed, and the boy allowed free use of the limb. At the end of six weeks the joint could be moved with the greatest freedom, and there was no appreciable deformity. CASE II.—An injury of the same kind was sustained by a boy, two years old, by falling down three steps and striking on his elbow. Two weeks had passed before he was placed under treatment. The same methods were employed, and at the end of three weeks the position was excellent and moderate freedom was allowed. CASE III.—A boy, four years old, fell from a table. He complained, at the time, only of his thumb, but subsequently the elbow swelled, and when the swelling had subsided, a week after the fall, deformity was noticed, and the boy was brought for treatment. The deformity was the same as in the two other cases. Under anæsthesia crepitus was detected, and the fracture was regarded as deviating somewhat from the epiphysial line near the outer condyle. Flexion was abruptly arrested at a right angle, but the power of extension was nearly complete.

Dr. Abbe added the following remarks:

' 1. Epiphysial and other fractures at the elbow are often treated as sprains, and leave impaired joint motion. 2. The deformity is not extreme, being chiefly an antero-posterior thickening above the joint, with rather a full ridge, parallel to and just above the flexure-crease caused by the lower edge of the shaft. There is usually no heel-like backward prominence of the elbow, as in dislocations. 3. There is impairment of flexion, but not so much of extension. The elbow can scarcely be bent to a right angle before flexion is stopped abruptly by the overhanging shaft, the lower end of which comes in contact with the radius. 4. Reduction can be accomplished several weeks after the injury, if the deformity is bad enough to call for it. 5. Sufficient manipulation to break up the callus at a late date is said to be dangerous to the integrity of the joint; but, while great force is required to loosen the fragments if applied so as to flex the elbow forcibly, less is needed to over-extend it, and much less when it is exerted laterally. Therefore backward and forward lateral bending, with some over-extension and only occasional violent flexion, succeed best in freeing the fragments with least risk to the joint. 6. The repair of the damage done to a child's joint by fracture in its vicinity, which leaves it in a state of so-called fibrous ankylosis, is best left to nature; as the free use of the arm is allowed, the mobility will usually be restored at least as quickly as by frequent passive motion.'

Bardenheüer resected a portion of the humerus with great improvement to the deformity in two cases of old standing separation, with displacement backwards and inwards of the epiphysis.

The author has performed the same operation three times in old separations of the lower epiphysis of the humerus, with good results.

In one case the edge of the humeral diaphysis pressed up the median nerve, with loss of sensation in the. fingers, the brachial artery being pushed by the diaphysis prominently forwards beneath, threatening to produce a rupture or aneurism on the slightest blow over the edge of the bone.   In a second case the inner angle of the diaphysis beneath the median nerve and brachial artery was removed with a chisel.   Hyperextension of the elbow existed in this instance.

Osteotomy of the shaft above the elbow-joint may be suitable in certain and well-selected deformities after separation.

A case of old separation of the lower epiphysis of the humerus, in which the bone was divided above the line of separation, is reported from the Hospital for Sick Children, Pendlebury (*Abstracts of Medical and Surgical Cases at the General Hospital for Sick Children*, Pendlebury, 1885, p. 173).   E. H., aged four years, was admitted October 14, 1885.   Eighteen months previously he broke his arm.   It was put in splints for three weeks ; when taken out it was crooked; he could do anything but carry weights with it. .On admission, he could flex, extend, pronate, and, with little difficulty, supinate ; in flexion the forearm was in same plane with the arm, but in extension there was much abduction ; there had been separation (supra-condylar) of the lower epiphysis of humerus, with displacement of the lower fragment and forearm inwards, and considerable wasting of muscles.   *October 23.*—Section with chisel just above line of separation ; antiseptic ; put up on inside angular splint.   *October 30.*—Tube removed.   *November 5.*—Stitches taken out, wound nearly healed ; arm almost straight in extension ; passive motion on splint. 16.—Slightly adducted in extension, owing to original deformity being over-corrected ; put up on straight back and inside splints ; flexion not quite perfect owing to callus.   18.—The splints left off. *December 4.*—Straight back splint at night only ; no rise of temperature since operation.   *December 16.*—Sent home.

CHAPTER V

SEPARATION OF THE LOWER EPIPHYSIS OF THE HUMERUS IN YOUTHS

SEPARATION of the lower epiphysis of the humerus after puberty— i.e. the articular and external epicondylar epiphyses—or separation of the articular epiphyses just before puberty, accompanied by *fracture of the cartilage* uniting the internal epicondyle to the trochlear portion of the epiphysis, is a much more rare form of injury than the one we have just considered in the last chapter. For details of the development we must refer the reader to it.

ANATOMY.—The lack of discrimination between the anatomical features of the lower end of the humerus at the different ages of infancy and youth has led to much confusion amongst authors.

The difference of opinion between Malgaigne and R. W. Smith in connection with lesions of this end of the humerus can be readily explained in this way.

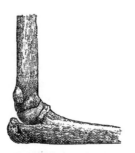 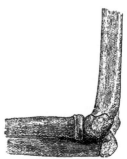

FIG. 86.—EPIPHYSES ABOUT THE LEFT ELBOW-JOINT AT FIFTEEN YEARS OF AGE. VIEW FROM THE INNER SIDE

FIG. 87.—SAME AS FIG. 86. VIEW FROM THE OUTER SIDE

To reconcile Dr. R. W. Smith's views of separation of the lower epiphysis of the humerus, which he published in 1850 ('Observations on Disjunction of the Lower Epiphysis of the Humerus,' *Dublin Quarterly Journal of Med. Science*, No. 9, N.S. 1850, p. 63), with precise anatomical facts would be impossible. He says ' *that the lower epiphysis of the humerus does not include the condyles, which belong entirely to the shaft of the bone,*' and, after alluding to the writings of Malgaigne, Dupuytren, Adams, and Vidal, he goes on:[1] 'The preceding extracts from the works of some of the most celebrated authors upon the subject of fractures are, I should think, sufficient to show that disjunction of the lower epiphysis of the humerus (of which I find no particular mention made either by

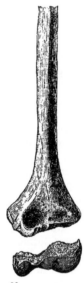

Borger or Sir Astley Cooper) is an accident which has hitherto been confounded with fracture immediately *above* the condyles, an error from which it may be inferred, I think, that the exact line of junction of the epiphysis with the shaft of the bone is not generally known to surgeons. At all events it is manifest that, by the authors from whose writings I have quoted, this line has been supposed to traverse the bone *above* the condyles, whereas the anatomical fact is, *that these processes belong exclusively to the shaft of the bone, and form no portion whatever of the epiphysis, which comprises nothing but the capitellum and the trochlea.* The line which marks its junction with the shaft is directed downwards and inwards, terminating below and external to the epicondyle, which, in the young subject,

FIG. 88. — LOWER EPIPHYSIS (PROPERLY SO CALLED) OF THE HUMERUS AT SIXTEEN AND A HALF YEARS OF AGE. SEPARATED BY MACERATION

The external epicondyle, the trochlea, and capitellum form one osseous mass. The internal epicondyle is still an isolated epiphysis, not yet united to the diaphysis. ⅔ size.

is distinct both from the epiphysis and from the shaft.'

After referring to the differences in the condition of the trochlea and capitellum in the young and adult, Dr. Smith says: 'The knowledge of this fact is not destitute of practical importance in the diagnosis of that embarrassing accident, fracture through the line of the epiphysis with the

shaft, or, in other words, fracture of the humerus immediately *below* the condyles.'

Again, after alluding to the signs he believes to be common to these lesions—dislocation backwards and fracture *above* the condyles —Dr. Smith writes thus : 'As the loss of the normal relation between the olecranon and the condyles renders the separation of the epiphysis peculiarly liable to be confounded with dislocation of the forearm backwards, and as it is obviously a matter of the utmost importance to distinguish carefully between these accidents, let us now consider the signs, by availing ourselves of which we materially diminish the chance of mistaking it either for luxation or for fracture above the condyles. In the case of fracture traversing the line of the epiphysis,

[1] The italics in the following passages are the author's.

the transverse diameter of the tumour which projects in front is equal to that of the opposite humerus, measured anteriorly from condyle to condyle ; in this respect the accident resembles the dislocation of both bones backwards, but differs from fracture *above* the condyles. The outline of this osseous tumour is rounded, presents to the feel none of the irregularities or sharpness of an ordinary fracture ; and upon its inferior surface, which is convex, and limited at either extremity by the condyles, neither trochlea nor capitellum can be distinguished. When the joint is viewed posteriorly, two osseous prominences are seen, and can be distinctly felt ; they are both placed above and behind the plane of the condyles, but are themselves situated (if the patient be not more than six or eight years of age) nearly upon the same level, the internal, however, being always a little higher up than the external. At a more advanced age the distance between these two prominences is observed to be greater, in consequence of the increased development of the internal, which is formed by the olecranon, the summit of which process grows by an epiphysis. At no period of life, however, at which it is possible for the accident in question to happen, is the distance between the two projections nearly as great as it is always found to be between those which, in cases of luxation of both bones of the forearm backwards, constitute so marked a feature of the injury. In the latter accident the distance averages about one inch and a half, while in the former it is seldom more than three-quarters of an inch ; the external tumour, in this case, being formed by *the capitellum of the humerus*, still surmounting the head of the radius, for which, in consequence of the concave form of its superior surface, it is extremely liable to be mistaken, if attention be not paid to the diagnostic sign which has just been mentioned.'

In the rough figure given by R. W. Smith the external condyle (external epicondyle) of the humerus is very distinct from the capitellum and the rest of the articular process, and produces a very erroneous impression of this portion of the lower epiphysis.

Farabeuf, in a paper in 1886 'On the Lower Epiphysis of the Humerus and its Traumatic Separation' (*Bulletins et Mémoires de la Société de Chirurg*. Paris, N.S. xii. p. 692 ; *Revue des Sciences Médicales*, No. 57, 15 January, 1887 ; *Le Progrès Médical*, second series, vol. iv. No. 32, 1886), agrees with Dr. Smith's observations, and states that in this separation the humerus, displaced forwards, carries with it its lateral eminences, the epitrochlea and epicondyle, whose lower part only remains with the condyle (capitellum), and *preserves its width* as in dislocation of the elbow, and that the signs differ considerably from those of supra-condyloid fractures. He, moreover, says that Dr. Smith's views were adopted by Giraldès in his clinics.

E. Bottini (' Note sur la disjonction de l'épiphyse inférieure de l'humérus et son traitement,' *Bullet. général de Thérapeutique*, Paris,

1850, xxxix. pp. 167–170) has reproduced and endorsed R. W. Smith's views as to the characters of this form of separation.

A recent writer in the *American Text-book of Surgery*, 1892, Part I., in speaking of separation of the lower epiphysis of the humerus, falls into a similar error. 'The lower fragment usually comprises,'. he says, 'the entire epiphysis, which is composed of several distinct pieces, but it is possible that either or both epicondyles may remain attached to the upper fragment.'

It is difficult to agree with R. W. Smith in believing that separation of the two articular processes alone is frequent while *both* epicondyles remain in contact with the diaphysis.

His observations are true with regard to the internal epicondyle after or just before the thirteenth year of life. About this period this process, by the natural growth of the diaphysis, is isolated from the rest of the lower epiphysial end, and may, and probably will, go with the diaphysis. But for the external epicondyle to remain attached to the shaft is inexplicable at any age. It appears as a small nodule towards the outer and upper aspect of the capitellum in the cartilage of the lower epiphysis about the thirteenth or fourteenth year, and very rapidly, generally about the fifteenth to sixteenth year, ossifies to the rest of the epiphysis. As seen at the fourteenth to fifteenth year, not more than a third of its upper end comes in contact with the diaphysis.

Now, as we shall see later on, the internal epicondyle usually does, after puberty, remain attached to the diaphysis in this accident, but from its anatomical condition it is difficult to understand how the external epicondyle can ever remain attached to the shaft.

While Bardenheuer calls all four pieces of the lower end of the humerus the whole epiphysis, he recognises a separation of the trochlea and capitellum together, without any reference to the external epicondyle. He says (*Deutsche Chirurgie*, 'Die Krankheiten der oberen Extremitäten, I. Theil, 1886, S. 729) that these may be displaced either backwards or forwards. He calls the injury 'separation of the trochlea and capitellum,' stating that Gurlt has collected five, and Bruns four, authentic cases; but, as the author has elsewhere mentioned, these are not clear cases of separation of these two processes alone.

If we take Dr. Smith's description, with the exception that the external epicondyle remains with the capitellum, we should have a good description of *complete separation of the lower epiphysis of the humerus at or beyond the age of puberty (thirteen or fourteen)*, the epiphysis comprising the articular processes and the external epicondyle. The epiphysial line of cartilage then passes from the outer edge of the diaphysis from *above* the external epicondyle, not transversely, but obliquely downwards and inwards towards the lower edge of the trochlea on the inner side.

Such a lesion is by no means infrequent, but rare in comparison with the complicated epiphysial injuries of the elbow ; for experience has shown that separations of this epiphysis after this age are usually partial and often complicated by other lesions.

The greater portion of the external condyle (of anatomists) in the adult is formed by the outer end of the diaphysis of the humerus and the very small external epicondylar epiphysis. After the formation of the latter in the cartilage adjoining the capitellar portion of the lower epiphysis, it very rapidly blends with it, so that its detachment from this part must be an occurrence of extreme rarity in the injury under consideration.

It is more than probable that separation of the true lower epiphysis just below the age of puberty, before the internal epicondyle is completely separated from the lower end of the bone, will in consequence be accompanied by a fracture through the small cartilaginous strip between the internal epicondylar and trochlear epiphyses. We then have a separation of the external epicondylar, capitellar, and trochlear epiphysial mass, associated with a fracture between the trochlea and internal epicondyle.

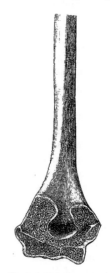

FIG. 89.—CORONAL SECTION OF THE LOWER END OF THE HUMERUS AT FOURTEEN AND A HALF YEARS OF AGE. ½ size.

In the adult, from an examination of museum specimens and from experimental research, these epiphysial processes are found to be frequently detached from the rest of the bone.

AGE.—Six published cases may be considered under this heading. In Mr. Heath's case of operation for deformity the age was eighteen years; in Smith's compound separation, about twelve years; in one simple case it was twelve years; and in three other simple cases, presumably accompanied by fracture of the lateral epicondylar strip on the inner side separating it from the rest of the cartilaginous epiphysis, the age was five years.

PATHOLOGICAL ANATOMY.—Displacement of the epiphysis may be backwards, forwards, or lateral.

The only specimen recorded is that of *displacement backwards and outwards.*

Professor Smith (*Proceedings of the Pathological Society of Dublin,* N.S. vol. iv. 1870, p. 111) has described it as follows in a case of compound separation, sent to him by Dr. F. E. Clarke, county of Donegal. It is also recorded (*Med. Press and Circular,* August 31, 1870, p. 157) by Dr. Clarke himself. The case was treated by a

z

bone-setter, and resulted in gangrene of the hand and forearm from the application of a tight bandage and splints, and in death on the eleventh day after the accident.

In 1868 a boy, in county Donegal, aged about twelve years, was thrown when wrestling with a companion, and sustained a compound fracture of the humerus through the line of junction of the epiphysis of the lower extremity with the shaft of the bone. It appeared that the lad, in falling, put out his right arm with a view of 'breaking his fall,' and that his antagonist fell across the extended arm. On his being brought home, the bone was seen to protrude through the skin. Ten hours after the accident he was seen by a bone-setter, who 'set' the broken limb with splints and bandages, after reduction of the displacement. Although the sufferings of the patient were great and the pain intense from the tightness of the apparatus, he was not seen by the bone-setter again for six days. Death ensued five days after his second visit, and eleven days after the receipt of the injury, gangrene having supervened. On the fifth day after death, and second after interment, the body was exhumed by order of the coroner for the purpose of having an inquest held and an autopsy made, a feeling of indignation having arisen against the bone-setter, to whose mismanagement the death of the boy was attributed. On superficial examination a large external wound was to be seen traversing the antecubital fossa, through which the lower end of the upper fragment could be felt projecting forwards, but it did not protrude beyond the edges of the wound. The edges of the wound had not been approximated nor the bone reduced. From upwards of an inch above, the entire forearm and hand were extensively gangrenous; so much so that it was impossible to make an accurate dissection of the soft parts or to determine the state of the vessels or nerves in the neighbourhood of the fracture. The body had, in addition, undergone great decomposition. When the wound was extended both above and below by incision, the continuity of the *entire shaft of the humerus was found to be complete, and contained the two condyles in an uninjured condition*; it was devoid, however, of the two eminences which form respectively the trochlea and capitellum and articulate with the two bones of the forearm. The upper fragment, then, was the entire humerus merely denuded of its inferior epiphyses; the lower, those epiphyses themselves. The lower end of the upper fragment was nearly at the external orifice of the wound, and directed forwards; and including, as it did, the two condyles, was broad, with an extremely roughened, jagged, and uneven extremity. The epiphyses alone constituted the lower fragment, and still continued united together in one piece and attached by the ligaments of the joint to the bones of the forearm; so that the articulation proper remained normal. The upper extremity of this fragment was directed backwards and outwards. On measuring the arm before dissection, there was found slight shortening as compared with the other, but the normal relation of the olecranon process to the condyles (epicondyles) was lost. The limb was gangrenous from an inch above the wound to the extremity of the hand.

Dr. Clarke says that the lesion was in all particulars similar to that described by Professor R. W. Smith.

In October 1897, Dr. F. B. Judge Baldwin, of Rotherham, an old friend of the author, mentioned to him a case of compound separation of the lower humeral epiphysis. It occurred in a boy aged seventeen years. The diaphysis, stripped anteriorly and posteriorly of periosteum, protruded for two inches through the wound on the anterior surface of the arm, just above the bend of the elbow. The joint was intact, and the brachial artery uninjured. A partial excision of the joint was performed—that is, only the olecranon process of the ulna was removed besides the humeral epiphysis. The internal epicondyle was found to be absent from the epiphysis, while the external was contused. Unfortunately this important specimen was not preserved.

Separation with fracture of the epiphysis.—Mr. Christopher Heath excised (Clinical Soc. of London, *British Medical Journal*, October 20, 1888, p. 879) the elbow-joint of a young man aged eighteen, which was ankylosed and distorted after injury. There was found to be much thickening of the lower end of the humerus around the fractured and separated epiphysis.

ETIOLOGY.—The direction of the force, whether it be direct or indirect, determines the form of the displacement.

Gurlt, in describing the mechanism of this form of fracture with *displacement forwards*, says that *à priori* it ought only to be possible in complete extension of the elbow. The violence, then, acting directly on the posterior aspect of the olecranon, causes this process to start forwards; and in support of this he observes that, in a specimen in the Vienna Museum, there is a small fracture of the olecranon.

Bardenheuer also believes that this form of injury is produced in children by falls upon the olecranon, and that the violence is more direct.

In several of the recorded cases of *displacement backwards* the injury was said to have been produced by a fall on the elbow.

It is more frequently caused by the violence being more indirect, as by a fall on the palmar surface of the outstretched hand during extension of the forearm, the violence being transmitted to the capitellum and trochlea.

According to Farabeuf, it is the result of a retro-humeral blow whilst the hand is in contact with the ground.

'La meilleure condition pour que le décollement de l'épiphyse inférieure de l'humérus se produise, c'est un choc rétro-huméral pendant que l'avant-bras est fléchi et la main appuyée sur une table ou sur le sol.'

'Le radius, fixé par la main, ne peut suivre le mouvement en avant imprimé par le choc à l'humérus ; la tête du radius fait sauter l'épiphyse condylienne, qui se détache suivant la ligne oblique inter-diaphyso-épiphysaire. L'action du cubitus est dans cette circon-stance toute différente de celle du radius ; le crochet coronoïdien accroche la partie diaphysaire de l'os et ne peut contribuer au décollement de l'épiphyse.'

Schüller's experiments prove that forcible abduction, adduction, flexion, extension, or pronation, or a combination of these, is pro-bably sufficient, by still more indirect violence, to cause a detachment of these processes.

SYMPTOMS.—R. W. Smith was the first to describe this form of injury.

Deformity. — This differs, as in other epiphysial separations, according to the direction of the displaced epiphysis.

DISPLACEMENT BACKWARDS.—The forearm is flexed, and in a position midway between pronation and supination.

The outline of the joint has much the appearance of dislocation of the radius and ulna backwards.

The signs of this injury as given by R. W. Smith (quoted in F. E. Clarke's case, *Med. Press and Circular*, 1870, p. 157) are : 'The great transverse breadth of the anterior tumour caused by the retention of the two condyles in the lower extremity of the upper fragment, and the two osseous tumours posteriorly, both of which signs serve to distinguish it from a supra-condyloid fracture of the humerus, which it much resembles, not only from the facts of shortening and anterior osseous tumours being present in both lesions, but also because the antero-posterior diameter of the arm is increased likewise by each form of injury. It is also to be borne in mind that the normal relation of the three bony projections at the back of the elbow was disturbed, the olecranon being above the condyles, a fact which also serves to distinguish this epiphysiary fracture from a supra-condyloid fracture, but which causes it to resemble much a luxation of both bones of the forearm backwards, a surgical lesion which Professor Smith likewise pointed out as liable to be confounded in diagnosis with this fracture of the humerus through the line of juncture with its lower epiphyses if the important differential signs of the latter be not accurately attended to. The two tumours posteriorly in an epiphysiary frac-ture, being the head of the olecranon and the end of the epiphyses, are nearly on a level, but those caused by a dislocation are fully an inch one above the other, as they are formed by the olecranon and of the radius respectively.'

Smith sums up by saying : 'It is manifest that (contrary to what the statement of authors would lead us to infer) implicit reliance is not to be placed upon the loss of the normal relation between the olecranon and the condyles of the humerus, as a means of distinguishing between luxation of the forearm back-wards, and fracture of the lower extremity of the humerus. It is evident that there is an accident of the elbow in which the bones of the forearm lose their natural relations to the condyles, and yet that accident is not necessarily a dislocation, but may be a fracture through the line of the lower epiphysis of the humerus, which line is situated *below* the condyles.

Bardenheuer also states that the distance of the *olecranon from the epicondyles is increased* in this injury. The epicondyles are in normal relation with one another and with the humerus, and immovable, but the olecranon is drawn considerably upwards and backwards by the triceps, which is curved. The antero-posterior diameter of the joint is increased, and the lower end of the humerus projects forwards, capped on the inner and outer sides by the epicondyles. This resemblance to dislocation has caused Pitha to term it *disjunctive dislocation.* Bardenheuer clearly describes epiphysial separation of the trochlea and capitellum.

Farabeuf also mentions this preservation of the natural breadth of the upper fragment in contradistinction to tranverse supra-condyloid fracture, where it is much smaller and the lateral processes are carried much further forwards than in fracture. But instead of feeling, as in dislocation, the radial cup on the outer side, and very much beneath the olecranon summit, the finger detects, in separation, the condyloid (capitellar) fragment in place, on the outer side of the olecranon but a slight distance only from the summit of this process.

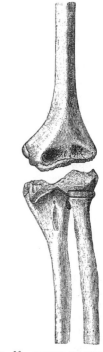

Fig. 90.—Diagram of separation of the lower epiphysis of the humerus at the age of fifteen and a half years. Usual form of injury. Front view

The internal epicondyle is quite distinct from the epiphysis, and is not detached. Its normal relation with the olecranon is lost; that of the external epicondyle to the radius is preserved.

To this description the author would add that the measurement from the internal epicondyle to the styloid process of the ulna will be greatly diminished, as in dislocation.

If the author's views are correct with regard to the external epicondyle remaining with the articular epiphysis, the distance between this epicondyle and the styloid process of the radius will not be diminished.

Dr. Smith concludes by quoting a case bearing out his views.

Michael F., aged twelve, was admitted on August 24, 1847, into Jervis Street Hospital under Dr. J. S. Hughes. He stated that he was thrown down by another boy with great violence, and in falling stretched out his arm to save himself, while the other boy fell with all his weight across the back of the extended limb. On being examined twenty minutes after the accident, before swelling occurred, the arm was found to be powerless, the forearm semiflexed, and the hand in position of half supination. The olecranon formed a remarkable projection above and behind the condyles of the humerus. A second osseous tumour—the upper surface of which was concave, and which was supposed at first to be the head of the radius—could be distinguished behind the outer condyle as the capitellum. The lower extremity of the humerus formed a considerable prominence in front. A moderate amount of flexion was permitted at the joint, and distinct crepitus was felt on grasping the arm and forearm in each hand and moving the fragments. The diagnosis was made of fracture through the line of junction of the epiphysis with the shaft, with displacement upwards and backwards of the epiphysis. The deformity was easily removed by extension and counter-extension, and the limb was secured by angular splints. . There was some difficulty in keeping the fragments in position, so that there was ultimately some projection forwards of the diaphysis, indicated by increase in the antero-posterior diameter of the elbow, but the boy recovered very considerable use of the limb ; he was able to extend the forearm perfectly, and could flex it beyond a right angle.

Mobility is a marked feature. Adduction, abduction, and extension and flexion of the forearm may produce mobility close to the joint.

Crepitus of the usual muffled character may often be detected, especially during the reduction of the displaced epiphysis, which is easily effected.

The following case of G. C., aged five years (for which he is indebted to Dr. Andrew Fullerton), came under the author's observation at the Miller Hospital, Greenwich, in August 1891. The left internal epicondyle was still attached to the humerus, but the remaining portion of the lower epiphysis of the humerus was detached and drawn backwards and somewhat outwards, forming a projection at the back of the lower part of arm. The distance between the internal condyle and the olecranon was greater than on the sound side. Muffled crepitus was readily felt. Active movements of all kinds were completely lost. Pain, mobility, &c. were also present.

In this instance, the child being below the age of puberty, the separation was accompanied by a fracture of the cartilage uniting the internal epicondylar portion to the rest of the lower end of the humerus.

Other symptoms of intra-articular fracture are often present, but effusion into the joint will always be more marked than in separation above the epicondyles in infancy, in which the articular lesions may be wholly absent.

Enlargement of antero-posterior diameter of elbow is present in both forms of backward displacement of the epiphysis, as well as in the forward variety.

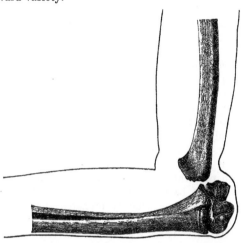

FIG. 91.—DIAGRAMMATIC VIEW (FROM THE OUTER SIDE) OF SEPARATION OF THE LOWER EPIPHYSIS OF THE HUMERUS AT THE AGE OF FIFTEEN AND A HALF YEARS. DISPLACEMENT OF DIAPHYSIS FORWARDS

The external epicondyle remains united to the capitellar portion of the epiphysis.

Passive movements of flexion and extension; pronation and supination may be effected in some degree, but never to the same extent as in separation of the whole lower end of the humerus during infancy.

Shortening of arm is very slight.

DISPLACEMENT FORWARDS.—The symptoms are almost the same as in separation of the whole cartilaginous epiphysis, and both epicondyles with displacement forwards.

Loss of flexure of elbow-joint in front, which is occupied by an osseous mass.

Increase of antero-posterior diameter of joint.

Measurement between epicondyles altered very slightly. The internal one is immovable, in normal relation with the diaphysis and on a level with the olecranon.

The olecranon does not project, and the triceps tendon is not curved.

There is **mobility of the forearm** with the epiphysis, especially in the antero-posterior direction.

DIFFERENTIAL DIAGNOSIS. Dislocation backwards of elbow.—This accident may be distinguished from a dislocation by the readiness with which the epiphysis is replaced and again recurs, also by the absence of the hollow of the sigmoid notch.

There is likewise a certain amount of lateral motion which is not met with in dislocation at the elbow-joint, and muffled crepitus is frequently present.

In this form of epiphysial separation, as in dislocation, the relative position of the internal epicondyle to the olecranon is altered.

Bardenheuer says that the absence of the trochlear process of the humerus in front of the joint is a symptom in favour of epiphysial separation.

Pitha (according to Bardenheuer) relates a case in which the epiphysis (*sic*) was broken off and displaced backwards, simulating a dislocation in this direction. A boy, aged five years, fell from a window on to the open hand. The elbow was greatly swollen and distorted, the triceps tendon concave, and the olecranon projected markedly an inch distant from the humerus. The flexure of the elbow was sharply defined, and immediately above it there was felt the sharp projecting edge of the humerus, which threatened to penetrate the skin. The separate portions forming the joint could not be made out on account of the swelling. The forearm, which was kept slightly pronated and flexed, could be more fully flexed, pronated, and supinated without difficulty and without crepitation. There was an inch shortening of the arm, and the diameter in depth increased by fourteen lines. Although the diagnosis was said to be clear, and the injury classed by Bardenheuer as one of epiphysial separation of trochlea and capitellum, it is by no means evident that it was not an example of separation of the whole lower end in infancy.

Smith epitomises the points of resemblance and dissimilarity between this form of separation of the lower end of the humerus and the two injuries with which it is most liable to be confounded—viz. fracture immediately *above* the condyles and luxation of both bones of the forearm backwards—but he says it is to the latter it bears the greatest resemblance.

'The symptoms which belong to it in common with fracture above the condyles are the following: shortening, crepitus, the removal of the deformity by extension, and its tendency to recur when the extending force is relaxed, the presence of an osseous tumour in front of the joint, and the increase in the antero-posterior diameter of the elbow.

'It differs from the supra-condyloid fracture in the greater transverse breadth and regular convex outline of the anterior tumour, in the existence of two tumours posteriorly, and in the loss of the normal relation of the olecranon to the condyles.

'It resembles dislocation of both bones of the forearm backwards in the following particulars: the transverse diameter of the anterior tumour is the same in each case; so also is the antero-posterior breadth of the elbow, and in both the olecranon ascends above the condyles, the limb is shortened, and two osseous prominences can be distinguished posteriorly. It differs, however, from luxation in the existence of crepitus, the tendency of the deformity to recur, in the anterior tumour being destitute of trochlea and capitellum, and in the circumstance of the two posterior tumours being nearly upon the same level.'

These remarks of Professor R. W. Smith are quoted again by him in his address to the British Medical Association in 1867 (*British Medical Journal*, August 17, 1867, p. 122) on 'Epiphysiary Disjunctions.'

Displacement of the epiphysis forwards simulates in like manner **dislocation of the radius and ulna forwards** at the elbow-joint.

Pitha (according to Bardenheuer) relates an instance where the separated trochlea and capitellum were displaced forwards, resembling dislocation of the forearm.

A child, aged five, sustained a fall upon its elbow. The flexure of the elbow was found to be obliterated, the biceps and brachialis anticus raised up by a rounded mass, and the diameter of the joint in its depth increased by eight lines, but the olecranon was not prominent, nor the triceps curved. The epicondyles were well marked and immovable, and on a level and in normal relation with the olecranon. Mobility of the trochlea and capitellum from before backwards was detected, with crepitus, when they were held by the hands and the olecranon fixed. Reduction was effected by means of pressure upon the trochlea and capitellum, and by increase of the flexion. Complete recovery took place.

From the age of this child it is difficult to understand how the epiphysis of the external epicondyle could have gone with the diaphysis, although on the inner side the cartilaginous process of the internal epicondyle might have been broken off from the rest of the lower, almost cartilaginous, end of the humerus.

Bardenheuer adds that the differential diagnosis of the injury from displacement through dislocation is the normal relation between the olecranon and the epicondyles (*sic*).

The **PROGNOSIS** and **TREATMENT** are precisely the same as for epiphysial separation below the age of puberty.

CHAPTER VI

SEPARATION OF INTERNAL EPICONDYLE
OF THE HUMERUS

ANATOMY.—It is preferable to restrict the terms 'internal' and 'external epicondyles' to the lateral epicondylar epiphyses, as being anatomically correct. They are placed upon—or, rather, comprise—a large portion of the abrupt lateral projections on the inner and outer sides of the lower end of the humerus; and for the projections themselves it is better to keep the names mostly known to English anatomists—viz. the 'internal' and 'external condyles.'

These condyles are thus formed in part by a prolongation of the inner and outer elevated margins of the diaphysis of the humerus, and in part from separate centres of ossification, which in early life are formed from the lateral elevated portions of the cartilaginous lower epiphysis.

The external condyle, in addition, is formed by a portion of the non-articular posterior part of the capitellar epiphysis.

They do not include any part of the articular surface, but American and some British surgeons speak of the internal and external condyles as including as much of the articular surface as belongs to the trochlea and capitellum.

As the lower end of the diaphysis develops and grows downwards, especially on the inner side, these lateral epiphyses or epicondyles overlie the diaphysis more than before. This is especially the case on the inner side, where the internal epicondyle becomes entirely separated from the rest of the lower epiphysis. It becomes a distinct epiphysis, the osseous nucleus of which unites with the inner aspect of the diaphysial projection; whereas the external epicondyle is seldom separated from the rest of the lower epiphysis, and overlaps the diaphysis to a very small extent.

The osseous epiphysis of the internal condyle, which develops in the upper portion of the primary cartilage of the end of the humerus at the inner side, has nothing to do with the fully formed lower epiphysis, properly so called—at any rate after the thirteenth year. From this time it is separated from the trochlea by a quarter of an inch and more of the lower end of the diaphysis of the humerus

which forms the inner aspect of this process, and its lower end is
$\frac{3}{16}$ inch above the synovial cavity on the inner side.

But from the time of the first appearance of this centre for
twelve years and more it may be detached.   In the first years its
separation must be accompanied by a
fracture of the thin cartilaginous strip
extending between it and the trochlear
portion of the lower epiphysis.   On
making a frontal section of the fully
developed lower end of the humerus,
this process is found to be nearly a
quarter of an inch above the epiphysial
line of junction (see fig. 89).

The centre for the internal epicondyle (epitrochlea) appears at about the
fifth year, and is the origin of its projection.   This process is almost separated from the rest of the lower epiphysis by the growing diaphysis about
the thirteenth year or a little later.   It
becomes a separate epiphysis and unites
with the lever-like process of the
humeral diaphysis at the eighteenth or
twentieth year.

The internal epicondyle is directed
a little backwards, and from its anterior
aspect arise five of the flexor muscles—
viz. the flexor carpi radialis, flexor carpi

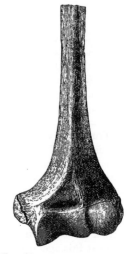

Fig. 92.—Epiphysis of the internal epicondyle at seventeen and a half years of age
All the other epiphyses of the
lower end of the humerus united.
$\frac{1}{2}$ size.

ulnaris; flexor sublimis digitorum, palmaris longus, and a small
portion of the pronator radii teres at the upper part.   The internal
lateral ligament is attached to its lower aspect, which spreads out in
a radiating manner, and connects it to the coronoid and inner border
of the olecranon process.

The ulnar nerve runs in a groove at the back of this process.
This relation is of great importance from the fact that injury to this
nerve is of frequent occurrence in epiphysial separations.   It should
be remembered that the fibro-osseous canal for this nerve is completed by the fibrous band which stretches from the epicondyle to the
inner border of the olecranon, and has fibres of the flexor carpi ulnaris
attached to it.

Although the base of this process is slightly curved, with the
convexity outwards, at the age of fourteen to fifteen years, it is
almost on a level with the inner border of the trochlea continued
upwards.   After this period, from the continued inward and downward growth of the diaphysis, its convex base is placed further
to the inner side of this, so that at the eighteenth year it is nearly
three-eighths of an inch from the same line.

At this age the epicondyle projects two·centimetres beyond the inner side of the trochlea; this measurement, therefore, corresponds now exactly to the length of the lower border of the process.

In its fully formed condition the epicondyle is five-eighths of an inch vertically, three-eighths of an inch· thick, and nearly half an inch wide in the antero-posterior direction; convex on its anterior aspect, concave and smooth on its posterior aspect. Its lower border is almost transverse and of some length, while its upper is not of any extent, it being the commencement of the inner or upper border of the internal condyle formed by the diaphysis of the humerus.

At fourteen years of age the apex of the internal epicondyle is 15 mm. from the inner margin of the olecranon when the elbow is bent at a right angle; at nineteen years of age it is 20 mm. distant.

True separations of the internal epicondyle are therefore limited to this epicondylar epiphysis, and can only occur in a pure form after the formation of the epiphysis, from about the thirteenth to the twentieth year—that is, before union has taken place to the humeral portion of the internal condyle—and will be extra-articular. Before this period the internal epicondyle is still part of the lower cartilaginous epiphysis, and its separation will be attended by a cartilaginous fracture detaching it from the rest of the lower end; while at this age it is probable that the synovial membrane will be opened on the inner side of the trochlea, but this need not of necessity occur.

The epicondylar epiphysis sometimes persists to the age of twenty-five years, according to Rambaud and Renault (*Développement des os*, Paris, 1864, p. 203), or even further into adult life, rendering an epiphysial separation possible in the adult.

The author will endeavour to omit as far as possible all discussion of fractures of the whole of the internal condyle (including in this term the diaphysial as well as the epiphysial portion), which are even more commonly met with in children than they are in adults, and draw a line of distinction between them and separation of the small epiphysial portion of this process.

Many surgeons reject this distinction, because 'practically there is no difference in the treatment or in the results; and, furthermore, they state that the differential diagnosis between the two cannot be made upon the living with anything like certainty.'

This opinion cannot any longer be held, since so many cases of fracture limited to the epiphysial line have now been verified in the recent state by direct examination.

ETIOLOGY. Muscular action.—Granger, who was the first to describe this injury in 1818 ('On a Particular Fracture of the Inner Condyle of the Humerus,' by Benjamin Granger, Burton-on-Trent; *Edinburgh Med. and Surgical Journal*, vol. xiv. p. 196, April 1818), attributed it solely to muscular action.

He says: 'A distinguishing circumstance attending this fracture'—which he calls a particular fracture of the internal condyle—'is that of its being occasioned by sudden and violent muscular exertion; and it will be recollected that from the inner condyle those powerful muscles which constitute the bulk of the fleshy substance of the ulnar aspect of the forearm have their principal origin. The way in which the muscles of the inner condyle are involuntarily thrown into sudden and excessive action I take to be this: the endeavour to prevent a fall by stretching out the arm, and thus receiving the percussion from the weight of the body on the hand.'

In only two of Granger's cases does he clearly establish that the fracture was caused by muscular action; but, on the contrary, as Hamilton says, from the violent inflammation which generally ensued in his cases, the frequency of ecchymosis, and the injury done to the ulnar nerve in at least three instances, one must rather believe that most of them were produced by direct blows from below in the fall upon the ground.

Denucé and César thought, like Granger, that this lesion could only be produced by muscular action or direct violence.

Certainly, in children muscular action alone is quite sufficient to effect a separation.

Hamilton relates (loc. cit. supra, p. 304) the case of a man, aged thirty-four, who, probably from muscular action, separated a portion of the internal condyle, presumably the epicondyle. It was displaced downwards, and was accompanied by a dislocation backwards of the forearm. He thought that delay in the epiphysial union might have been present in this case.

Poinsot refers to one case, mentioned by M. E. Hirtz, in which the accident was declared to be plainly the result of muscular action, it being occasioned in a little boy aged nine years by the act of raising himself by his arms while suspended from a trapeze.

Clement Dukes (British Medical Journal, 1874, vol. ii. p. 403) reports the case of T., aged sixteen. For three months he had had a little pain at the inner side of the arm at the elbow when exercising in the gymnasium. On July 4, 1874, he injured his elbow through a fall from the horizontal bar while performing the exercise called 'back away.' He says that he kept hold of the bar with his hands too long, so that, instead of alighting on his feet as usual, he fell on 'all fours,' with his arms extended; but the force was sufficient to make the left arm suddenly flex outwards. He felt something crack and cause him pain at the elbow and a feeling of faintness. On examination the arm was held stiff, neither flexed nor extended. There was a swelling over the internal condyle of the humerus like a swollen bursa, making the condyle appear very prominent. Immediately below this, instead of the usual convex contour on the inner side of the forearm, there was a considerable

hollow or concave outline, with slight extra thickness of the
muscles of the forearm antero-posteriorly. Owing to this the outer
contour of the forearm seemed increased in convexity, but was in
reality normal when the two arms were compared, thus dispelling
the idea of a dislocation of the radius and ulna outwards, which it
resembled at first from the prominent inner condyle with the
depression below. On manipulation, flexion and extension were
perfect and almost painless, also rotation internally and externally ;
but when the palm of the left hand was placed over the inner
condyle and the arm moved, great pain was elicited. Over the
inner condyle a free, movable morsel of bone could be felt, causing
no crepitus, but moving easily and smoothly, and distinctly external
to the joint, being a separation of the internal epicondyle of the
humerus, caused by muscular action through the forcible flexion
of the forearm on the arm. There was no injury of the ulnar
nerve. A rectangular splint was applied, with a figure-of-eight
bandage and a pad on the elbow. Position and union were effected
well.

Direct violence.—This injury is frequently occasioned by a direct
fall upon the inner side of the elbow, although in adults direct
violence is much more commonly a cause of fracture of the internal
condyle than in children, where the internal epicondyle is less
prominent and therefore less liable to be injured by direct violence.
The marked projection of this process in adults might almost make
it regarded as a predisposing cause of the injury.

Separation of the internal epicondyle before twelve or thirteen
years of age will be more adequately produced by direct violence,
which will also detach it from the trochlear portion of the lower
epiphysis, and the synovial membrane of the joint will become more
liable to injury, as has already been said.

Out of fourteen cases collected by M. César (A. César, Thèse,
Essai sur la fract. de l'épitrochlée, Paris 1876), four being in adults,
at least eight were said to have been produced by a direct cause.[1]

A lad, aged eleven, was brought to Hamilton, in October 1848.
He had just fallen upon his elbow, the blow having been received—
as he affirmed and as the ecchymosis showed pretty conclusively—
directly upon the inner condyle. The fragment was quite loose,
and crepitus was distinct. He could flex and extend the arm and
rotate the forearm without pain or inconvenience. Hamilton was
quite sure the fracture did not extend into the joint. The result
seemed also to confirm this opinion, for in three months from the
time of the accident the motions of the elbow-joint were almost
completely restored.

Indirect violence.—In several instances it has been produced by a
fall upon the wrist or palm of the hand, the arm being extended.

---

[1] It must be stated that two of these are Granger's cases, in which the cause of the
injury is but vaguely given.

In these the result may sometimes be due to the action of the internal lateral ligament, the epiphysis being torn away by the stress thrown upon this ligament during the over-extension rather than by muscular action (Packard, Pingaud, Bouilly, and others).

Two of Granger's cases were due to falls on the hand, and this author thought that such falls were a common mode of injury, the epiphysis being torn off by violent contraction of the muscles in the act of the patient putting out his hand in falling; but this theory is hardly borne out by the recorded cases. In five out of ten instances, complicated with dislocation (two in adults), collected by G. Fallier, the fracture was produced by a fall upon the palm of the hand, in two by a fall on the elbow, and in one by a fall on the dorsal aspect of the wrist. The remaining few were caused by direct violence, showing that in these complicated cases the violence is usually indirect.

In *separations accompanied by dislocation* the injury is less indirect. Forcible adduction, abduction, and powerful rotation of the forearm are common modes of violence.

In two of Fallier's cases caused by a fall on the elbow, the one (Richet's) case was complicated by a dislocation of the elbow backwards and inwards; the other, also inwards, was in an adult.

It will be seen hereafter that separations produced by indirect violence, from the tearing away of this process by the resisting internal lateral ligament and other ligamentous structures attached to it, are usually accompanied by dislocation backwards or outwards of the elbow—a mechanism sufficiently obvious when we see how firmly the epicondyle is bound to the ulna.

The force of the fall upon the palm of the hand produces over-extension of the forearm, with forcible lateral flexion towards the outer side, causing the natural inclination of the forearm outwards to become greatly exaggerated and the internal lateral ligament violently put on the stretch.

Hence it cannot be wondered that some surgeons, especially in Germany, regard the separation of this process as the usual complication of outward dislocation of the elbow.

In Berthomier's experiments lateral flexion, with or without torsion, produced epiphysial separation of the internal epicondyle (epitrochlea) or of the external epicondyle (epicondyle), according to the direction of the flexion. He thought that the latter injury was sometimes mistaken in very young children for the injury called ' subluxation of the head of the radius.'

AGE.—Detachment of the internal condyle is much more frequent in children than in adults, whether it be a pure separation of this epiphysis or a true fracture of its diaphysial portion.

Malgaigne treated a fracture of the epitrochlea in a boy of ten. M. Pézerat had also seen (1832) one in a boy aged ten ('Sur la fract. de l'épitrochlée, *Journal Complémentaire*, t. xlii. p. 418).

Denucé considered all fractures of the epitrochlea in subjects below eighteen years of age as epiphysial separations.

In an instance just quoted Hamilton has gone so far as to assume that a fracture of the internal epicondyle in a man aged thirty-four, the result of muscular action, must have been due to delay in the union of this epiphysis.

Coulson, in a discussion at the Royal Medical and Chirurgical Society, January 11, 1859, gave three instances—two in boys aged ten and a half and eleven, respectively; and one in a girl aged three and a half.

Stimson mentions two cases, one in a girl aged thirteen, and the other in a boy aged eleven.

M. César describes ten cases in children out of a total of fourteen. Two were from eight to ten years old, five from eleven to twelve, and three from fifteen to sixteen (César, *Essai sur la fract. de l'épitrochlée*, Thèse de Paris, 1876).

Out of five cases mentioned by Hamilton four occurred in children between two and fifteen years of age.

In Fallier's eight cases, complicated with dislocation, one was at nineteen years of age, one at eighteen, three at fifteen, and one each at fourteen, twelve, and eleven; that is, six cases between eleven and fifteen years.

In thirty-eight cases of detachment of the internal epicondyle collected by Mr. Jonathan Hutchinson junior (*British Medical Journal*, December 30, 1893, p. 1419) 'the age ranged between eight and eighteen years.'

In the author's collection of cases, amounting to sixty-one, the ages in the five *operation cases* were : one at eighteen years, one at thirteen, one at eleven, and one at ten and a half; while in one the age was not stated.

In the five *pathological specimens* the age was undeterminable.

Among the *simple cases* the age is not given in six; in three others it occurred in young boys; of the remaining forty-two no less than thirty-one ranged from ten years to sixteen; only one above this age, at seventeen years; and ten cases from three to nine years of age.

SEX.—In César's fourteen subjects only one was of the female sex, and that was an adult.

The ten cases recorded by M. Fallier—which were all complicated with dislocation, and two of them in adults—were all of the male sex. He thinks that, besides the occupation of the male sex rendering these subjects especially liable to this as to other forms of fracture, the presence of the adipose tissue which surrounds and protects this process in the female from direct violence, the lesser power of the epitrochlear muscles, and the smaller projection of the process in women than in men, may account for the greater preponderance in men of this form of injury, which is even greater than in ordinary fractures.

Fallier collected forty-eight cases of fracture of the internal epicondyle, simple or with dislocation, including adults. Of these, nineteen were complicated with dislocation of the elbow.

Although the author has been able to collect only sixty-one authentic examples of separation of this process in children, it cannot be doubted that this injury must be vastly more frequent than these figures would lead us to suppose.

PATHOLOGICAL ANATOMY.—Specimens showing the existence of a diastasis of the epiphysial internal epicondyle are few in number, although it must be admitted that it is a very frequent injury in the living subject.

With the exception of the dissecting-room specimens, most have been accompanied by other serious complications.

It is probable that separation of this small epiphysis is even more frequent than separation of the whole lower epiphysis of the humerus. Bardenheuer puts it next to the lower epiphysis of the humerus in order of frequency.

Malgaigne, in speaking of fracture of the epitrochlea, or the whole of the internal epicondyle, says 'there is good ground for supposing that, in some cases at least, it is a disjunction of the epiphysis.' Yet no drawing of one is to be found in Malgaigne's 'Atlas.'

Gurlt also states (*Handbuch der Lehre von den Knochenbrüchen*, Hamm. 1862, pp. 796, 797) that clinical experience shows that both the inner and outer epiphyses are sometimes broken, however difficult it may be to demonstrate the fact anatomically.

Displacement downwards.—Hamilton gives (*loc. cit. supra*, 305) a full description and a figure of a specimen sent to him by Dr. Zuckerkandl—demonstrator of anatomy in the University of Vienna—but without a clinical history. The following is Zuckerkandl's account of the specimen:

'The separation of the internal epicondyle I found on the left arm of a strong-boned man. After the removal of the flexors, the epicondyle appeared projecting forwards tumour-like, but immovable, so that at first sight I thought of a fracture healed by callus. As I removed the dense connective tissue which surrounded the epicondyle, there appeared a furrow, which encircled the irregular bony prominence, and formed a sharp line of demarcation between it and the humeral epicondyle. The tumour-like bony prominence, therefore, represented the epiphysial epicondyle. On further examination it was seen that the epiphysial was connected with the humeral epicondyle only by dense tissue, was irregularly formed on its uneven upper surface, slightly concave on its superior attached side, and of about the size of an os lunatum. In the figure is plainly seen the intact humeral epicondyle, the epiphysial epicondyle, and between them the above-described furrow, which was filled with fibrous tissue. The separated epicondyle does not

A A

correspond in form to that of a youthful person, nor to the inferior part of the flexor condyle in the adult. Its long axis in the latter is parallel with that of the humerus; in our preparation, however, it is sagittal, twisted, as it were, on its axis. The inferior portion of the epicondyle is, in the adult, about one-half centimetre distant from the edge of the trochlea, but it is more than one centimetre removed in this preparation, so that the lateral surface of the trochlea is very deep.'

However, Hamilton adds that 'the bone is from an adult, as stated by Dr. Zuckerkandl, but he has omitted to mention that the coronoid fossa is small and the olecranon fossa nearly obliterated, indicating that for a long time before death the motions of the joint were limited. The presumption is, therefore, that this was an old

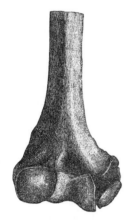

FIG. 93.—DETACHMENT AND DIS-PLACEMENT DOWNWARDS OF IN-TERNAL EPICONDYLE

fracture, a fact which increases greatly the difficulty of determining precisely the original character of the accident. There is a broad, vertical, and remarkable facet mentioned by Dr. Zuckerkandl on the inner side of the trochlea; the outer condyle is probably not normal in its shape, and altogether there are indications that the bone has at some time suffered a very severe and perhaps complicated injury. Perhaps there was more than one line of fracture, possibly a transverse fracture through the shaft at the base of the condyles, or through the line of the epiphysial junction. If such were the fact, the specimen does not illustrate a simple fracture of the epicondyle; but these are points which the ancient character of the fracture does not permit us to determine positively. We think, however, this may properly be called a separation of the epiphysial portion of the internal epicondyle, but whether it was a simple fracture or separation, uncomplicated with any other lesion of the bone, cannot now be determined.'

This is presumably the specimen from a fully developed man figured and alluded to by Dr. Zuckerkandl (*Allgemeine Wiener medizinische Zeitung*, February 1878) as a true epiphysiary disjunction united by fibrous material to the shaft.

A specimen is here figured of separation of the internal epicondyle removed by the author from the body of an adult in the dissecting room of Guy's Hospital in 1888.

The displacement is directly downwards and a little forwards; it is completely off the internal condyle, to which it is still connected at its lower and posterior part by a thick band of fibrous tissue. The process of bone is almost exactly the shape of the normal epiphysis, and is in contact with the inner side of the trochlea of the humerus, between which there was some fibrous tissue. There are no other signs of fracture in the bone (see fig. 93).

M. Paulet found by dissection on a dead subject the epicondyle ' carried downwards and lodged on the inner border of the great sigmoid cavity of the ulna, over which it played and looked like a kind of independent sesamoid bone adhering by its inner aspect alone to the lateral ligament.'

Dr. Kammerer showed, before the New York Surgical Society on October 24, 1888 (*New York Medical Journal*, January 26, 1889, p. 109), a specimen of separation of the internal epicondyle that he had removed in resecting the elbow of a man aged sixty-one. He found the epicondyle separated from the humerus, and attached to it by fibrous tissue. There were no other injuries of the bone. On section of both portions across the line of separation the inner fragment was found to be lined with hyaline articular cartilage. It was doubtful whether the epicondyle had been united to the humerus at all, or had been separated by a fracture, a new joint forming subsequently.

Gurlt figures (*Lehre von den Knochenbrüchen*, II. Theil, II. Lieferung, S. 797, fig. 109) a specimen of fracture of the internal condyle in the museum of Würzburg. The fragment is displaced directly downwards a little beyond the lower border of the trochlea, to the inner side of which it has become united. This was the only specimen of united fracture known to Gurlt. From the figure it appears probable that the epitrochlear fragment included also a small portion of the shaft above it. Such a specimen cannot be regarded as a non-union of the normal epiphysis: on account, first, of the dissimilarity with the normal epiphysis, and, secondly, its displaced position downwards.

In Mr. Hutchinson junior's excised specimen it was proved on section to include the whole of the small epiphysis for the internal epicondyle.

Displacement backwards.—A notable example of this form of displacement came under the author's care at the Miller Hospital on December 18, 1893, in which there was pressure upon the ulnar nerve by backward displacement of the fragment.

E. J., aged eleven years, was running along the street when he fell and struck his left elbow against the pavement. On admission the arm was semiflexed and midway between pronation and supination. Any attempt at movement caused the greatest pain. There was great swelling and extravasation of blood over the posterior and outer aspects of the arm and elbow; less on the inner side, so that the outline of the olecranon was not much obscured. The deformity on the inner side was very marked. The internal epicondyle was very prominent and movable on the inner and posterior aspects of the joint in the position in which the patient held it ; but when the elbow was more extended the inner side of the olecranon tip came in contact with this process, so that in extension merely a wrinkled fold of skin was left between these two points. The internal epicondyle was also above the normal inter-epicondylar line crossing the tip of the olecranon posteriorly. All measurements showed the close approximation of the internal epicondyle to the inner side of the olecranon process, while the external epicondyle, olecranon, &c., held their normal relation one with another. There was some loss of sensation on the inner side of the hand. The elbow was put up on an anterior rectangular splint, and the epicondyle

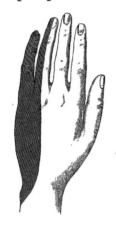

placed in position. However, the loss of sensation, with some weakness of the muscles of the little finger, continued, while at the end of a fortnight the internal epicondyle did not appear to be so much displaced backwards as it had been previously. As the condition had its possible origin in direct injury to the ulnar nerve at the time of the injury, operative measures were delayed till January 5, 1894. The loss of sensation then extended over the whole of the little finger, and the inner half of the ring finger, and inner side of the hand. Flexion, extension, and pronation and supination were limited. Under chloroform, January 5 (eighteenth day after the accident), a small incision was made through the skin over the internal epicondyle, which was found to be almost quite loose, i.e. with the exception of a slight process of fibro-cartilaginous tissue at the lower part. The periosteum and the muscular and tendinous attachments were completely stripped from off its apex, leaving the bone quite bare. The epicondyle was rotated backwards on its vertical axis, so that the sharp anterior edge where it joined the internal condylar portion of the humeral diaphysis was directed backwards and inwards, and the fractured surface, which still presented a very small amount of unossified cartilage, looked inwards and forwards. Its size was, after removal, 13 centimetres vertically and 10 centimetres antero-posteriorly (see fig. 95).

Fig. 94.—SEPARATION OF INTERNAL EPICONDYLE, WITH DISPLACEMENT BACKWARDS AND PRESSURE UPON ULNAR NERVE. DIAGRAM OF AREA OF LOSS OF SENSATION BEFORE OPERATION

After removal of the epicondyle, three silk sutures closed the wound, without drainage ; a rectangular splint was again applied for ten days. On the following day, January 6, the loss of sensation in the parts supplied by the ulnar nerve had almost entirely disappeared. On January 10 the wound had healed by primary union.

Sensation had entirely recovered two days previously; the sutures were removed. On January 20 passive movement was begun. When the author saw the patient again on May 4, 1894, the functions of the elbow were almost perfect; extension was the only movement that could not be carried out to its fullest extent; this was so slight as to be quite inappreciable to the patient. An interesting feature was now present in marked prominence at the site of the original epicondyle; in fact, a new epicondyle had been formed, the base of it no doubt by the continued growth of the diaphysis of the humerus, but the bulk of it by the periosteal covering of the epicondyle. This, as well as the complete return of function of the muscles attached to the epicondyle, is probably accounted for by the fact that the periosteum was completely stripped with the muscles from off the epiphysis.

Two months later the elbow was completely restored to its normal range of movement.

FIG. 95.—INTERNAL EPICONDYLE OF HUMERUS REMOVED BY OPERATION

a, Under or separated surface of conjugal cartilage, with a few granules of the diaphysis adherent to it. *b*, Upper or superficial aspect; osseous nucleus exposed. *c*, Section showing cartilage and osseous nucleus.

COMPLICATIONS are numerous and frequent; so much so that separations of the internal epicondyle appear to be insignificant compared with other concomitant lesions.

Articular lesion.—The articulation is not so likely to be primarily involved after thirteen years of age.

Although in these instances the separation may be at first extra-articular, the epiphysis, being displaced downwards on the inner side of the trochlea and placed against the synovial membrane, the latter will ultimately become adherent to the epicondyle, and, if an attempt be made to remove this process by operation, it will lead to opening of the articular cavity.

In younger children—from the fifth to the twelfth year—the internal epicondyle being still part of the cartilaginous epiphysis, its separation is much more likely to be intra-articular, but opening of the articulation need not, of necessity, occur; the earlier the age the greater the probability of its occurrence.

The author cannot agree with J. Hutchinson junior, that 'when the epicondyle is separated, the elbow-joint is probably always opened.'

Comminution of the epicondyle is the result of direct violence.

An example which came under the author's observation at the Miller Hospital in May 1893 was compound, and caused by direct crushing violence. Some small comminuted fragments were removed, and a most successful recovery obtained.

Dislocation of elbow is one of the most frequent complications, especially in the outward direction.

Professor Humphry's specimen of detachment of this process with fracture of the olecranon preserved in the Cambridge Museum, and figured by Mr. Jonathan Hutchinson junior (*British Medical Journal*, January 16, 1892), was also complicated with forward dislocation of the elbow-joint.

An interesting case of detachment of a portion of the internal epicondyle, associated with dislocation of the elbow backwards and outwards, is quoted by M. Fallier from M. Debruyn's memoir on luxations of the elbow ('Mémoire sur les luxations du coude,' *Annales de la Chirurgie*, ix. 1843):

In 1841 a lad (F. V.), aged eighteen, while descending a ladder quickly, slipped and fell to the ground, a distance of twelve feet. The whole weight of the body was received upon the palm of the left hand, the arm being stretched out in front of the body. The forearm was found to be slightly flexed, pronated, and somewhat shortened. The deformity of the elbow was very considerable, and the articular lower end of the humerus was readily recognised at the bend of the elbow; the olecranon, displaced upwards and backwards, was situated near the outer border of the humerus. Directly below and behind the external epicondyle the head of the radius could be felt and rotated, while below the epitrochlea (internal epicondyle), which was very prominent on the inner side, a very distinct depression was noticeable. Repeated attempts at reduction were unsuccessful, and gangrene of the forearm supervened, which necessitated amputation at the lower part of the arm on the eighth day.

On dissection of the limb, the tendons of the brachialis anticus and biceps were seen to be displaced behind the external epicondyle, and the ulna and radius were situated on the outer and posterior aspect of the humerus. The brachial artery was ruptured, and on the inner side of the elbow there was a portion of bone which had been detached from the internal epicondyle, and to which the muscles were still attached.

Langenbeck quotes (Lücke, Langenbeck's *Archiv für klin. Chir.* Bd. 3, 1862, S. 311, No. 139, 1858) a case recorded and figured by H. Senftleben, in which ankylosis followed, the bones of the forearm being *displaced backwards and outwards*. Resection of the whole elbow-joint was performed seven months after the injury, when the internal epicondyle was found lying in the olecranon fossa

attached by fibrous tissue. The bones were completely dislocated
backwards and outwards. The trochlea and capitellum were intact.
Death occurred on the thirteenth day from pyæmia.

Paralysis of ulnar nerve.— The paralysis may be immediate, from
direct contusion or injury to the nerve or from pressure of the
displaced epiphysis.

In the author's case, just related, the paralysis was noticed immediately after the injury. As it was considered that it might be due
to direct injury to the nerve, the epicondyle was not removed until the
eighteenth day. The nerve was then found to be directly pressed
upon by the displaced epiphysis.

Paralysis may be observed *later* from pressure of displaced
fragment or excessive callus.

Denucé excised the internal epicondyle of a man for intense
neuralgia of the ulnar nerve caused by the displaced fragment
having united in a false position. The man had fallen upon his
elbow three months previously.

In 1887 Professor Kocher (*Beiträge practisch wichtiger Fracturformen*, 1896, S. 158) successfully excised the internal epicondyle four
months after the accident in a boy aged seventeen and a half years.
The elbow had been dislocated backwards, but was immediately
reduced. For three weeks sensibility over the distribution of the ulnar
nerve to the ring and little fingers was diminished. The left forearm
being thinner, and the interossei muscles of the hand, especially
between the thumb and index finger, weaker than the right, and as
extension was limited and the detached epicondyle felt in contact
with the side of the olecranon, the operation was undertaken. The
epicondyle was found displaced downwards and forwards, and firmly
fixed by fibrous tissue between the coronoid process and olecranon.
The joint was not opened.

In many of the simple cases the separation was only detected
after the dislocation had been reduced.

SYMPTOMS.—In spite of the well-recognised fact that separation
of the internal epicondyle is so common an accident in children,
few authentic cases have been published.

Little attention seems to have been given to it before Granger's
time, but it has been followed up to some extent by César, Denucé,
Hamilton, Pingaud, Pézerat, Malgaigne, Fallier, and a few others.

Packard says : ' With regard to separations of the outer and inner
angles of the lower extremity of the humerus, of the epicondyle or
epitrochlea, or of the epiphysis, it is impossible to lay down any
distinct and definite statements, partly because of the small number
of recorded cases, and partly because of the obscurity of the conditions attending these lesions.' Like many other writers, he makes
no attempt to differentiate these injuries, and places fractures of the
internal epicondyle with those accompanied by fracture of the
trochlea as well.

Cheever dismisses the subject of separation of the epicondyles (*Boston Medical and Surgical Journal*, cxxvii. p. 588) as follows:

' The most common accident that happens to little children is separation of the epicondyles, and inasmuch as the internal epicondyle is by far the more prominent of the two, this is the one that ordinarily breaks. Why it does not occur universally is probably because, being carried next the body, it is not quite so apt to receive blows as the outer one, on which the child falls more frequently. The latter is a small affair, and, if broken off, it is drawn down by the muscles, and mobility can be felt. The internal epicondyle is quite large, and gives perceptible widening if broken, and mobility is obtained.'

SEPARATION WITHOUT DISPLACEMENT.—If the violence be slight, it is improbable that there will be any displacement of the epiphysis, but it is seldom that, when quite detached, it is not displaced by the action of the internal lateral ligament attached to its lower surface and of the powerful muscles attached to its apex.

In Hamilton's case, already quoted, that of the lad aged eleven years, with epiphysial separation from a direct blow, the motions of pronation, with flexion, were not at all impaired, either immediately or at any subsequent period, whilst the fragment was never sensibly, or only very slightly, displaced.

The same surgeon has seen other cases in which the fragment did not seem to be displaced.

Dr. Powers, of New York, showed the following as an example of eight cases which he had observed in children:

P. B., a boy, aged eight, fell three feet, striking the inner aspect of the left elbow. Examination revealed tenderness over the inner condyle, together with moderate swelling. Active movements at the elbow were feeble and painful. The internal epicondyle was freely movable, and on moving it crepitus was elicited. In full extension of the forearm it slipped a little downwards, but on flexing the elbow to a right angle it was easily replaced. The forearm was placed, midway between pronation and supination, at an angle of 90 degrees, in a plaster-of-Paris splint. The splint was removed at the end of ten days, then re-applied, and finally removed on the twenty-eighth day. The joint was free from pain and swelling ; the epicondyle was in place, but moderately thickened. The patient could flex the forearm to 75 degrees, and could extend it to 135 degrees. Pronation and supination were nearly perfect. The functions quickly improved, and on the sixtieth day they were completely restored, but moderate thickening persisted at the seat of the fracture.

On the other hand, Granger believed that displacement was always present.

DISPLACEMENT OF EPIPHYSIS.—Displacement of the epiphysis is one of the principal signs of this diastasis.

Downwards.—The detached portion is usually, or nearly always, drawn somewhat downwards towards the hand, or downwards and a little forwards, by the action and in the direction of the fibres of some of the superficial flexors and pronators, especially the pronator radii teres, attached to this process.

The extent of the displacement downwards is variable, in some cases from two to four centimetres.

In some instances it may be displaced as far downwards as the inner side of the trochlea, but in others the displacement is more gradual before the time of formation of callus.

When the separation is the result of muscular action, this direction of the displaced epiphysis is the only one possible.

Hamilton says that he had seen what he supposed to be this epiphysis displaced in the direction of the hand, or downwards, very manifestly, twice, and in two other examples a careful measurement showed a slight displacement in the same direction.

Granger also found in his cases the epicondyle carried towards the hand, with more or less variation in its lateral position, so that while in some instances it touched the olecranon, in others it was removed an inch or more in the opposite direction.

Fallier, in ten cases of fracture of the internal epicondyle accompanied with dislocation (adults and children), noted that in nine there was this form of displacement.

Careful measurement should be made from the internal epicondyle to the apex of the styloid process of the ulna on the two sides. The internal epicondyle will also be absent from the normal transverse line which passes through the apex of the epicondyles and olecranon during the extended position of the elbow.

The following case of disjunction of the epiphysis of the internal epicondyle was treated in July 1891 at the Miller Hospital. The patient, a lad (Wm. C.), aged ten years, had fallen on his left elbow. On examination the inner side of his left elbow was found to be swollen and painful; however, a small nodule of bone, the epiphysis of the internal epicondyle, could be moved up and down in a vertical direction on the inner side of the humerus. This process of bone was displaced downwards by the muscles attached to it. There was pain on pronation and on flexion and extension of the forearm. The epicondyle was replaced, and the elbow fixed in a rectangular splint. Union, apparently bony, occurred in the normal position, with no restriction of any of the movements of the joint.

The internal supra-condyloid ridge is often felt to be abruptly terminated below, and in the position of the normal internal epicondyle the finger may feel a somewhat *rugged surface* or elevation, never so prominent, however, as the epicondyle itself. Below this, if the displacement has been great and the contusion slight, the finger may feel the flat inner side of the trochlea, and then, a little in front of this, the displaced fragment.

Mr. Jonathan Hutchinson mentions (*Medical-Press and Circular*, November 18, 1885) the case of a young medical student who had fallen at a football match and had knocked off the internal condyle, which had been displaced downwards close to the side of the olecranon. The condyle was absent from its proper position.

Displacement backwards.—Displacement of the epiphysis directly backwards is largely due to the direction of the violence, for it is difficult to understand how such a displacement could be effected by muscular action alone. In these cases, therefore, the ulnar nerve is very liable to be injured from the direct violence which caused the separation.

The author's own case is a good example of this form of displacement.

In other instances the displacement may be more downwards and but slightly backwards, so that the fragment becomes lodged in the groove between the trochlea of the humerus and olecranon. In the adult the fractured piece of bone has been found firmly wedged in this position between the two osseous projections.

Displacement upwards can only be produced by direct violence, this being directed from below upwards, as in a fall on the ground.

Some portions of the triceps and brachialis anticus remain untorn, and act upon the fragment above, whilst the muscles attached to this process below are torn across.

It will probably be found to be complicated by some other lesion in the elbow-joint.

Granger found this form of displacement in one case of fracture of the internal condyle in the adult.

In one of Fallier's cases, in a boy aged fifteen, the fragment was displaced one and a half centimetres upwards. This was complicated with dislocation, and the epicondyle was thought to have been displaced into this position during reduction and the application of the apparatus. It was felt by the finger which examined the inner edge of the humerus, being arrested by it.

Another instance is quoted by Troschel (*Medicin. Zeitg. des Vereins für Heilk. in Preussen*, 1839, Gurlt, ii. Theil, S. 820) of a youth, aged twelve, who was pushed by his comrades and fell on the pavement, the arm being in a flexed position against the side of the body.

The epitrochlea (internal epicondyle) was broken off and displaced one centimetre upwards, and could be moved both backwards and forwards without giving rise to any pain. A splint was applied to the limb in the semiflexed position, and at the end of eight days the fragment was already found to be fixed and firmly adherent, without any articular rigidity.

Out of four cases of fracture of the epitrochlea in children recorded by Hamilton ('Report on Deformities after Fractures,' *Trans. of Amer. Med. Association*, vol. ix. 1856, p. 133), in one instance only was the 'epiphysis' displaced three lines upwards and two backwards towards the olecranon (*vide infra*).

Displacement forwards.—Some authors, including Mr. Hutchinson, think that the displacement of this process is usually forwards in front of the joint.

In Sturrock's case (quoted below) the epicondyle was displaced forwards and outwards, i.e. the prominence was situate in front and to the outer side of the normal site of the internal epicondyle.

Size and form of fragment.—Unless accompanied by much swelling—which in all probability will occur if the lesion is due to muscular action—or if seen before swelling has set in, the piece of bone, although small, will in such cases be readily felt by the examining finger and thumb.

The detached process can sometimes be felt lying over the ulnar nerve.

In one case related by M. César the internal epicondyloid fragment was comminuted.

Mobility of the epiphysis.—In nearly all the published cases this has been a well-marked sign. It is rare to find the epiphysis fixed, without any mobility.

The epiphysis will usually be found an inch or more below and in front of its normal position at the level of the articulation, and rarely, as we have seen, in other positions, above or behind. It is especially mobile in an antero-posterior direction, less so in the vertical direction.

Its extent is influenced by the position of the elbow, being most marked when the forearm is slightly flexed and supinated in order to relax the epicondylar muscles, and being more fixed in the incompletely extended and pronated position, which exists in some cases complicated with dislocation.

In other examples it has been found movable in every direction, vertically as well as in the antero-posterior direction. It depends also in some measure upon the swelling of the soft parts and the extent of separation of the periosteum.

Coulon, in his *Traité des fractures chez les enfants*, describes these injuries under the title of extra-articular fractures of the epitrochlea, and quotes three cases in children, three and a half, ten and a half, and eleven years respectively, the two last being characterised by the crepitus and mobility of the small fragment of this process. All were caused by falls upon the elbow.

Gurlt was undoubtedly right in considering such examples as separations of the internal epicondylar epiphysis.

M. Pézerat noted (*loc. cit. supra*) this mobility of the fractured internal epicondyle, both forwards and backwards as well as upwards and downwards, in the case of a child, aged twelve, who had fallen upon the inner side of his elbow. Graduated compresses were applied in front and behind, consolidation took place by the twentieth day; and by the thirtieth day the natural movements were completely restored.

In the following case, which came under the author's notice at the Miller Hospital, the mobility of the epiphysis was most marked in the antero-posterior direction; less so from above downwards.

Ethel G., aged three years and four months, was brought to the hospital by her father. About half an hour previously she had fallen and struck her elbow against the edge of a drinking-fountain. She was a well-nourished, healthy-looking child, without any appearance of syphilis or rickets. Over the situation of the internal epicondyle of the left elbow there was a well-marked prominence, and the skin over it was slightly contused. This was found to be the epiphysis itself, which was movable readily from before backwards, the motion being accompanied by pain and soft crepitus. There was little or no displacement, for the epicondyles were found to be in their normal position, as well as the radius and ulna. Pronation and supination were painless, but on extreme flexion and extension the child cried. There was no evidence of any other epiphysial separation of the lower end of the humerus. The injury was treated by a rectangular splint and a short posterior one. When the author saw her ten days later there was still evidence of considerable bruising over the inner side of the elbow, extending upwards for two inches, and great thickening over the internal condyle, extending laterally about one inch and upwards a little over an inch, also a little outwards towards the olecranon. There was also some synovitis of the elbow-joint.

Muffled crepitus is characteristic, even if the injury occurs in the first few years of life, and is associated with the inevitable fracture through the cartilaginous strip which unites it in one mass with the cartilaginous lower end, separating it from the trochlea. The soft character of the crepitus will not, therefore, be obscured by this cartilaginous fracture.

If there is much displacement it will be detected in replacing the fragment in position—viz. by pressing it upwards and backwards whilst the forearm is semiflexed and pronated. But crepitus, though distinct at first, may be subsequently lost from the gradual separation of the epiphysis by muscular action.

When displacement is absent, or but little marked, slight movement of the epiphysis will readily produce it.

Impaired movement.—There is frequently some hindrance to the free movements of the elbow-joint. This may be partly accounted for by the swelling present, partly by the separation of the epiphysis —to which some of the principal flexors and pronators of the arm are attached—and partly by the tearing off of the periosteum from the diaphysis, together with important muscles.

Gurlt, however, states that in these extra-articular fractures 'the patient can, in spite of the pain, move his arm in flexion and extension, as well as in pronation and supination.'

For the forearm the common position is semiflexed and semipronated. It may be abducted to a greater extent than is normal.

Swelling and pain.—In a young subject, swelling and ecchymosis on the inner side of the elbow, accompanied by acute pain in the position of the internal epicondyle, and following a blow in this situation or a fall upon the hand or elbow, are quite sufficient to suggest the occurrence of a separation of the epiphysis of the internal condyle. The ecchymosis may be very extensive, extending up the inner side of the arm and downwards towards the antéro-internal aspect of the forearm.

The pain, although persistent at this spot, is never excessive; it may be felt in the little finger from bruising of the ulnar nerve.

In many cases the swelling is so great as to prevent a thorough examination and exact diagnosis being made. It may extend in the course of a few days down the inner aspect of the forearm in the direction of the sheath of the muscles attached to the epiphysis (César), and assist by the course it takes in diagnosing the lesion from a simple contusion of the elbow.

In Malgaigne's case, of a boy aged ten (quoted below), the pain and swelling made him suspect fracture; but the mobility was doubtful, and no crepitus was perceptible. It was not until eight days afterwards, when the swelling had subsided, that all doubt was removed by the occurrence of distinct crepitus. There was no appreciable displacement.

COMPLICATIONS. **Injury to the ulnar nerve.**—The ulnar nerve, from its close proximity to the epiphysis, is exceedingly liable to be injured by the direct violence which caused the separation or by the displacement of the epiphysis—especially if this is carried in a backward and downward direction by the force of the violence. Granger believed that the paralysis is always due to compression by the displaced fragment. In Fallier's case the violence was certainly indirect, the patient having fallen on the palm of his hand.

But indirect violence may cause injury to the nerve, not by *pressure* of the displaced fragment, but rather by *dragging* upon it and lacerating its sheath or fibres, or by mere stretching.

César and Hamilton thought it exclusively due to direct injury to the nerve inflicted at the same time as the process is broken off. Direct contusion of the nerve probably happened in Richet's case, in which the elbow violently struck the ground.

The paralysis of the nerve may be partial or complete at the time of the accident.

An accompanying dislocation will probably injure the ulnar nerve much more readily than a simple separation of this process.

Granger (*loc. cit. supra*) describes the following remarkable case: A boy, eight years old, fell with violence, and broke off completely the whole of the inner epicondyle of the right humerus. The lad said he had fallen on his hand. The fragment was displaced towards the hand, and severe inflammation followed, but he recovered the free and entire use of the elbow-joint in three months after the accident. No splints or bandages were ever employed. From the moment of the accident, the little finger, the inner side of the ring finger, and the skin on the ulnar side of the hand lost all sensation. The abductor minimi digiti and two contiguous muscles of the little finger were also paralysed. This condition lasted eight or ten years, after

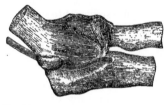

Fig. 96.—DIAGRAM OF RELATION OF ULNAR NERVE TO INTERNAL EPICONDYLE

which sensation and motion were gradually restored to these parts. As a consequence of this paralysed condition of the ulnar nerve, successive crops of vesications, about the size of a split horse-bean, commenced to form on the little finger and ulnar edge of the hand some weeks after the accident, leaving troublesome excoriations. This eruption did not entirely cease for two or three months.

In two other cases Granger states that he found 'the same paralysis of the small muscles of the little finger, the same loss of feeling in the integuments, and the same succession of crops of vesicles on the affected part of the hand, as had occurred in the preceding case.'

The trophic changes were probably the result of neuritis due to the direct contusion of the nerve against the internal condyle. Both cases were said to have ultimately recovered.

Richet's case of detachment of the epitrochlea, accompanied by dislocation of the elbow inwards and complete paralysis of the ulnar nerve, is quoted below.

Dislocation of the elbow.—Dislocation of the elbow combined with separation of the internal epicondyle is not an uncommon accident. Granger, in 1818, was the first to indicate this complication. It may be produced by a direct blow upon the elbow or a fall upon the hand. It will be found to be more common from thirteen to nineteen years of age. Out of forty-eight cases of fracture of the epicondyle, nineteen were complicated with dislocation of the elbow (Fallier).

One of Granger's patients, a boy, aged eleven, had also a luxation of the elbow, which was reduced, but by reason of neglect he failed to recover flexion and extension in the joint. When the swelling, which was exceedingly great, had gone down, the forearm was found immovably fixed at right angles with the humerus. By means of passive motion considerable use of the elbow had been regained at the end of three weeks. The patient neglected the elbow for a considerable time, and the elbow was then fixed in a position of complete extension, and remained immovable as before. However, some improvement in flexion subsequently took place.

The dislocation may be *backwards*, as in Fallier's, Debruyn's, and Kocher's examples.

Seeing that the chief connections between the humerus and forearm—namely, the powerful muscles and internal lateral ligaments—are set free when the internal epicondyle is detached, it is surprising to find that dislocation is not more frequently present. In two or three separated internal epicondyles under his care the author has demonstrated very clearly the facility with which a dislocation may be produced.

In all separations of the internal epicondyle, undue mobility of the ulna with the forearm is a very noticeable feature, especially in a lateral direction.

Hutchinson recorded (*British Medical Journal*, vol. ii. 1866 ; *Medical Times and Gazette*, January 1884, p. 3) an example of this complication. A young gentleman, aged sixteen, whilst playing racquets, fell and struck his elbow against a wall. He was found to have ' a dislocation,' and within an hour a surgeon reduced it. Nothing further was recognised at the time, but some months later his father, who was a surgeon, but did not see him in the first instance, found that the inner condyle had been fractured. He was brought to Mr. Hutchinson six weeks later, and it was then quite evident that the inner epicondyle was broken off and displaced downwards, so as to rest against the inner side of the olecranon, where it was fixed a year later. The elbow being examined on a subsequent occasion, the condition of things was found to be exactly as before. On the side of the olecranon was a lump of bone, nearly as large as the end of one's thumb. · If not ankylosed to the olecranon, it was certainly very firmly fixed, as no movement could be obtained. The origin of the flexor carpi radialis, and also, Mr. Hutchinson thought, a part of the pronator radii teres, could be distinctly traced to this bone. That it was the inner condyle there could not be the slightest doubt, for the part of the humerus from which it had been broken still presented a rough edge, and the condyle had disappeared. When seen two years later the patient had regained almost perfect use of the joint. Mr. Hutchinson adds : ' In what manner the displacement of this fragment downwards is effected it is difficult to conjecture, but I have since seen another case which was, in this feature, exactly like the one which I have described. Possibly such a displacement can occur only when there is dislocation at the joint as well as detachment of the epicondyle. Dislocation might be productive of considerable laceration of the soft structures, and be attended by dragging of the epicondyle downwards. The usual position of the fragment in this accident is, I think, forward in front of the joint, and this is where a knowledge of the muscular attachments would lead us to expect it.'

Manoury has recorded a case complicated by backward dislocation which he called a fracture by muscular action.

Gurlt quotes a case of Senftleben's (Gurlt, *Lehre von den Knochenbrüchen*, II. Theil, II. Lieferung, S. 823, Case 305). A boy, aged eleven years, fell and struck his right elbow. There was dislocation backwards and outwards of the elbow, with the characteristic deformity, accompanied by displacement backwards of the internal epicondyle into the olecranon fossa. The dislocation was reduced under chloroform, and the fragment easily replaced. The fragment firmly united by the fourteenth day, and all movements of the elbow-joint were ultimately perfectly free.

L. Fallier has published (*Revue des Sciences Médicales*, 1890, p. 265; 'Contribution à l'étude des fractures de l'épitrochlée, Thèse de Paris, 1889) a number of cases of fracture of the epitrochlea in addition to those already recorded, and finds that they are almost exclusively observed in the male sex. He also shows that when they are complicated with dislocation of the elbow they are as often caused by indirect as by direct violence. When the violence is indirect the fracture is the result of detachment of the internal lateral ligament of the elbow, and the fracture ought always to be considered as a complication of the dislocation; but, on the contrary, in the rare cases where the fracture is due to muscular action, the dislocation should be considered as the complication of the fracture.

Dislocation inwards.—Dislocation inwards is much more rarely met with than dislocation outwards. Richet has recorded a case in the adult complicated with dislocation backwards and inwards, but it is probable that in this instance the trochlea itself was fractured.

The following case was communicated to Dr. A. César by Professor Richet.

A youth, aged about fifteen years, slipped on some ice and fell upon the inner side of the elbow, the arm being away from the body. M. Richet found a fracture of the epitrochlea, with dislocation of the elbow backwards and inwards. After the dislocation had been immediately reduced, it was found that the ulnar nerve had been so seriously contused that it was entirely paralysed, the little finger being completely insensitive. At the end of a few days the arm was enclosed in a splint, which was removed by M. Richet at the end of twenty days for fear of ankylosis resulting from the dislocation. The insensibility remained as complete as before, and was so marked that a month later the patient was able to hold his finger for more than a minute in a candle flame, to the astonishment of his companions, without feeling the least pain. The burn was so great that the skin frizzled and cracked and the nail ignited. It took several weeks to heal, and left traces which were still recognisable ; but after this violent cauterisation sensibility re-appeared in a progressive and rapid manner.   There was no vesicular eruption such as Granger speaks of.

As regards the movements of the elbow, they almost completely returned, with the exception of full flexion and extension.

Hamilton records ('Report on Deformities after Fractures,' *Trans. of Amer. Med. Association*, vol. ix. 1856, p. 112 ; and *Treatise on Fractures and Dislocations*) the case of a boy (F. C.), aged fifteen years, who had fallen upon his arm in wrestling, and the surgeon found a dislocation inwards of the bones of the elbow-joint, which he immediately reduced.   The diastasis of the epicondyle was not at that time detected, the arm being greatly swollen.   No splints were applied.   It was three months after the accident when Hamilton saw him, at which time he found the internal epicondyle removed downwards towards the hand one inch and a quarter, and at this point it had become immovably fixed.

Partial ankylosis existed at the elbow-joint, but pronation and supination were perfect.

Dislocation outwards is readily explained by the attachment of the internal lateral ligament to the epicondyle. It is most correctly considered as a variety of dislocation backwards, for in many instances, the muscles on the inner side having lost their attachment through the fracture of the internal epicondyle, the muscles on the outer side continue to act upon the forearm, and so tend to displace the bones of the forearm outwards.

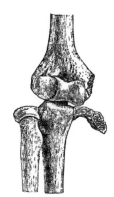

FIG. 97.—DIAGRAM OF DISLOCATION OF ELBOW OUTWARDS, WITH SEPARATION OF THE INTERNAL EPICONDYLE. (HELFERICH)

Dislocation directly outwards is of occasional occurrence.

Fig. 97 is from an experimental preparation by Helferich (*Atlas der traumatischen Fracturen und Luxationen*, 1895, Tab. 33, Fig. 1). The ulna is in contact with the side of the capitellum and outer portion of the trochlea, whilst the radial head stands out free on the outer side.   By means of the internal lateral ligament the internal epicondyle is torn off and remains still connected with the ulna.

Fig. 98 (Helferich, *ibid.* Tab. 33, Fig. 2) represents a case observed by Helferich during life, displaying the lesion just figured, in which the characteristic projection of the olecranon in dislocation backwards was entirely absent, and the other contours of the elbow little altered.   But on the outer side the radial head could readily

B B

be seen, and, in lifetime, felt, especially during supination and pronation.

Dislocation of the elbow forwards is extremely rare. It is remark-able that in all the four cases of simple dislocation forwards of the

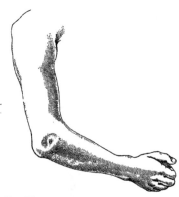

elbow collected by Denucé in 1869 the injury was due to a fall upon the elbow, while in the following case it was caused by a fall upon the hand.

Poinsot has recorded this case as seen by W. Dale, in which a child of fourteen years fell on to the palm of its hand, which caused an incomplete dislocation of the elbow for-wards. It was noticed after reduction, which was readily accomplished, that the epi-trochlea had been torn off at its base. Recovery took place

FIG. 98.—DISLOCATION OUTWARDS OF ELBOW ACCOMPANYING SEPARATION OF THE INTERNAL EPICONDYLE. · (HELFERICH)

without any mishap, and with absolute restoration of all movements.

M. Poinsot thought that this form of dislocation with the fracture had been brought about by torsion and lateral bending outwards of the forearm.

Dislocation of ulna backwards is produced in much the same manner as dislocation of both bones backwards—viz. by over-exten-sion of the forearm and lateral flexion outwards, as in a fall on the palm of the hand.

A case of *dislocation of the ulna backwards,* complicated by fracture of the internal epicondyle, is quoted by M. L. Fallier, seen by Beaurieux, of Orleans ('Note sur un cas de luxation isolée et complète du cubitus en arrière, compliqué d'une fracture de l'épi-trochlée,' *France Médicale,* 25 Août 1880).

A youth (O.), aged twelve years, had fallen (1880), while at gym-nastics, upon the palm of his left hand, and had lost almost the entire use of the limb. On examination two hours after the accident, the forearm was found in the pronated position, the elbow semiflexed, and the hand flexed at the wrist and adducted. There was only a moderate amount of swelling around the elbow-joint. Active and passive motion, especially flexion, were very painful and restricted. The deformity of the joint was very distinct, for its internal angle was obliterated, whilst its external angle, on the contrary, projected more than is normal. On the posterior aspect of the arm, about two inches above the lower end of the humerus, the upper end of the ulna made a considerable projection, which was easily distin-guished. The head of the radius preserved its normal relations with the external epicondyle, and moved freely during pronation and supination of the forearm. The internal epicondyle could not, however, be made out, and it was only during reduction of the dislocated ulna that the epitrochlea (internal epicondyle) was found to be detached from the humerus. The elbow was kept flexed on a splint at a right angle until the sixth day, when the apparatus was removed, as there was no displacement or swelling, but merely slight discoloration. All movements were easily carried out, with little impediment, and the fractured epitrochlea appeared to be consolidating, for neither mobility nor crepitus was present. Fifteen days later the child had completely recovered, with full use of its limb.

Another previously unpublished case of dislocation of the ulna backwards with fracture of the internal epicondyle is recorded by M. Fallier.

On August 21, 1885, the patient (A. S.), aged fifteen, an iron-platework apprentice, fell, whilst running, on the dorsal aspect of his left wrist, the hand being bent on the forearm and the forearm but slightly on the arm. He was seen by M. Depasse immediately after the accident, and the ulna alone was found to be completely dislocated backwards. The humeral trochlea projected forwards in the flexure of the elbow, and the epitrochlea was detached and freely movable in every direction. The head of the radius rotated in its normal position. Reduction was easily effected by extension and supination of the forearm and manipulation of the displaced bones, and a splint was applied. On his admission to the Maine Hospital at Brest, Professor Fontan found, on removing the apparatus, that the epitrochlea (internal epicondyle) was elevated about one and a half centimetres, and all movements of the elbow-joint could be carried out, the head of the radius still rotating in its normal position. It was noted that with the forearm slightly flexed on the arm, and the hand on the forearm, the epitrochlea approached its normal site; the limb was therefore put up in this position. On August 25 a dorsal splint was applied, and on September 1 replaced by one of gutta-percha. On October 1 the patient left the hospital cured, to resume his work.

It is not necessary here to describe in detail the symptoms of each kind of dislocation which may complicate the detachment of the internal epicondyle. It will suffice to say that, any of these forms of dislocation having been diagnosed, it is essential that the presence or absence of a detached internal epicondyle should be determined from the symptoms already related.

However, in many instances complicated with dislocation it has been found difficult to recognise the displacement of the fragment, or any mobility or crepitus, before reduction, and it is only after this has been accomplished that they have been observed. This has been noticed to be the case even where little or no swelling was present.

After reduction of the dislocation and before any great swelling has taken place, it has been found possible to make out some impediment to the movements of the elbow caused by the detached epicondyle. The fragment dragged downwards and forwards by the epitrochlear muscles may limit *flexion*, but more often *pronation* is incomplete, partly from the acute pain experienced by the patient at the seat of fracture during any attempt at this movement, and partly from the loss of power due to the attachment of a portion of the pronator muscles to the epicondyle, and to the neighbouring periosteum, which is detached from the diaphysis.

Fallier ascertained, in ten cases of dislocation, that in only three was this fracture detected, although present. All three were dislocations backwards (one at the age of eleven, and two at fifteen years).

Although a separated internal condyle has sometimes been recognised in dislocation backwards before reduction, it is essential that in all cases of apparently uncomplicated dislocation of the elbow in children careful examination of the epicondylar regions should be made after reduction.

Fracture of the olecranon.—In Sir Astley Cooper's case of separation of the internal epicondyle the injury was complicated with a fracture of the olecranon.

Fracture of the coronoid process.—This has occurred in one instance.

Wounds.—It is interesting to note that the author has only been able to obtain one example of separation complicated with a wound—viz. his own case, already quoted.

Acute synovitis.—Synovitis is often met with as the result of implication of the synovial membrane in the laceration, or from the extension of the inflammation about the epiphysial separation. If not properly treated it will give rise to ankylosis later on.

Intra-articular separations are most likely to occur before the age of twelve to thirteen years. The fracture, separating the internal epicondyle from the rest of the cartilaginous epiphysis at this early age, will probably open the synovial cavity on the inner side, close to the trochlea.

Although the elbow-joint may be opened during the first few years of childhood, it usually escapes injury after about the twelfth year.

Synovitis was present in the author's case of the girl aged three years and four months, described above. In one of Granger's cases, complicated with dislocation of the elbow, the fracture must certainly have entered the joint.

Gurlt believed that all epiphysial separations of the internal epicondyle must necessarily be extra-capsular, but of this he had no anatomical proof.

Berthomier thinks (*Mécanisme des fractures du coude chez les enfants*, Paris, 1875) that the occurrence of extra-articular fracture of the internal epicondyle has not been sufficiently proved, and states that he was unable to produce extra-capsular fracture of either the internal or external epicondyle.

D. W. Cheever, Professor of Surgery of Harvard University, speaks (*Boston Med. and Surg. Journal*, cxxviii. p. 589) of epicondylar separations as very unimportant injuries, and as having nothing to do with the joint. 'Separation of the internal epicondyle is a matter of little consequence, speedily unites, and ought not to make any stiffness of the elbow, because it does not go into the joint.'

Some authors believe that when the fracture is complicated with dislocation of the bones of the forearm backwards and outwards it communicates with the joint.

Severe inflammation is apt to take place around the seat of separation when the injury has been caused by severe direct violence.

Granger has carefully noted severe inflammation about the elbow and forearm, involving the muscles attached to the epicondyle, and producing such extensive swelling as to prevent almost completely all movement at the elbow.

DIFFERENTIAL DIAGNOSIS. Fracture of the internal condyle.— The character of the *crepitus*, the size and shape of the separated epiphysis, and its causation from muscular action alone in many cases—with, consequently, less swelling and ecchymosis present—are the only guides we have to distinguish it from fracture of the internal condyle.

Where the injury is complicated by dislocation, &c., in which there is great swelling and laceration of the soft parts, the diagnosis from fracture is rendered even more difficult.

Severe contusion on the inner side of the elbow may completely prevent a minute examination of the epicondylar region, thus causing a separation of this process to be unrecognised. This may be especially true when a dislocation complicates the case.

Until the dislocation has been reduced no precise diagnosis can, as a rule, be made; and even then it may be undetected for some days or weeks, on account of the peri-articular inflammation. It should, however, be recognised as soon after reduction as possible, on account of the consequences that may follow.

If no dislocation be present, the swelling, pain, and bruising will disappear in a few days, and permit a complete exploration of this region.

In all cases for an exact diagnosis to be made an anæsthetic must be given, although in many of the uncomplicated cases it is quite evident that one, more or less satisfactory, might be arrived at without its use.

PROGNOSIS AND RESULTS. Rigidity and impairment of movement.—Where there is no displacement of the epiphysis, and the separation is therefore *extra-articular*, the rigidity is likely to be only temporary and the movements of the joint completely restored in a short time, provided that proper treatment is adopted and the arm not confined too long in the flexed position.

Granger, César, and Hamilton agree that it is rare to find much articular rigidity in simple fracture of the epicondyle.

In one out of four cases of separation of the internal epicondyle recorded by Hamilton (*Trans. of Amer. Med. Association,* vol. ix. 1856, p. 111) the result was perfect.

A boy (C. F.), aged eleven, fell and struck the internal condyle of the left humerus. He was seen immediately, when the internal condyle was found to be loose and motion produced a distinct crepitus. Hamilton did not think the fracture extended into the joint. The patient could flex and extend the arm perfectly, and rotate the forearm. A right-angled splint was applied for five weeks. Three months afterwards he could nearly straighten the arm, and all movements were almost perfect.

Even where displacement exists and the deformity is permanent, as in some of Granger's cases, flexion and extension of the elbow have been perfect. In others the movements of the elbow have been but little interfered with. The muscles attached to the displaced epiphysis soon regain their natural power, and are seldom permanently affected. In all of Coulson's cases the movements of the joint were almost perfectly recovered. Gurlt also mentions another similar example observed by Troschel.

César believed that the epicondyle was often imperfectly united by fibrous tissue, and it is probably true that in the majority of cases in which displacement of this process has taken place the union is a fibrous one.

In the more uncommon cases of separation, with little or no displacement, union by bone is probably not an unusual result.

Stimson saw two cases : one in a girl aged thirteen, and the other in a boy aged eleven years. In both the internal epicondyle was movable, and ended in complete recovery without interference with the movements of the joint. In the latter case the fragment united, with displacement downwards to the distance of a quarter of an inch, and it was thought that the lesion was associated with a separation of a part of the lower epiphysis of the humerus or of its trochlear portion.

Mr. Jonathan Hutchinson junior mentions (*British Med. Journal,* January 16, 1892, p. 111) five cases, and alludes to others, in which practically complete recovery of power in the elbow took place, although the epicondyle remained united to the humerus only by fibrous tissue.

CASE I. E. R., a boy aged ten, fell on the curbstone, the point of his right elbow striking the ground. A backward and outward dislocation of the radius and ulna was thus produced, with detachment of the internal epicondyle. Reduction was effected and an outside angular splint applied. Three weeks later the epicondyle was found displaced slightly downwards and backwards. Both flexion and extension were somewhat limited, but the patient recovered completely under passive motion.

CASE II. H. T., aged eleven, had his epicondyle detached by a fall on to the hand; he was positive that the elbow had not been struck. The epicondyle could be readily felt and moved laterally; full relaxation of the flexor muscles had no effect upon the displacement, which was chiefly downwards. An outside angular splint was applied with a circular pad over the fractured part. Ultimately fibrous union, but with almost perfect use of the joint, was obtained.

CASES III. and IV. In both these cases (young boys) the forearm was dislocated outwards at the same time that the epicondyle was dragged off by the traction on the internal lateral ligament. In both, the small fragment of bone was drawn under the trochlear surface, and was not detected in one until the dislocation had been reduced.

CASE V. B. B., aged fourteen ; one arm 'gave way' as he was crawling on hands and knees. Dislocation of the forearm outwards resulted, with detachment of the epicondyle. At the end of four weeks' treatment the latter remained in a position close to the coronoid process, united only by fibrous tissue to the humerus. Extension was less by 15 degrees than on the other side. Eighteen months later, on carefully examining the elbow again, the epicondyle was found (two centimetres in long diameter) still quite movable. The elbow was considered as strong as the other one, but in lifting weights the patient felt occasional pain in the region. Out of ten cases under this surgeon's observation (*Brit. Med. Journal*, December 30, 1893), ' almost perfect range of movement in the elbow-joint was ultimately secured in the seven which were followed up long enough to decide upon. Perseverance in the performance of passive motion was required in nearly all for some weeks.'

Dr. C. A. Sturrock records (*Edinburgh Hospital Reports*, vol. ii. 1894, p. 599) an instance of perfect recovery, with bony union, fourteen months after the accident.

H. Y., æt. ten, was admitted to the Royal Infirmary, Edinburgh, on June 6, 1892, giving a history of having fallen on his elbow, and of having lost the power of his arm immediately. A deficiency was noticed in the region of the internal condyle, and a prominence in front and to the outer side of the normal site of the interna condyle, due apparently to the displaced internal condyle, which was immovable when the hand and forearm were extended. The fragment could be manipulated into position, and the so-called cartilaginous crepitus elicited. On flexing the pronated forearm to less than a right angle, it was found that little or no trace of the displacement remained, and the arm was accordingly retained in splints in this position for fourteen days, after which gentle passive movements were commenced and continued for two months. By this time free and complete movements at the elbow-joint were readily performed, and, when the last observation was made, fourteen months after the accident, these had been maintained, the only trace of the injury being a slight amount of thickening at the base of the internal condyle, which had apparently united to the shaft by bony union.

In several instances of separation of the internal epicondyle which have come under the author's observation at the Miller Hospital, the same good result has always ultimately resulted. In a few cases flexion and extension were a little limited for some time, of which the following case is an example.

R. S., aged eleven, was pushed down in the road, November 11, 1893, and struck the inner side of his right arm. He was seen at the hospital half an hour afterwards, when there was found to be swelling over the situation of the epicondyle, with some flexion and pronation of the forearm. On fixing the shaft of the humerus, the epicondyle could be grasped and moved, especially from above downwards, with velvety crepitus. A rectangular splint was the form of splint adopted. By December 28, 1893, supination and pronation were quite perfect, and extension almost complete. Flexion was not quite so good, but still this could be carried beyond·a right angle.

If there has been much extra-articular inflammation, the muscles attached to the internal epicondyle are likely to become much shortened, rendering the displacement of this process quite impossible to be reduced, and considerable deformity and hindrance to the proper functions of the limb will result.

Rigidity not amounting to ankylosis is due to the prolonged fixation of the elbow. It must be distinguished from articular ankylosis due to synovitis of the articulation, and will rapidly disappear under treatment.

Ankylosis of the joint.—Severe inflammation in the neighbourhood of the articulation, with contraction of the muscles and tendons and deposit of new bone, caused by stripping up of the periosteum, will all tend to produce more or less ankylosis.

In one of Hamilton's cases there was partial ankylosis three months after the accident, but pronation and supination were perfect.

Even when the injury has been complicated with a dislocation, the impairment of the movements of the joint has not been permanent to any great extent.

Hamilton remarks that ' we might, therefore, reasonably conclude that, where the accident has been properly treated, permanent ankylosis would be the exception, and not the rule.' On the other hand, Malgaigne and others have thought that articular rigidity with serious impairment of movement is almost inevitable—even ankylosis in many cases. It is certain that in many of the recorded cases the diminished extent of range of movement is very disproportionate to the apparently small amount of injury.

Malgaigne (*Treatise on Fractures*) mentions the case of a boy, aged ten, who fell on the path, the inner side of his elbow being driven into the gravel. No crepitus was at first present, and owing to the swelling no diagnosis was made until the eighth day, when the epitrochlea was plainly made out to be broken off, but without marked displacement. The forearm was kept flexed on a splint, and some pressure made on the epitrochlea; passive motion was begun at the end of a fortnight. Little inflammation was present; yet, after two months and a half had elapsed, Malgaigne states that flexion could only be obtained between 80 and 140 degrees.

Without going so far as this surgeon, it must be said that ankylosis, partial or complete, is inevitable in certain cases. Especially when the articulation of the elbow-joint is involved in the injury, the results are very grave.

In one of Granger's cases, the patient, through neglect, never recovered flexion or extension of the elbow-joint, and Hamilton says that he had only once found any considerable ankylosis of the joint after the lapse of a few years.

Jonathan Hutchinson junior also records (*loc. cit. supra*) another example of partial ankylosis.

W. W., aged seven, fell on the right arm, and separated the internal epicondyle, dislocating the forearm backwards. He came to the clinic two days later, when the swelling was very great. Under anæsthesia, however, the diagnosis could be effected and reduction made. A plaster-of-Paris bandage was employed. He was sent out of hospital, and told to return in a fortnight; unfortunately he did not do so for several weeks, by which time movement in the joint had become much impaired, and it did not improve greatly.

Union of epiphysis.—If the epiphysis is but little displaced, there is every reason to believe that it will unite by osseous material, for of this the author has seen several instances. Sturrock's case (quoted above) illustrates this point.

Still, it is somewhat surprising that in the larger proportion of cases of detachment with displacement, this epiphysis, unlike most of the other epiphyses in the body, does not unite by bone, but by fibrous tissue.

There is frequently no large amount of callus about the detached epicondyle, such as we find in other epiphysial separations. This is probably due not so much to the displacement as to the laceration of the periosteum connecting it with the rest of the internal condyle.

Deformity.—According to some surgeons, no deformity should be expected, although Gross says of this form of fracture that 'few cases recover without a certain degree of deformity, or even ankylosis.'

Of ten cases recorded by Dr. C. A. Powers (*New York Medical Record*, December 22, 1888)—eight in children and two in adults— nine regained the functions perfectly ; the other was lost sight of at the end of the second month. In none was there resulting deformity. On the removal of the splint, the average range of motion found was 35 degrees, and this generally improved in direct proportion to the intelligence and faithfulness with which the patient followed directions.

The epicondyle was found by Hamilton in one case displaced *downwards* for a distance of one inch and a quarter, and immovably fixed, three months after the accident.

In M. Paulet's specimen, and in M. Fallier's case, the fragment was still displaced downwards and freely movable eight months after the accident.

In others it has remained fixed in its displaced position.

Displacement downwards and backwards.—In another case of Hutchinson's it was found after a year displaced downwards and backwards, and very firmly fixed against the inner side of the olecranon. This case had been originally complicated with a dis- location.

Packard has (*International Cyclopædia of Surgery*, vol. iv. p. 137) unfortunately placed under fractures of the epitrochlea (internal epicondyle)· eleven cases of fracture of the trochlea and internal condyle recorded by Hamilton. The following is what Hamilton says of these cases in his 'Report on Deformities after Frac- tures' (*Trans. Amer. Med. Association*, vol. ix. 1856, pp. 114, 133) :

'The eleven fractures of the internal condyle (' trochlea and epi- trochlea' of Chaussier) occurred in children between the ages of six years and eighteen. Of the whole number, four are known to have been fractures of the condyle outside of the joint, or fractures of the apo- physis (' epitrochlea '), and four are known to have entered the joint (fractures of the 'trochlea'). Of the fractures of the apophyses, two are recorded as imperfect, because there remains a partial ankylosis, and two as perfect, because no ankylosis exists. In three of the four cases there was, however, a permanent displacement of the apophysis. In one instance it was displaced slightly upwards and backwards,. and in two cases it was very much displaced downwards.'

The two cases of displacement downwards were :

I. Boy (F. C.), aged fifteen (case reported above). Three months after accident the apophysis of the internal condyle was found to be broken off and removed downwards towards the wrist one inch and a quarter, where it was immovably fixed. The elbow was partially ankylosed, so that it could not be straightened completely nor flexed to a right angle. Pronation and supination were perfect.

II. 'Boy (F. B.), aged nine, fell and broke left internal condyle.

Six years after the accident, when the patient was a student of medicine, the internal condyle was found to be displaced downwards towards the wrist half an inch. Cannot straighten the arm completely. Can only flex it slightly, the elbow being fixed at an obtuse angle. The power of pronation and supination imperfect. He thinks the arm is as strong as before.'

In 1859 Coulson stated at the Royal Medical Chirurgical Society that he had seen a great many cases of fracture of the internal condyle in boys, and thought that they were almost always followed by deformity. He quoted the case of a boy in which Mr. Key refractured the part for fixation of the elbow. The boy ultimately recovered good movement.

Displacement forwards.—If the epiphysis be displaced forwards it may unite with the lower end of the shaft, and very considerably hamper the proper movements of the joint.

Mr. Hutchinson describes. (*Brit. Med. Journal*, 1886, July 24) a case in which he found this epicondyle displaced forwards twenty months after the injury. A girl, aged four years, fell while in the care of a nurse, but it was not known precisely of what kind the violence had been. The elbow was bruised and swollen for some time. She was treated by means of a plaster-of-Paris case, and subsequently by a hinged splint. On examination twenty months afterwards the elbow could not be flexed quite to a right angle, nor could it be straightened. Slight flexion only was permitted, but pronation and supination were quite free. The arm was strong, and the child used it for almost anything, yet could not raise it to the mouth. It appeared probable that the injury had been complicated. The head of the radius projected strongly, as if almost, though not quite, free from the external condyle, so that the finger could be placed in the outer two-thirds of the cup of the radius ; still, it certainly had not wholly left the condyle. The distance between the radius and ulna was much increased, and no doubt the articular ligament was completely torn. The inner condyle was lost, the inner side of the ulna being in the same plane, or nearly so, as the inner edge of the humerus. There was thickening in front of the humerus in this position, making it seem possible that the epicondyle had been broken off and displaced forwards. The thickening in front of the lower part of the humerus was, however, not nearly so great as is usual in separation of the whole lower epiphysis. Under an anæsthetic the elbow was bent up to an angle of 45 degrees, and very nearly straightened. Systematic and vigorous movements of the joint were advised, and in the course of a few years its use would be almost perfect.

Displacement upwards.—In only one instance out of four recorded by Hamilton was the fragment displaced permanently upwards and backwards. A boy (G. B.), 'aged six, fell and separated the apophysis from the internal condyle of the right humerus. The

fracture did not extend into the joint.   When examined seven
years after the accident the arm was perfect in every respect, except
that the apophysis was carried backwards about two lines, and
upwards towards the shoulder about three lines ; and it was a little
more prominent than the apophysis on the opposite arm, the right
elbow measuring three and three-quarter inches in its transverse
diameter, and the left three and a half.'

Injury to the ulnar nerve, paralysis, &c.—In Granger's case loss of
sensation over the distribution of the ulnar nerve, and paralysis of
the abductor minimi digiti and two contiguous muscles of the little
finger, lasted for eight or ten years, after which sensation and motion
were gradually restored to these parts.   As a consequence of the
paralysis of the ulnar nerve, trophic changes took place in the skin,
and successive crops of vesications formed on the little finger and
ulnar edge of the hand some weeks after the accident, leaving
troublesome excoriations, and did not entirely cease for two or three
months.

These vesications, noticed by Granger in his three cases, on the
inner side of the hand have not been found in any of the other
examples of paralysis of the ulnar nerve subsequently met with.

In one of César's cases the injury to the ulnar nerve was complicated with dislocation inwards of the elbow, but the sensibility of
the nerve gradually returned.

Compression of the ulnar nerve may be produced by the
pressure of the epicondyle united in a bad position.   In one instance
it is stated that the nerve was found ' hypertrophied and in contact
with an osseous spine, produced by the epicondyle consolidated in
faulty position.'

In a case of Denucé's, resection of the projecting spine-like
process of bone, for neuralgia produced by pressure upon the ulnar
nerve, was followed by loss of the nerve symptoms.   It occurred to
a man who had fallen upon his elbow three months previously.

Sir Astley Cooper (*Fractures and Dislocations*, 1842, p. 466) relates
the case of a girl who, by a fall upon her elbow, had fractured the
olecranon, and also the internal epicondyle of the humerus.   The
point of the broken bone had almost penetrated the skin.   The
cubital nerve had also been injured, for the little finger and half the
ring finger were benumbed.

Mr. Jonathan Hutchinson junior publishes (*Transactions of the
Hunterian Society*, 1891, p. 110) a parallel case where flexion was
limited to 10 degrees, and the muscles supplied by this nerve were
wasted with anæsthesia.   He removed the epicondyle after opening
the elbow-joint ; sensation returned, and flexion was increased to 50
degrees, with a useful arm.   The following are the particulars of the
case (*Brit. Med. Journal*, January 16, 1892, p. 113) :

H. W., aged thirteen, whilst ' turning cart wheels ' on his hands,
fell and detached the epicondyle of one humerus.   He was treated

at Guy's Hospital in the most thorough manner, and from particulars which Mr. Hutchinson junior was fortunate enough to obtain from one of the dressers who had attended to him, it was ascertained that passive motion was tried for long, and that he was twice anæsthetised with the view of overcoming the rigid extension of the elbow. When he came to the London Hospital at the end of some four or five months, the condition was as follows: his left arm was practically useless, since he could not bend the elbow more than a few degrees, and he complained of great pain if any attempt were made to increase this limit. Further, there was evidence of serious injury to the ulnar nerve. The little finger and half the ring finger were anæsthetic, there was wasting of the short muscles of the former and of the adductor pollicis, and the interossei would hardly act at all. The epicondyle was readily felt to be drawn downwards and a little backwards, and that region was very tender to palpation. Seeing that all ordinary means had failed and that the muscles were wasting, it was thought advisable to relieve the condition by operation, to which the parents readily consented. Under antiseptic precautions the epicondyle was cut down upon and found to be firmly fixed in the position described, with the ulnar nerve stretched over its posterior and outer surface. The nerve was not distinctly made out to be inflamed. It seemed unadvisable to fix the epicondyle in position, as it would have been necessary to divide all the muscles and ligaments attached to it; so it was carefully excised. The elbow-joint was, of necessity, opened. The boy made a good recovery, with the exception that a small abscess (probably not in the joint) formed and had to be drained. The ultimate functional result was very satisfactory. Sensation returned in the anæsthetic area within a few weeks; power was regained over the interossei, &c., and he was able to bend the elbow to about 50 degrees. Some six months later, although slight limitation of both flexion and extension remained, the arm was thoroughly useful, all pain on movement had disappeared, and the patient considered the arm practically as strong as the other.

A second almost identical case was operated upon by the same surgeon with an equally satisfactory result (*Brit. Med. Journal*, December 30, 1893, p. 1419):

W. E., aged ten years and six months, fell on his right elbow across a bar; he stated that he struck the outer side, but this was doubtful. The result was that the internal epicondyle was separated; an internal angular splint was applied. On examination twelve days later complete absence of the normal projection of the epicondyle was extremely marked. The detached piece of bone was displaced backwards and downwards, and was fairly fixed in its new position. The elbow had been kept at a right angle, and the patient resisted efforts to extend it further than a few degrees beyond this. As he had considerable pain during the last few days (the splint having been left off, and the imperfectly fixed fragment no doubt irritating the ulnar nerve), it seemed best to re-apply the splint for a short time longer before beginning passive motion. At the end of three weeks passive motion was instituted, but the boy would not move the elbow at all himself, and as it was very stiff, he was anæsthetised for the purpose of breaking down any adhesions that might be present. It was interesting to note that the greater part of the stiffness was purely due to tonic muscular contraction ; for whilst the range of flexion had before been limited to about 15 degrees, under the anæsthetic a range of at least 90 degrees was at once obtained without the least force. Evidently, however, some fibrous adhesions (? extra-articular) were responsible for some of the limitation, as when the arm was fully extended or flexed they were felt to give way. The epicondyle, as previously noted, was drawn downwards and fairly fixed ; its lower point must have been close to the coronoid process. A regular course of passive motion was instituted, but great difficulty was experienced in obtaining the power of flexion, any attempt at this causing pain. Mr. Hutchinson was not able to state that this patient perfectly recovered. His case made it quite clear that the chief difficulty to be met lay in the pressure on the ulnar nerve, for nothing else would account for such reflex spasm disappearing almost entirely under the anæsthetic. In another subsequent case, under the same surgeon, the cause was still more obvious ; indeed he believes that the difficulty in obtaining good movement after this accident was largely due to the fact that every attempt at flexion of the joint increased the pressure upon the nerve.

The following example of atrophy of muscles and loss of sensation of the parts supplied by the ulnar nerve is recorded by M. Fallier. The injury was complicated by dislocation backwards and outwards of the elbow, which occurred twice.

J. P., a mechanical workman, fell on October 22, 1888, on board ship, with his hands carried forwards against the bridge. There was a complete dislocation of the left elbow backwards and outwards, whilst there was considerable projection forwards and inwards of the humeral trochlea, with backward and outward displacement of the olecranon and head of the radius. The forearm was semipronate. Reduction was easily effected, and the arm kept in a sling. Three weeks later the sling was removed and passive motion commenced ; the ship's doctor then recognised a fracture of the epitrochlea and disturbances in function of the ulnar nerve, and the patient experienced acute pain in the epitrochleo-olecranon hollow. Treatment by electricity was now commenced, and by the end of a month the pain had quite disappeared and the movements of the forearm had become almost complete, there being but slight weakness of limb and loss of sensation on the inner border of the hand and little finger ; also, the little and ring fingers were contracted in a clawlike manner. The patient resumed his occupation; but two days afterwards, in lifting a large piece of wood, he experienced severe pain on the inner side of the elbow, which again became dislocated. The dislocation was readily reduced, but the patient was unable to resume work on account of the loss of power of the arm and the paralytic condition of the ulnar nerve, which increased in spite of the continued electrical treatment. On April 1 he was sent to the Maritime Hospital at Brest, under the care of Professor Guyot. A transverse fracture of the epitrochlea was immediately detected, the upper fourth remaining as a sharp projection attached to the humerus, corresponding to the upper angle of this process, and the lower three-fourths, nearly two centimetres in diameter, had been dragged downwards and inwards by the epitrochlear muscles. Between these two fragments a depression a finger's breadth in width could be felt, with the trochlear surface of the humerus at its bottom. The lower fragment was lying more than one and a half centimetres to the front and inner side of the lowest part of the inner border of the olecranon, freely movable from before backwards—especially when the forearm was semiflexed and semipronate—and also slightly movable from below upwards, when distinct crepitus was elicited. Flexion of the forearm was complete, while extension could only be carried to 140 degrees. Pronation and supination were normal. Flexion of the hand could not be effected to a right angle, and its adduction caused slight pain at the inner aspect of the elbow. The epitrochlear muscles attached to the displaced fragment were clearly atrophied, and the forearm diminished in muscular power. The inner border of the forearm, which was said by the patient to have been insensitive at the commencement, was now normal; however, there was some loss of sensation at the inner side of the wrist, and complete anæsthesia on the palmar aspect of the hand over the hypothenar eminence and all the palmar aspect of the little finger. Around this area was a zone of diminished sensibility, and the dorsal and lateral aspects of the little finger were completely insensitive. The little and ring fingers were both in a claw-shaped position (the first phalanges extended and the second flexed), and the only voluntary movements these were capable of effecting were flexion and extension of the first phalanges upon the metacarpus. The separation of the middle and index fingers from their neighbours could not be carried out, and adduction of the thumb was weak. The rest of the movements of the fingers appeared to be normal. Atrophy of the muscles of the hypothenar eminence was also very evident, as well as that of the interosseous muscles and of the adductor of the thumb. At the end of May the portion of the epitrochlea attached to the humerus appeared to be rounding off gradually, and the lower fragment became more and more fixed, with loss of the crepitus. The Faradaic current was employed without any great improvement in the paralytic condition of the ulnar nerve up to June 15. The termination of the case has not been published.

This case was rather a fracture than an epiphysial detachment, for the inner and lower borders of this process were believed to have been alone torn off, leaving the rest of the epicondyle projecting the same as on the opposite side, although it was sharp and pointed and smaller in its other dimensions.

The paralytic condition may be of considerable duration, but is very variable.

In one of Granger's cases sensibility and contractility only commenced to appear at the end of seven years, in Fallier's case at the end of eight months, and in Richet's case at the end of several months.

Atrophy of epicondylar muscles.—César mentions this *atrophy of muscles* connected with the epicondyle in three of his cases: indeed he was the first to draw attention to this condition, and discusses at length in his thesis the causes which may produce it. In all three the fragment consolidated without displacement.

M. Richet observed in two cases *rapid atrophy and paralysis of the muscles* attached to the inner condyle. One of them was the case mentioned above, in which the trochlea was also fractured and the joint became ankylosed. He attributed the paralysis to contusion of the ulnar nerve at the time of the accident. But in none of these was there any known lesion of the ulnar nerve, nor did the muscular atrophy include the flexor profundus and flexor carpi ulnaris supplied by this nerve.

Separation with dislocation of elbow-joint.—Unfortunately, it has occasionally happened that the dislocation has been immediately reduced but the detachment of the epicondyle overlooked. In Hamilton's case (boy aged fifteen) the fracture had remained unrecognised for three months, when he came under his care; and in Fallier's case it was only noticed on removing the splint after more than three weeks.

Where the fracture has been entirely overlooked, the displacement of the fragment becomes greater, the articulation more or less stiff and weak or useless, and there may even occur a fresh dislocation.

Under these complicated circumstances the swelling will diminish rapidly and complete consolidation quickly follow, provided the fracture has been recognised at the time of the accident, or immediately after reduction. If properly treated, complete recovery of the function of the arm will follow. Consolidation has taken place even after some delay in the recognition of the fracture. Yet in other instances incomplete movements of flexion and extension may be the result, as in Granger's and Richet's cases.

In a case of Langenbeck's quoted by Gurlt (Langenbeck's *Archiv für klin. Chir.* Bd. iii. 1862, S. 123, No. 3), ankylosis with partial displacement backwards of the elbow, associated with separation of internal condyle, was seen in a boy aged sixteen years. The elbow had been injured by a fall on the ground six months previously. Some improvement in the movement of the joint took place after forcible flexion under chloroform.

TREATMENT.—An attempt should be made to replace the displaced epiphysis; but this can seldom be retained perfectly in position, on account of its small size and the numerous muscles attached which tend to displace it. The elbow, as well as the wrist and fingers, should be semiflexed to relax these muscles as completely as possible, and the epicondyle replaced in its position, as

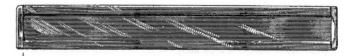

Fig. 99.—FLEXIBLE METAL SPLINT WITH FOLDED EDGES FOR SEPARATED INTERNAL EPICONDYLE OR OTHER MILDER CASES OF INJURY NEAR THE ELBOW-JOINT [1]

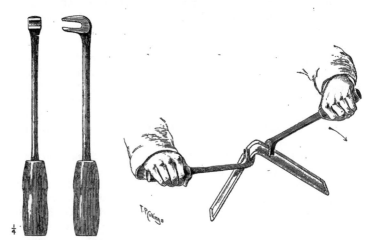

Fig. 100.—WRENCHES USED AT THE CITY ORTHOPÆDIC HOSPITAL

Fig. 101.—METHOD OF APPLYING WRENCHES FOR BENDING METAL SPLINTS OF ALL KINDS TO FIT ACCURATELY THE SHAPE OF THE JOINTS IN ANY POSITION

far as practicable, by the fingers. An anterior angular splint of wood, metal, or other material should then be put on to maintain the parts at rest, and a bandage carefully applied. Any subsequent inflammation of the joint or injured structures should be treated by

[1] This splint when bent into the required position may be applied to the front or back of the elbow, or be combined with a short wooden splint on the opposite side of the arm or forearm. Ordinary flexible band or hoop iron, one and a half to two inches wide, such as may be obtained at any ironmonger's or blacksmith's, is equally serviceable. With the use of a file, hammer, and ordinary wrenches, almost any form of splint for the upper extremity can be readily made.

appropriate evaporating lotions. Especial care should be taken that
the bandage is not applied too tightly, for fear of gangrene or of
increasing the inflammation.

The elbow should always be put up in a semiflexed position, as
that is the most useful position of the joint should ankylosis subsequently take place. Malgaigne recommended this position.

In César's thesis, in 1876, Malgaigne's view is supported, inasmuch as the trochlear muscles are flexors—viz. that the forearm
should be flexed upon the arm, and the fingers also flexed, so that
the displaced fragment may be more readily replaced.

Granger's observations in 1818 as to the difficulty of maintaining the fragment in position are very accurate. He says: "I have
purposely avoided saying one word about replacing the detached
condyle, and for these reasons: during the state of tumefaction of
the limb, no means could be adopted for confining the retracted condyle in its place beyond that of the relaxation of the muscles;
and both before the tumefaction has commenced, and after it has
subsided, all endeavours to replace the condyle, or even change the
position of it, have failed.' He discarded the use of all splints and
bandages, following his predecessors from the earliest history of
medicine.

However, a cone-shaped compress of lint or cotton-wool placed
over the epicondyle will often assist materially in maintaining this
process in position, or a horseshoe-shaped piece of wadding placed
below it, after reduction, according to Richet's plan, and kept in
position by strapping; or a moulded inside splint of poroplastic felt
or other material may be employed, with a gap over the situation of
the internal epicondyle.

Pingaud (art. 'Coude,' *Dictionnaire encyclopédique des sciences
médicales*, 1878) agrees with Granger's views that no attempt at
fixation should be made, but that the limb should be placed in a
simple trough splint, on account of the danger of articular ankylosis.

As to the rest of the treatment advocated by Granger, it is
impossible to agree with him in recommending passive movement
to be commenced from the time of the accident. He says that
'while attention ought to be given to the reduction of the inflammation by appropriate means, we ought, nevertheless, to instruct the
patient to flex and extend the arm daily from the moment the
accident occurs until the cure is completed, and without any regard
to the consolidation of the fragment.' 'The exercise of the joint in
this manner must constitute the principal occupation of the patient
for several weeks, and should it be remitted during the formation
and consolidation of the callus, much of the benefit which may
have been derived from this practice will be lost, and will with
difficulty be regained.'

Granger's views in considering that it was of no consequence
whether the internal epicondyle united or not will hardly be accepted

by the majority of British surgeons, even though in many cases the union be a fibrous one.

Another plan is for the forearm to be secured in the semiflexed and semipronate position by means of pasteboard splints secured with a roller bandage and a pad of cotton wool or tow below the epicondyle after reduction. The fingers may be also semiflexed on a pad of tow. Other surgeons prefer an outside angular splint.

M. Coulon (*Traité clinique et pratique des fractures chez les enfants*, Paris, 1861) in all his cases fixed the arm in the bent position, but in only two out of eight was the result very successful, and these he believed were of the extra-articular variety.

The following is an example of many others which have come under the author's own observation at the Miller Hospital, treated by rectangular splints with excellent results. It was one of displacement downwards and forwards of the internal epicondyle.

J. F., aged seventeen, on June 10, 1894, whilst riding a bicycle, fell, striking his elbow and side. He came to the hospital soon after, holding the injured arm with the other. On examination, flexion and extension could be carried out without much pain, but pronation and supination were much more painful. There was considerable extravasation of blood over the situation of the normal internal condyle, extending down the inner side of the forearm. The small movable fragment of the internal epicondyle could be distinctly felt below and in front of the normal situation of this epiphysis. By means of manipulation in the flexed position, the detached epiphysis could be brought into accurate apposition with the internal condyle. The elbow was therefore put up in the flexed position on a posterior rectangular splint. On the second day the splint was re-adjusted, and the bone found to have retained its excellent position. On the fifth day the swelling began to diminish, and five days later passive movements were commenced, and so successfully that on the eighteenth day active and passive movements were almost perfect. By July 7th the functions of the elbow were perfect; there was no deformity, and the epicondyle had united by osseous union.

The author thinks that a separated epicondyle is best replaced by flexion to within a right angle, and treated in this position according to the plan advocated above – at any rate, all those cases in which the displacement is downwards and forwards—so as to relax the epitrochlear muscles. The fingers and hand may also be flexed with advantage, in order to relax the flexors attached to the epiphysis.

M. Pézerat, in 1832, was one of the first to reintroduce the *extended position*, but at that time his views were severely criticised by Malgaigne and others. Recently Dr. L. C. Lane, of San Francisco, Dr. Bardenheuer, and Dr. Frere have insisted upon it.

Berthomier, in an article on the mechanism of fractures about the elbow in children (*Gazette des hôpitaux*, 1876, p. 21), also recommends treatment of separation of the epitrochlea by extension, combined or not, according to the case, with moderate traction. In fact, he thinks that all fractures about the elbow should be fixed in the extended position, with the exception of separation of the epiphysis of the epicondyle (external epicondyle).

This writer treated several cases of fracture of the internal epicondyle, and obtained much better results than by the flexed position. He says that accurate adaptation of the fragments can only be obtained by the straight position.

In three cases seen by Hamilton, a displacement of the fragment, either forwards or backwards, occurred whenever the arm was flexed, and it was necessary, therefore, to treat the case with the arm in a straight position.

A. Hanbury Frere, of Frizinghall, advocates (*Brit. Med. Journal*, January 23, 1892, p. 195) the extended position in the following words :

' I may,' he says, ' perhaps be permitted to point out that, with the arm at a right angle, it is possible for the detached fragment to move about in many directions ; in fact, we have no control over it whatever. At the same time, the ulnar nerve is almost certain to become entangled in the effusions or the callus. On the other hand, with the arm extended, we can see and feel in what direction the fragment is displaced. We can more easily manipulate it into its proper place ; and when once we have got the fragment into good position, it can easily be retained there by an immovable dressing. With the arm straight, the skin and tissues around the fragment, being somewhat tense, would of themselves almost keep it in place. At any rate, the only possible movement would be downwards from the action of muscles ; but I believe that, in elbow fracture, muscular action has not nearly so much to do with displacement of the fragments as is generally believed. If in this way the fragment is kept in proper position, there is no reason why bony union should not take place. I suppose the chief fear of downward displacement would be from the action of the pronator, and therefore, I say, dress the limb in the extended position, with the forearm prone. Berthomier dressed the arm in the extended and supine position, and I consider his results are better than any that have been obtained in the bent position ; and therefore I wish to take this opportunity of suggesting that our hospital surgeons should give the straight position a fair trial, seeing that those who have done so have found that by dressing the limb straight they can be certain of accurate coaptation. and they therefore obtain a much earlier return to usefulness ; and, above all, obviate deformity, which is so common after the present treatment of elbow fracture in the bent position.'

Guedeney relates (*Du traitement des fractures du coude chez l'enfant*, Lyon, 1893) nine cases from M. Vincent's clinic at Lyons, six of which were treated successfully by fixation in the extended position alternating with flexion, both in the supine position.

(1) Boy, aged thirteen and a half; internal epicondyle displaced backwards and a little downwards, with a depression at side of epicondyle. Fall from height on elbow. (2) Boy, aged (?). Detachment of internal epicondyle; swelling on inner side of elbow. (3) Boy, aged twelve. Detachment of the internal epicondyle, with displacement of ulna backwards and outwards and laceration of internal lateral ligament. Epicondyle felt below the trochlea movable with crepitus, but the apex of the olecranon on the outer side a little above the capitellum. (4) Boy. Fall on right elbow. Detachment of external epicondyle. (5) Boy, aged thirteen years. Swelling of elbow. Detachment of internal epicondyle. Great looseness of joint. (6) Boy, aged ten and a half. Fall on elbow. Detachment of internal epicondyle, which was movable, and laceration of external lateral ligament. (7) Boy, aged ten. Fall on left elbow (treated by flexion). (8) Boy, aged thirteen. Fall on elbow. Treated for eight days by bone-setter. Extensive ecchymosis and internal epicondyle separated from humerus for one centimetre. Deformity and loss of movement remained in spite of treatment in the extended position. (9) Girl, aged six. Two months before fell from a donkey. The detachment of the internal epicondyle was accompanied by subluxation and a deposit of vicious callus in the bend of the elbow, which limited movements. After manipulation, the elbow was kept fixed in the flexed position. Child still under treatment.

Passive motion.—This should be commenced from the seventh to tenth day and carried out daily for some weeks. If delayed later, ankylosis or articular rigidity may ensue. As already stated, Granger trusted entirely to passive motion without the use of splints.

Some modern surgeons, however, have thought not only that early passive motion is unnecessary to prevent stiffness of the joint, but that it may be actually harmful by increasing the amount of inflammation. It should always be of the gentlest kind, and so slight as not to cause pain.

At the end of a fortnight the arm may be carried in a sling without any splint.

The splints should be removed and flexion and extension carried out thoroughly every day and the patient be kept under observation for some months.

Complications.—A separated epicondyle will only render a *dislocation* difficult of reduction when it has become impacted between the articular surfaces. When this is recognised, resection of the epiphysis should be performed immediately.

The rules for reduction of dislocation in the more simple cases need not be alluded to in this place. After its accomplishment some surgeons recommend the arm to be simply placed in a sling until the swelling has subsided in a week's time, when the displaced fragment may be brought into position as advocated above. As far as children are concerned, this is not to be recommended, consolidation commencing in them within a few days ; the fragment should be replaced at once.

Articular rigidity.—The slight articular rigidity which remains will usually yield to gentle massage, exercises, and shampooing. These, with the addition of the Faradaic current, will be found beneficial in preventing the wasting of the muscles.

Should the ulnar nerve be paralysed, the continuous current must be used.

Primary operation for displacement.—It has been suggested to fix the epiphysis in good position after displacement in order to obtain osseous union. As yet this plan has not been attempted. The pin should be removed in about two weeks.

Excision of epicondyle.—When the displaced epiphysis appears to be the cause of the limitation of the movements of the elbow, or when there are symptoms of pressure upon the ulnar nerve— especially if it is believed that such is not due to recent callus and that the pressure symptoms are not likely to disappear— excision of this process should be carried out under strict antiseptic precautions on account of the probability of opening the joint.

In Mr. Hutchinson junior's case quoted above (*loc. cit. supra*) a useful arm resulted after excision of the epicondyle had been performed, although the joint was opened. He alludes to the fact that Bardenheuer and other German surgeons have excised the whole elbow for conditions similar to that which his patient presented, an operation he considers quite unjustifiable.

Richet successfully resected a portion of the epicondyle in a man for intolerable neuralgia due to pressure upon the ulnar nerve, the result of union in a bad position after a fracture of this process.

Pauly has also (*Centralblatt für Chirurgie*, 1882, p. 157) removed the epicondyle in the hope of diminishing the risk of excessive formation of callus.

In Debruyn's case of a boy, aged eighteen, the dislocation could not be reduced, the repeated attempts at reduction only rendering the peri-articular swelling greater ; gangrene ensued, which necessitated amputation, when a detachment of the internal epicondyle was discovered. This did not of itself lead to the disastrous result. Therefore, in complicated irreducible dislocations, or ankylosis from a similar cause, resection should be performed. In some complicated dislocations the internal epicondyle may be the cause of the impossibility of reduction, by being wedged between the trochlea and sigmoid cavity of the ulna, and then resection is rendered necessary.

COMPOUND SEPARATIONS.—In these very rare cases excision of the epicondyle will be necessary.

As regards fixation, surrounding the joint and limb with the usual dressings will, as in other compound injuries about the joint, give a sufficient support to the joint.

Early passive movement must be instituted as soon as the condition of the wound will permit. It may be commenced in some instances a few days after the operation.

CHAPTER VII

**SEPARATION OF THE EXTERNAL EPICONDYLE
OF THE HUMERUS**

ANATOMY.—The osseous nucleus of the external epicondyle appears about the thirteenth or fourteenth year in the cartilage of the lower epiphysis, towards the upper and outer aspect of the capitellum.

The epiphysis, when completely osseous, very rapidly joins on to the capitellar portion of the articular surface—viz. about the sixteenth year—and only a small portion of its upper part overlaps the diaphysis.

The external epicondyle, in association with the rest of the articular portions, unites with the diaphysis about the seventeenth year.

Sometimes, but rarely, this process forms a separate epiphysis, which joins on to the diaphysis as a distinct process.

This process, which is curved slightly forwards, is so small that, with the exception just mentioned, it is impossible for a traumatic separation to occur without a fracture of the cartilage or bone which unites it to the epiphysis, detaching it from the capitellum. The synovial membrane will most probably be implicated. This diastasis may therefore be said to be intra-articular.

The size of the external epicondyle is five millimetres in the fully developed condition.

Its posterior aspect can just be detected in the child, being subcutaneous and covered only by the superficial fascia and deep aponeurosis of the arm and forearm, which blend together here.

It presents neither such a pyramidal shape, rough appearance, nor anterior cavity as is met with in the adult.

At the fourteenth year its apex is nearly one and a half centimetres above the radial cup, and projects outwards and slightly downwards and forwards.

In the adult the external condyle (of English writers) is formed partly of the external epicondylar epiphysis, partly of a slight projection of the diaphysis of the humerus, and a small part of its lower end by the non-articular posterior part of the capitellar portion of the lower epiphysis.

Its upper limit is the attachment of the fibres of the extensor carpi radialis brevior and the commencement of the outer supra-condyloid ridge, but below and behind it extends beyond the capitellum, and quite posteriorly is separated from the outer lip of the trochlear groove; so that, as M. Austric puts it, it is as much post-condyloid as epi-condyloid (i.e. the condyle or capitellum).

In the adult it only projects half a centimetre beyond the level of the capitellum.

To the external epicondyle are attached the extensor communis digitorum (to its lower part), the extensor carpi radialis brevior, the extensor carpi ulnaris, and the anconeus muscles (to its back part, above the attachment of the external lateral ligament); also the external lateral ligament and supinator brevis (at extreme lower and back part).

The extensor minimi digiti is only attached to the external epicondyle by means of the fascial aponeurosis between it and the extensor carpi ulnaris and extensor communis digitorum on either side of it.

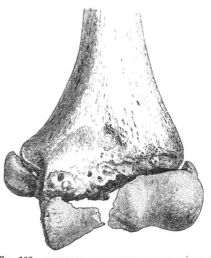

FIG. 102.—EPIPHYSES OF CAPITELLUM, TROCHLEA, INTERNAL AND EXTERNAL EPICONDYLES, AT THE END OF THE FOURTEENTH YEAR AFTER MACERATION. (ROYAL COLLEGE OF SURGEONS MUSEUM)

The fibres of the capsular ligament in front extend quite up to the base of the external epicondyle in front, beneath the fibres of the extensor carpi radialis brevior.

Relation with synovial membrane.—There is only the thickness of the fibres of the external lateral ligament and the capsular ligament (anterior ligament) separating the epiphysis from the synovial membrane below and in front. Behind, the posterior *cul-de-sac* of the synovial membrane passes over the humeral portion of the external condyle of the adult, which intervenes between the external epicondylar epiphysis and the outer lip of the trochlea. In the child, however, the synovial membrane on this aspect is at a considerable distance from the epiphysis.

Of the synovial bursæ in relation with the external epicondyle, those found in the adult are enumerated by M. Poirier, and quoted by M. Gabriel Austric (Thèse de Paris, 1889, No. 13, *Les fractures expérimentales de l'épicondyle*) as follows:

1. Subcutaneous bursa.—Very rare, but may be developed pathologically from pressure.

2. Bursa beneath the anconeus muscle, often (always, according to Henle) communicating with the joint, was found in one out of three or four cases.

3. Bursa of the extensors of the hand, between the supinator brevis and radial head and the superficial extensors covering them. It was discovered in about fifty per cent. of cases, and occurred more often on the right than on the left side. It never communicates with the joint, but may be divided into two compartments.

These bursæ are important, inasmuch as they may complicate separations of this epiphysis.

Effusions into the third or last bursa mentioned might be detected by pronating and supinating the forearm whilst the hand is placed over the situation of the bursa—viz. the radial head.

AGE.—True separation of the osseous epiphysis of the external condyle can only occur from the thirteenth to about the seventeenth year. Below this age this process may be detached by a fracture of the cartilaginous tissue uniting it with the capitellar portion of the lower epiphysis of the humerus.

The three or four pathological specimens alluded to below were from the dissecting room, and can throw no light upon the question of age.

Out of the six clinical cases, in one the age is not given, one was aged fourteen years, one eleven and a half, two were ten, and one three and a half.

ETIOLOGY. Indirect violence.—Forcible adduction of the arm is believed to be the most common manner of violence indirectly to the epicondyle.

M. Berthomier has experimentally produced a detachment of the external epicondyle by torsion combined with traction of the forearm, and also by violent flexion inwards, showing the great strength of the external lateral ligament.

M. Barros has also produced a fracture of the lower part of the external epicondyle still attached to the external lateral ligament, and combined with dislocation of the radius outwards, in a child aged fourteen, by means of violence applied to the palm of the hand, whilst the arm was in a straight position.

Direct violence.—It has been stated that direct violence is almost always the cause of detachment of the external epicondyle. This is probably true in the case of the adult; but in children, the external epicondyle being so little developed before the age of eight or ten years, it is impossible that direct violence can come into play—at any rate, from its posterior aspect.

In 1842 M. Huguier, in a thesis on the diagnosis of diseases about the elbow-joint, gave special attention to fractures of the epitrochlea and epicondyle, and he thought that such were produced by a cause which acted directly or solely on these two processes. He believed that mobility was easier to obtain in these than in fractures of the trochlea or capitellum, because in them the ulna or radius is not compelled to be moved. The smallness of the fracture he imagined would very likely lead to an error in diagnosis, were it not for the fact that the articulation is not deformed, and its movements free and painless comparatively to those fractures which involve the joint.

In none of Berthomier's experiments at the elbow-joint in children by direct violence was he able to produce a fracture of the external epicondyle alone ; yet he does not deny either the possibility or the frequency of such an injury.

MM. Charvot and Franchet ('Note clinique sur les Fractures de l'Épicondyle,' *Archives de Médecine et de Pharmacie militaires,* Nov. 1888, p. 334), in relating two cases in adults, think that the essential condition for the production of the fracture (which occurred in the person of one of them) was one of semiflexion of the forearm during a fall, for in this position the external epicondyle is sub-cutaneous and uncovered by the supinator longus and extensor carpi radialis longior. The external epicondyle is caught and broken off backwards and displaced downwards by the action of the extensor muscles of the forearm inserted into it.

In the second case the fractured epicondyle was displaced down-wards and forwards, and complicated a dislocation of the bones of the forearm backwards, and reduction could not be effected. It was thought to be due to indirect violence (*par arrachement*).

But M. Austric thinks that, on anatomical grounds, this is hardly possible from the traction alone of the external lateral ligament, and certainly not from muscular action in adults, while muscular action alone cannot displace the fragment—at any rate, if it is only the apex which is detached, only a few tendinous fibres being attached to it.

PATHOLOGICAL ANATOMY.—Separation of the external epi-condylar epiphysis is a very much rarer form of injury than separation of the internal epicondyle.

Traumatic separation of the external epicondyle can only be possible before the sixteenth year.

Gurlt thinks that this injury is possible up to the eighteenth or twentieth year, and that it lies entirely outside the articulation.

Malgaigne, in his treatise in 1847, denied the existence of these lesions in adults : ' Quelques écrivains modernes ont parlé d'une fracture qui ne pénétrerait pas dans l'articulation et qui n'affecte-rait que l'épicondyle ; mais personne jusqu'à présent n'en a cité d'exemple.'

Marjolin recognised fractures of the external epicondyle, but Denucé, in the *Nouv. Dictionnaire de Médecine et de Chirurgie pra-tiques,* 1868, classified them under those of the lower end of the humerus, and Pingaud with those of the capitellum and external condyle.

The latter thought that the thickening of the humerus met with in these cases indicates that the original injury has been more extensive. He had never met with a detachment of the epicondyle alone.

M. Berthomier (Thèse de Paris, 1875), in eighty experiments on the elbows of children, never produced a fracture of the external epicondyle alone ; but in those cases where he only perceived abnormal mobility of the external epicondyle after simulating a fall upon the elbow, and where the examination of the part was neces- sarily more easy than in the living subject, he always found a transverse fracture passing more or less exactly through the diaphyso- epiphysial line.

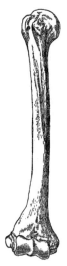

Sir Astley Cooper was the first, in 1823 (*Treatise on Fractures and Dis- locations*, London 1823), to allude to this class of injury.

In the case figured by Sir Astley Cooper the injury doubtless occurred in an adult. It was taken from a specimen in St. Thomas's Hospital, and is described by him as follows : 'The preparation is a specimen of the transverse fracture of the extremity of the condyle [Sir A. Cooper com- bines under this term the external epicondyle and the capitellum] within the capsular ligament, and not the least attempt at ossific union can be detected.' He continues : 'It is obvious, therefore, that this principle of ligamentous union extends to all detached portions within a capsular ligament, the vitality of the bone being supported merely by the ligament within the joint.'

FIG. 103.—FRACTURE OF THE EXTER- NAL EPICONDYLE AND A SMALL PART OF CAPITELLUM. (ST. THOMAS'S HOSPITAL MUSEUM. SIR ASTLEY COOPER'S 'FRACTURES AND DISLOCA- TIONS ')

According to the figure here reproduced (fig. 103), the external outer limit of the capitellum appears to have been involved. Whether this was the extent of the original injury it is difficult to say.

There is no authentic specimen of separation of the external epi- condyle alone in any of the London hospital museums.

Hamilton figures (*loc. cit. supra*, fig. 87) a supposed fracture of the entire external epicondyle—a specimen sent to him by Dr. E. Zuckerkandl, of Vienna. 'It was found in the dissecting room, and is unaccompanied with any clinical history ; but it is evidently from a person near the twentieth year of life. There is, indeed, an apparent absence of a portion of the external epicondyle, and there are two ossicula, situated in the external lateral ligament, with smooth, slightly bossellated surfaces. Dr. Zuckerkandl explains the presence of two by supposing it was an exceptional process of development; but it is more difficult to explain how the epiphysis should have found its way into the lower or distal portion of the external lateral ligament, where he correctly states that it is situated. The supposed original seat is covered in by perfectly formed lamellated tissue, and underneath the situation in which the ossicula are found is a deep fossa fitted exactly to receive them.'

The specimen is undoubtedly one of fracture involving the diaphysis, from the appearance of the drawing which Hamilton gives.

The case is described and figured by Dr. Zuckerkandl (*Allgemeine Wiener medizinische Zeitung*, Feb. 1878), and considered by him as a real epiphysiary fracture or separation in an adult.

Gurlt also figures (*Handbuch der Lehre der Knochenbrüchen*, 1860, II. Theil, S. 798) another similar specimen, in the Museum of Giessen, in which the fracture—an old, consolidated one—is almost strictly limited to the external epicondyle. The fracture being close up to the capitellum, indicates clearly that the articulation must have been involved. He remarks that the existence of this injury had always hitherto been doubted, and describes another specimen at Berlin. The detached epicondyle in this, like the other specimen, had united with considerable downward displacement.

Bardeleben has also verified the existence of this fracture.

McBurney (Stimson, *Practical Treatise on Fractures*, p. 395) states that 'he had found in the dissecting room isolated pieces of bone resembling detached epicondyles, and existing symmetrically at both elbows.'

This rendered very unlikely the idea that they were the result of injury.

Hamilton says: 'It is not difficult to admit, however, the possibility of a detachment of the epiphysial portion prior to its consolidation with the shaft of the humerus; and, indeed, the occurrence of such an accident would seem quite probable, yet we lack any absolutely conclusive evidence that it has ever taken place.'

He distinctly separates in this way disjunction of the external epicondylar epiphysis from fracture of the external condyle (of English anatomists) which involves the diaphysis of the humerus forming part of this process in the adult. He thinks the lesion quite impossible as a simple uncomplicated fracture ' unless the line of fracture includes a portion of the joint, and in that case it is to be designated as a fracture of the condyle (capitellum) and not of the epicondyle (external condyle). At least I may say that no satisfactory clinical example or anatomical specimen has ever been presented.'

However, one of the two cases described by Bardenheuer

(*Deutsche Chirurgie*, von Billroth und Lücke, 1888) proves conclusively that this form of fracture may occur in the adult. Direct inspection of the fracture (in a woman aged sixty-eight) proved that it was extra-capsular and appeared as if detached from the capitellum by a gouge.

M. Gabriel Austric (*Les fractures expérimentales de l'épicondyle étudiées chez l'enfant et chez l'adulte*, Thèse de Paris, 1889) in some experiments found that in the bodies of adults a fracture of this process by direct violence may be confined to it or combined with a fracture of the capitellum or outer edge or anterior aspect of the humerus; but even in the latter the greater part always belonged to the external condyle. In some instances the articular edge of the outer aspect of the capitellum was scarcely involved for a quarter of a centimetre, which agrees with Sir Astley Cooper's and Gurlt's cases.

In similar experiments on seven children (from four to fourteen and a half years) application of direct force in the same way from without inwards produced a similar division of the fractures into simple separation of this process (cartilaginous or bony) or combined with a fracture of parts of the humerus similar to those in the adult. The bony particles in children were very frequently attached to the lower aspect of the detached epiphysis. In one case in a child fourteen and a half years the epiphysial fragment was split into two pieces. More commonly he found that scales or small portions of the diaphysis adhered to the epicondylar fragment, and moreover he states that this fracture (from his experiments) is only intra-articular when it involves the capitellum, as in the adult.

Injury to the joint.—Although the synovial membrane extends almost up to the external epicondyle, it is probable that in a number of cases the joint may escape injury, and the separation remain an extra-articular one.

No direct proof of injury to the joint has yet been furnished in the case of pure separation of the external epicondyle.

SYMPTOMS.—Very little has been written upon fracture of the external epicondyle; indeed, Hamilton did not think it possible to diagnose the existence of a fracture of the external epicondyle.

Coulon, who was the first to clinically study fracture of the external epicondyle (*Thèse sur les fractures du coude chez les enfants*, 1861), quotes Marjolin as having observed several cases (one or more each year) all produced by direct injury, and mentions the following case of Marjolin's, in which a boy aged three and a half years fell from a chair to the pavement. The very small broken piece of the external epicondyle was distinctly felt, and could be moved by seizing it between the finger and thumb. There was no displacement of the fragments, but great swelling of the whole elbow with ecchymosis on the outer side. The arm was simply kept on a pillow, and compresses soaked in arnica applied; consolidation had taken place by the twentieth day, and all movements of the elbow joint were perfect when the patient left the hospital three weeks later. The external epicondyle was somewhat bulky, more rounded, and less prominent than that of the opposite side.

According to Coulon, abnormal mobility and crepitus are the chief signs to be relied upon.

Absence of articular rigidity after consolidation also confirmed the diagnosis in Coulon's case.

Small size of fragment.—It is possible where there is little displacement or swelling that this small nodule may be seized between the finger and thumb, and moved from before backwards.

Absence of great articular pain on movement.—The pain is mostly about the external epicondylar region on active or passive movement.

Considerable swelling of the postero-external aspect of the elbow may be so extensive as to render a diagnosis impossible for the first few days.

Crepitus will be of the usual soft character.

Forearm semiflexed and slightly pronated, and the hand perhaps held in front of the chest.

Voluntary movements will be almost entirely absent.

Passive supination will be very painful, while pronation is free; but flexion and (especially) extension somewhat limited on account of the pain experienced on the outer side of the elbow.

Displacement will probably not be so great as in the adult, from the thickness of the periosteum attaching the epiphysis to the diaphysis.

The fragment may not be felt for some eight days or more until the swelling has disappeared. It is possible in some cases that a *depression* may be felt at the normal prominence of the external epicondyle.

Displacement of the epiphysis may be *inwards and forwards,* as in M. Marchand's case; *outwards and backwards,* or *downwards and outwards,* as in Zuckerkandl's case, the fragment being lodged in the external lateral ligament, or even displaced still lower below the cup of the radius, or simply *downwards,* as in Gurlt's case. In one of M. Lannelongue's and Coudray's cases the most prominent symptoms were some thickening about the external epicondyle and some displacement downwards of this process.

A similar case was communicated to M. Austric by M. Coudray (*loc. cit. supra*) of a boy, aged ten years, who had fallen (May 1889) on to his left elbow while alighting from a carriage. No diagnosis was made at the time. When seen by M. Coudray, fifteen days after the accident, the swelling of the elbow had completely disappeared, but pain was still present and the forearm semiflexed; in this position, measuring at the posterior part of the elbow, the distance from the internal epicondyle to the external epicondyle on the left side was fully eight centimetres, while on the right side it was only from six and a quarter to six and a half centimetres.

The antero-posterior width of the external epicondyle, which was placed a little lower than its normal position, was 0·03 on the left and only 0·02 centimetre on the right.

The left olecranon appeared to be brought a little inwards, in consequence perhaps of a slight separation of the bones of the forearm. Flexion was limited to a right angle, and extension was not permitted beyond 45°. Pronation and supination were fairly normal. Forcible movement was the treatment adopted, but the subsequent history of the case was not recorded.

Articular effusion was observed after two hours in the following case under M. Lannelongue's care (quoted by Austric).

A girl, aged eleven and a half years, whilst wrestling with a little boy (April 1889), fell on to the palm of her left hand stretched forwards, and at the same time the boy fell against the limb supporting her in this position. She fell down and experienced acute pain in the elbow and upper part of the forearm, which she kept semiflexed and supported in front of the body. Two hours afterwards it was found there was swelling on the whole of the outer side of the elbow without any ecchymosis. The external epicondyle was very painful, increased in bulk, and somewhat lower than usual, but there was no abnormal mobility or crepitation. There was also a little effusion into the elbow-joint. The rest of the humerus and the bones of the forearm were normal. Flexion could not be effected beyond a right angle, and *extension was quite impossible*, whereas pronation and supination were almost natural. The limb was placed in the semiflexed position in a sling, with a layer of cotton wool and bandage round the elbow. The next day active movements were commenced and were carried out twice a day for the four following days, when massage was used. A month later a displacement downwards of the epicondyle for half to three-quarters of a centimetre was noted, and an enlargement of nearly a centimetre. The movements of the elbow were absolutely normal, and the functions of the limb and muscles were perfect when seen later.

DETACHMENT WITHOUT DISPLACEMENT.—Displacement may not occur if the periosteum remains uninjured, as in Sir Astley Cooper's and M. Marchand's cases.

Swelling about the epicondyle and *mobility of fragment*, with the joint slightly *movable* in a lateral direction, may be the only signs that will assist in making a diagnosis.

COMPLICATIONS. **Dislocation.**—In many cases separation of the external epicondyle will be complicated with a dislocation of the elbow, as has been frequently found in adults (backwards or laterally). Such a complication of dislocation of the elbow gives rise to great obscurity of diagnosis as well as to great difficulty of reduction.

Subluxation of the elbow outwards.—Some surgeons affirm that pure luxation of the elbow cannot take place without fracture of the epicondyle. This is questionable, although no doubt in lateral dislocation fracture of the external epicondyle exists, though un-recognised.

Guedeney records, in his collection of cases, the following case of fracture of the external epicondyle complicated with a dislocation backwards of the elbow.

A boy (J. G.) (age not stated), while climbing on a weaving frame, fell (July 1890) to the ground on to his left elbow. Although there was marked swelling and bruising about the elbow, the deformity was very perceptible. The humerus projected in a marked manner; the ulna was very prominent behind, and the radial cup free. As there was no crepitus, simple dislocation backwards was diagnosed. Reduction being effected under an anæsthetic, the joint was put up in the flexed position in a plaster-trough splint. On August 12 osseous crepitus was perceived about the epicondyle, and the limb put up again in extension. On September 12 cure is said to have occurred, and the epicondyle completely united. When seen on February 11, 1893, the movements of the elbow were perfectly recovered, extension being even a little exaggerated. There was no shortening of the limb, but the epicondyle and olecranon still projected very much. Pronation and supination were normal, and there was no loss of muscular power. Whilst in the hospital the patient had some trophic changes—shedding of the nails and insensibility of the fingers—which had now completely disappeared.

Dislocation of the radius.—Guedeney in his thesis (*Du traitement des fractures du coude chez l'enfant, &c.*, Lyon, 1893) relates a case of fracture of the external epicondyle with dislocation of the radius, diagnosed as such by M. Vincent.

A boy (P.), aged two years, was admitted April 25, 1885. About a month previously he had fallen a distance about his own height, and had been treated by a bone-setter unsuccessfully. Under an anæsthetic an oblique fracture of the epicondyle was made out with clear crepitus and displacement; this displacement was accompanied by dislocation of the radial head. The dislocation was reduced, the fragments placed in apposition, and the arm fixed in the extended position. There was neither bruising nor swelling. On May 5 fresh dressings were applied, the arm being still in extension. On May 21 the dressing was removed, and the fracture found to be well con-solidated. Child discharged cured.

It is probable that in this case the epicondyle was detached with a slight portion of the capitellum, and displaced with the radius.

The difficulties of diagnosis are very great in consequence of the small projection which this epiphysis presents in children. Berthomier states that separation of the external epicondyle may sometimes, in very young children, be mistaken for subluxation of the head of the radius.

PROGNOSIS.—The epiphyses will unite by fibrous tissue if dis-placed; probably by bone where there is no displacement. Coulon thinks the prognosis good, and that patients should get well in fifteen to thirty days. In a case treated by M. Coudray the child regained the complete function of its arm a month after the accident.

Supination may be limited for some time and give rise to some hindrance to free movements from peri-articular inflammation, or even from some localised inflammation of the radio-humeral articulations. But it was entirely absent in Coulon's case.

The small triangular fragment may be felt in its abnormal position under the skin; but, as the articulation is not usually opened, recovery with free movement of the elbow should result.

When dislocation or other lesion complicates the separation of the epicondyle, the ultimate condition of the elbow appears to be a more serious matter.

In M. Lannelongue's second case (quoted by Austric), which he saw seven months after the accident, all movements of extension were absolutely impossible, and flexion and supination were very limited, but pronation was nearly normal.

A boy, aged fourteen years, fell from a trapeze (October 1889) with his left upper extremity beneath him, receiving the whole weight of the body. A dislocation was diagnosed, and attempts at reduction made. The swelling increased during the following days, and a month later, on removing the sling supporting the elbow, it was found to be almost impossible to effect any movement of extension and flexion. Thirty-five days after the accident massage and forcible movements were attempted, for there was now considerable stiffness about the elbow-joint. Seven months after the accident (April 1890) M. Lannelongue saw the case; the wasting of the left upper extremity was then very marked, the muscles of the forearm, arm, and shoulder being in an atrophied condition. The forearm was semiflexed, and the elbow held in a sling in consequence of the loss of function of the limb. The rigidity of the articulation was so considerable that extension was quite impossible, and flexion could only be carried out up to a right angle. Supination was very limited, and pronation was the only movement which was fairly extensive. The deformity consisted especially in a widening of the elbow, and the antero-posterior diameter of the epicondyloid projection was on the left 0·03 and on the right only 0·02 centimetre. Forcible movement gradually increased, and electricity and massage improved the condition considerably, so that at the end of fifteen days active flexion passed beyond a right angle, and extension was almost complete. Pronation and supination were also nearly normal and accomplished without pain. When the patient was seen later the condition of the limb was perfect.

M. Marchand records (Th. de Lartet, 1889 ; M. Marchand, quoted by Austric, *loc. cit. supra*) a case of fracture of the external epicondyle in which flexion of the arm was limited by an osseous mass.

A boy (A. R.), aged ten years, had fallen (September 1887) on his elbow from a height of two metres. The doctor who saw the case applied traction to the arm. Fifteen days after the accident the forearm was found fixed in a position midway between semiflexion and complete extension, and the hand semi-pronated. Pronation and supination of the limb were painful; all the osseous prominences about the elbow were in their normal relations, with the one exception of the external epicondyle, which was displaced a little forwards, thickened, and painful on pressure. A very distinct depression was found in the epicondyle's normal position. The diagnosis of detachment of the prominence of the external epicondyle was confirmed under chloroform when the elbow was forcibly flexed and extended, with sensation of cartilaginous crepitus. During flexion the radial head could now pass freely in front of the osseous mass, which before was not possible, as it kept the radial head back. The arm was put up in an immovable apparatus, the forearm being flexed to an acute angle. This was removed after fifteen days; the movements, though fairly free, were very painful. Eight days after, some muscular contraction having occurred, an anæsthetic was again administered, and the elbow freely moved. Continual movement and massage were recommended.

Muscular malnutrition and atrophy, as in M. Lannelongue's case, may involve all the upper extremity. They should therefore be carefully guarded against by appropriate treatment.

TREATMENT.—As in the corresponding fracture of the internal epicondyle, the fragment should be replaced in its normal position, and a horseshoe-shaped pad of lint or other soft material, as recommended first by M. Richet, placed and fixed below it, while the elbow should be fixed by an internal lateral splint in the semiflexed position.

The **extended position** for three or four weeks is recommended by Dr. L. C. Lane.

Seven cases are said by Guedeney to have been diagnosed in M. Vincent's clinic at Lyons as fracture or detachment of the external epicondyle, and treated by fixation in the extended position. An eighth case in a boy, one and a half years old, although placed under this form of injury, appears to have been clearly accompanied by a fracture in the capitellum as well; indeed, considering the age of the patients recorded—viz. below eight years—the small size of the cartilaginous nodule representing the epiphysial process in later childhood, and its intimate connection with the rest of the cartilaginous lower end of the humerus at this age, all render it extremely unlikely that these cases were instances of this rare form of injury—viz. simple detachment or fracture of the external epicondyle. The ages were respectively: (1) three and a half years; (2) not stated; (3) five years; (4) not stated; (5) eight years; (6) not stated; (7) six and a half years.

The presence of *dislocation* complicating this separation is of grave importance, for if the fragment be displaced forwards towards the bend of the elbow, reduction of the dislocation and flexion of the elbow will be rendered so much more difficult.

This difficulty of flexion from the abnormal position of the external epicondyle was noted in M. Marchand's case.

Primary resection.—Should the freedom of movement of the joint be greatly interfered with on account of some dislocation accompanying it, or on account of the great displacement of the epicondyle, the epiphysis should be resected and the parts replaced in their normal position under strict antiseptic precautions. In *compound separations* immediate resection of the epiphysis should be performed. The epiphysis will probably be found in one or more

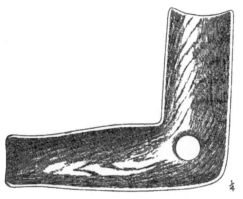

Fig. 104.—INTERNAL RECTANGULAR SPLINT HOLLOWED FOR RIGHT ELBOW

pieces; or the small epiphysis, under aseptic measures, may be fixed to the diaphysis by means of a steel pin driven through it into the latter.

Passive movement should be commenced very early—on the seventh or tenth day. In M. Lannelongue's patient movement of the elbow was commenced on the day after the accident.

Massage and electricity, and forcible movement gradually increased will tend to counteract any tendency to muscular atrophy.

Should the formation of callus prevent complete flexion of the joint, the ankylosis must be carefully broken down and the joint moved with caution.

Operative treatment of faulty union.—Brun-Bourgeret, in a recent thesis (Thèse de Bordeaux, 1892), recommends linear osteotomy as a treatment for vicious consolidation of fractures of the external epicondyle.

CHAPTER VIII

SEPARATION OF THE TROCHLEA WITH INTERNAL EPICONDYLE (EPICONDYLO-TROCHLEAR SEPARATION) OF THE HUMERUS

AND

SEPARATION OF THE TROCHLEA WITH FRACTURE OF INTERNAL CONDYLE (CONDYLO-TROCHLEAR FRACTURE) OF THE HUMERUS

A TRUE separation of the trochlear and internal epicondylar epiphyses of the humerus in one piece can only take place before the period at which the internal epicondyle becomes a distinct epiphysis.

The line of separation will pass through the base of the internal epicondyle, obliquely downwards and outwards, through the lower limit of the coronoid and olecranon fossæ to the middle of the trochlear articular surface.

Such a separation is rare compared with *separation of the trochlear portion, combined with fracture of the internal condyle.* In this case it is a partial separation accompanied by intra-articular fracture and fracture of the diaphysial portion of the internal condyle.

ETIOLOGY.—Direct blows upon the elbow are the most frequent cause.

It is quite possible that **muscular violence**, which can tear off the internal epicondyle, may also detach the trochlear epiphysis with it, by means of the leverage of the upper end of the ulna.

Indirect violence is often noted, from falls upon the hand or elbow.

In the typical 'oblique internal trochlear fracture,' indirect violence is almost invariably the cause.

In a fall upon the elbow the posterior aspect of the upper end of the ulna strikes the ground, the violence being transmitted to the bottom of the trochlear surface by the articular convex ridge of the sigmoid cavity, which acts as a wedge, the internal lateral ligament also playing an important part through its attachment to the internal condyle.

The violence, again, may act in the long axis of the ulna, thereby displacing the trochlear fragment upwards or upwards and backwards.

Finally, the violence acting upon the ulna may be more lateral, acting upon its outer or inner side. If in the latter direction, the forearm is thrust towards the ulnar side; the powerful internal lateral ligament will cause detachment of the condylo-trochlear fragment, which is thus displaced downwards, and probably accompanied by a complete or partial dislocation of the bones of the forearm described below.

AGE.—Among eight clinical cases of condylo- and epicondylo-trochlear fracture in children, one was stated to be at twelve years of age, one at eleven, two at ten years, one at nine, one at four, and in two cases the age was not stated.

PATHOLOGICAL ANATOMY.—There is no authentic specimen of separation of the epicondylo-trochlear epiphyses.

The lesion would correspond exactly to the simultaneous fracture of the internal condyle and inner half of the trochlea, which is not infrequently met with in adults. Such cases have been recorded by Sir Astley Cooper, Th. Markoe, Hugo Senftleben, Gurlt, Ch. Bell, Desault, Malgaigne, and Gueneau de Mussy in 1837, and specimens are to be seen in several museums, e.g. the Museum of the Edinburgh University and Musée Dupuytren.

Sir A. Cooper adds in his description that these fractures were especially frequent in children. Malgaigne, however, thought they were exceedingly rare.

Out of eight cases observed by Markoe and Senftleben, five were in children—one at ten, another at eleven, another at fourteen, and two at sixteen years of age, and all in male subjects.

The 'fracture trochléenne oblique interne' of Denucé, in which the inner half of the trochlear articular surface and more or less

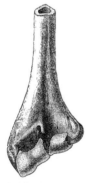

of the internal condyle of the humerus are detached in one piece, crosses the outer portion of the olecranon fossa, and terminates on the outer side of the trochlear groove. So that in the adult a considerable portion of the diaphysis is always detached, and the line of fracture may even traverse the coronoid and olecranon fossæ.

The authors, Markoe, Senftleben, and Astley Cooper, have noted *displacement backwards* of the fragment in these cases, and with it the ulna and radius.

The ulna is firmly bound to the epiphysial fragment in its normal relation especially by means of the internal lateral ligament, and the radius will also accompany the ulna if the orbicular

FIG. 105.—FRACTURE OF THE INTERNAL CONDYLE AND TROCHLEA; DISPLACEMENT UPWARDS OF FRAGMENT. BRESLAU MUSEUM. (AFTER GURLT)

ligament be not torn across; the ulna, with the forearm, consequently being displaced with this fragment. So that it is more than probable that a dislocation either backwards or backwards and inwards will be immediately diagnosed, and the fracture or separation overlooked.

A condylo-trochlear fracture is figured by Gurlt, from the Anatomical Museum of Breslau. The fractured part, composed of the internal condyle and a portion of the trochlear surface of the humerus, has been displaced *upwards*, and united in this position, so that the lower end of the humerus is very oblique (see fig. 105).

SYMPTOMS.—The symptoms of separation of the epicondylo-trochlear epiphyses are almost identical with those of fracture of the internal condyle traversing the diaphysis from above the base of this process, obliquely downwards and outwards through the olecranon and coronoid fossæ to the groove of the trochlea. The latter is a very common accident in children.

Out of twenty cases of this fracture seen by Hamilton, only two were after the eighteenth year of life. Malgaigne, Sir Astley Cooper, South, Gurlt, R. Adams, have all recorded cases in children.

Crepitus is of the characteristic muffled character when the separation is pure, but is more likely to be of a rougher character if the separation traverses any part of the diaphysis.

It may be felt either on grasping the portions of the lower end of the humerus on either side and imparting some lateral motion, or on grasping the internal condyle and trochlea with one hand and flexing and extending the forearm with the other.

Mobility of the internal condyle, especially in the antero-posterior direction, may be detected when this process is grasped between the finger and thumb whilst the rest of the elbow is fixed. It can also be felt on flexion and extension of the elbow-joint.

If there is displacement of either or both bones of the forearm, unnatural mobility will be felt on reduction; in this case the displacement will be found to be readily reproduced.

Displacement.—There may be little or no deformity, from the fragment being held in position by the periosteum and other ligamentous structures.

The precise appearance of the elbow will be determined by the position of the displaced fragment, so that the forearm may be adducted or abducted, pronated or supinated.

Upwards and backwards, and perhaps a little inwards, will be the usual form of displacement.

It will be recognised by carefully ascertaining the relations of the internal epicondyle with the olecranon and with the external epicondyle, as compared with the uninjured side. This relationship should be determined both before and after reduction of the displacement.

It should be also remembered that, normally, in full extension of the elbow, a line joining the two epicondyles behind will cross the tip of the olecranon.

Increase of breadth between the epicondyles of the humerus.—This increase in the transverse diameter of the lower end of the humerus may be masked, to a great extent, by the swelling and ecchymosis present.

Prominence of ulna behind when the forearm is extended, so that it appears dislocated, the ulna projecting backwards with the fractured portion of the humerus, and *the relation between the olecranon and the internal epicondyle being altered* as compared with the opposite side. The ulna is restored to its normal position on again flexing the forearm. The distance is widened or shortened according to the form and degree of displacement.

Projection of lower end of humerus in front, upon the anterior aspect of the elbow-joint, on extreme extension.

Forearm deflected to ulnar side, in extreme extension, when the fragment has been displaced upwards.

The deformity is immediately reproduced when the parts are left to themselves after reduction.

The displacement may be *downwards*, from indirect violence, or even directly *forwards*.

Swelling.—The amount of extravasated blood in the surrounding tissue and the distension of the joint may be so excessive as to render an accurate diagnosis impossible until these have subsided.

COMPLICATIONS.—**Dislocations of elbow**, either backwards or backwards and inwards, are frequent complications. If the trochlea and internal condyle be displaced, the ulna at any rate will follow the fragment; but it may occasionally happen that both bones of the forearm will be displaced.

Dislocation of radius backwards, in association with the analogous fracture in adults, has been especially noted by Gurlt (*Handbuch der Lehre von den Knochenbrüchen*, 1863, S. 822), Markoe, Hamilton, and others, and presents a most serious complication. Dr. Markoe, indeed, believes that dislocation of the radius seldom or never occurs without a fracture of the internal condyle (i.e. internal condyle with trochlea). He claims to have been the first, in 1855, to have directed attention to the importance of this complication.

In this complication the radius, ulna, and internal condylar fragment of the humerus preserve their normal relation to one another.

It will closely resemble simple dislocation of both bones backwards, with this difference—that the internal epicondyle preserves its normal relation with the olecranon, and that mobility of the fragment is present, accompanied by crepitus; but in both the head of the radius will be felt behind and below the external epicondyle.

The reduction in this form of separation with dislocation of the radius will be easily effected, but is immediately reproduced.

To these signs Markoe (*New York Medical Record*, 1880, vol. xviii. p. 119, 'On Fracture of the Internal Condyle of the

Humerus, with Dislocation of the Head of the Radius') adds the following, viz. that on the anterior aspect of the joint a somewhat sharp protuberance can be felt, which is the end of the humerus from which the internal condyle has been detached.

This surgeon gives the following case from his notebook :

' M. L., aged ten, was admitted to the New York Hospital, October 11, 1859. Five days before he had fallen from a horse, striking his left side, with his arm twisted behind him. Great swelling and ecchymosis took place immediately, so that a thorough examination could not be made. On the 17th the swelling had so far subsided as to give us a chance to examine the fracture. The internal condyle and the olecranon were in proper relation to one another, while the head of the radius had left the external condyle and was easily felt rotating behind and to the outside of it. The whole aspect of the elbow was that of dislocation backwards, the end of the olecranon projecting about an inch backwards, and the end of the humerus making a rounded projection on the anterior aspect of the joint. The parts were so easily movable that it could further be distinctly made out that a considerable fragment of the internal condyle, broken from the shaft of the bone, remained attached to the olecranon and moved with it. The whole displacement could be easily reduced and the deformity removed, while on letting go the limb it was immediately reproduced. Dr. Van Buren saw the case, and agreed in the diagnosis of fracture of the internal condyle, involving so much of the basis of support of the olecranon as to allow of its displacement backwards to a sufficient extent to permit the head of the radius to be also backwards, as in ordinary luxation. The displacement was reduced, and the arm placed at an angle less than a right angle, and so retained by an angular tin splint, a firm pad being placed on the prominent end of the humerus to keep it in place. On the 30th the apparatus was removed, and it was reported that union of the detached fragment was firm and the joint in good shape. The patient was discharged the following day.'

Stripping of periosteum from the diaphysis gives rise to great swelling around and above the joint.

Acute synovitis, more or less intense, is inevitable from the separation involving the articular surface.

Injury to the ulnar nerve.—The ulnar nerve may be pressed upon and injured by displacement of the fragment, giving rise to paralysis or impaired motion on the inner side of the forearm and hand, or to loss of sensation in the same parts, or pain or numbness of the little finger.

Senftleben once observed paralytic symptoms from injury to the ulnar nerve follow violent attempts to place the limb in the flexed position. They, however, gradually disappeared.

Sir Astley Cooper saw a girl who, by a fall upon her elbow, had fractured the olecranon, and also broken the internal condyle (i.e.

trochlea and internal condyle) of the humerus, the point of the broken bone having penetrated the skin; the cubital nerve had also been injured, for the little finger and half the ring finger were benumbed. Cooper says : 'The cause of this accident is a fall upon the point of the elbow. It usually occurs in youth before the epiphysis is completely ossified; although I have seen it, but less frequently, in old age. It is often mistaken for dislocation.'

The precise lesion in this instance is obscure, for Packard places it under the heading of fracture of the epitrochlea; while Sir Astley Cooper places it under fracture of the internal condyle (i.e. epicondyle and trochlea), and presents a diagram of the lesion.

Rupture of brachial artery.—A case of oblique fracture through the lower epiphysis of the left humerus into the elbow-joint (involving the internal condyle, trochlea, and capitellum), with rupture of the brachial artery, is given by Mr. George Lawson (*Lancet*, December 1, 1894, p. 1277). At first no fracture was detected; but at the end of a fortnight, when the swelling from the extravasated blood began to subside, the deformity about the elbow became manifest, and the arm was found shortened three quarters of an inch, measuring from the coracoid process to the olecranon, and a shortening, though to a less extent, from the coracoid to the internal condyle; but none was discovered from the coracoid process to the external condyle. Flexion and extension were very considerably impaired, whilst pronation and supination were not interfered with. At the end of seven weeks flexion could be carried out to a right angle, whilst extension was nearly perfect. The swelling from the ruptured vessel had then completely subsided.

DIAGNOSIS. Fracture of the coronoid process of the ulna with dislocation backwards will simulate in some respects epicondylo-trochlear separation complicated with dislocation of the radius. For in both there may be some lateral inclination of the forearm on forcible extension with lateral mobility and crepitus.

But in the former the precautions necessary to effect the reduction of the dislocation backwards, the ease with which the displacement is immediately reproduced, together with the loss of the proper relations of the olecranon to *both* the epicondyles, are quite sufficient to distinguish it from the latter.

PROGNOSIS AND RESULTS.—In the more simple cases, without much displacement, a good and useful joint may be expected in five or six weeks, provided careful treatment has been carried out and passive motion commenced early.

There is sure to be a good deal of new periosteal deposit around the condyle and lower end of the humerus from the stripping up of the periosteum, but this will mould in the course of years to the natural shape of the limb, and almost perfect restoration of utility of the limb may be expected.

Impaired movement will be inevitable in certain cases where complication exists, and has resulted at times in apparently more simple cases.

The lesion is always of a serious nature, inasmuch as the fracture extends into the joint, and is therefore attended with more or less inflammation and consequent impairment of the mobility of the articulation.   Moreover, articular extravasation of blood will also tend to ankylosis, whilst the callus may be excessive and occur in a position likely to greatly restrict the movements of the joint.

Besides, as the humero-ulnar articulation forms the principal physiological portion of the elbow-joint, any interference with the relation or normal position of its humeral portion, such as we find in this injury, must result in impairment of function of this joint.

The epiphysial fragment will usually unite firmly with the shaft, although in a displaced position.   Coulon (*Fractures chez les enfants*, Paris, 1861, p. 159) gives the following example of this injury, which is scarcely typical, in a child, four years old, who was brought to the hospital two hours after she had fallen down a staircase. The elbow was swollen, the forearm slightly flexed upon the arm, and the relations between the olecranon and epicondyles normal.   Pressure upon the epitrochlea produced crepitus, but the swelling made it impossible to recognise the size of the fragment or the extent of the mobility.   Flexion and extension were rendered almost impossible by the swelling and pain.   The limb was partly flexed and fastened on a cushion, and on the fifth day placed in a gutta-percha splint. . On the twenty-first day passive motion was commenced.   At the end of the month the patient left the hospital ; the arm could then be flexed to a right angle, and extended to an angle of 140° ; the epitrochlea was displaced inwards and forwards, and the fragment could be felt to be voluminous.   Two and a half months later the condition was said to be the same.

Mr. Durham had under his care at Guy's Hospital in October, 1885, a case of considerable deformity of the elbow-joint after partial separation of the trochlea.

John S., aged ten, while running along the top of a wall, fell off and injured his elbow.   There was considerable swelling, great pain, and loss of power in the elbow.   He had been treated for three weeks with a gutta-percha splint.   This was removed at the end of this time, and the arm was found to be useless.   There was considerable deformity of the left elbow, and flexion and extension were both incompletely performed.   The head of the radius rotated on the capitellum, but the external condyle appeared to be much more prominent than usual.   The relations of the radius and ulna were not disturbed. The distance between the inner border of the olecranon and the inner side of the inner condyle was increased by nearly half an inch as compared with the right side.   It seemed certain that the original injury was one of separation of the trochlear epiphysis with displacement inwards of this process.

Powers relates the case of a boy (T. D.), aged nine years, who fell forcibly on the sidewalk, striking the left elbow. Examination revealed all the evidences of fracture through the internal condyle and trochlea. There was no tendency to posterior displacement of the condyle, but when the forearm was in extension it made the normal angle with the arm. The elbow was placed at 90 degrees, midway between pronation and supination, and the condyle drawn a little forward to correct its displacement. A plaster splint was applied for twelve days, and then re-applied and left on till the twenty-eighth day, when the elbow was painless and but slightly enlarged. The range of motion was from 80° to 150°, pronation and supination were all but perfect, and there was no apparent deformity. At the end of the third month the functions were completely restored. There was moderate thickening at the side of the fracture, but no real deformity.

Gurlt quotes a case from Senftleben, in which the result is said to have been good: it was that of a boy, aged eleven. In four other cases ankylosis ensued; one was at an angle of 140°, in which death ensued after resection by Langenbeck. In another case complicated by dislocation ankylosis followed (Langenbeck's *Archiv*, Bd. iii., 1862, S. 311, No. 139); excision was performed seven months afterwards, and this direct examination showed the fragment of the internal condyle lying in the olecranon fossa.

At the Société de Chirurgie, Paris, in 1861 (Langenbeck's *Archiv*, Bd. xxi. S. 237) M. Marjolin showed a boy, aged twelve, in whom rectangular ankylosis of the elbow occurred after detachment and displacement forwards of the trochlea with the internal condyle (internal condyloid fracture of the French). Passive motion under an anæsthetic was proposed.

Deformity will probably be great where the separation has been complicated with dislocation.

Displacement upwards.—In severe cases a reversal of the normal elbow obliquity has been found. This is known in America as the 'gunstock' deformity, from the elevation of the internal condyloid fragment and inward deflection of the normal axis of the extended forearm. The normal humero-ulnar or 'carrying angle' becomes reversed, giving rise to the deformity known as cubitus varus.

G. A. Wright, of Manchester, figures (Ashby and Wright, *Diseases of Children*, 3rd edition, 1896, p. 754) an example of separation of the trochlear epiphysis of the humerus, showing adduction of the forearm with loss of this 'carrying angle' (see fig. 106).

Out of twelve cases of fracture of the internal condyle entering the joint seen by Powers in children and adults, nine perfectly recovered their functions; in one all motions became complete except extension, this being five degrees short; one was perfect, and one was still under treatment. In none was there deformity. From the brief account Powers gives of these cases they appear to have been unusually mild. But little of the articular surface could have been involved to leave such a complete restoration of function without deformity.

The displacement of the epiphysial fragment should never be permitted to be permanently so great as to prevent complete or almost complete loss of movement of the elbow-joint due to the locking of the radius or ulna against the displaced fragment. Such deformity ought never to be met with; the instances in which it occurred ought to have been operated upon and reduced.

It is well to repeat here that deformity at the elbow cannot be accurately judged when the joint is flexed; it is only in an extended position that its presence can be made out with any accuracy.

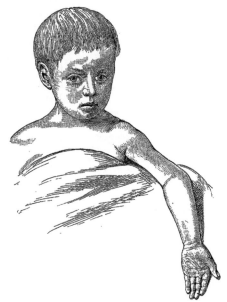

FIG. 106.—CUBITUS VARUS FOLLOWING SEPARATION OF THE TROCHLEAR EPIPHYSIS OF THE HUMERUS. (ASHBY AND WRIGHT)

Osseous ankylosis has ensued in cases of fracture in this position from improper treatment.

Exuberant callus.—The danger from an excessive production of callus is very great. Seeing that the separation is an intra-articular one, the movements of the joint are in great danger of being much restricted from this cause alone.

Paralysis or neuralgia of ulnar nerve.—From pressure of exuberant callus in conjunction or not with displacement of the condylar fragment.

Agnew has recorded a case of the kind in the adult, and Weir Mitchell has added a second, occurring seven years after a fracture.

·**Arrest of growth.**—A slight amount. of arrest of growth of the end óf the humerus may result, and give rise to permanent and very singular alterations in the form of the limb.

TREATMENT.—Where there is little or no displacement the elbow should be fixed at once at a right angle by means of a posterior angular splint. This should extend along the back of the arm and forearm as far as the wrist. The splint should not as a rule be applied on the front or the side. The posterior splint presses the olecranon forwards and helps to support the separated fragment. Evaporating lotions, lead and opium lotions, &c., should be applied to allay the inevitable inflammation and synovitis of the elbow.

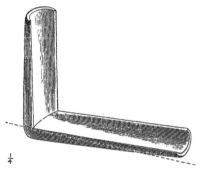

Fig. 107.—POSTERIOR RECTANGULAR AND HOLLOWED SPLINT FOR LEFT ELBOW, AS USED BY AUTHOR. THE ANGLE IS OBLIQUE AND THE FOREARM PIECE DEFLECTED OUTWARDS

After the swelling has subsided the elbow should be put up in the rectangular position, with the hand supine, in a plaster-of-Paris, leather, poroplastic, or other form of casing until a week or ten days has elapsed from the time of the accident. Gentle passive movement should then be commenced. For the first day or two only movements of pronation and supination should be performed, and later on flexion and extension. The utmost care should be taken to prevent any. yielding of the soft material uniting the fragment to the shaft. It should be repeated daily for several weeks to lessen the stiffness which always follows this injury.

The plaster-of-Paris splint in the form known as 'Croft's' is superior to all other splints ; the effusion, both intra- and extra-articular, subsiding more rapidly when it is employed. It makes equal pressure all over the joint, and keeps the joint and fragments absolutely at rest. Plaster-of-Paris bandages should never be employed.

The lower forearm piece should not be in a line with the upper arm piece, but make with it an angle outwards, which should vary according to the age of the child, so as to preserve the normal oblique direction of the axis of the joint.

Hamilton's rules for treating similar fractures in this situation apply with equal force to epiphysial separations. 'Considerable swelling is almost certain to follow, and no surgeon ought to hazard the chances of vesications, ulcerations, &c., by neglecting to open or completely remove the dressings every day. Within seven days, and, perhaps earlier, passive motion must be commenced, and perseveringly employed from day to day until the cure is accomplished; indeed, in many cases it is better not to resume the use of splints after this period, for although no bony union has taken place, yet the effusions have somewhat steadied the fragments, and the danger of displacement is lessened, while the prevention of ankylosis demands very early and continued motion.'

To this it may be added that all violent movements should be carefully avoided; passive motion should only be undertaken by skilful hands.

Displacement.—The reduction of the displaced epiphyses should be immediately effected, as well as that of any associated dislocation, and the arm and forearm fixed in an internal or posterior rectangular position, as recommended above, taking care to preserve the outward deflection of the forearm, and the hand in the supine position.

But many modern writers now agree that the results from the flexed position are not satisfactory in a large proportion of cases, on account of the malposition of the fragment and more or less loss of function of the joint.

Dr. O. H. Allis, of Philadelphia, goes so far as to say that with the splint at this angle the ulna and the attached condyloid fragment are actually pressed out of position in an upward direction and give rise when the forearm is fully extended to deviation inwards of the latter, and to gunstock deformity.

In the case of similar fractures in adults Stephen Smith recommends the elbow to be kept fixed (in the straight position) until union is complete, when passive motion is to be commenced, and voluntary efforts of the patient gently attempted, under the influence of fomentations.

At any rate, in the case of children, where union is more rapid, so prolonged a time is not only unnecessary, but rather tends to fixation and ankylosis of the joint, which will cause the usefulness of the joint to be regained only at the expenditure of a considerable amount of time and treatment on the part of the surgeon.

The bad results of many cases treated in the rectangular position are probably due to the fact that the elbow has not been placed in its normal position. The axis of the joint is not perpendicular to the long axis of the humerus, but is inclined to it at an angle which varies with the age and with the individual. This is best observed when the arm is extended, when the forearm is seen to be directed away from the side of the trunk, as in carrying. The anterior crease in the flexure of the elbow corresponds in direction and obliquity with the axis of the joint.

The ulna remaining attached to the epiphysial fragment of the forearm is not placed in its normal position with the axis of the joint oblique; it will, if put up with this at right angles to the long axis of the humerus, as is the case with the common rectangular splints, cause displacement upwards of the fragment, or tend to keep up this displacement if it has already occurred. The hand and

forearm should therefore be slightly directed outwards. By means of
Physick's rectangular splint, or of those devised by the author with an
angle opening outwards, the normal oblique direction of the articular
surface of the humerus to that of the vertical axis of the shaft is
well preserved.

J. S. Dorsey, in 1823 (*Elements of Surgery*, vol. i. 1823,
p. 168), was one of the first to describe accurately this *angular projection of the elbow outwards*, resulting from fracture of
either condyle penetrating the elbow-joint.   In the cases now
under consideration it is this internal condyloid fragment with the
trochlea which ascends and causes the axis of the forearm to be
displaced inwards.   He recommended treatment by the flexed
position at a right angle, which, he said, was completely successful
in preventing deformity.

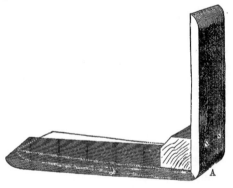

FIG. 103.—ANTERIOR RECTANGULAR SPLINT FOR LEFT ELBOW AS USED BY
AUTHOR. DEFLECTION OUTWARDS.   THE DOTTED LINES INDICATE THE
FOREARM PIECE IN A STRAIGHT LINE WITH THAT OF THE ARM. THE
ANGLE AT A SLOPES OBLIQUELY DOWNWARDS AND INWARDS, CORRESPONDING
WITH THE AXIS OF THE JOINT. THE POSTERIOR RECTANGULAR SPLINT HAS
THE SAME DEFLECTION OUTWARDS OF THE FOREARM PIECE AND THE SAME
OBLIQUITY CORRESPONDING TO THE FLEXURE OF THE JOINT (see fig. 107)

Normally, the axis of the elbow-joint is not perpendicular to
that of the axis of the arm, but forms an angle with it, so that the
forearm is deflected outwards away from the trunk at a varying
angle; 170° (Denucé).

Packard says (Keating's *Cyclopædia of Diseases of Children,*
vol. iii., part ii., p. 1073) : ' One point should never be overlooked in
any case of fracture at the lower end of the humerus, but especially
in separation of the trochlea; there is apt to be caused a change in
the relation of the arm with the forearm, which seriously impairs not
only the shape, but also the usefulness, of the limb.   Normally, if
the elbow is extended with the hand in supination, the forearm
forms with the arm an obtuse angle salient inwards, towards the
median line of the body, and the fold of the elbow in front curves
obliquely downwards and inwards.   The reason of this is the

obliquity of the trochlea.   If, now, a splint is applied which presses
straight across, it pushes up the lower and more movable fragment,
and the result is that the forearm either comes into a straight line
with the arm, or even makes with it an angle salient outward.
Union taking place under such circumstances—as pointed out long
ago by Dorsey, and later very forcibly by Allis (*Annals of the
Brooklyn Anatomical and Surgical Society,* August 1880)—there
will be at all times a very notable awkwardness in the limb, besides
marked interference with its strength and usefulness in many of its
functions.   In order to obviate this difficulty, Allis and others have
proposed treating these fractures with the limb in the straight
position.   I think the better plan is to make a splint which' shall
conform to the normal shape of the joint, and to keep the hand
away from the body.   This is not always easy to do, and indeed

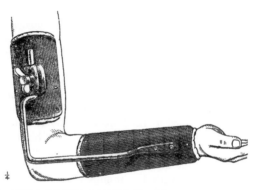

FIG. 109.--LATERAL EXTERNAL TIN SPLINT FOR THE RIGHT ELBOW.   TREATMENT
N THE FIXED RECTANGULAR POSITION.   INTERRUPTION AT ELBOW-JOINT WITH
LATERAL MOVEMENT OF FOREARM UPON ARMPIECE TO PRESERVE THE NATURAL
OBLIQUITY OF THE FOREARM OUTWARDS

one may often see these fractures dressed not with the hand
in supination, but with the forearm carefully drawn forward and slung
as close to the front of the body as possible.'
    The truth of these remarks must be evident to every one, viz. that
unless properly guarded against, as Packard suggests, the trochlea
will be forced upwards beyond the separated surface on the end
of the diaphysis.
    Deformity in this respect, it must be admitted, will be consider-
ably lessened, if not entirely avoided, by the extended position, for in
this way the elbow may be made to assume any degree of obliquity.
    Straight position of limb with forearm away from side.—Complete
extension of the elbow has been much employed of late years for
these as well as for other forms of injury to the elbow-joint.
    It is said by the advocates of the extended position that, with
the head of the radius resting firmly against the capitellum, the

E E

internal condylar fragment can be brought fully down by fixing the arm and drawing the wrist gently outwards, and that so long as the forearm is kept in this position the internal condyle cannot rise. At the same time it is admitted that the forward and backward displacement is not corrected by this means.

Stephen Smith adds to the same effect: 'A fact of much importance in the treatment of fractures of the condyles (internal oblique trochlear and capitellar fractures) relates to the preservation of the normal angle of the forearm with the arm, which gives to the entire limb its "carrying function." This angle is such as to give an outward position of the hand when carrying a weight, the elbow resting naturally on the thigh. This angle may be lost either by the ascent of the internal condyle (sic), or by the descent of the external condyle (sic), and constitutes, in the opinion of Dr. Allis, the usual deformity after fractures of the condyles (sic). To prevent or overcome this displacement, which Dr. Allis attributes in part to the flexed elbow and the bandages and splints ordinarily used, he places the whole limb in a straight position. The radius and ulna at the elbow-joint then tend to bring the internal condyle into position and retain it there, the internal lateral ligament attached to the condyle and ulna aiding much to effect this result. The dressings are now applied, it being borne in mind that "the perfection of the cure will depend wholly upon the natural position assumed by the limb while the dressing is applied." Dr. Allis advises that the patient be placed on his back and both arms stripped, in order that the sound arm may be a guide in fixing the final position of the injured arm. The sound arm is to be placed in a supine position, with the thumb looking outwards, and the injured arm is to be placed in the same position. The forearm of the injured limb must form the same obtuse angle with the arm at the elbow as is noticed in the sound arm. In that position, constantly maintained, the dressings are to be applied, and, if plastic, allowed to become firm. Dr. Allis prefers immovable dressings or a moulded splint. He applies a temporary dressing for a week, the patient being in a recumbent position; then he proceeds to the permanent dressing, as follows: (1) an envelope of cotton, an inch thick, extends from the shoulder to the wrist, thickest at the bend of the arm; (2) a layer of bandages applied sufficiently tight to compress the cotton and afford support; (3) the stiffening material selected—starch, plaster of Paris, &c.—is rubbed in, and a second and third layer of bandage is applied in the same way. The arm is kept in an easy position until the dressing is perfectly hard. He gives a simpler form of dressing as a substitute. Envelop the arm with cotton and then apply a single covering of bandage; cover the whole of this with adhesive plaster. This dressing may be applied from first to last; it has the advantage that it permits the patient to flex the joint a little.'

Dr. L. C. Lane, of San Francisco, also recommends (*Trans. American Surgical Association*, vol. ix., 1891) the extended position secured by a straight splint of pasteboard, felt, or tin. On the second day passive motion with rotation of the forearm should, he holds, be commenced, and 'it should be continued with scrupulous fidelity for many weeks.'

. One disadvantage of the extended position is that if the extension be too great the epiphysial fragment will be tilted and thrown forwards by the olecranon impinging upon it from behind. Another is that the limb, which is usually in a dependent position, has a tendency to swell and cause great discomfort to the patient.

Incomplete extension.—Some surgeons prefer incomplete extension—that is to say, 30° or 40° short of full extension—while others *modify the extended position* by putting the elbow in this position for a limited period, ten to fourteen days, when it is put up again in the rectangular position. It is said that, the displacement having been corrected, the amount of union which has then taken place is sufficient to prevent any recurrence of the deviation from the natural position.

. **Passive motion.**—In 1848 Dr. J. C. Warren, of Boston, U.S.A. (*Trans. of American Med. Association*, vol. i. 1848, p. 174), and some modern French surgeons more recently, in order to prevent ankylosis after treatment by angular splints, in fractures of the condyles of the humerus, recommend early and daily passive movements without the application of any splints.

The former probably hits the right mark when he adds that the accomplishment of this process is so very painful that few patients have courage to submit to it, and few surgeons firmness to prosecute it.

Passive motion should be commenced on the twelfth or fourteenth day, and should be of the most gentle character.

It should be carried out daily, and increased on each occasion, provided it is painless and accomplished without difficulty; anything like forcible movement at this early stage is to be strongly condemned. Movements of pronation and supination should be commenced before those of flexion and extension.

After the lapse of four weeks the movements should be more extensive. If, however, the movement be carried out early and gently, there will be no necessity for the very violent efforts which are sometimes resorted to in the later stages to break down the intra-articular adhesions which have formed.

Objections have been raised to passive motion being undertaken in the early stages on account of the possibility of increasing and prolonging the articular inflammation, and thereby causing ankylosis of the joint. These are not borne out in practice, provided the movement be of the most gentle description, while on the contrary there are plenty of cases on record where rigidity has resulted, although no passive movement was carried out in the earlier stages.

Massage will do much towards hastening the absorption of excessive inflammatory material and promoting the functional activity of the limb.

COMPLICATIONS.—Where dislocation complicates the separation great difficulty will be experienced, not only in replacing the bones in their normal relations, but also in retaining them in this position after reduction.

In nearly all instances it may be found impossible to satis: factorily treat them except in the semiflexed position, in order to prevent the constant recurrence of the dislocation and deformity. Even the advocates of the extended position do not recommend this position when dislocation is present.

A well-moulded posterior splint is the best kind of dressing.

Passive motion should be delayed a little longer in these complicated cases. It may be attempted in a very gentle manner about the third week.

RECENT IRREDUCIBILITY OF DEFORMITY FROM DISPLACEMENT OF FRAGMENTS.—The displacement of the fragments must be reduced *immediately*. It is a mistake to suppose that the fracture may be put up temporarily, and that as time goes on the displaced fragment may be gradually pushed into position.

In all cases where the fragments are so misplaced that they cannot be reduced by manipulation, an incision should be made under strict aseptic precautions, and the fragments reduced and wired in position.

Resection of part or the whole of the elbow-joint.—After all the ordinary means of reduction have been attempted and have failed, in severe displacements and complicated injuries, this last operative resource will be the best and safest for the future welfare of the limb. In many cases removal of the separated fragment or fragments with the rest of the lower end of the humerus will be all that is required. It should be performed at once. It will not be desirable, as a rule, to wait until the swelling and inflammation have subsided.

The same treatment may be found necessary where the parts after reduction cannot be maintained in position.

COMPOUND SEPARATIONS should be carefully explored by means of an incision, the fragments wired in position, or, if necessary, the fragments removed and the joint partly or *wholly excised*.

The author, in conclusion, quotes the trite remarks of Dr. H. R. Wharton, of Philadelphia (*International Clinics*, 2nd Series, 1892, vol. iv. p. 217), when describing an intercondyloid fracture of the humerus in a young patient: 'There is probably no class of cases that has caused surgeons as much trouble as these injuries at the elbow-joint, for these are the cases which are constantly brought into the courts for damages from the attending surgeon for maltreatment. It is very important on taking charge of any case with this injury that the surgeon should be extremely careful as to the examination and the prognosis.'

CHAPTER IX

SEPARATION OF THE CAPITELLAR AND EXTERNAL EPI-CONDYLAR EPIPHYSES AND EPICONDYLO-CAPITELLAR AND CONDYLO-CAPITELLAR FRACTURES

ANATOMY.—The anatomy of the capitellar and external epicondylar epiphyses has already been sufficiently described when speaking of the lower epiphyses of the humerus and its epicondylar epiphyses (see Chapter IV. of Part II.).

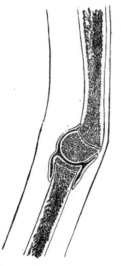

Fig. 110.—SAGITTAL SECTION THROUGH THE OUTER PORTION OF THE ELBOW-JOINT, SHOWING THE RELATION OF THE SYNOVIAL MEMBRANE TO THE EPIPHYSIAL LINES OF THE BONES (RADIO-HUMERAL ARTICULATION), IN A YOUTH AGED FIFTEEN AND A HALF YEARS

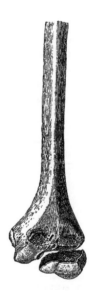

Fig. 111.—DETACHMENT OF THE CAPITELLAR AND EXTERNAL EPICONDYLAR EPIPHYSES PRODUCED BY MACERATION AT THE FIFTEENTH YEAR. (½ SIZE)

The synovial membrane extends for a short distance above the epiphysial junction of the capitellum with diaphysis in front, while behind it does not reach up to this level. On the outer side the synovial sac just gains the lower limit of the external epicondyle.

ETIOLOGY.—From the records it appears that separations of these epiphyses are a much more common injury than the corresponding separations on the inner side.

They have been experimentally produced by H. Senftleben.

Indirect violence.—Indirect violence is the most frequent cause. For in *falls upon the hand* it is clear that the force of the concussion would be carried from the wrist mainly by the radius to the capitellum.

Again, if the forearm is flexed upon the arm *and a blow* is received upon the lower part of the *back of the arm*, these processes may be detached and displaced backwards by the head of the radius, for during flexion of the forearm the capitellum receives from in front backwards the direct thrust of the radius when a retro-humeral blow is made.

Again, in forcible bending inwards of the forearm upon the arm it is possible to produce this fracture, from the attachment to the external epicondyle of the muscles tending to drag off this process, combined with the pressure of the concave ridge of the sigmoid cavity on the bottom of the trochlear groove—a fracture '*par pression et arrachement*' of the French writers.

More **direct violence** may also cause this separation, generally by a fall upon the elbow on the inner and posterior aspect, the ulna being driven from within outwards and impinging against the outer portion of trochlea and capitellum, as in the corresponding separation of the trochlea together with the internal epicondyle or internal condyle. But here, the violence being received on the posterior aspect of the ulna, the arm is at the time of the accident close to the body (Malgaigne), whilst in the case of the trochlea and internal condyle the arm is, on the contrary, away from the trunk in the position of abduction, according to Bernard and Denucé.

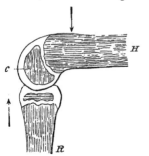

FIG. 112.—VERTICAL ANTERO-POSTERIOR SECTION OF THE FLEXED HUMERO-RADIAL ARTICULATION AT THE AGE OF THIRTEEN YEARS. TWO FORCES ACTING IN OPPOSITE DIRECTIONS (LIKE THE ARROWS) PRODUCE SEPARATION OF THE CONDYLOID EPIPHYSIS *C*. (AFTER FARABEUF)

H, humerus ; *R*, radius

Pingaud produced this fracture many times in attempting, on the dead subject, to dislocate the bones of the forearm directly inwards.

Farabeuf says that the best way to produce this lesion, which he places under the head of separation of the lower epiphysis of the humerus, is by a retro-humeral blow whilst the forearm is flexed, with the hand resting on a table or on the ground as in the accompanying sketch, by which he shows how he succeeded in his experiment on the body of a boy aged thirteen years. The radius causes the capitellar epiphysis to be detached obliquely, carrying with it more or less of the epicondyle and of the cartilaginous substance of the trochlea.

He continues: 'Although the radius, when flexed and supported, can effectually contribute to separation of the epiphysis, it is not the same with the ulna, whose coronoid hook, during flexion, advances · in such a manner as to support itself against the diaphysial part of the trochlea.'

M. Champenois has reported a case of this fracture in a child aged nine years, who had fallen from a horse on to the left side with the forearm entangled behind the back. The fracture was accompanied by incomplete dislocation of the bones of the forearm inwards.

Sir Astley Cooper, in describing this form of injury, says: 'This accident usually happens in children by falls upon the elbow; at least, in my observation, a very large proportion of them have been in young persons. I have seen it occur in the adult, but very rarely in advanced age.'

AGE.—In the *two pathological specimens of old date* the age is not stated; in one complicated *recent one* it is given as ten. Of the eight *simple* cases two were at eleven, one at seven, one at five and a half, two at five, and two at four years of age.

PATHOLOGICAL ANATOMY.—The line of separation in a pure example passes from just above the base of the external epicondyle downwards and inwards, skirting the lower edge of the radial and outer part of the olecranon fossa, and terminating at the middle of the trochlear surface, thereby separating the outer part of the trochlear surface which belongs to the capitellar epiphysis.

In this true form it can only occur before the fifteenth to sixteenth year, the period of junction of this epiphysis with the rest of the trochlea.

In early years there may be a fracture through the cartilaginous epiphysis, and in later years one in the same position, i.e. where the junction takes place.

Several specimens show the exact nature of this injury.

The analogous fracture in the adult (*fracture oblique externe*) was well recognised and described by Malgaigne. Malgaigne, Bernard, Sir Astley Cooper, F. Schmitz, and others give figures of this injury.

Gurlt figures a specimen from the Giessen collection—more a fracture than an epiphysial separation, for the detached portion comprises the external epicondyle and a portion only of the capitellum. There was considerable loss of function of the limb; the only possible movements were those of rotation of the radius, and the forearm was immovably fixed at an obtuse angle.

According to Giraldès, in a considerable number of cases of injury to the lower end of the humerus, 'the trochlea is seen, on the one hand, to be still attached to the lower extremity of the diaphysis, and its proper relationship preserved with the ulna, whilst the condyle (capitellum), the epicondyle (external epicondyle), and the radius are detached and displaced. The radius, with the epiphysial fragment which it supports, is displaced either forwards or backwards according to the direction of the violence causing the injury.'

Displacement.—Judging by the description which Gurlt gives of more than one specimen, displacement usually takes place, and the periosteum is only partially lacerated.

It will be found that according as the periosteum remains intact or is appreciably lacerated, so will the detached capitellar epiphysis remain in position or be displaced to a greater or less extent. The epiphysial fragment may be displaced in any direction and rotated on any one of its axes.

Displacement upwards and outwards is the most common direction for the separated epiphyses to take.

In the Museum of the Royal College of Surgeons there is a specimen, No. 945A, of the articular ends of bones forming the elbow-joint removed by excision (*Catalogue of the Museum of the Royal College of Surgeons*, Appendix I., p. 30) presented by Mr John Wood (1885).

It shows a separation of the epiphyses of the capitellum and external epicondyle in one piece, which has been displaced outwards,

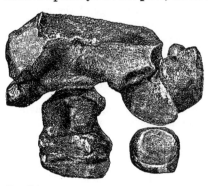

and is united to the shaft in that position. The head of the radius is still in contact with the capitellum, and the articular surface of the ulna, being carried with it, lies in a rough saddle-shaped surface intervening between the displaced capitellum and trochlea. The ulna was fixed in a semiflexed position, movement being prevented by ridges of callus in front and behind it.

FIG. 113.—SEPARATION OF EPIPHYSES OF CAPITELLUM AND EXTERNAL EPICONDYLE. (ROYAL COLLEGE OF SURGEONS MUSEUM)

In other instances the separation does not pass through the epiphysial junction of the external epicondyle, but *as a fracture traversing the diaphysial portion* of the external condyle. The fracture in this injury will commence above at the lower part of the external supra-condyloid ridge, through the coronoid and outer part of the olecranon fossa, traversing the epiphysial line of the capitellar epiphysis.

It is by far the more common form of injury, and is identical with a pure fracture of the external condyle and capitellum and outer part of the trochlea—so commonly met with in children.

Writing in 1884, Hamilton says of twenty-nine fractures of the external condyle (external condyle and capitellar and outer trochlear portions of the articular surface) of which he had a record, twenty-seven were in patients under fifteen years of age.

Sir Astley Cooper figures (*Fractures and Dislocations*, 2nd edition, 1823, p. 491) an excellent specimen of this kind from the Museum of St. Thomas's Hospital.

'In this preparation, in which the external condyle (i.e. the external condyle and capitellum) is split obliquely, the bone is somewhat thickened ; but although this accident had obviously happened long before death, no union but that by ligament had been produced.'

A well-marked specimen which was found on a skeleton supplied to the author by an anatomical dealer in Vienna shows this injury in a very clear light. The skeleton was of a well-made and evidently muscular youth, aged eighteen. Unfortunately, no clinical history could be obtained ; but from the condition of the bones and the considerable remodelling of the parts, it could fairly be presumed that the injury had taken place some years before death. The capitellar epiphysis and outer part of the trochlear surface had evidently been separated through the epiphysial line. This portion of the articular surface with the external condyle was displaced slightly *outwards* and *upwards*, and *rotated* somewhat on its transverse axis, so that the groove between the capitellar and trochlear surfaces, instead of being vertical, ran obliquely downwards and outwards. The line of union of the fracture through the diaphysis could be traced through the radial and outer part of the olecranon fossæ, which were thereby almost obliterated. Between the capitellar epiphysis and the inner margin of the trochlea was a huge gap $\frac{3}{4}$ inch deep, and about the same size in width ; with this the sigmoid cavity and coronoid process of the ulna articulated. The remaining horizontal portion of the trochlear surface had quite disappeared, probably from the pressure of the ulna, leaving the inner edge of the trochlea very prominent.

This remaining portion of the trochlea, by means of a large facet on its outer side, articulated with a similar facet on the inner side of the coronoid process, and its lower margin nearly reached ($\frac{1}{4}$ inch distant) the posterior border of the ulna when the elbow was placed at a right angle.

The movements were very restricted even in the dried condition of the bones ; extension could only be effected to an angle of 125 degrees on account of the olecranon coming in contact with the posterior aspect of the humerus. It was the upward displacement of the whole of the ulna which prevented full extension, as well as some osseous deposit, which partially filled the upper and outer portion of the olecranon fossa. Flexion was impossible beyond an angle of fifty degrees, the coronoid process of the ulna coming in contact with some deposit of new bone just below the coronoid fossa, which was not obliterated. A facet was situated immediately above the outer margin of the trochlea for articulation with the inner side of the coronoid process.

There was *increase of width* of the lower end of the humerus; the distance between the two epicondyles on the left side being 3¼ inches, and on the right side nearly 2⅛ inches.

There was a diminution of rather less than ⅛ inch in the distance between the internal epicondyle and the inner side of the olecranon as compared with the sound side; whereas between the external epicondyle and the outer side of the olecranon there was an increased difference of ¼ inch, the left side measuring 1½ inches and the right 1¼ inches. In each case the elbow was flexed to a right angle.

The head of the radius had clearly accompanied the fragment.

The inner part of the humerus and the inner aspect of the trochlea were quite normal.

Another sign was present which the author has not seen alluded to by any writer, either in recent or old injuries, viz. the *upward displacement of the whole upper end of the ulna*. In this specimen it was a very marked feature. Although a considerable amount of this displacement was probably caused by the subsequent absorption of the remaining horizontal portion of the trochlea, yet this portion of the trochlear epiphysis from its small size cannot prevent this displacement in recent injuries when such a gap is produced between the two portions of the trochlea by the displacement upwards and outwards of the capitellar epiphysis, which the ulna accompanies to some extent.

On comparing the measurement between different points of bone the upward displacement of the ulna was found to be ⅜ inch.

The distance round the lower part of the elbow over the olecranon from one epicondyle to the other on the right side was 4⅜ inches, and on the left 4 inches, the forearm being at right angles. Measuring from the lowest margin of the trochlear surface to the posterior border of the olecranon (the elbow at right angles), on the left side it was ¼ inch, on the right ⅝ inch.

The forearm being in the same position, the distance from the outer limit of the upper epiphysial line of the humerus to the posterior border of the olecranon, on the right side, was 14 inches, on the left 13⅝ inches. There was no deflection to the radial side on extension.

On testing by Wright's line (*Guy's Hospital Reports*, 3rd Series, vol. xxiv., 1879), the elbow being in the extended position—that is, by a line drawn from the most prominent point of the internal epicondyle, obliquely downwards and outwards to the head of the radius—the upper border of the olecranon, instead of being on a level with it, was ¾ inch above it.

Again, when a horizontal line was drawn across the back of the joint in full extension (as far as it was possible) from the external to the internal epicondyle, the upper border of the olecranon was ¼ inch above this line, which in the normal condition passes just above the olecranon.

There was no difference on the two sides, measuring from the epicondyles to the styloid process of the ulna and radius respectively.

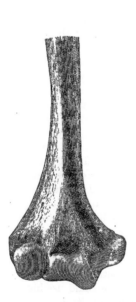
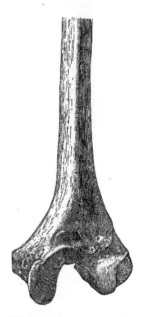

FIG. 114.—LOWER END OF RIGHT HUMERUS; UNINJURED. SAME SUBJECT AS THE NEXT FIGURE. (½ NATURAL SIZE)

FIG. 115.—DISPLACEMENT OF THE CAPITELLAR AND EXTERNAL EPICONDYLAR EPIPHYSIS OF LEFT HUMERUS, WITH FRACTURE OF SMALL PART OF DIAPHYSIS. UNITED. FROM A LAD AGED EIGHTEEN YEARS. (½ NATURAL SIZE)

On the posterior aspect of the humerus towards the outer side there was some evidence of old osseous deposit for two inches upwards, probably the result of periosteal detachment.

The inner remaining portion of the trochlea and the articular surfaces of the ulna and radius, and contiguous portions of these bones, appear to be somewhat hypertrophied. A similar enlargement in this form of fracture is noted and figured by Malgaigne.

Franz Schmitz gives (*Ein Beitrag zur chirurgischen Pathologie des Elbogengelenks*, Munich, 1880, S. 27) drawings, after dissection, of two cases (in adults) in which there was extreme displacement outwards and upwards. In one the outer condyle (condyle and capitellum) was ununited. Flexion and extension limited to the arc between 105° and 140°; pronation and supination perfect. A neuritis of the ulnar nerve had been excited by its overstretching and had led to paralysis of the corresponding muscles. The second case was found in the dissecting room, with no history, and no appearance of nerve trouble.

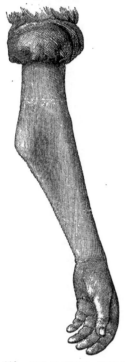

An exactly similar lesion was under the author's care at the City Orthopædic Hospital in April 1895. The fragment, consisting of the capitellar portion of the lower epiphysis and a portion of the outer part of the diaphysis, remained connected with the radius, but quite ununited to the diaphysis.

The boy (W. T.) was at this time aged nine years. Six years before he had slipped down indoors, and fell on to his left elbow. He was treated at the German Hospital, London, and the limb put up in plaster-of-Paris bandages for six weeks. Passive motion was then commenced; after a week the elbow could be used, but stiffly. When the patient came under observation he could use his arm very well, but it was weaker than the other. Flexion, extension, pronation, and supination were good. From the front as well as the back the elbow looked widened. On the outer side there was a fragment of the outer portion of the lower end of the humerus freely movable on the shaft. With this the radius was still connected, and on this it rotated. The distance between the epicondyles behind was an inch and a quarter more than on the uninjured side. During flexion the olecranon was in the same plane as the epicondyles, having passed upwards and outwards between the two fragments of the lower end of the humerus; so that when the elbow was placed in this position on a table, each of these osseous projections touched the surface of the table.

Fig. 116.—CUBITUS VALGUS, WITH UNUNITED CONDYLO-CAPITELLAR FRACTURE.   AUTHOR'S CASE

The accompanying skiagraph, kindly taken by Mr. Thos. Moore in December 1896, shows clearly the condition of the bones, as well

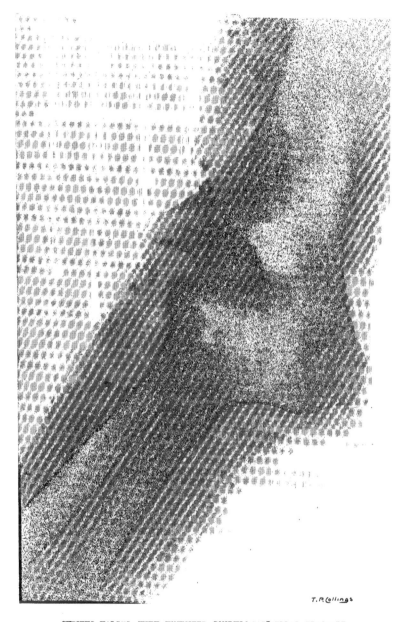

T. R. Collings

CUBITUS VALGUS, WITH UNUNITED CONDYLO-CAPITELLAR FRACTURE.

AUTHOR'S case.   Taken by Mr. THOMAS MOORE.

as some dark spots, which represent calcareous nodules in the subcutaneous tissue.[1]

That the head of the radius does not always accompany the fragment in its displacement is proved by a specimen in Professor Annandale's collection in Edinburgh, which he kindly gave the author the opportunity of examining. There was **displacement backwards** of the outer half of the epiphysis; but the head of the radius was in contact in front with the lower end of the diaphysis. There was a considerable deposit of new bone round the lower end of the humerus, especially in the olecranon fossa. The condition of the elbow rendered excision necessary.

Annandale ('On some Injuries implicating the Elbow-joint,' *Edinburgh Medical Journal*, Feb. 1885, p. 685) subsequently published the case. A boy, about six years old, injured his elbow by a fall, and this was followed by ankylosis, making the arm very useless. Excision of the joint was performed, and an examination of the parts excised disclosed an oblique fracture through the condyles of the humerus, completely separating the outer half of the epiphysis, together with the external condyle. This portion of bone was displaced upwards and backwards, and also slightly rotated outwards, and was attached by osseous material to the posterior aspect of the humerus immediately above the articular surface. The olecranon fossa was filled up by osseous material, and the olecranon itself was displaced slightly backwards from its normal position by this new material. The posterior margin of the head of the radius was displaced a little upwards and forwards, its posterior margin resting against the epiphysial line from which the external condyle had been separated.

COMPLICATIONS.—**Dislocation of elbow** is one of the most common lesions accompanying this injury. It might be laid down as a rule that dislocations at the elbow in children are almost all complicated, the complication usually being a partial separation of the lower epiphysis of the humerus.

Dislocation of the elbow outwards or outwards and backwards has been observed in the six specimens of this fracture recorded by Gurlt.

There is in the Guy's Hospital Museum a specimen, No. 1306[12], showing the portions of bone forming the elbow removed by excision. On carefully dissecting out the parts, and removing the fibrous tissue which united the ends of the bone, the author was able to make out the precise condition of the fragments, which he notes below. For the opportunity thus afforded the author, he is indebted

[1] These nodules were very numerous all over the body, but most marked on the forearms and legs, and felt like shot, freely movable beneath the skin. The skin was generally atrophied and extensible. The nodules were probably phlebolites, for there were traces of a congenital and universal nævoid condition. The author removed a pendulous mass of nævoid tissue at the back of each heel, which had undergone cystic and fatty degeneration, and prevented the boy wearing boots.

to Mr. Bryant.   The specimen is figured by Mr. Bryant (*Practice of
Surgery*, 1884, vol. ii. p. 425, fig. 486A).

G. L. S., aged ten years, fell from a horse on to his right side,
with his arm extended under him, and he then rolled over on to his
face.   There was mobility about the lower end of the humerus, and
it was considered by the surgeon as a T-shaped fracture and treated
with splints.   When admitted under the care of Mr. Bryant at
Guy's Hospital in August 1883, six weeks after the injury, a dislocation of the elbow was detected, and great impairment of movement.   The elbow was kept flexed at an angle of 145 degrees, and
active and passive movement of flexion could only be effected through
10 degrees from that point.   Pronation and supination were good.
The distance between the external epicondyle and the outer edge of
the olecranon was 1¾ inches, and on the left side 1 inch.   The articular
cup of the head of the radius could be felt behind and somewhat

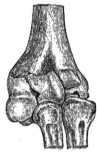

below the level of the external
condyle, and it rotated freely.
There was a remarkable prominence of the olecranon on the
inner side, looking not unlike
the internal epicondyle.   After
an unsuccessful attempt to replace the bones, excision was
performed.   The capitellar epiphysis, including the outer part
of the trochlea, was found to be
separated, and had undergone
rotation into an almost vertical
position, the capitellar portion
being the lower part.   The
radius and ulna were dislocated
inwards and locked in that

position, the coronoid process being in contact with the lower aspect
of the internal condyle, and its outer edge lying against the inner
margin of the trochlea.   The head of the radius was in contact with
the inner portion of the trochlear surface, and the internal epicondyle
was completely detached, displaced forwards, and united by fibrous
tissue on to the front of the humerus, to the outer side of the
trochlea.   Complete recovery with good movement ensued.

In other instances the dislocation may be only a partial one.

Dislocation of the radius alone may be present, especially in the
outward direction.   However, of this there is no specimen recorded.

Detachment of periosteum.—The periosteum will probably not be
torn to any serious extent, except when the displacement is very great.

Wounds.—This fracture may be complicated, though very rarely,
by a wound.

Gurlt relates the case of a child, eleven years old, whose arm was caught by a machine in motion and extensively lacerated from the middle of the forearm to the insertion of the deltoid. Through one of the lacerations the capitellar (external condylar) portion of the humerus was seen to be detached, but still adherent by some muscular or aponeurotic fibres. The osseous fragment was drawn up into position, and the limb fixed at a right angle, with the result that at the end of four months recovery took place, with the forearm ankylosed at a right angle, but the movements of pronation and supination were preserved.

Desault also has reported a case of this fracture complicated with a wound and terminating in recovery.

SYMPTOMS. SEPARATION WITHOUT DISPLACEMENT.—In many instances of this injury there will be found no displacement, or so little displacement as to be quite inappreciable, the periosteum being but little torn.

The injury may then be detected by the following signs :

Mobility.—Before swelling has occurred the external epicondyle may be grasped between the finger and thumb, and this process, with the separated capitellar epiphysis, moved in a forward and backward direction. Some mobility of the fragment will occasionally be detected on extreme pronation, through the action of the supinators and carpal extensors; this is likely to be the case if the separation is really at its upper limit a fracture of the lower part of the supracondyloid ridge of the diaphysis.

Muffled crepitus will usually be perceived during the manipulation just mentioned, and is very distinct.

It can also be easily obtained on rotating the radius and on extreme pronation.

Pain is usually considerable over the seat of injury, and on extreme flexion and extension of the elbow.

Swelling rapidly ensues, from the bruising of the soft structures and the injury to the articulation. It may sometimes be so great as to render the osseous prominences quite indistinguishable.

Occasionally an opportunity is afforded of examining the elbow a few minutes or directly after the accident, and even then some fulness may be found over the synovial membrane on either side of the olecranon, indicating the presence of blood in the joint.

Impaired movement of joint.—The movements of the elbow-joint are more or less restricted, and executed with great pain. The forearm is in a semiflexed and pronate position.

The two following cases, which came under the author's care, are good examples of this form of injury.

No. 1.—Walter E., seven years old, was knocked down by another boy, and fell on his left elbow. On examination, within half an hour of the accident (May 7, 1887), there was no deformity, but soft crepitus on flexion and extension, most marked on extreme extension. Slight mobility of the external epicondyle was detected on grasping this process between the finger and thumb, and also on pronation and supination. The greatest pain experienced was during extreme extension. The prominences about the elbow-joint were in normal relationship, and the radius and ulna intact. The elbow was put up in a plaster-of-Paris dressing in the semiflexed position, and complete recovery subsequently ensued.

No. 2.—Amelia H., aged five years and six months, had been knocked down and had fallen upon her left elbow. She was brought to the Miller Hospital twenty minutes later, and the following signs were found : mobility and soft crepitus on seizing the external epicondyle, the movement taking place from before backwards. There was no appreciable displacement; the external epicondyle appeared to project very slightly backwards. Rotation of the radius produced the characteristic crepitus, without pain. Pain was experienced on extending the elbow beyond an angle of 125 degrees, and on extreme flexion. There was considerable swelling over the lower end of the humerus, especially towards the outer side, and on either side of the olecranon, from effusion of blood into the synovial cavity.

Of fractures generally of the external condyle and capitellum Sir Astley Cooper states that the ' accident is readily detected by the following symptoms : there is some degree of swelling upon the external condyle [i.e. external condyle and capitellum], and pain upon pressure; the motions of the elbow-joint, both of extension and flexion, are performed with pain ; but the principal diagnostic sign is the crepitus produced by the rotatory motion of the hand and radius. If the portion of the fractured condyle be large, it is drawn a little backwards, and carries the radius with it ; but if the portion be small, this circumstance does not exist.'

It is only by carefully examining the relationships of the various osseous projections that a diagnosis can be made with any certainty, but the discrimination of these points about the joint often becomes a matter of great difficulty, on account of the amount of blood extravasated into the articulation, as well as into the tissues surrounding it.

SEPARATION WITH DISPLACEMENT.—Although, as a rule, the displacement is very inconsiderable, the fragment and with it the head of the radius are very liable to be displaced backwards, backwards and outwards, or forwards.

Displacement backwards.—When the epiphysial fragment is displaced backwards the head of the radius will usually accompany it. The forearm is placed in the prone position. Even if the displacement is great, there will be no difference in the distance on the two sides between the external epicondyle and styloid process of the radius so characteristic of dislocation.

Projection of lower end of diaphysis.—On extreme extension of the elbow with the forearm pronated, the lower end of part of the diaphysis or upper fragment may be felt in front of the joint; that is, when the epiphysial fragment is much displaced backwards. This may persist even after consolidation. At other times it is so slight that it disappears when the elbow is flexed.

It is possible for the *olecranon and ulna to be displaced backwards* to a slight extent, along with the epiphysial fragment and radius. It is best detected by extending the forearm on the arm; the olecranon will then become prominent behind.

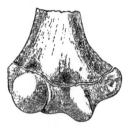 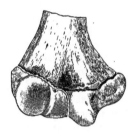

FIG. 118.—LINE OF FRACTURE THROUGH EPIPHYSIAL LINE

FIG. 119.—SEPARATION OF EXTERNAL EPICON-DYLAR AND CAPITELLAR EPIPHYSES

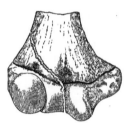 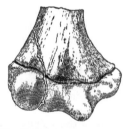

FIG. 120.—EXTERNAL DIAPHYSIO-TROCHLEAR FRACTURE. SEPARATION OF CAPITELLAR EPIPHYSIS WITH FRACTURE OF EXTERNAL CONDYLE OR DIAPHYSIS THROUGH SUPRA-CONDYLOID RIDGE

FIG. 121.—DIAPHYSIO-CAPITELLAR FRACTURE. FRACTURE BETWEEN CAPITELLUM AND TROCHLEA AND THROUGH DIAPHYSIS, TRAVERSING OR PASSING ABOVE RADIAL FOSSA

DIAGRAMS OF THE MORE COMMON FORMS OF FRACTURE ON THE OUTER SIDE OF THE LOWER END OF THE HUMERUS

The whole ulna is also *displaced upwards* in the direction of the axis of the humerus, so that there will be more or less diminution in the distance from one epicondyle to the other over the posterior aspect of the olecranon, the forearm being held at right angles. This displacement is brought about by the direction of the violence, which is applied directly to the olecranon, and by the action of the triceps, biceps, brachialis anticus, and other powerful muscles passing from the arm to the forearm.

Sir A. Cooper says that the appearance presented in this injury is similar to that of dislocation of the radius backwards.

Displacement upwards and outwards, and inclined slightly backwards,

F F

is the more common form of displacement of the fragment. The prominent signs are as follows :

Loss of relation of the external epicondyle and the olecranon.

Slight displacement of olecranon backwards, so that when the forearm is fully extended the ulna projects behind the humerus.

Displacement of ulna upwards as measured by the distance from epicondyle to epicondyle, as in the last-mentioned form of displacement.

This upward and backward displacement of the ulna can readily be ascertained also by Wright's line passing from one epicondyle to another. The upper border of the olecranon, which should normally be on a level with this, will be considerably above it.

Widening between the epicondyles of the humerus. The transverse measurement between the epicondyles is increased from the displacement outwards of the fragment.

Displacement forwards.—This displacement of the epiphysial fragment is accompanied by *supination of the forearm* and *loss of relation of external epicondyle and olecranon.* The epicondyle preserves its normal relation with the head of the radius, and the radial head may be felt, if the swelling be not too great, to rotate at the normal distance below the external epicondyle.

Displacement downwards is rarely met with, although Hamilton and others think this the more common form of displacement in adults, on account of the action of the supinator and extensor muscles attached to the fragment. This, however, does not apply to pure epicondylo-capitellar separations in children.

Some *deflection of forearm* inwards will probably exist.

The following signs are common to all the varieties of displacement :

Mobility of the epiphysial fragment, whilst the remainder of the joint is fixed even after the fragment has been replaced. Pronation and supination of the forearm will, through the radius, cause some movement of the fragment with crepitus.

Soft crepitus is found when the separation is pure, but is of a bony character when the separation is accompanied with a fracture of the supracondyloid ridge of the diaphysis. It is readily felt in detecting mobility, or on rotating radius, or on pronation.

Pain is very great on the slightest movement. Sometimes it is limited to the region just above the external epicondyle.

Swelling from injury to the joint is very great.

Ecchymosis.—Extravasation of blood into the interior of the joint as well as into all the tissues round the joint is very considerable.

Impaired movement of elbow.

Deflection of forearm to radial or to the ulnar side when the forearm is fully extended on the arm. This is in accordance with the severity of the displacement of the epiphysial fragment upwards or downwards.

Hamilton met with deflection downwards three times in children under three years of age; in one of whom he could not discover that the condyle (capitellum and external epicondyle) was carried towards the shoulder, but only outwards; in each of the other cases the fragment had united by ligament.

Reproduction of deformity is particularly marked when much displacement is present with partial or complete dislocation of the bones of the forearm backwards and outwards, the deformity being reproduced with the greatest ease directly after it has been corrected.

Indeed, in dislocations backwards and outwards in children which at first appear to be simple, but which are immediately reproduced after reduction, the surgeon should consider the probability of the occurrence of this form of epiphysial separation. A careful examination of the various prominences will probably reveal one or other form of displacement of the epiphysial fragment.

COMPLICATIONS.—**Dislocation of elbow** *outwards or backwards and outwards* is the most usual complication.

Dislocation of elbow inwards has only been met with in a few instances, e.g. Champenois's and Bryant's, already described.

Dislocation of the radius.—This complication has only been observed once by Hamilton, the radius being completely separated from the capitellar fragment. It must be considered quite an exceptional instance; for the head of the radius always goes with the fragment, which includes the external epicondyle, and is therefore in normal relation with it.

'A boy (F. K.), aged eleven, fell from a load of hay, and he is confident that he struck the ground with the back of his elbow. When seen, six hours after the accident, the arm was much swollen, and the external condyle (i.e. external epicondyle and capitellum) could not be distinctly felt; but when pressure was made directly upon it, crepitus and motion became manifest. The head of the radius was at the same time dislocated backwards, and separated entirely from the condyle, its smooth buttonlike head being very prominent. It is difficult to conceive how a blow from behind should leave the head of the radius dislocated backwards, or how the radius could have separated from the broken condyle; but as the examination was repeated several times and while the patient was under the influence of ether, Hamilton had no doubt of the fact. The dislocation of the radius was reduced, but it would not remain in place a moment when pressure or support was removed. The lad recovered with a very useful arm, the motions of flexion and extension, with pronation and supination, after the lapse of a year, being nearly as complete as before the accident, the radius remaining unreduced.'

DIFFERENTIAL DIAGNOSIS.—A pure separation of the capitellar and epicondylar epiphyses is distinguished from vertical or oblique fracture of the external condyle into the trochlear or capitellar surface by (1) the projection forwards of the lower end of diaphysis on extension of the elbow, and (2) the muffled crepitus.

Separation of the capitellum with fracture of the external condyle is indistinguishable from true fracture traversing the parts mentioned, inasmuch as the tracks are almost exactly the same.

G. A. Wright gives (*Guy's Hospital Reports*, 1879, p. 55) two useful test lines in the diagnosis of injuries about the elbow. He says : ' It will be found that a line can be drawn in all positions of the joint, from the most prominent point of the internal condyle, through the upper border of the olecranon, obliquely downwards and outwards to the head of the radius, and that such line is bisected at a point corresponding to the superior and external angle of the olecranon. Hence any displacement of any one of these points will be manifested along this line.'

As to the second test he says : ' If also a line be drawn across the back of the joint in full extension, from the external to the internal condyle, or *vice versâ*, that line will lie above the upper border of the olecranon, or, in other words, the angle it forms with the first test line will be on the distal side of the intercondyloid line. This line is most conveniently taken by extending the arm horizontally, with the humerus rotated so that the bicipital or anterior aspect looks towards the middle line of the body, and by then dropping a perpendicular through the condyles.'

PROGNOSIS AND RESULTS.—Like all other epiphysial separations, this injury without displacement, or with only slight displacement, will readily unite firmly by callus under appropriate treatment, although many cases of ununited fracture or fibrous union only are recorded in the case of adults. The functions of the limb, except in cases of great displacement and with complications, are not likely to be permanently affected.

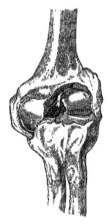

Even when displacement is considerable, union will still take place, though at a later period.

FIG. 122.—FRACTURE OF THE OUTER CONDYLOID (CAPITELLAR) PORTION OF THE HUMERUS. UNUNITED. (AFTER SIR ASTLEY COOPER.) (ST. THOMAS'S HOSPITAL MUSEUM)

Speaking of this form of fracture, Sir Astley Cooper says that if the fracture be very oblique, a considerable portion being external to the capsular ligament, a steady and long-continued support of the part will occasion it to unite, but that if the whole extent of the fracture be within the ligament it does not unite by bone, whatever may be the means employed.

In two out of three cases of fracture in this position in children under three years of age Hamilton found the fragment united by ligament.

A girl, aged three, fell and broke the external condyle (i.e. capitellum and external epicondyle) of the left humerus, the fracture extending freely into the joint; crepitus was distinct, and the forearm slightly flexed and prone. The lesser fragment was displaced outwards and a little backwards, carrying with it the radius. On the second day Hamilton was dismissed on account of the unfavourable prognosis which he gave—or, rather, because he refused to guarantee a perfect limb—and a quack was called in. Several months after the accident the father brought the patient for examination. There was no ankylosis, but the lesser fragment had never united, unless by ligament, moving freely with the head of the radius. When the forearm was straightened upon the arm it fell strongly to the radial side, but resumed its natural relation again when the elbow was flexed.

Deformity.—Where there has been but little displacement the slight deformity will be quite indistinguishable in the course of a year or more, from the remoulding of the parts.

In other cases the deformity will be very noticeable, when the fragment has united in a bad position and the bones of the forearm have remained somewhat displaced.

In a case shown by L. A. Bidwell (*Lancet*, May 4, 1889; *Hunterian Society's Transactions*, 1890, p. 62) to the Hunterian Society, a boy, aged five, had had a fall on the hand thirteen weeks previously. He was said to have dislocated the elbow, and splints were applied for a few days only. There was deformity, increase in circumference of the elbow by $\frac{3}{8}$ inch, wasting of the arm, and very little motion—extension not being permitted at all. There was an increase in the width of $\frac{3}{4}$ inch between the condyles of the humerus. The outer half of the articular surface of the humerus, displaced somewhat forwards and outwards, was firmly united, and the ulna was in normal relation to the humerus. The probable injury consisted in a fall upon the radial side of the hand, pushing up the radius against the capitellum and causing a fracture running from just above the external condyle to the middle of the articular surface. Excision of the joint was proposed.

The author's case, already narrated, is a notable example of cubitus valgus due to an ununited condylo-capitellar fracture.

Hamilton has noted in several instances of fracture of the capitellum and external condyle in children the existence of lateral inclination towards the radial side on extending the arm, its natural relation nevertheless being resumed when the elbow was flexed.

In one case, however, the deflection was towards the opposite

side. Hamilton examined the child one year after the accident, the
patient being then five years old, and found the external condyle (i.e.
capitellum and external condyle) very prominent and firmly united,
but not apparently displaced in any direction except outwards. The
radius and ulna had evidently suffered a diastasis at their upper
ends, but all the motions of the joint were free and perfect.

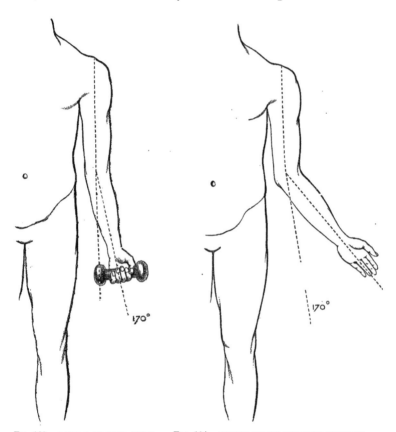

FIG. 123.—NATURAL CARRYING ANGLE   FIG. 124.—CUBITUS VALGUS FOLLOWING FRACTURE
OF ELBOW. 170° OUTWARDS   INTO ELBOW-JOINT. EXCESS OF CARRYING ANGLE

Coulon reports two other instances of what he calls intra-
articular fractures of the epicondyle, one in a boy six years old,
another in a boy of fourteen.   Both these cases resulted in serious
deformity and disability.
Descent of the external condyloid fragment with the capitellum
will cause the normal axis of the forearm outwards in the extended
position to be substituted for a more inward position, so that the
elbow will then project outwards. The deformity will, in this case,

be precisely similar to that so frequently met with after separation of the trochlea and internal condyle.

Sir William MacCormac, in speaking of injuries involving the elbow-joint (*Clinical Journal*, October 10, 1894, p. 383), says : ' In many of these cases the change in the shape of the surface of the articulation as the result of fracture in itself greatly militates against a satisfactory result as regards function, and in many cases, whatever the treatment be, a great deal of alteration in the shape of the joint may ensue.'

Cubitus varus and valgus may also be brought about by irregular growth at the epiphysial line of the humerus without any displacement of the epiphysis having occurred.

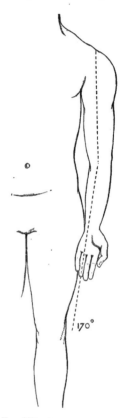

An injury to the conjugal cartilage in early childhood may cause an early ossification or destruction of the conjugal cartilage and arrest of growth of a part of the growing end of the bone, and thereby produce considerable deformity of the joint in after years.

Ankylosis.—From the intra-articular nature of the injury some degree of *temporary ankylosis* must result, but it will usually disappear entirely at the end of some months under proper treatment.

The permanent stiffness which is met with does not arise so much from arthritis as from the intervention of the separated fragment, or the improper reduction of the fragment, giving rise to alteration of the normal articular surfaces.

In some instances the *olecranon fossa* may be filled up with *inflammatory or osseous* material, and greatly hamper or entirely prevent the movements of

Fig. 125.—CUBITUS VARUS. AN ANGLE OF 170° INWARDS

the joint. This has led the advocates of the treatment by the extended position to insist upon this method, as in the flexed position this great hollow is left unoccupied by the olecranon.

In other instances, as in the author's, there will be, from the nature of the lesion and from the obliteration of the articular cavity by inflammation, some permanent ankylosis. In Bidwell's case no extension of the arm was permitted.

Malgaigne saw, in consultation with M. Amussat, a child of

twelve years, who for nearly two months had had a fracture of the external condyle (i.e. capitellar epiphysis and external epicondyle), and as yet no consolidation. The space between the two tuberosities was increased by six or seven millimetres; the upper end of the fragment projected forwards, its lower part about two millimetres backwards; motion was much impeded, and there was still pain in the elbow; it was thought that the joint would never wholly

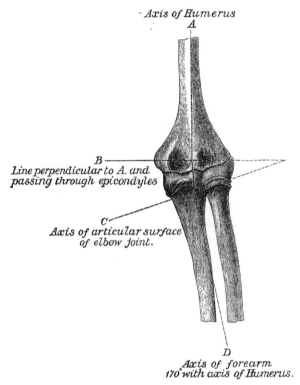

- Axis of Humerus
A

B ——
Line perpendicular to A. and
passing through epicondyles

C
Axis of articular surface
of elbow joint.

D
Axis of forearm
170° with axis of Humerus.

Fig. 126.—DIAGRAM SHOWING THE NATURAL DEVIATION OF THE LEFT FOREARM OUTWARDS, AND THE RELATION OF THE AXIS *C* OF THE ELBOW-JOINT TO THAT OF AXIS *A* OF THE HUMERUS

B, a line drawn at right angles to *A* through the epicondyles (fifteen years of age);
D, axis of forearm at an angle of 170° with *A*

recover its mobility. However, by carefully directed exercise the movement gradually increased, and when Malgaigne again saw the child, nearly two years afterwards, flexion, pronation, and supination were complete, extension was only to the amount of a few degrees, and there was every promise of its full restoration. The only remaining annoyances from the fracture were the persistent deformity of the elbow, a slight displacement of the head of the

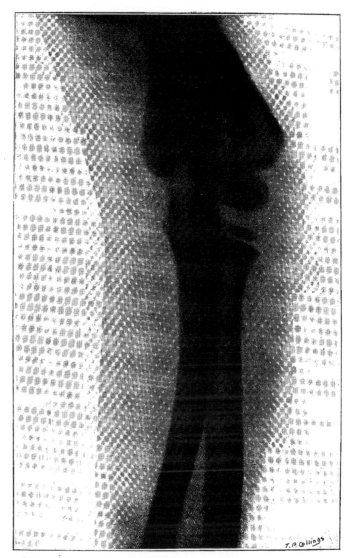

SEPARATION OF THE CAPITELLAR AND EXTERNAL EPICONDYLAR PORTION OF THE
LOWER HUMERAL EPIPHYSIS WITH DISPLACEMENT DOWNWARDS AND INWARDS.

Severe cubitus varus three and a half years after a fall on the right elbow.
Movements of the elbow joint perfect.

Mr. T. F. RAVEN'S case.   Taken by Mr. A. F. STANLEY KENT.

radius backwards during extreme extension, and occasional pain about the elbow.

Pingaud has stated that the ultimate result of this form of fracture differs entirely from that of the corresponding internal trochlear fracture on the inner side, and that the latter frequently ends in ankylosis, whilst the former frequently terminates in the formation of a false joint.

The greater difficulty in rendering immovable the capitellar fragment—which is moreover connected with a very movable bone (the radius)—no doubt, in the adult, renders these fractures more liable to be followed by a false joint, but in the case of children such circumstances do not carry so great weight. In fact the author knows of no case of this kind followed by a false joint in children which has been recognised and undergone appropriate treatment. In children the ultimate result, as regards the function at any rate, may be said to be good. Even if stiffness of the joint has remained for several months, it will in the majority of cases, with appropriate treatment by massage, &c., gradually become less, and at the end of a year or two completely disappear.

In the case of a boy, aged five years, seen by Powers, a fracture of the external condyle extending to the trochlear surface, and exhibiting all the usual signs and slight posterior displacement, was treated by plaster-of-Paris splint, with the result that all the motions of the elbow were satisfactory and union was complete, with thickening and widening of the condyles. The forearm, however, was more nearly in a straight line with the arm than on the opposite side.

Of fifteen cases of this form of fracture in adults and children, Powers found that nearly all presented some deformity, due to the marked prominence of the condyle and its slight backward displacement; but the functions were a very little short of complete.

Mr. Hutchinson relates (*British Medical Journal*, July 24, 1886) the case of a boy, aged ten, in whom full freedom of all motion had been rapidly restored. It was only nine weeks since the accident, yet there was not the slightest swelling, and he could flex and extend almost perfectly, and pronation and supination were equally free. The external condyle, together with the articular surface for the radius, was visibly displaced, and very conspicuous. Some surgeons who examined it thought that it was still movable. The internal condyle was almost, if not quite, in due relation with the olecranon; but there was some thickening of the humerus, and the olecranon did not seem to project so much as usual. Mr. Hutchinson's impression was that the end of the shaft was displaced a little backwards, but he had not an opportunity for forming a deliberate opinion. The wonder was that there could be such displacement with perfect motion.

Irregular growth of the humerus from injury to this part of the epiphysial junction may subsequently ensue, but will be trifling compared with the deformity from displacement.

TREATMENT.—The elbow should be flexed to a right angle, with the forearm in the position of supination, an anterior or posterior rectangular splint applied from the shoulder to the wrist, and the fragment, if displaced, restored to its proper position. The posterior splint with outward deviation of the forearm piece is the most efficient. A cotton pad over the detached fragment will assist in

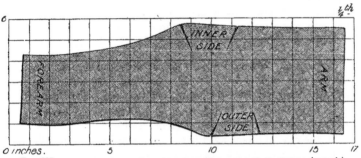

FIG. 127.—PATTERN FOR POSTERIOR PIECES OF ANTERO-POSTERIOR SPLINTS (CROFT'S) WITH ELBOW AT A RIGHT ANGLE. FOR A BOY OF FIFTEEN YEARS

Reduced to one quarter size on scale of inches

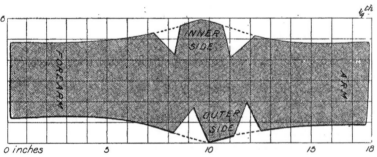

FIG. 128.—PATTERN FOR ANTERIOR PIECES OF ANTERO-POSTERIOR SPLINTS

Size as above

keeping it in position ; or one may be necessary over the lower end of the upper fragment of the diaphysis, which tends to be thrown forwards.

At all times there is but little hold to be obtained on the capitellar fragment, so that it would appear to be impossible to secure much direct pressure upon it. Care should therefore be taken to fix the radius securely. When the fragment is clearly displaced in a downward direction, the forearm should be extended and abducted into its normal outward deviation, and, with some manipulation of the fragment, the reduction of the displacement will usually be effected.

At the end of ten to fourteen days, or earlier, a modified 'Croft's' splint, consisting of anterior and posterior pieces of plaster of Paris, will be found of the greatest service, and allow the daily examination of the elbow without the risk of displacing the fragment. It is often preferable from the commencement of treatment to apply this splint instead of wooden ones on the anterior or posterior aspect. A poroplastic, leather, gutta-percha, or other moulded splint may, like the latter, be applied directly after the accident. The limb should under these circumstances be in the semiflexed position, midway between pronation and supination.

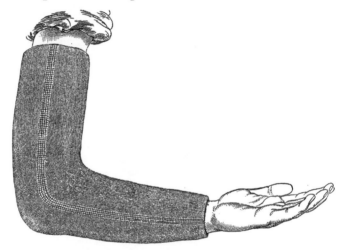

Fig. 129.—CROFT'S ANTERO-POSTERIOR SPLINTS OF PLASTER OF PARIS
APPLIED TO LEFT FOREARM

In cases of slight displacement the treatment merely consists in keeping the elbow semiflexed with a starch, plaster-of-Paris, or other immovable apparatus.

Malgaigne treated a case of slight displacement in a boy nine years old by applying a starch bandage, and putting a graduated compress in front of the elbow, to push backwards the upper end of the fragment, which tended to start forwards. The union was easy and perfect.

Sir Astley Cooper recommends for this injury in children an angular splint to be applied to the back of the arm, elbow, and forearm. He says: ' It may be made of stiff pasteboard bent to the shape of the elbow; but the best mode for its application is to dip it in hot water and apply it wet, so that it may exactly adapt itself to the form of the limb.'

Hamilton says : ' Generally the forearm ought to be flexed upon the arm, especially with a view to overcome the usual tendency in the upper end of the lower fragment to pitch forwards, which form of displacement is greatly increased by straightening the arm.' He mentions an exception (one of two cases which he had seen) to this rule.

J. C., a boy aged six, was brought to him, having, a few minutes before, fallen from a height of four or five feet to the ground. His father said the elbow had been broken at the same point two years before, and from that time had remained stiff and crooked. The

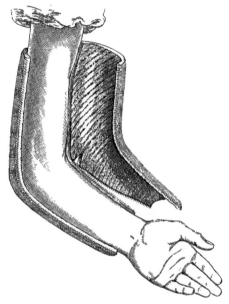

Fig. 130.—THE SAME, WITH THE ANTERIOR PIECE LAID TO THE OUTER SIDE AFTER CUTTING THROUGH THE MUSLIN ALONG THE WHOLE OF THE GAP ON THE INNER SIDE AND THROUGH PART OF THE GAP ON THE OUTER SIDE

external condyle (i.e. capitellum and external condyle) was found to be broken off, and, with the head of the radius, carried backwards. This was the position which it occupied constantly, although it was easily restored and maintained in position when the arm was straight, but not by any possible means when the elbow was flexed. The arm was therefore put up in the extended position in a long felt splint, and the fragments remained well in place till a cure was accomplished.

Mason's elbow splint, as used for excision, has sometimes been employed, as it enables not only flexion and extension, but also pronation and supination, to be carried out while it is on the limb.

The extended position is recommended by Dr. L. C. Lane for fractures in this situation :

'Adjustment and co-aptation must first be carefully done, and then the splint applied while the arm is extended in supination. In the supine and straight position the biceps and pronator radii teres muscles tend to prevent the radius and its fragment from deviating backward, in which direction displacement normally occurs. Should there be a tendency to displacement of the fragment or of the head of the radius after they have been reduced to their proper site, then compresses should be so placed as to correct and prevent such displacement. Passive motion must be commenced early and continued until satisfactory motion is obtained ; and the guide should not be the number of weeks occupied, but the work should be continued until freedom of movement is obtained.'

Guedeney briefly records (*Du traitement des fractures du coude chez l'enfant*, Lyon, 1893) two cases of fracture of the external epicondyle with fracture of the capitellum (condyle). Both occurred in girls aged four years, who had fallen their own height on to the elbow. There was slight swelling and clear crepitus in each. In one there was pain on moving the forearm laterally. A diagnosis of fracture of the humeral external epicondyle and of the capitellum was made. The latter remained fixed to the radius in both cases. Both were treated by fixation in the extended position. Some weeks later, on removal of the bandage, there was found to be complete consolidation, and the movements of the limb were entirely preserved in both cases.

Allis also recommends this position. For a further description of this subject the author must refer the reader to Chapters IV. and VI. of Part II.

Yet it must not be forgotten that if an ankylosed joint follows treatment in the extended position, the limb will be rendered almost useless.

When a dislocation is also present, the greatest difficulty is to maintain the bones in position after reduction. The displaced capitellar fragment, in its position backwards, forwards, or outwards, may then be detected for the first time. An attempt should be made to replace it by pushing it back by its apex into its normal position.

The extended position is quite unsuited to cases complicated by dislocation, for in these the dislocation will be reproduced in this position.

Passive motion should be commenced early—on the eighth to tenth day—and performed daily with great gentleness.

Sir Astley Cooper recommends the 'splint to be worn for three weeks, when passive motion is to be begun ; it must be very gentle at first, and may be gradually increased as the pain and inconvenience attending it subside.'

Passive movement and massage should be commenced early, on account of the damage to the joint. Hitherto it has been the practice to delay these for fear of non-union of the fracture.

Rigid and stiff limbs and joints are far more frequent than non-union of fracture; indeed, the latter in children are exceedingly rare.

Inflammation of the joint and surrounding structures is to be treated by the use of lead, spirit, or other suitable application.

Resection of the whole joint, or partial resection, i.e. of the humeral fragment alone, may be rendered necessary in exceptionally complicated cases of great and irreducible displacement or rotation of the epiphysial fragment or dislocation of the elbow. It is always best, if possible, to leave the radius and ulna intact. The resection may be performed at the time of the accident, or preferably at a later period.

But where reduction simply cannot be efficiently and fully carried out, then **incision and replacement and wiring or suturing of the fragments** in position should be undertaken with proper aseptic precautions. Indeed, in all cases in which it is found to be impossible to reduce the displacement by manipulation, it may be carried out in hospital practice.

Partial resection in old cases of dislocation backwards of forearm.— F. Fischer has recorded (*Deutsche Zeitschr. f. Chir.*, 1889, T. 29, 370, and *Archives Générales de Médecine*, 1889, vol. ii. p. 235) three cases, two of them in girls, aged sixteen and ten years, and one in a boy, aged fifteen years, from Lücke's clinic at Strasburg. In each case the joint was fixed at an angle of 170° to 180°; flexion impossible. Pronation and supination only slightly marked in one case. Partial resection, consisting of removal of the olecranon and a small portion of the radius, was followed by very satisfactory results. The girl, aged sixteen, could follow her occupation of domestic servant, and extension of the arm was the only movement that might have been more complete. In the other two patients the elbow could be used perfectly, all active movements being very easily carried out. In all these cases the dislocation of the bones of the forearm backwards was complicated with a fracture of the epicondyle, the track of which extended obliquely from the posterior aspect of this process towards the outer side of the trochlea.

Fischer adds some remarks upon the mechanism of this injury, experimental and otherwise. The injury, he says, is usually produced by forcible over-extension of the forearm whilst in the pronate and abducted position, and at the same time the arm is brought nearer to the trunk, producing a violent twisting force at the elbow. Direct violence—viz. a kick on the elbow—was added to the other etiological conditions in the case of the boy aged fifteen. Fischer thinks that the dislocation occurs first during the accident, and that the fracture of the epicondyle is caused by the impingement of the radial head against the posterior aspect of this process while the forearm is abducted and the arm adducted.   On the other hand, in experiments on the dead body, fracturing first the epicondyle by direct violence or by abduction and forcible pronation of the forearm, he never succeeded in producing a dislocation backwards, but always outwards.

CHAPTER X

SEPARATION OF THE TROCHLEA

ANATOMY.—Between the eleventh and twelfth years the nucleus
or nuclei, for there are often two, appear first towards the prominent
part of the inner edge of the trochlea.

About the thirteenth year the internal epicondyle is completely
separated from the trochlear surface by the growth downwards and
inwards of the diaphysis, and becomes a distinct epiphysis.   This
inner portion of the trochlea, when fully ossified, unites with the rest
of the articular surface about the fifteenth to sixteenth year.

M. Mayet describes (*Bulletins de la Société anatomique de Paris,*
Avril–Mai 1895, p. 375) accessory points of ossification occasionally
met with in addition to the chief centre of the trochlea : one an
inner marginal (appearing at twelve years of age), situated on the
inner aspect of the trochlear projection and blending with the diaphysis, and the others, two or three in number, at the bottom of the
trochlear groove (appearing at twelve and a half years of age, and
joining at fourteen to fifteen with the neighbouring centres).

AGE.—In one old and doubtful pathological specimen the age was
stated to be ten years.

Of the two clinical cases, one was aged eleven years and the
other seventeen—the latter age certainly the utmost limit at which the
trochlear portion of the epiphysis remains a distinct portion uncon-
nected with the rest of the trochlear surface.

PATHOLOGICAL ANATOMY.—A pure separation of the trochlear
epiphysis can only, on anatomical grounds, occur between the
thirteenth, sixteenth, and seventeenth years ; for before this period
the internal epicondyle is still connected with it, and after the
sixteenth year it is blended with the rest of the articular surface.
However, before or after this period, separation with a fracture
detaching it from either of these parts is even more likely to
occur than a pure separation.

Professor Laugier was the first, in 1853, to assert the possibility
of a fracture in the adult involving the trochlea alone, but he was
unable to furnish any proof of his statement.

Pingaud states that there exists in the Museum of Breslau a specimen (No. 1116) of an old fracture of the lower extremity of the humerus, in which the principal lesion appears to have been in the trochlea, which was atrophied and displaced upwards.

The only uncomplicated case the author can find verified by actual inspection is the case of a boy aged ten years, quoted by Gurlt from Langenbeck. The elbow was ankylosed, and on resection the broken condyle (trochlea) was found in the olecranon fossa. Death ensued from pyæmia.

COMPLICATIONS.—**Dislocation of the elbow** *backwards, backwards and inwards*, or *backwards and outwards*, is very likely to complicate a separation of the trochlear epiphysis.

Packard, writing in Keating's *Cyclopædia of Diseases of Children* (vol. iii., part ii., p. 1072), states that in the Warren Museum (Catalogue, p. 172) there is a specimen from a girl aged sixteen, who had a fracture of the inner condyle (trochlea) with dislocation backwards and outwards of the elbow. Sloughing ensued, and amputation was performed on the forty-sixth day. 'The condyle is seen to have undergone considerable change, as have also the other bones, more or less.'

ETIOLOGY.—But little is known of the etiology and mechanism of this separation.

Direct blows, such as a fall upon the elbow.

Indirect violence. — Falls upon the palm of the hand, as in Laugier's case, in which there was entire absence of evidence of direct injury to the elbow—the forearm being semiflexed, and the ulnar hook formed by the coronoid process dragging off this process.

SYMPTOMS.—It is possible for the trochlea to be separated *without any displacement*, the detached portion remaining entirely within the joint.

Some *pain* on movement of the joint, with *impaired use* of the limb, and possibly *crepitus*, will assist in forming a correct diagnosis.

The injury will often be rendered more obscure by the *swelling* which rapidly ensues after the accident between the internal epicondyle and the inner side of the olecranon, where the injury has been caused by more direct violence to the elbow.

Mobility of a loose body on the inner side of the elbow-joint.

Lateral movement inwards of trochlea with the ulna when the ulna is held firmly at the level of the coronoid process.

Ulna and epicondyles intact, and no loss of relationship between these processes. The epicondyles are not movable on the humerus or between one another, and there is no displacement of the ulna backwards or inwards.

Laugier sums up the signs of this fracture by the following characteristics :

G G

1. Passive movements of flexion and extension of the elbow to their full extent, and there is even the possibility of passive mobility beyond the physiological limits.

2. The internal lateral inclination of the forearm in extension of the limb, the forearm forming with the arm an angle, opening inwards, whose apex is below the epitrochlea.

3. The possibility of detecting abnormal lateral mobility on forcible extension, and at the same time producing crepitus.

4. The immobility of the different osseous processes and the preservation of their normal relations.

5. No mobility of the epicondyles, either on the humerus or between themselves.

J. H. Packard, in speaking (Ashhurst's *International Encyclopædia of Surgery*, 'Injuries of Bones,' p. 138) of disjunction of the lower epiphysis of the humerus, says : 'I think the fracture may concern a portion only of the epiphysis, and then be entirely within the joint. The cases of this kind which have come under my notice have been in children, and the mechanism of their production was not known. On passive motion of the elbow, distinct crepitus was elicited, and no other sign of fracture existed except loss of power in the limb and pain, aggravated by handling ; there was no perceptible deformity.   In the two cases of which I have kept notes, complete recovery ensued in about six weeks.'

An example was seen by M. S. Laugier (*Arch. Gén. de Médecine*, 1853, vol. i. p. 45, ' Sur une variété de la fracture de la trochlée humérale') in a girl seventeen years old, who had fallen upon the palm of her hand, without directly injuring the elbow itself.   It was not followed by swelling or bruising about the elbow, or by effusion into the joint.   Laugier considered it undoubtedly a fracture of the trochlea alone ; but the exact line of separation does not appear to have been clearly established.

Voluntary movements were painful, and therefore difficult ; but passive flexion and extension, pronation and supination, could be carried out to their fullest extent, though accompanied by pain. The rotation of the radius during pronation and supination was at times accompanied by intra-articular crepitus, but this was most evident on inclining the forearm inwards while it was fully extended on the arm ; and in bending it in the same position and direction, viz. inwards towards the ulnar side, a very obtuse angle was produced on the inner side at the elbow-joint.   Together with the crepitus, some lateral mobility was always felt in these movements, caused by the gliding of the trochlea upon the humeral diaphysis, in an inward and outward direction, and produced by means of the ulna.

The epitrochlea and epicondyle were quite immovable on the humeral diaphysis, as well as between themselves.

The treatment consisted in rest, the forearm being slightly

flexed and pronated. In a few weeks recovery took place, with complete restoration of the functions of the arm. A slight greenish discoloration on the inner and posterior aspect of the elbow was the only evidence of injury to the joint, there being no effusion into it.

Dr. Charles A. Powers (*New York Medical Record*, March 17, 1888, p. 311) diagnosed the following case of separation of the trochlear epiphysis of the humerus:

The boy, aged eleven, fell from a wagon, striking the inner aspect of the left elbow. Immediately after there was found to be almost complete disability at the elbow, very much pain, and moderate swelling at the inner aspect of the joint. There was no fracture through either condyle, or through their bases, and the ulna was intact. There was no difference in the contour of the epicondyles on comparison with the opposite side. Between the internal epicondyle and the inner aspect of the olecranon lay a loose body about the size of a bean; it was freely movable, and could be made to grate on the adjacent bone. When the ulna was firmly grasped antero-posteriorly at the coronoid process, it could be made to slip internally on the humeral trochlea, and in so doing carried with it the loose fragment. The inner edge of the trochlear surface could not be felt. The examination was made under ether. From the preservation of the contour of the internal condyle, and the free lateral movement of the ulna, Dr. Powers concluded that this fragment could come only from the inner trochlear surface of the humerus.

The forearm was flexed at ninety degrees, midway between pronation and supination, and a plaster-of-Paris splint was applied and kept in place four weeks, at the end of which time the condition noted was as follows : ' Moderate thickening at the inner aspect of the humerus below and without the internal epicondyle; flexion to 80 degrees, extension to 120 degrees; pronation and supination almost complete.

' The functions gradually returned, and six months later all were complete except extension, which was ten degrees short of normal.'

COMPLICATIONS.—**Dislocation of elbow.** Gurlt reports the case of a boy, aged seven, in whom the luxation was reduced, but the joint was permanently stiffened.

DIAGNOSIS.—Separation of the trochlea alone has a close relationship with **separation of the trochlear and internal epicondylar epiphyses,** or with a **separated trochlea accompanied by a fracture of the internal condyle.** But both the latter have very marked differences which should prevent them being confused—viz. the mobility of the internal condylar process, projection of the olecranon backwards, the ulna being displaced backwards with the detached fragment, simulating dislocation (Sir A. Cooper), and projection of the upper or humeral fragment forwards.

None of these are present in separation of the trochlea alone.

There is no mobility of the epicondyle, or appearance of dislocation of the ulna backwards or inwards.

On the other hand, in both injuries the forearm will incline inwards during forcible extension of the limb, and at the same time some lateral mobility and crepitus may be felt.

TREATMENT.—Evaporating lotions are recommended by some to be applied for the first few days, with or without the use of a splint, especially when great swelling and ecchymosis exist.

If displaced, the epiphysis should always, if possible, be replaced at once. The elbow should then be put up in the flexed position in a leather or other moulded splint for the next ten days, after which time passive movement should be resorted to and gently carried out every day.

A posterior angular splint, if preferred, will tend to support the olecranon and prevent any displacement backwards of the trochlea.

SEPARATION OF THE CAPITELLUM

·**ANATOMY.**—The nucleus of the capitellum is the first of the osseous centres of the lower end of the humerus to appear. It does so during the third year, and rapidly spreads throughout the whole of this process, and extends inwards to form the outer half of the trochlea— that is, as far as the trochlear groove. About the fifteenth or six-teenth year the capitellar surface, including the outer half of the trochlea, unites with the inner part of the trochlea, and soon afterwards the external epicondyle, now completely osseous, joins the upper and outer aspect of the capitellar epiphysis.

The entire lower epiphysis of the humerus thus formed joins the shaft at the seventeenth year.

The fully formed epiphysis is somewhat triangular in shape; its upper, slightly concave, surface sloping downwards and inwards. The base of the triangle on the outer side is almost as thick as the whole transverse length of the capitellum; it is thin on the inner side, where the diaphysial end has penetrated the inner portion of the cartila-ginous end of the humerus.

From the anatomical condition of the bone, the external epi-condyle being so largely connected with the capitellar epiphysis, it is improbable that separation of the capitellum alone will be a frequent accident. The external epicondyle, when fully ossified, is only in contact with the diaphysis of the humerus to a very small extent, and very rapidly after its complete formation blends with the capitellar epiphysis. Before the thirteenth or fourteenth year, when this centre of the external epicondyle appears, this cartilaginous process is merely a part of the cartilaginous lower end of the humerus.

AGE.—In the only clinical case recorded, and it is a doubtful one, the age is given as seven years.

PATHOLOGICAL ANATOMY.—From pathological specimens which have been recently recorded, it is quite possible for the capitellum to be alone separated.

The separation of this epiphysis will be entirely within the capsule.

Hahn, of Stuttgart, has recorded an interesting fracture of this process in an old woman, aged sixty-seven. The elbow had been injured four years previously, when she was in a state of intoxication, so that no account could be obtained of the circumstances of the accident.

The olecranon and coronoid fossæ were filled up by new osseous material. The capitellum was separated at its base from the epicondyle and from the external aspect of the trochlea; it was displaced forwards and upwards, and formed with the epicondyle an almost right angle; at its upper border it adhered and became blended with the osseous mass which filled the radial depression of the humerus. The anterior aspect of the epicondyle and the posterior aspect of the detached fragment limited an excavation in which the radial head lodged. The latter was in its normal position, and was held in relation with the lesser sigmoid cavity of the ulna by means of the annular (orbicular) ligament. The humerus was also in contact with the great sigmoid cavity of the ulna. From the anterior aspect of the epicondyle there projected an osseous plate (lamella), which passed in front and to the inner side of the capitellum without touching it. A similar plate stood out from the anterior aspect of the epitrochlea, and extended downwards and inwards towards the coronoid process.

Gurlt also met with a specimen in an adult in which the capitellum was broken off, displaced upwards, and united to the radial depression. The injury was not diagnosed during life.

In a case recorded by G. A. Wright (*Guy's Hospital Reports*, 1879, 3rd Series, vol. xxiv. p. 53) a strumous boy, aged twelve, had a fracture detaching the capitellum. He had fallen down, striking the right elbow against a wall in his fall, the arm at the time being in a flexed position. No fracture or dislocation was discovered. There ensued pulpy degeneration of the joint, which demanded excision. On opening the joint it was discovered that there had been a fracture of the capitellum, which had been chipped off; the part separated appeared from its size to represent only a portion of the epiphysis developed from the capitellar centre of ossification. It was, therefore, a true fracture, and not analogous to the separation of an epiphysis.

The capitellum may be rotated round its vertical or transverse axis, as well as displaced in either direction, as in Mr. Bryant's case of separation of external epicondyle and capitellum complicated with dislocation. Mr. Jonathan Hutchinson junior, assisted at an operation on a case of this kind performed by Mr. Treves several months after the accident (*Brit. Med. Journ.*, November 3, 1894, p. 967) in which the capitellum was found to be completely turned round, so that its normal lower surface faced upwards, and in which considerable improvement followed its removal.'

ETIOLOGY.—The *violence* may be **direct** or **indirect**, as in falls upon the radial side of the hand.

Hahn attributed to a fall upon the hand, when the forearm was flexed, his specimen of fracture of the condyle (capitellum) ; but it is difficult to see how the fragment could have been driven upwards by the radius unless the forearm was in the extended position at the time of the accident.

SYMPTOMS.—When the epiphysis is but little displaced, an exact diagnosis is almost impossible, as there is no deformity.

Crepitus on rotation of the radius or during extreme pronation and supination will be the most constant sign ; indeed, this, together with pain, especially on manipulation, and some loss of active movement of the elbow, are the only immediate signs of fracture.

Pain on rotation of the radius is often considerable.

Swelling and **synovitis** rapidly ensue, as the injury is entirely within the joint, while **impaired movement of limb** is a noticeable sign.

In Hahn's case the symptoms presented by the patient the day after the accident were as follows: Voluntary movements absent ; passive movements limited and very painful ; forearm bent almost to a right angle ; distinct crepitus below the external condyle (epicondyle). The olecranon, coronoid, epicondyle, and epitrochlea were in their proper position and immovable. In front of the external condyle (epicondyle) there was an abnormal and rounded projection, which at first was taken for the dislocated head of the radius ; but as this projection remained immovable during pronation and supination of the forearm, and when, in displacing it with the fingers, crepitus could be detected, the diagnosis of fracture of the neck of the radius was made out. The patient recovered very well, with only some hampering of movements of flexion and extension of the forearm. The exact condition of the parts was disclosed by the autopsy four years later (see above).

Mr. L. A. Dunn showed, at the Clinical Society, November 25, 1892 (*Lancet*, December 3, 1892, p. 1273), a boy, aged seven, who had a piece of loose bone in his elbow-joint. He had fallen down and injured the elbow three years previously. The part separated seemed to be the capitellum of the humerus, which had become loosely attached to the head of the radius. It was situated between the head of the radius and the lower extremity of the humerus. It was somewhat disc-shaped, and measured $1\frac{1}{4}$ inches in diameter and $\frac{1}{2}$ inch in depth, quite movable apart from both humerus and radius, although more nearly connected with the latter. All the movements of the normal elbow could be perfectly performed.

Rotation of the capitellar fragment in this injury, as well as in epicondylo-capitellar fracture, is probably more frequent than is generally supposed. It is caused by extreme flexion of the forearm in the semipronate position.

COMPLICATIONS.—**Dislocation of elbow** is probably not an uncommon.complication.

In Wright's case the inflammation of the elbow-joint led to a more serious result—viz. pulpy disease, for which excision of the joint was performed.

PROGNOSIS.—**Deformity** may not be great, yet **ankylosis** will be inevitable if sufficient and appropriate treatment be not employed, while **arrest of growth of the outer part of the humerus** will be slight.

TREATMENT.—The flexed position of the elbow is the best after reduction of the displaced capitellum. Anterior or posterior angular wooden splints or moulded casing are equally serviceable. Inflammation of the joint should be subdued by appropriate applications.

Passive motion should be commenced early, about the tenth day, and gently continued each day until the cure is effected.

SEPARATION OF THE CAPITELLAR AND TROCHLEAR EPIPHYSES OF THE HUMERUS (INFRA-EPICONDYLOID SEPARATION OF THE LOWER EPIPHYSIS OF THE HUMERUS)

It cannot be supposed that such a diastasis entirely within the joint could occur without being accompanied by that of the external epicondylar epiphysis. This would then be a separation of the lower epiphysis after puberty.

By the time the internal epicondyle is completely separated from the rest of the lower end of the humerus, the external epicondyle is firmly blended with the capitellum, but a small portion of the latter is in relation with the outer part of the humeral diaphysis.

Pingaud states that the Pathological Museum of Josephine in Vienna possesses a very remarkable specimen of simultaneous fracture of the trochlea and condyle (capitellum), which have been carried in one mass forwards and upwards; but the detached fragment, instead of slipping upwards parallel to its great axis, has rotated for almost a quarter of an inch, so that the articular cylindrical mass was almost parallel to the general direction of the humerus.

In this position the condyle (capitellum) was joined above to the coronoid fossa, whilst the trochlea, which was free below, chiefly covered it without adhering to it.

Gurlt has had such a specimen in an adult.

Holmes says: 'It is quite conceivable, and may be true, that fracture might occur through the line of junction of the trochlea and capitellum below with the shaft and condyles above, but in order to prove the reality of this injury, anatomical examination is absolutely necessary.'

Other writers also mention that, exceptionally, the capitellum and trochlea alone are separated, the condyles remaining *in situ*, and designate it *infra-condyloid separation of the epiphysis*.

This lesion corresponds to Professor R. W. Smith's separation of the lower epiphysis of the humerus. It is only necessary, therefore, to refer the reader to Chapter V., Part II.

CHAPTER XI

SEPARATION OF THE UPPER EPIPHYSIS OF THE ULNA

ANATOMY.—The cartilaginous upper end of the ulna at birth, and for the first few years of life, is seen to include nearly the upper half of the olecranon process, and a strip of cartilage passes down the front articular aspect of the olecranon, covering the upper aspect of the coronoid process as a thin lamella.

This strip of cartilage gradually disappears by the upward growth of the olecranon and shaft of the ulna, so that by the eighth year almost all that remains is the epiphysis of the olecranon process. The greater part of the olecranon is thus formed by the upward growth of the shaft. But often as late as the tenth year, and later, a portion of cartilage may still be found forming the summit of the coronoid process; it disappears during the growth and development of the coronoid, without, as a rule, undergoing any ossification.

Some anatomists have described a separate nucleus for the coronoid process, but this has not been generally confirmed nor has the author met with it.

The olecranon epiphysis is but a small process, occupying little more than a third of the whole olecranon at about the tenth year. In this cartilage ossification appears at the summit of the olecranon as a single nucleus usually at this period—in rare cases a year or two sooner, more often a little later— and rapidly invades the whole.

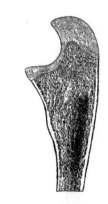

FIG. 131.—SAGITTAL SECTION OF UPPER END OF ULNA AT THE AGE OF SEVEN YEARS. THE OSSEOUS CENTRE FOR THE SUMMIT OF THE OLECRANON HAS NOT YET APPEARED

A second nucleus is very often seen, it may be as early as the fifth year, and forms the outer side of the upper part of the sigmoid cavity and the tip or beak of the olecranon, and a small portion of the inner side of the sigmoid cavity (upper part). This nucleus

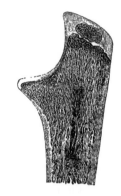

encroaches but little on the posterior aspect, and unites with the rest of the epiphysis soon after the commencement of the ninth year.

In the fully ossified state, at the fifteenth year, the epiphysis comprises the upper aspect of the olecranon with the insertion of the triceps, part of the attachment of the posterior ligament of the elbow-joint, and a small portion of the upper part (less than a quarter of an inch) of the triangular subcutaneous surface posteriorly; on the inner side it is above the tubercle for the

Fig. 132.—UPPER END OF ULNA AT ABOUT THE TWELFTH YEAR. (AFTER RAMBAUD AND RENAULT)

flexor carpi ulnaris.

This epiphysis, with its forward projection, enters very little into the formation of the elbow-joint.

The chief part of the olecranon is formed by the upward extension of the diaphysis, so that it is quite incorrect to state, as most text-

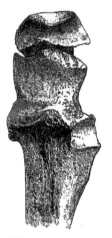

books do, that the union of this epiphysis with the shaft is marked by a constriction below the centre, at the base, of the olecranon—the usual situation of fracture of the olecranon.

The epiphysial line slopes obliquely downwards and backwards from the articular surface in front—viz. the upper part of the sigmoid cavity. At the age of fourteen and a half years the whole of the olecranon is about one-inch long, and the epiphysis, which is now largely composed of osseous tissue, is rather more than three-eighths of an inch long (ten millimetres), so that this process forms slightly more than a third of the whole olecranon. The epiphysis at

Fig. 133.—OSSIFICATION OF OLECRANON EPIPHYSIS ALMOST COMPLETE, AT THE FOURTEENTH YEAR

(Specimen, Royal College of Surgeons Museum)

this age is fifteen millimetres in width laterally, and thirteen millimetres thick antero-posteriorly.

This epiphysis unites with the shaft at the seventeenth year. Some anatomists state that it may remain disconnected throughout life, but the author has been unable to find any specimen to confirm this. The union is generally effected before that of the lower end of the humerus.

The anterior surface of the olecranon epiphysis—viz. the extreme upper part of the sigmoid cavity—forms but a small part of the articular surface. A small process of the synovial membrane overlaps its upper edge in front of the attachment of the posterior ligament of the elbow-joint.

The epiphyses of the bones of the arm and forearm at the elbow-joint commence to ossify *later*, but join their respective diaphyses *earlier*, than the epiphyses at the opposite ends of these bones; while the epiphyses of the femur and tibia (the upper epiphysis of the fibula being exceptional) at the knee-joint are the earliest to ossify and the latest to join with their diaphyses.

Bérard's law is thus verified, as in the humerus, radius, and ulna the nutrient canals are directed *towards* the elbow; in the femur and bones of the leg they are directed *away* from the knee.

PATHOLOGICAL ANATOMY.
Separation of the olecranon epiphysis is one of the rarest forms of epiphysial detachment. The only specimens in the London museums occurred in infancy, while this epiphysis is still cartilaginous, and both were the results of direct violence.

In the one, the whole cartilaginous end was detached; in the other, only the olecranon portion.

The specimen in St. Mary's Hospital Museum, No. 97 (*Catalogue of Pathological Museum of St. Mary's Hospital*, 1891, p. 10), shows a separation of the whole cartilaginous upper end of the ulna, including the upper surface of the coronoid process, in one piece.

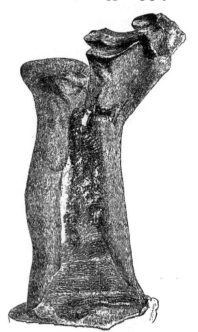

Fig. 134.—COMPLETE SEPARATION OF THE WHOLE CARTILAGINOUS UPPER END OF THE ULNA IN A CHILD AGED THREE YEARS (St. Mary's Hospital Museum. Natural size)

It was held to the diaphysis merely by a tag of periosteum at the posterior part, and there was present also a greenstick fracture of the shaft one and a quarter inch below the coronoid process.

The child, aged about three years, was admitted with compound dislocation of the elbow-joint. There was also much laceration of the soft parts, and division of the ulnar artery and nerve, in addition to the fractures just mentioned. Amputation was performed at the elbow-joint by Mr. Owen, and the patient made a good recovery.

The other specimen in St. George's Hospital Museum, Series 1, No. 110 (*Catalogue of St. George's Hospital Museum*, 1866, p. 37), is figured by Holmes (*Surgical Diseases of Children*, 1868, p. 264, fig. 48), and shows the line of fracture traversing the cartilaginous base of the olecranon in a child aged two years. There was also a compound dislocation of the radius forwards (the head of the bone lying exposed in a large lacerated wound), but the shaft was entire. The ulna was fractured below its middle. The injury, which had been caused by a carriage-wheel passing over the arm, proved fatal from pyæmia.

In the author's case, which occurred at the Miller Hospital in 1893, the specimen is probably a unique one. The separation of the olecranon process was a pure one, and took place at the age of six years; it was accompanied by fracture immediately above the lower epiphysial line of the humerus, whose lower epiphysis was displaced forwards (see Part II., Chap. IV., page 280, and fig. 71). The olecranon epiphysis is seen (three months after the accident) to be displaced backwards off the ulna and firmly united to the posterior aspect of the lower end of the humeral diaphysis.

Helferich represents a separation of the olecranon epiphysis with longitudinal fracture of the upper end of the ulna, which complicated a partial separation of the lower epiphysis of the humerus, the result of a severe machine accident (see page 275).

Once, in his experiments, Cruveilhier detached the olecranon epiphysis with the cartilaginous upper end of the coronoid process, to the latter of which some osseous granules adhered.

Berthomier found, in his experiments on the elbows of children, that displacement of the epiphysis of the olecranon was excessively rare on account of its being held in position by the triceps and internal lateral ligament.

The author has, however, on more than one occasion detached and displaced this process on the dead subject, by extreme extension of the elbow.

Compound separation of olecranon epiphysis without displacement.—In October 1883 a case came under the care of Mr. Bryant at Guy's Hospital in which the author had the opportunity of dissecting the specimen. He (the author) came to the conclusion that it was a case of partial separation without displacement, but complicated with a wound leading to suppuration of the joint and destruction of part of the cartilaginous portion of the epiphysis.

Jas. F., aged fourteen, slipped and fell with some violence on his right elbow, causing a small wound over the olecranon, which bled profusely at the time. Two days later he was admitted into the hospital with suppuration of the wound and extensive inflammation of elbow and forearm. Suppuration of the joint ensued, and an incision was made, evacuating pus and revealing the presence of necrosis about the olecranon. Two months after the accident excision was performed on account of disorganisation of the joint. The olecranon epiphysis was then quite loose, the cartilage surrounding the exposed osseous nucleus much eroded, and over the olecranon a deposit had been made of new bone from the periosteum.

AGE.—Separation of the whole cartilaginous upper end of the ulna is possible only before the eighth year or thereabouts, and pure separation of the olecranon epiphysis can only occur from about the tenth year to the seventeenth or eighteenth, the time of junction with the epiphysis.

Of the nine cases recorded, three recent *pathological specimens* occurred in patients at the age of two, three, and six respectively, while in one somewhat older pathological specimen the injury occurred about the sixteenth year.

Of the two *compound separations* the age is given only in one— viz. at fourteen years.

Of the three *simple cases* one was at eight, one at seven, and one at four years of age.

ETIOLOGY.—The rarity of this injury in children, as compared with fractures of the olecranon process in adults, may be accounted for, to some extent, by the small size and less prominent projection of this process in the former.

The posterior aspect of this epiphysis in children before the fourteenth year is on a plane anterior to that of the epicondyles and posterior aspect of the diaphysis of the humerus when the elbow is at a right angle. Consequently, in falls upon the elbow and in other injuries the force of the blow is much more likely to be received by the epicondyles than by the olecranon.

Cheever says that ' the olecranon epiphysis is easily separated in childhood.'

Guéretin was able to separate this epiphysis on the dead subject only by forcible hyperextension, but the lower epiphysis of the humerus usually gave way in this manner.

Colignon was unable to produce a separation of this epiphysis.

Direct violence.—The injury is commonly caused by a fall upon the back of the elbow while the elbow is in a flexed position, or by some other direct blow.

Direct violence was the cause of separation in Eames's case.

In 1885 at Guy's Hospital Mr. Davies-Colley diagnosed a separation of the point of the olecranon, which was also broken in two, in the case of a boy, aged eight, who had fallen a distance of forty feet from a bridge over a railway line. There was also separation of the lower epiphysis of each radius. The patient did well, but flexion and extension of the elbow were somewhat limited.

At this early age the epiphysis has not any trace of ossification; it is more usual for its osseous nucleus to appear after the tenth year than at an earlier period. In this instance, therefore, it is more probable that the upper cartilaginous end was much com-

minuted by direct violence than that a true fracture of this process
had occurred combined with separation.

Indirect violence.—*Extreme flexion of the elbow* may cause separation.

In Hamilton's case of old dislocation of the elbow in a boy, aged
seven, forcible flexion produced this lesion.

Hyperextension may likewise produce it, as shown by the post-
mortem experiments of Salmon and many observers. The author has
readily effected it in this way on three occasions. During this over-
extension the apex of the olecranon impinges against the posterior
aspect of the lower end of the humerus and breaks off the epiphysis
of this portion of the bone.

An experimental specimen in the Royal College of Surgeons
Museum (No. 946A), by Mr. Jonathan Hutchinson junior, 1889,
gives the posterior view of the elbow-joint of a child, aged nineteen
months, in whom forcible hyperextension after death resulted in
separation and backward displacement of the olecranon epiphysis,
which is seen by section to be wholly cartilaginous. The attachment of the triceps to the epiphysis is shown, and the periosteum is
stripped off the shaft for about an inch.

Lonsdale was the first to suggest this mode of fracture of the
olecranon in the adult.

Muscular action.—It has been supposed that separation may also be
occasioned by the violent contraction of the triceps during extension
of the forearm. It is, however, questionable whether in children
the action of this muscle is sufficiently powerful to detach this
process, unless it be combined with one or other of the causes mentioned above.

SYMPTOMS.—The symptoms are almost the same as those of
fracture of the olecranon. As in fractured olecranon, the thick
periosteum and tendinous structure prevent any extensive displacement.

SEPARATION WITHOUT DISPLACEMENT.—In some instances there
may be no displacement of the fragment whatever, from its being
held in position by the periosteum and ligamentous structures,
and by the tendinous expansion of the triceps being attached to the
lateral margins and posterior aspect of the olecranon process, as
well as (the thick part of its tendon) fixed into the posterior part
of its upper surface, not into the beak-like tip of this process.

Pain, swelling, and **mobility** are the chief signs, while **crepitus** may
be often perceptible.

Surgeon William Eames records (*British Medical Journal*, July
16, 1887, p. 124) a fracture of the olecranon in a child of four years
which was doubtless one of separation of this epiphysis. The boy
(P. A.), whilst walking, slipped and fell with the whole weight of
his body on the point of his right elbow. On examination there
was some fulness over the olecranon, and a fracture of the upper

half of the olecranon was found, the upper fragment being freely movable, with soft cartilaginous crepitus in a lateral direction, but with no separation to be detected between the fragments. There was inability to extend the arm, and flexion was partially impaired. The limb was treated by being placed in a long splint in the fully extended position.

SEPARATION WITH DISPLACEMENT. **Deformity.**—In other instances the *displacement* of the epiphysis may be considerable and *upwards*, not so much owing to the action of the triceps muscle as to the displacement of the lower fragment away from the upper. Below the detached epiphysis a *depression* will be felt at the back of the elbow-joint, which can be rendered more distinct on flexing the forearm, and be diminished by extending it.

Hamilton relates the case of a boy, aged seven years, who had an unreduced dislocation of the radius and ulna backwards of nine weeks' standing. While reducing this dislocation, it became necessary to flex the arm forcibly. The epiphysis constituting the olecranon process gave way, and became separated from one half to three quarters of an inch. This is the only example of separation of this epiphysis which had come to his knowledge.

A case of fractured olecranon in a young girl recorded by Sir Astley Cooper has been quoted on insufficient grounds as a case of separation of the olecranon epiphysis.

Marked displacement may not be present directly after the injury. A mere chink or depression just sufficient to admit the finger-nail is all that may be detected at first at the back of the elbow. After the lapse of a day or two we may detect the separation and place the finger between the fragments.

The action of the triceps in causing separation of the epiphysis is even less efficient than in fracture in adults. It is, however, a very important factor in maintaining the displacement of the epiphysis when once this has taken place.

Mobility of epiphysis.—This epiphysis is so small a shell of bone that it can be grasped with difficulty if much swelling be present. It will be found to be movable from side to side. If it has been displaced, it will be discovered immediately above the depression at the upper end of the triangular subcutaneous surface of the olecranon by extending the forearm, which will bring the fragments together.

Muffled crepitus.—This will be easily detected during the lateral movement of the epiphysis, but when displacement has taken place it can only be discovered by extending the forearm and approximating the fragments.

Ecchymosis and swelling.—The former is less marked in cases caused by indirect violence than direct violence ; but at times the swelling about the elbow will be so great as to entirely obscure the outline of the olecranon and the gap between the fragments. In such cases it will be better to wait till this has subsided before expressing a definite opinion on the character of the injury—i.e. if an examination under an anæsthetic has been refused.

Pain.—The pain is not very great, except when the patient or surgeon attempts to flex or extend the elbow. It is most acute over the upper end of the olecranon process.

Synovitis.—There is sure to be more or less effusion into the joint as the separation passes into the articular cavity. It will be considerable when the joint is freely opened in displacement of the epiphysis, which lacerates the synovial membrane at the posterior part.

When the effusion of blood and fluid in the joint is great, it may tend to keep the fragments from being brought together.

Loss of power of the forearm, especially in extension by the patient, will be present to a greater or less extent according to the amount of displacement, whereas flexion can be readily effected. In many instances where the displacement is slight and the triceps expansion incompletely lacerated, the power of extension will be retained to a considerable degree.

Flexion of the elbow gives rise to great pain at the seat of the disjunction.

DIFFERENTIAL DIAGNOSIS. Fracture of the olecranon.—In epiphysial separation the character of the *crepitus* and the *form and situation* of the separated fragment are sufficient to render it distinguishable from fracture of the olecranon.

Hamilton falls into the common error in supposing that the place where the epiphysis joins the shaft is below the centre of the olecranon, the most common situation for fracture ; he says : ' Fractures of the middle (of the olecranon) are generally transverse, and only slightly oblique, occurring in the line of the junction of the epiphysis with the diaphysis.'

On the other hand, the annual surgical reports of several of the London hospitals mention in their statistics numerous cases of fracture of the olecranon before adolescence, many of which were probably examples of epiphysial separation.

Guedeney (*Du traitement des fractures du coude chez l'enfant*, &c., Lyon, 1893), while stating that fracture (*sic*) of the olecranon is rare in children, was able to record four cases out of sixty injuries to the elbow-joint in these young subjects. A fifth is classed as a separation of the olecranon epiphysis with laceration of the internal lateral ligament, but neither the age nor any other details are given of this case. Of the four cases of fracture, the first was a boy (J. B.), aged ten and a half. There was enormous swelling and great extravasation of blood even into the joint, with abnormal mobility and crepitus. The joint could be moved laterally, showing that the internal lateral ligament had been lacerated. In the second, a girl (J. M.), aged eight and a half, had a blow against a door a month previously. The fracture of the olecranon was accompanied by juxta-epiphysial sprain of the radius with periostitis; also great swelling of the forearm.   In the third case, of a boy (F. T.) aged (?), the fracture of the olecranon was incomplete and accompanied by laceration of the internal lateral ligament.   In the fourth case, of a boy (C. D.), eleven and a half years, the detachment of the olecranon was complicated by complete dislocation backwards of the bones of the forearm.   Crepitus was clearly made out.   There were, besides, fracture (*sic*) of the lower end of the radius, with 'back of fork' deformity, detachment of the styloid process of the ulna, and abnormal mobility of the wrist.   These lesions had been caused by a simple fall from the boy's own height on to the dorsal aspect of the hand.

All the above five cases were treated by a plaster splint in the extended position with a successful result, especially as regards the free movement of the joint.

The *age* of the patient will not assist us greatly; for although Hulke (Holmes's *System of Surgery*, 1882, vol. i. p. 961) says that fracture of the olecranon is almost unknown before the age of fifteen, cases have been recorded by Hamilton in a boy aged fourteen years, and in the Warren Museum, according to Packard, there is a specimen removed by excision of the elbow from a patient at the age of twenty-three years who had injured his elbow when eight years old.

Fletcher has reported (*Medical Times and Gazette*, 1851, vol. ii. p. 173) a case of complete osseous union of fracture of both olecranons in a boy aged sixteen years, who had fallen over some timber a short time before.   There was separation to the extent of a finger's breadth on both sides.   Swelling not great.   Fragments loose and movable in any direction.   Full use of both arms took place after treatment in the extended position.   Death occurred ten months later from phthisis.   On dissection the signs of fracture were an irregular furrow on the surface of each sigmoid cavity two lines wide, along which the articular cavity was entirely wanting.   On the right olecranon this furrow was three-eighths and on the left five-eighths of an inch from the humeral end.   Posteriorly there was no furrow or projection, but a slight deviation from the normal line beginning about an inch from the humeral extremity.   On section, the cancellated structure above the line of fracture 'was slightly condensed, but all remains of the callus seem to have been removed.'

Professor Annandale (' On some Injuries implicating the Elbow-joint,' *Edinburgh Medical Journal*, February 1885, vol. xxx. part ii. p. 688) records another instance of fractured olecranon in a boy aged sixteen in which he resected the ends of the fragments and successfully wired them together.   The elbow had received a kick from a horse five months previously.

PROGNOSIS.—**Bony union** should always be expected when the fragment has been properly reduced, and if passive movements

H H

be carried out at an early period the limb will entirely recover its functions.

Should **fibrous union** occur from the displacement of the upper fragment, and leave only a short gap between the fragments, the utility of the elbow will be but little impaired.

In one case out of three of fracture of the olecranon process Hamilton found osseous union. A boy (P. C.), aged fourteen, fractured his olecranon. Sixty-nine years after the accident—he being then eighty-three years old—the olecranon process united by bone. He could not, however, straighten the arm completely nor supine it freely. In the other two cases the bond of union was ligamentous. J. C., aged eighteen, fractured his right olecranon process. It was treated with a straight splint. Nine years later the process was united by a ligament half an inch in length, and he could nearly, but not entirely, straighten the arm. In all other respects the functions and motions of the arm were perfect. The other case was a lad aged fifteen, whose olecranon process had been broken by a fall six months previously, and at the same time the head of the radius had been dislocated forwards. Hamilton found the radius in place, and the olecranon process united by a ligament about half an inch in length. The patient was not able to straighten the arm completely, the forearm remaining at an angle of forty-five degrees with the arm.

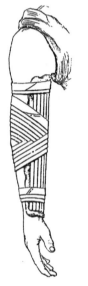

IG. 135.—STRAIGHT ANTERIOR SPLINT (GOOCH'S SPLINTING) FROM SHOULDER TO WRIST FOR SEPARATION OF THE OLECRANON

A bandage is applied in oblique turns to the elbow-joint above and below the olecranon to prevent displacement of its epiphysis. (After Spence)

Ankylosis is a serious occurrence, from adhesions taking place within the joint. It may occur from neglect to move the joint. Permanent ankylosis is unlikely to result when this has been properly performed, whether the elbow be kept in the extended or flexed position

TREATMENT.—All cases should be put up at once in the completely **extended position**, and maintained in that position by a long anterior straight splint, or other suitable apparatus, extending from the shoulder to the end of the metacarpal bones. The olecranon must be secured in its natural position.

We must not wait until swelling has subsided, as recommended by some surgeons, for it will be found very much more difficult to straighten the forearm subsequently than it would have been at first, and there will be the risk of the olecranon becoming displaced, if this had not occurred already. Should displacement of the olecranon have taken place, it will be still further drawn up and fixed in that position. The synovial fluid, being in contact with the fractured ends of the bone, will not only tend to prevent the accurate apposition of the fragments, but, by lining the surfaces with synovial lymph, may entirely stop the formation of osseous union between the fragments.

This position has been almost universally adopted for fractured olecranon in England since the time of Sir A. Cooper, and in France also—following the authority of Roux, Malgaigne, and Dupuytren.

Where *displacement* has occurred, the exact apposition of the fragments—the most important factor in the treatment, which should be aimed at in all cases—can only be brought about by extension of the arm. In this position only can the triceps be relaxed, and the descent of the epiphysis permitted.

The circular and transverse bandages of Sir Astley Cooper, above and below the olecranon, with lateral tapes to draw them together, to which also a straight anterior splint is added, will be found sufficient in some cases to bring the fragments into contact where there is little displacement.

The descent of the olecranon may be aided by the fingers, and a pad of lint placed above the process.

In the eighteenth century, Camper was the first to try fixation of the fragments in fracture of the olecranon, but he appears to have soon abandoned this method and followed all his early predecessors by treating these injuries without any immobilisation.

Some modern surgeons have recommended the limb to be placed in a **semiflexed position,** in the opinion that, should ankylosis occur, the arm will be in its best position for the performance of all its functions. This is met by the statement that ankylosis is rarely observed when the arm is treated by extension or flexion in a proper manner, and that it is only in exceptionally severe and complicated cases, or where the proper movement of the joint has been neglected, that ankylosis has been met with in the adult.

Aspiration of the joint.—This may be necessary when the effusion of blood and serum due to the lacerated synovial membrane of the joint prevents the fragments being brought together. It should be performed only in exceptional cases to secure exact apposition of the fragments : the intra-articular effusion in this case being so great as to prevent the fragments being brought together.

The splint described as follows by Hamilton for fractures of the olecranon with great displacement appears to be at once effectual and simple.

'The surgeon will prepare—extemporaneously always, for no single pattern will fit two arms—a splint from a piece of thin light board. This must be long enough to reach from near the wrist-joint

to within three or four inches of the shoulder, and of a width nearly
or quite equal to the widest part of the limb. Its width must be
uniform throughout, except that, at a point corresponding to a point
three inches, or thereabouts, below the top of the olecranon process,
there shall be a notch on each side, or a slight narrowing of the
splint. One surface of the splint is now to be thickly padded with
hair or cotton-batting, so as to fit all the irregularities of the arm,
forearm, and elbow, and the whole covered neatly with a piece of
cotton cloth, stitched together upon the back of the splint. Thus
prepared, it is to be laid upon the palmar surface of the limb, and a
roller is to be applied, commencing at the hand and covering the
splint, by successive circular turns, until the notch is reached, from
which point the roller is to pass upwards and backwards behind the
olecranon process and down again to the same point on the opposite
side of the splint; after making a second oblique turn above the
olecranon, to render it more secure, the roller may begin gradually
to descend, each turn being less oblique, and passing through the
same notch, until the whole of the back of the elbow-joint is covered.
This completes the adjustment of the fragments, and it only remains
to carry the roller again upwards, by circular turns, until the whole
arm is covered as high as the top of the splint. The advantages of
this method are apparent.

'It leaves, on each side of the splint, a space upon which neither
the splint nor bandage can make pressure, and the circulation of the
limb is therefore unembarrassed, while it is equally effective in
retaining the olecranon in place, and much less liable to become
disarranged.

'We must always keep in mind the fact that, the fracture being
usually the result of a direct blow, considerable inflammation and
swelling around the joint are about to follow rapidly; and on each
successive day, or oftener if necessary, the bandages must be examined
carefully and promptly loosened whenever it seems to be necessary.
For this purpose it is better not to unroll the bandages, but to cut
them with a pair of scissors along the face of the splint, cutting only
a small portion at a time, and, as they draw back, stitch them together
again lightly; and thus proceed until the whole has been rendered
sufficiently loose.'

Plaster-of-Paris bandages should be avoided if possible.

Extension of the arm by a weight in bed has been advocated, but
has not proved very satisfactory, in fracture of the olecranon.

Passive motion.—Passive motion should be commenced about the
fourteenth day. If there is much effusion into the joint, this may be
delayed a little longer. The finger and thumb should be placed above
the olecranon epiphysis, and pressure made upon it downwards. The
elbow should then be gently flexed to a very slight extent, and the
limb replaced on the straight splint. This should be continued daily
until the third week, when the straight splint should be replaced by

an angular one, or by an immovable moulded splint flexed to a right angle or less.   From this time the flexion may be daily increased until consolidation has taken place, or, at least, it may be carried as far as the inflammatory condition will permit.

The angle of the splint should be changed from time to time.

After the fragment has firmly united, and all fear of separating the epiphysis has vanished, the patient should commence to use the limb, and passive motion should be continued for a considerable time.

Extra-articular suture.—Mr. Mayo-Robson's plan of fixing (*Clinical Society's Transactions*, 1889, p. 286) the fragments in position by means of extra-articular pins is at once simple and effectual in certain cases when other means have failed to bring the fragments into apposition.

Carefully cleansed steel pins are passed, under antiseptic precautions, through the skin and triceps above the upper fragment, and another below the upper end of the lower fragment through the skin and dense structures over the back of the olecranon, and a figure-of-eight asepticised silk is passed over the ends of the pins (not over the olecranon, the pins being drawn together by gentle traction) and an anterior straight splint applied.   Antiseptic dressings are then applied and left on for about two weeks.

By this method Mr. Robson, in a case of fractured olecranon, apparently secured bony union without any stiffness of the elbow-joint.

Wiring of the fragments in position.—This should only be undertaken in cases of *compound separation* under strict antiseptic precautions, and in other *extreme and quite exceptional cases of non-union* of the epiphysis in childhood, the patient being thereby incapacitated from using his arm and unable to gain his livelihood in later life.

This operation may also be necessary after ununited fractures of the olecranon in older subjects just about the time of union of the epiphysis with the upper end of the bone.

Dr. A. E. Morison (*Lancet*, November 23, 1896, p. 1531) wired the olecranon of a boy, aged sixteen, who had fallen on his elbow five months previously.   The olecranon was freely movable, and separated three-quarters of an inch from the upper end of the ulna. There being inability to extend the forearm, with much weakness and wasting of the muscles, especially the triceps, a longitudinal incision was made over the elbow posteriorly, and the ends of the upper and lower fragments were sawn off, opening the elbow-joint. The bones were brought into apposition by two strands of silver wire passed through a hole drilled in each, and the wound closed without drainage.   In ten days it was entirely healed.   The movements of the arm were now perfect, but the joint a little weak.   The union was so firm that it would have been regarded as bony if skiagraphs had not shown a clear line at the junction of the apposed surfaces.

This was considered to be cartilage, and would ultimately become bone.

Mr. G. A. Wright, of Manchester, once wired (Ashby and Wright, *Diseases of Children, Medical and Surgical*, 2nd edit., 1892, p. 707) a case of compound separation of the upper epiphysis of the ulna with a good result.

COMPOUND SEPARATIONS.—The wound must be thoroughly cleansed, and all portions of soiled tissue removed.

The joint should be carefully washed out with some antiseptic lotion, and the fragments brought together with wire or carbolised silk.

Ankylosis should be very carefully guarded against, and measures taken to combat the articular inflammation which must result from the opening of the joint.

Should the bone be much comminuted, or the wound improperly treated from the first, and asepticism neglected, *excision of the joint*, as probably affording a better and more speedy recovery, should not be delayed as a secondary procedure. To secure a useful limb is certainly preferable to risking a patient's life from prolonged suppuration of the joint, or even from pyæmia. The operation unperformed would involve, at the best, a very protracted recovery, with the certainty of ankylosis ensuing.

SEPARATION OF THE UPPER EPIPHYSIS (HEAD) OF THE RADIUS

ANATOMY.—The osseous nucleus for the head of the radius appears in the centre of the cartilaginous upper end at the commencement of the sixth year.

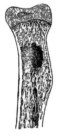

At the tenth year it is of a circular shape, about a centimetre in diameter, and placed rather to the outer and posterior side of the centre of the diaphysis, towards the part where the upper end of the diaphysis somewhat projects.

Rambaud and Renault describe a number of accessory osseous nuclei which are placed in a remarkable manner round the principal central plate, and, when joined together and to the central

FIG. 136.—UPPER END OF RADIUS AT THE SIXTH YEAR; MOSTLY CARTILAGE. ONE ELONGATED OSSEOUS NUCLEUS ONLY VISIBLE. (ACTUAL SIZE)

portion, form the characteristic concavity of the epiphysis. These pieces have each a triangular shape; their bases are turned outwards and constitute the rim of the cup; and together they make up an osseous crown bevelled off inwards. This part insinuates itself beneath the median disc, which is completely plane on both sides, and finally blends with it, forming one osseous mass.

About the sixteenth year the upper epiphysis is fully ossified, and towards the end of this, or the early part of the seventeenth, year joins the diaphysis; at times a little later. The upper extremity of the radius is there-fore remarkable as being, of all the epiphyses of the long bones, the last to become osseous and the first to unite with the shaft. The outer portion being the part to synostose first, the inner half of the epiphysial line, cor-responding to the lesser sigmoid cavity of the ulna, often remains distinct for a considerable time after the outer portion is quite obliterated.

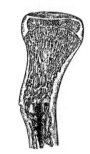

Fig. 137.—UPPER END OF RADIUS AT THE SIXTEENTH YEAR, AFTER RAMBAUD AND RENAULT

This epiphysis is of a bi-concave shape, narrower on the outer than the inner side, and includes only the upper part of the head— viz. the whole of the cartilage-clad area, part of which, round the inner edge, articulates with the lesser sigmoid cavity of the ulna, while the rest of the edge, the narrower portion, is surrounded by and rotates within the orbicular ligament.

The lower part of the head and the neck are ossified from the shaft.

In the fully formed epiphysis the depth (vertically) in the centre is only two millimetres, on the outer side five millimetres, while on the inner side it is one centimetre. At the fourteenth year it is three and a half millimetres on the outer side, and five and a half millimetres on the inner side.

In width laterally, at the fourteenth year it is sixteen milli-metres, and at the time of union with the shaft twenty-one millimetres.

The epiphysis is completely intra-articular.

The synovial membrane of the elbow-joint extends far beyond the epiphysial boundary of the head of the radius; completely lining the entire inner surface of the orbicular ligament, it passes off to blend above with the epiphysis of the head by a funnel-shaped process, being attached to the radius only by weak areolar tissue. Although highly probable, it is not absolutely necessary, that lacera-tion of the synovial membrane should accompany epiphysial separa-tion, since this synovial sac is so readily detached from the neck of the bone; yet by reason of its extent it must be especially liable to injury.

This epiphysis has no ligaments or tendons attached to it.

ETIOLOGY.   Direct violence.—It might at first be supposed that separation of this epiphysis could only occur as the result of direct violence, as in Mr. Mayo-Robson's and Mr. Mansell Moullin's cases.   Yet from the record of other cases it appears that **indirect violence** is more frequent, such as occurs in seizing the hand or forearm of a child when falling, and twisting it.

Dr. A. Foulerton gives (*Lancet*, October 2, 1886, p. 627, and October 30, p. 846) a note of a double fracture of the upper limb of a child by indirect violence.   One fracture was through the upper epiphysial line of the radius, and the other through the clavicle.

'A child, aged nineteen months, was being led along the street by his mother, who was holding his right hand.   The child stumbled, fell with a jerk, and was dragged up again—roughly, probably— by his mother, who, however, never let go his hand.   She then noticed that the boy's arm was quite powerless, and hung loosely by his side.   Shortly afterwards the child was brought to the Royal Isle of Wight Infirmary, where it was found that two fractures had occurred, one through the upper epiphysial line of the right radius, the other at the junction of the middle with the acromial third of the right clavicle.   One would certainly have expected dislocation rather than fracture as the result of such an accident occurring in so young a child, and Dr. Foulerton was unable to offer any exact explanation as to the mechanics of the lesion.

The signs upon which Dr. Foulerton based his diagnosis of epiphysial separation were as follows : genuine crepitus; some slight displacement of the upper end of the shaft, which displacement, having been once reduced, could without the exercise of any force be reproduced; non-participation of the head of the radius in movement communicated to the lower end.   Beyond this, when the fracture apparatus was removed, there was an irregular thickening around the upper end of the bone, which was believed to be callus.

Dr. Foulerton says that the age of the patient (nineteen months) and the nature of the accident (forcible traction on the arm) were both, it is true, against the *probability* of the lesion having been a fracture, but after careful examination no doubt was entertained as to the accuracy of the diagnosis.

AGE.—Of the two recent **pathological specimens**, in only one is the age stated—namely, at thirteen years.

Of the five **simple cases** the age is given in four—at twelve, eight, six years, and nineteen months of age.

PATHOLOGICAL ANATOMY.—The only specimen known to the author is in the London Hospital Museum (*London Hospital Museum Catalogue*, 1890, p. 96), No. 404A.   It is a compound separation caused by direct violence.   The upper epiphysis of the radius is clearly detached at the epiphysial line, and remains partly within the grasp of the orbicular ligament, the diaphysis projecting somewhat behind it.   The diaphysis is otherwise not injured, though the orbicular ligament is torn away. The synovial membrane of the joint still retains its connection to the head of the radius. The epiphysial disc remains with the epiphysis. The outer side of the elbow-joint has evidently borne the whole of the violence, as the capitellum is partially divided by a line of fracture passing downwards and inwards, in addition to the small epiphysis of the outer epicondyle and the adjoining part of the capitellum being torn off. The periosteum is only slightly detached at the anterior margin of the end of the shaft.

The patient was a lad aged thirteen years, who fell between a train and the platform, tearing off the skin of the forearm and lacerating the muscles. Primary amputation above the elbow-joint was performed, and he rapidly recovered. The case is reported by Mr. C. Mansell-Moullin in the Pathological Transactions for 1888, p. 242, and the specimen is figured by this surgeon (Mansell-Moullin, *Surgery*, 1891, fig. 118, p. 444).

Mr. Hutchinson junior, however, says (*British Medical Journal*, March 31, 1894, p. 669) there was another case at the London Hospital under his father (also from severe crushing force).

In both these instances the epiphysis lay loose in the elbow-joint.

SYMPTOMS. Impaired movements of elbow-joint.—When there is no displacement, all the movements of the joint will be found to be free.

When displacement has occurred, pronation and supination will be imperfectly performed, and complete extension and flexion not permitted.

Poucel ('Considérations sur les Disjonctions épiphysaires à propos d'une Observation de Disjonction traumatique de l'Épiphyse radiale supérieure;' *Marseille Méd.* 1869, vi. 847–858) has published a case of this injury, while Portal, in his *Anatomie médicale*, 1803, t. i. p. 424, alludes to separation of the upper epiphysis of the radius as of frequent occurrence and often mistaken for fracture. This author (*Anat. Méd.* t. ii. p. 31) has also recorded an example.

Yet Hamilton (*Fractures and Dislocations*, 1884, 7th edit. p. 355) says that he had not met with any recorded examples of separation of the upper epiphysis of the radius.

SEPARATION WITHOUT DISPLACEMENT.—There need be no deformity in any case if there has been no displacement.

The following example came under the author's treatment at the Miller Hospital in 1889.

Charles H., eight years old, had fallen down on his back with his right arm twisted behind. On lifting the child up, his mother heard a distinct crackle at the elbow.

On examination a few days after the injury, there was much effusion into the right elbow-joint, which considerably limited extension and to some extent flexion. The epicondyles were in normal relation with the olecranon, but on grasping with the finger and thumb the small head of the radius, which was in the normal position, and rotating the radius with the opposite hand, the head did not rotate with the diaphysis. This movement was accompanied by the usual muffled crepitus. On further examination, some unnatural mobility was detected between the epiphysis and shaft. There was no displacement of the bone. The patient could only slightly pronate the forearm, but not supinate in the slightest degree on account of the great pain which it caused him. Great pain was produced by pressure over the situation of the epiphysial line.

DISPLACEMENT OF THE DIAPHYSIS FORWARDS.—This is the most likely form of displacement to occur: a gap will then be felt below the *head of the radius*, which retains its *normal position* with the external epicondyle and capitellum. The shaft of the radius will be directed somewhat forwards, and will be felt to be somewhat closer than natural to that of the ulna.

When the diaphysis has completely cleared the epiphysis, the latter will be loose in the joint, being held only by the thin periosteum and synovial membrane covering the head and neck of the bone.

Unnatural mobility will be felt, but in the lateral direction, on seizing the small epiphysial head of the radius and grasping the shaft of the radius, also on rotation the former will be found to be motionless.

Pressure may likewise displace the separated head.

Muffled crepitus may be felt on bringing the diaphysis into its normal position with the head.

Pain on extreme extension and flexion, and on pressure over the situation of the head, will be found to be a constant sign.

Effusion into the elbow-joint will ensue with great rapidity, on account of the intra-articular character of the lesion.

PROGNOSIS.—If properly treated, all movements of the limb will be entirely recovered.

Mr. A. W. Mayo-Robson, however, gives (*Lancet*, March 21, 1885, p. 518) the following account of a boy, aged six, who was admitted into the Leeds General Infirmary with loss of supination, although the other movements of the forearm were perfect and the diaphysis greatly displaced. The parents stated that they had noticed impaired movement in the arm during the last four months, but on closer inquiry it was elicited that he had been run over by a cart four years before, and had been treated at the time for a bruise of the arm. On examination he complained of no pain, could flex, extend, and pronate the forearm completely, but could not supinate more than to place the hand vertical with the floor. The ulna could be traced along its whole length, and the olecranon bore a proper relation to the condyles, which were normal. The head of the radius was in position, but immediately below it was a hollow. The radius could be traced obliquely across the front of the forearm, from below upwards and inwards, ending in a hard bossy mass, apparently callus,

in front of and below the internal condyle of the humerus, where it
rotated in its new position. It was diagnosed from dislocation of
the head of the radius forwards by the detached head being felt in
its normal position, and by the ability to completely flex the forearm.
No treatment was recommended.—

DIFFERENTIAL DIAGNOSIS.—**Partial dislocation of the head cf
the radius in infants, or subluxation of the orbicular ligament.** Incomplete dislocation has been recently brought forward by several
writers as a new form of injury, though Nélaton, Sir Astley Cooper,
Goyrand, Malgaigne, Hamilton, and others have described and discussed cases of this kind in children.

As long ago as 1837 M. G. Goyrand (*Gazette Médicale de Paris,*
Février 1837, t. v. p. 115) treated of incomplete dislocation of the
upper end of the radius forwards, and its accompanying signs and
treatment. He moreover states that it is by no means a rare
accident from eighteen months to three years of age.

M. Pingaud has given (*Dict. Encycl. des Sc. Méd.* 1ère section, t. xxi.
1878, p. 575) a very exhaustive account of these injuries in children,
and figures the displacements which may occur to the head of the
radius from the slipping upwards of the orbicular ligament.

In this country Mr. Jonathan Hutchinson junior has again
drawn attention (*Annals of Surgery,* vol. ii. 1885, p. 91) to these
cases, which he calls ' elbow sprain ' or ' pulled elbow,' in infants and
young children. They are caused by the child being dragged along
by the arm, lifted by the hand or wrist, and swung round by the
arm, or may be the result of a fall. The head of the radius slips
below from beneath the orbicular ligament, and is partially displaced
forwards. The ligament rests in the angle between the radius and
capitellum.

This injury, he says, in the majority of cases is diagnosed as separation of the upper epiphysis of the radius, or fracture of the radial neck,
on account of the snapping sound produced either on reduction or at
the time of the accident, but this error is hardly possible if sufficient
care be taken, as in this injury the head of the radius lies free, and
can be felt in its abnormal position. All movements are free except
complete extension and supination, and a distinct click is heard at
the time of injury and on reduction. The forearm is generally
pronated and semiflexed. The subluxation is easily reduced by
flexion and full pronation of the forearm, and is accompanied by a
sound which might easily be mistaken for the cartilaginous crepitus
of the epiphysis upon the shaft.

This injury, Mr. Hutchinson thinks, never happens after five years
of age, because the head of the radius then becomes bony, and is no
longer elastic.

Van Arsdale reports (*Annals of Surgery,* 1889, vol. ix. p. 401)
one hundred cases of subluxation of the head of the radius in
children, and draws the following conclusions :

(1) The injury frequently occurring in childhood and called subluxation of the head, or displacement by elongation of the radius, is a well-defined typical injury, with well marked constant symptoms, and is due to the same anatomical lesion in every case.

(2) The frequency is over one per cent. of surgical injuries in children.

(3) It occurs in children under nine years of age.

(4) The most frequent exciting cause is sudden traction by the hand or forearm, or more rarely a fall.

(5) The principal symptoms of the injury are absence of appreciable deformity; loss of function of the arm; localised pain over the head of the radius on pressure; pronation of the hand; slight flexion of the elbow; crepitation or snapping upon forced supination, with restoration of function.

(6) Treatment with a splint is advisable, in order to prevent recurrence.

(7) The anatomical lesion causing the injury is not yet satisfactorily established.

In these cases this false crepitus may also be obtained by alternately pronating and supinating the forearm. The diagnosis will be made clear by the fact that the head of the radius will rotate with the shaft in cases of subluxation.

Again, in subluxation, after the reduction of the displacement, pain will be sooner removed and the joint become more quickly movable than in epiphysial separation, and in a short space of time little or no trace of the injury will be detected after subluxation.

Fracture of neck of radius may closely simulate epiphysial separation, especially if it be broken at its upper part.

The skiagram here reproduced of a fracture of the neck of the radius, complicated with a dislocation of the ulna backwards, was kindly placed at the author's disposal by Mr. Thomas Moore, of Blackheath, under whose care the patient was in June 1896. There was great displacement and rotation of the upper fragment of the radius. Another skiagram was taken by Mr. Moore after reduction of the dislocated ulna, which showed most clearly this bone in position, but the displacement of the head of the radius was then even more marked.

TREATMENT.—Replace the diaphysis and place the forearm in the flexed position by means of an anterior angular splint, to prevent the biceps displacing the diaphysis forwards. Antiphlogistic measures should be taken to subdue the inflammation of the elbow-joint.

Bardenheuer and Dr. L. C. Lane recommend extension for fractures of the upper end of the radius.

Passive motion at the end of the fourteenth day should be very cautiously commenced, on account of the contracted condition of the biceps.

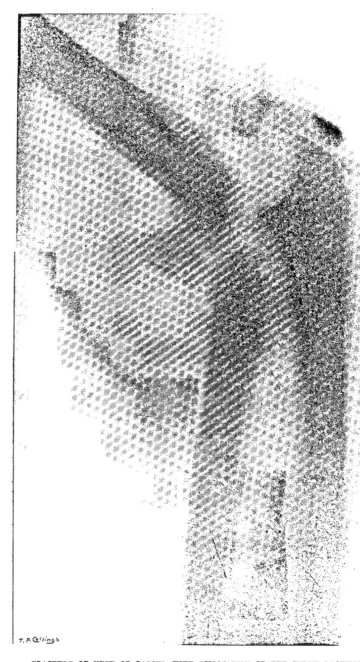

T. P. Collings

FRACTURE OF NECK OF RADIUS, WITH DISLOCATION OF THE ELBOW BACKWARDS.

The upper fragment of the radius, consisting of the epiphysis head and of the upper part of the neck of the bone, is greatly displaced and rotated.

Mr. THOMAS MOORE's case.

Taken by Mr. THOMAS MOORE.

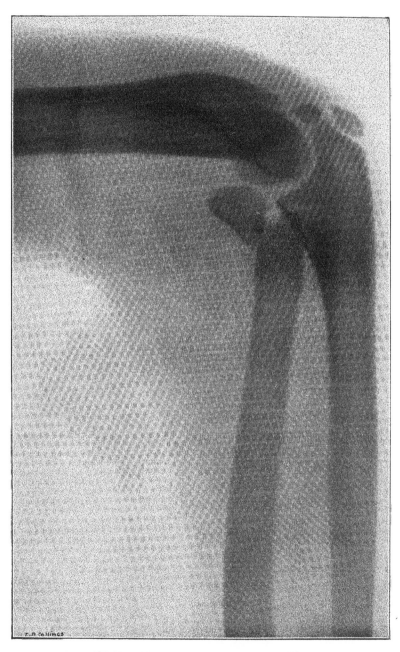

THE SAME CASE AFTER REDUCTION OF THE DISLOCATION OF ELBOW.

Taken by Mr. THOMAS MOORE.

Guedeney records (*Du traitement des fractures du coude chez l'enfant*, Lyon, 1893) the two following cases which were diagnosed by M. Vincent as separation of the upper epiphysis of the radius, and treated by fixation in the extended position.

I. A boy (J. G.), aged (?). Separation of the upper epiphysis of the right radius. The part was painful and swollen, and crepitus was present. Pronation and supination could not be effected, while the other movements of the joint were free. The ulna and humerus were intact. The radius was replaced in its normal position, and the limb fixed in the completely extended and supine position by means of a plaster splint. Four months later tuberculous disease developed, and flexion in a silicate splint was employed for two months after. At the end of thirteen months the movements were still imperfect, and a fistulous track remained with enlargement of the end of the bone.

II. Epiphysial fracture of the upper end of the radius, with dislocation of the elbow. A boy (L. O.), aged twelve years, fell from a crossbar on to the left arm, which was bent back. This was immediately followed by pain and loss of power. The child was admitted into hospital at the end of sixteen days, when extension was found to be free, while flexion was limited to a right angle. Pronation and supination could not be effected without pain, being prevented by muscular contraction. There was considerable increase in thickness at the level of the radial head—two centimetres thick on the right and three and a half on the left. This increased bulk was due to the diaphysial fragment causing a projection of the orbicular ligament, in which the radial cup still remained engaged. The swollen and puffy condition of the part was considerable, and interfered with examination. Reduction was effected under chloroform, and the limb put up in the complete extended and supine position. The ulterior results were unknown.

SEPARATION OF THE BICIPITAL EPIPHYSIS OF THE RADIUS

About the sixteenth year a small epiphysial plate is developed, which rapidly joins with the tuberosity.

It might be supposed that violent muscular action of the biceps would be sufficient to cause separation of this epiphysis, but as yet no case has been observed.

In the adult the biceps tendon has been torn from the radius and successfully wired to the periosteum on either side of the tuberosity (Johnson, *New York Medical Journal*, August 21, 1897, p. 261).

CHAPTER XII

SEPARATION OF THE LOWER EPIPHYSIS OF THE RADIUS

ANATOMY.—Towards the end of the second year the osseous nucleus of the lower epiphysis of the radius appears above the scaphoid facet. Sometimes two granules appear, which rapidly blend together and form a plate projecting towards the borders of the epiphysis. This becomes much thicker towards the outer part, where it extends from about the sixth year to form the styloid process. By the tenth year the styloid process and lower epiphysis are almost entirely invaded by the osseous centre. Between the fourteenth and fifteenth years the external, middle, and internal thecal tubercles begin to project and extend upwards from the posterior aspect of the epiphysis.

This epiphysis is not united to the shaft till the nineteenth or twentieth year. Union takes place first towards the middle of the epiphysis—its thinnest part.

M. Voillemier has quoted instances in which the conjugal cartilage still persisted in subjects aged twenty-four and twenty-five years.

The fully formed epiphysis is of an irregular quadrilateral shape, concave at the articular surface, which is formed into an outer triangular facet for the scaphoid and an inner quadrate facet for the semilunar bone. Its upper mamillated surface is also slightly concave, but more flattened than most of the diaphysial surfaces of the epiphyses, and accurately fits the quadrilateral convex end of the diaphysis.

Upwards it is limited in front by the anterior epiphysiary crest, and between this crest and the border of the scaphoid facet is a rough area—of a triangular shape for the attachment of the anterior ligament of the wrist-joint, and somewhat bevelled off to permit of flexion of the scaphoid.

On the inner side it forms the whole of the sigmoid cavity or sinus lunatus, which is transversely concave, coated with cartilage for the convex articular head of the ulna.

The lower margin of this is separated from the inferior articular surface by a thin edge, to which is attached the thin base of the triangular fibro-cartilage of the wrist-joint.

The anterior epiphysiary crest ends at the outer side towards the base of the styloid process in a sharp tubercle, which is the lower end of the pronator crest on the diaphysis, and which limits the lower and outer part of the pronator quadratus. Posterior to this is a shallow groove divided into two for the tendons of the extensor ossis metacarpi pollicis and the extensor primi internodii pollicis.

Behind the groove is a ridge, the external thecal tubercle, passing downwards to the apex of the styloid process. Into the lower end of the pronator crest, and the surface of bone running backwards to this ridge, the supinator longus is inserted. Posterior to the external thecal tubercle is another broad shallow groove, divided into two by a slight ridge, for the transmission of the tendons of the extensor carpi radialis longior and extensor carpi radialis brevior. Still more internal to this on the posterior surface of the epiphysis is the prominent middle thecal tubercle, on the inner side of which is a deep oblique narrow groove for the extensor secundi internodii pollicis tendon. This prominent ridge, therefore, forms a good guide to the epiphysial line on this aspect of the bone, the line running across the bone an eighth of an inch below the posterior end of the ridge. The inner ridge of this groove is the less prominent internal thecal tubercle. Between this and the posterior extremity of the sigmoid surface is the wide groove for the tendons of the extensor indicis and the extensor communis digitorum.

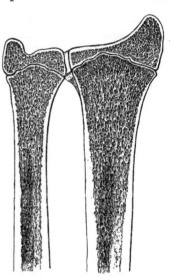

Fig. 138.—SECTION OF RADIUS AND ULNA AT THE EIGHTEENTH YEAR. RELATION OF THE EPIPHYSES AND EPIPHYSIAL LINES. STRUCTURE OF THE ENDS OF THE BONES. (ACTUAL SIZE)

The epiphysis, as seen at the seventeenth to eighteenth year of age, is $1\frac{1}{4}$ inch (3 centimetres 2 millimetres) in width from side to side, and rather more than $\frac{3}{4}$ inch (2 centimetres) in width antero-posteriorly ; $\frac{5}{16}$ inch in thickness about its centre. Its anterior lip is rather less than $\frac{1}{4}$ inch (6 millimetres) in depth about the middle, and the posterior lip more than $\frac{3}{8}$ inch (10 millimetres) at the same point; in the centre it is 5 millimetres thick vertically. On the outer side from the epiphysial line of cartilage to the apex of the styloid process it measures rather more than $\frac{3}{4}$ inch (2 centimetres). At its ulnar border, the sigmoid cavity, it is nearly $\frac{1}{4}$ inch (6 millimetres) thick vertically.

At fourteen years of age the vertical measurements are from the epiphysial cartilage, outer side, to apex of styloid process, 7 millimetres; ulnar border, 4½ millimetres; anterior lip, 6 millimetres; posterior lip, 9 millimetres, each about the middle.

To the apex of the styloid process is attached the external lateral ligament of the wrist-joint, and to the posterior border of the epiphysis the posterior ligament of the wrist.

De Paoli gives the following table of measurements of the lower epiphysis of the radius and ulna at different ages:

| Age | RADIUS | | | | ULNA | |
| | Height | | | Breadth | Height | Breadth |
	Styloid Process	About the middle	Internal edge			
Before birth	5 mm.	4 mm.	3 mm.	10	6·5	6
Twenty months	8 ,,	5 ,,	4 ,,	12	7	11
Two years	.4 ,,	4 ,,	3·5 ,,	12	6	—
Four years	8 ,,	5 ,,	3 ,,	21	5	13
	12 ,,	6 ,,	3 ,,	22	6	14
Five years	11 ,,	5 ,,	3 ,,	24	5	14
Six years	12 ,,	5·5 ,,	4 ,,	22	5	12
Seven years	7 ,,	3·5 ,,	4 ,,	16	5	—
Nine years	13 ,,	6 ,,	5 ,,	—	5	—
	11 ,,	5 ,,	4 ,,	—	5	—
	14 ,,	6 ,,	4 ,,	23	6	14
Ten years	14 ,,	5 ,,	4 ,,	21	8	13
Fourteen years	15 ,,	7 ,,	6 ,,	26	8	—
Fifteen years	16 ,,	7 ,,	6 ,,	29	8	—
Sixteen years	15 ,,	5 ,,	4 ,,	29	8	16
Seventeen years	17 ,,	7 ,,	5 ,,	27	8	12
Nineteen years	16 ,,	8 ,,	5 ,,	28	7	15

The synovial membrane of the wrist-joint does not come into relationship with the epiphysial line of the radius, nor with that of the ulna, which forms no part of the articulation.

From the margin of the articular surface of the epiphysis springs the synovial membrane of the wrist-joint, but it does not pass upwards either on the anterior or posterior aspects.

Although the synovial membrane of the inferior radio-ulnar articulation forms a loose pocket—the membrana succiformis—upwards between the radius and ulna above their epiphysial boundaries, it is but loosely connected with the diaphyses. Below, it is firmly connected with the epiphyses.

Laceration of the synovial pouch is possible, but not absolutely inevitable, in epiphysial separations.

ETIOLOGY. Indirect violence.—Separation of this epiphysis is nearly always produced by indirect violence, such as *falls from a height on to the outstretched hand.*

In analysing the cases the author has collected, we find that of the *thirteen museum specimens* the cause of the injury is given in nine. In all of these the lesion was produced in precisely the same manner—viz. a fall from a height, in some instances a distance of fifty-five, thirty, and twelve feet on to the ground, in others a fall from a second or third story window or a fall from a tree. In two cases it is noted that the fall was probably upon the outstretched hand.

Again, we find the cause given in eight out of *ten cases of compound separation* with the same uniformity — viz. a fall from a height in seven cases, as follows :

Fall from a tree, twenty-six feet ; off a parapet, fifteen feet ; fall from crags ; from third story (one) and from fourth story (one) ; and down a flight of stairs. In one instance only entanglement of the arm in the band of a machine.

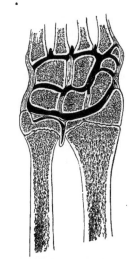

Fig. 139.—Frontal section through the bones of the wrist and hand in a youth aged eighteen years. (⅔ size.) Relation of the synovial membranes to the epiphysial junctions

In nineteen cases out of thirty-five inspected anatomically De Paoli found the same cause—a fall from a great height, from second and third floors, in one a distance of forty feet. In two cases only it was a simple fall to the ground while walking, in one case a fall from a horse.

Colignon notes that one half of his cases were due to a fall from a height upon the hand.

In eight out of nine cases of simple separation verified by an autopsy, and in which the cause is recorded, all were due to the same accident—viz. a fall from a considerable height, thirty to forty feet, from a scaffold or tree (two instances), or from a second story, third story, &c.

In fourteen out of sixteen simple cases the cause is noted, and, with one exception, all were from a fall upon the outstretched hand. In some the fall was from a height, as from a trapeze, balcony, tree, or out of a warehouse window, but in many of these instances the fall was a shorter distance. Thus in two cases the youths fell from a cart on to some grass, and in a few cases there had been only a simple fall, as in slipping whilst walking.

I I

In these falls from a height the whole weight of the body is received upon the palmar aspect of the outstretched and pronated hand, and by the direction of the violence through the ball of the thumb nearly the whole of it is sustained by the lower end of the radius. The muscles assist very materially by their contraction in giving fixation to the bones, and allow the greater portion of the impulse of the violence to be received on the posterior border of the epiphysis, which is forced backwards. The epiphysis is thus displaced in a backward direction. The numerous strong anterior carpal ligaments and flexor tendons on the front, binding the epiphysis to carpus, are put violently on the stretch. The epiphysis is consequently wrenched off and tilted backwards, so that the aspect of its carpal surface, and with it the carpus and hand, is altered in a greater or less degree, and a gap is left between the fragments in front.

M. J. Cloquet (*loc. cit. infra*) dissected a separation of the lower epiphysis of the radius in a child of twelve years, who had fallen from the top of a tree.

M. Rognetta gives (*loc. cit. supra*) a similar case, occurring in a subject fifteen years old.

Cruveilhier, in his experiments on the dead body, almost always produced separation of this epiphysis by acting upon the carpus, either from the weight of the whole body or by a sharp blow from a hammer. In this way sometimes the lower epiphysis of the ulna was detached at the same time, but more frequently the epiphysis of the radius was separated alone.

Packard, writing in 1890, says that ' when the radius is broken near its lower extremity, it is almost invariably by a fall on the hand. These fractures are generally said to be infrequent in early life, but I recently had, at the Pennsylvania Hospital, within forty-eight hours four cases of Colles's fracture in patients between five and twelve years of age. All these were from simple ordinary falls on the hand ; there was no ice (it was in October) or any other circumstance to account for the coincidence. I have repeatedly seen this injury on both sides, from falls from greater or less heights. In one case, many years ago, a boy, about ten years old, fell five stories, with no other damage ; he made a good recovery. Sometimes, no doubt, the portion separated is the epiphysis, but I think this is very rare.'

This lesion, like Colles's fracture, may be brought about, as mentioned by Malgaigne, by backward *over-extension* of the hand at the wrist-joint ; the carpus being thrust violently backwards puts the anterior ligaments of the wrist-joint on the stretch, and these, by their forcible traction on the epiphysis, produce separation by ' cross strain ' (*arrachement*).

This was probably the cause of the separation in Ozenne's case mentioned below, and it has evidently been the mode of production in other instances.

Experimentally, it is very easy to produce this separation by forcible extension of the hand, also by torsion of the hand.

Bähr concludes, however, from his recent experiments (*Central-blatt für Chir.* 1894, No. 36) that this, as well as many other typical forms of fracture of the radius, may be explained by the impact of the upper carpal row upon the lower end of the radius.

Sir A. Cooper, in 1833, made experiments on the dead body, carrying the hand into extreme extension; the radius gave way, in one instance, at the epiphysis, in the other just above that point.

Rognetta produced the lesion by violent traction, and Anger by torsion or rotation of the hand.

M. L. Voillemier was the first to clearly point out (*Clinique Chirurgicale*, 1861, p. 33) the occurrence of separation of the lower epiphysis of the radius by cross strain (*par arrachement*) during over-extension, as in falls upon the hand. He believed that these separations only took place in this manner. Previous to M. Anger's similar experiments on the dead subject, M. Voillemier produced separation by forcible flexion and extension of the wrist, not only in young subjects, but also on a man, aged twenty-four, with a powerful physique.

This mode of production is supported by records of many clinical cases.

In nine out of seventeen cases, chiefly of incomplete separation, De Paoli noted that the cause of the injury was a simple fall, met with in running or walking, but that in seven others the violence was greater—viz. a fall from a height. In sixteen cases the cause was indirect, and acted upon the hand; in one only—a fall from a height of four metres on to the rung of a ladder—the force seems to have acted directly on the epiphysis, which was displaced forwards.

Bruns, in speaking of the lesser degree of violence sufficient to detach the epiphysis in simpler cases, alludes to the case of a boy, aged (?), in whom he recognised an undoubted separation of the lower end of the radius after a fall from a low ladder.

The following case, under the care of Mr. Howse at Guy's Hospital in 1888, was probably due to indirect violence or separation by 'cross strain.'

The boy (Michael G.), aged fifteen years, whilst swinging on a chain, fell off on to the ground, his head striking the ground, and his left arm doubling up under and behind him. Separation of the lower epiphysis of the left radius was found with the usual deformity. A Carr's splint was applied after reduction, and he was able to leave the hospital after seventeen days with the wrist and forearm in good position.

Packard, in an excellent article on 'Fractures of the Lower End of the Radius' (*American Journal of Medical Science*, Hays, N.S., Philadelphia, 1879, p. 123), states that the great majority of these fractures are more or less transverse and are produced by *leverage*.

Coulon, in his work on *Fractures in Children*, while discussing the rarity of fractures of the lower end of the radius in children as compared with the adult, says that a fall upon the palm of the hand in a child usually produces a fracture of the forearm, and not, as in the adult, a fracture of the lower end of the radius. However, he makes an important statement that when such a fracture does occur, it is almost always in children thirteen or fourteen years of age and but rarely before the tenth year.

He quotes three cases in children, twelve, twelve, and thirteen years respectively, with the characteristic deformity.

In one of the cases recorded by Rognetta this lesion was produced in a child, aged five years, by its being dragged violently about by the hand. In this case, however, there was apparently very little displacement of the fragments.

M. B. Anger mentions the case of a separation of the lower end of the radius in a young man whose hand had been seized in a machine.

In many instances it is probable that the mechanism of the injury is one composed of both factors—viz. a combination of cross strain or hyper-extension, and of the direct thrust of the violence displacing the epiphysis backwards, the bone yielding at its weakest point.

Separation of this epiphysis is very unlikely to be the result of **muscular action** alone, although it is a very important factor in maintaining the deformity or displacing the epiphysis after it has been separated at the time of the accident.

After reduction of the displaced epiphysis the muscles have but little tendency to reproduce the deformity.

Callender has recorded a case of fracture of both radii just above the epiphysis in a boy, aged fourteen years, which was produced by violent muscular efforts excited by a strong galvanic current.

Direct violence from a blow or passage of a wheel over the wrist.

The epiphysis in one of the London Hospital specimens was probably torn off by a toothed machine.

J. Hutchinson junior relates (*British Medical Journal*, March 31, 1894, p. 670) the curious case of a lad who was incautiously lying on the ground resting his head upon his hand underneath a lift. He happened to raise his head, and at that moment the lift descended, striking the front of his hand and forcing backwards his radial epiphysis.

SEPARATION WITH DISPLACEMENT FORWARDS.—Professor J. B. Roberts (*A Clinical, Pathological, and Experimental Study of Fracture of the Lower End of the Radius, with Displacement of the Carpal Fragment towards the Flexor or Anterior Surface of the Wrist*, Philadelphia, 1897, p. 42) has experimentally, in one instance, produced epiphysial separation with anterior displacement by extreme flexion of the wrist. He did this on the amputated forearm of a boy of fourteen years.

AGE.—In analysing the cases in which the age is recorded in the *forty pathological specimens*, we must exclude twelve in which it is not stated, two in young men, and one in a lad below 20 years. The age is definitely given in twenty-eight. In four the separation occurred at 18 years of age, four at 16, four at 15, five at 14, one at $13\frac{1}{2}$, one at 13, four at 12, one at 9, one at 8, one at 7, and one at 3 years of age, and one doubtful case of detachment of only a small part of the epiphysis at 1 year. Of these, the larger number, twenty-three, occurred between 18 and 12 years of age.

In *six pathological specimens*, showing dwarfing, &c., in three the age is not given, in one it is said to have occurred in boyhood, and in one case some years prior to the twentieth; in one case at 5 years.

Taking the fourteen cases of *compound separation*, the age is not stated in three, but is noted in eleven, one at 18, one at 17, one at 16, one at 15, three at 14, two at 12, one at 8, and one at 6; nine of these, therefore, were between 12 and 18 years of age.

Putting *all the cases together which were verified by direct examination*, sixty in number, we find that the age is stated in forty; the remainder are too inaccurately stated to be of any use. Five were at 18, one at 17, five at 16, five at 15, eight at 14, one at $13\frac{1}{2}$, one at 13, six at 12, one at 9, two at 8, one at 7, one at 6, one at 5 years, one at 3, and one at 1 year.

Of these forty, by far the greater number, thirty-two, were from 18 to 12 years of age; out of these thirty-two, twenty-six were between 16 and 12 years of age.

The average age of the cases must be just about the fourteenth year.

In De Paoli's figures, the age of the patients was in one case 7 years, in three 13, in two 15, in five 18, and in one 20; in ten it was unknown.

Among the *clinical cases*, of which there are fifty-two, the age is omitted in nine; two were said to have taken place in infancy, another in a child, one in a young man, and one in a youth, and in the other four it is not stated at all. Of the remaining forty-three cases in which the age is recorded, one was at 20, one at 19, one at $18\frac{1}{2}$, one at 18, three at 17, three at 16, one at $15\frac{1}{2}$, three at 15, four at 14, two at 13, two at 12, three at 11, six at 10, one between 10 and 12, two at 9, four at 8, one between 7 and 8, one at 5, two at 4, and one at 3 years of age. The greatest number, eighteen, were between 17 and 12 years of age.

Putting together the whole total, 112 cases of injury to the lower epiphysis of the radius, the age is not given in twenty-nine. Of the remaining total, eighty-three, no less than fifty-one occurred between the ages of 12 and 18 years, and of these thirty-nine were between 14 and 18.

From the notes which De Paoli took of seventeen cases under his care, his experience was the same—viz. that they occur much more frequently in the second decade of life, and represent about one half of the solutions of continuity of the bones which occur between the ages of ten and twenty.

Manquat puts the most frequent period for this separation at ten to fifteen years, but he adds that it is very often met with still later.

Among the fifty-four cases of separation of this epiphysis collected by Jonathan Hutchinson junior, seventeen of which were under his own observation, the age of the patient ranged from three years to twenty, the majority being over ten years, and quite a number of them seventeen or eighteen years.

D'Arcy Power (*Surgical Diseases of Children*, 1895, p. 182) thinks that with the increase of bicycling it is becoming rather more frequent in young adults.

SEX.—The sex is stated in nineteen of the thirty-two pathological cases, eighteen being boys and one a girl; but of the remaining cases, from the occupation in which the patients were engaged at the time of the accident, it is probable that the greater proportion were males. But in the total *sixty cases verified by anatomical examination*, the sex is given in forty-five—viz. forty-one in males and four in females. All the girls were at or below five years of age.

Out of sixteen clinical cases, thirteen are recorded as having occurred in boys and two in girls, and in one the sex is not stated. But in the total *fifty-two simple cases*, the sex is stated in forty-four. Of these, thirty-eight occurred in males and only six in females. All the girls were below fourteen years of age.

Out of the grand total of 112 cases, the sex is given in eighty-nine instances as seventy-nine in males and ten in girls—the whole of the latter being at or below fourteen years of age.

PATHOLOGICAL ANATOMY.—From the number of cases of traumatic separation of the lower epiphysis of the radius in which a direct anatomical examination was practicable, it would appear that they are more numerous than those of any of the other epiphyses.

Yet Hamilton, writing in 1884, says: 'The examples of separation of the lower epiphysis of the radius have seldom been clearly made out.'

Gurlt, in his treatise on fractures (*Handbuch der Lehre von den Knochenbrüchen*, Hamm. 1862), collected all the known cases of epiphysial separation to the number of eighteen, four of which were of the lower end of the radius; and Bruns collected twenty-five cases of separation of the lower end of the radius—verified by direct inspection—out of a total of eighty cases of epiphysial detachment. Since that time, 1882, the author has been able, as we have just seen, to bring together a considerable number.

Malgaigne observed that it was perhaps the most common of all epiphysial separations, but he has not given any description of its pathological characters or of its symptoms, dismissing the subject by saying that the causes, symptoms, and treatment are identical with those of fracture. He merely alluded to the cases described by J. Cloquet, Roux, and Johnston. Although Roux ascertained the existence of the lesion in his case, he did not give the age of the child.

Dupuytren was the first to point out, 1834 (*Leçons orales de clinique chirurgicale*, 1834, t. iv. p. 183), that in young subjects epiphysial separation was more likely to occur than fracture of the lower end of the radius.

Colignon, in his thesis, 1868, commences a chapter on traumatic separation of the lower epiphysis of the radius by stating that all authors agree in recognising this form of epiphysial separation as the most common.

From De Paoli's statistics (*Del distacco traumatico delle epifisi*, Torino, 1882, p. 105) of thirty-five cases directly examined, it appears that the separation was complete in twenty-three cases, incomplete in one only, and in four cases bilateral.

In eight cases small fragments of the cortical substance of the diaphysis adhered to the epiphysis; in twenty cases the separation had occurred above the conjugal cartilage; in three cases only, small strips of this cartilage adhered to the lower surface of the diaphysis; and in one the epiphysial separation was accompanied by a fracture of the epiphysis penetrating into the articulation.

J. Colignon was able to collect eighteen cases in his thesis (*loc. cit. supra*).

Bardenheuer (*Deutsche Chirurgie*, Billroth und Lücke, 1888, II. Theil, S. 238) agrees with Bruns in believing that it is the most common epiphysial injury after that of the lower end of the femur.

Gurlt thought the frequency of separation of the lower radial epiphysis in children beyond infancy was due to the fact that this epiphysis does not diminish in size, relatively to the rest of the growing bone, to such an extent as other bones—those, for instance, at the lower end of the humerus.

The great frequency is rather due, in all probability, to the anatomical characteristics of the epiphysis, and to its situation in the skeleton. Besides, this epiphysis is one of the last bones to join on to its diaphysis.

Its superficial position also renders separation more easy of detection than is the case with many of the other epiphyses.

Bardenheuer (*loc. cit. supra*) figures a specimen from a child one year old, which he gives as an example of epiphysial separation, although only portions of the epiphysial end were torn away. The styloid process, and the whole of the marginal portion of the articular surface of the radius, were separated, leaving the central portion uninjured. There were also fractures of the cuneiform bone and of the styloid process of the ulna.

In Bœckel's case the separation appears to have passed through the midst of the conjugal cartilage, for the protruding diaphysial end of the radius was said to have been covered with a layer of cartilage, which led the doctor who first saw the case to mistake it for a dislocation, and reduce it.

Displacement backwards.—Displacement in the backward direction has occurred in all the museum specimens. On carefully examining the condition of the bones it is seen to vary much in its degree ; thus, in one of the specimens in St. George's Hospital and in one at the Royal College of Surgeons the epiphysis is almost completely displaced off the diaphysis ; and Professor R. W. Smith found the epiphysis in one of his cases displaced directly backwards so far as to have nearly cleared the extremity of the upper fragment, and in another of his cases it was carried backwards for three-eighths of an inch. In the Guy's Hospital specimen, and in that of Professor Annandale, it was more than halfway off the diaphysis, and in one of the St. Bartholomew's Hospital specimens two-thirds of the way. In the specimen in King's College Hospital, and in one of those in St. George's Hospital, there is only very slight displacement backwards. In Mr. Shattock's specimen the epiphysis is described as being displaced backwards and forming an obtuse angle with the shaft.

Displacement backwards, without fracture of the diaphysis.—Several specimens in the London museums show the occurrence of pure separations through the epiphysial junction.

The conjugal cartilage in nearly every instance has remained with the epiphysis, but in some rare examples it is probable that the separation has taken place through the cartilage itself.

In Richet's case the end of the radius, after removal, was found to be covered with several thin lamellæ of the epiphysial cartilage, so that the separation was thought to have occurred through the epiphysial layer. The same condition is mentioned by M. Manquat in Péan's case. In one of the London Hospital museum specimens two small patches of the epiphysial cartilage remain on the extremity of the shaft, and in the compound diastasis mentioned by Gripat the diaphysial end presented some small particles of cartilage.

In the museum of King's College Hospital is a specimen, No. 644, from a child, aged twelve, presented by Professor Partridge. The lower radial epiphysis is separated exactly at the epiphysial line, and displaced slightly towards the dorsal aspect of the shaft, so that the anterior margin of the lower end of the latter projects but little. The periosteum is torn upwards from the front of the shaft for three-quarters of an inch. The styloid process of the ulna and triangular fibro-cartilage are uninjured. Death resulted from fracture of the skull.

M. Jules Cloquet ascertained by dissection (*Diction. de Médecine*, vol. ix. 1824, p. 448) the existence of a complete separation in a boy aged twelve years. Death occurred from fracture of the skull three days after a fall from a tree. The epiphysis of the right radius was completely separated, and a quantity of blood extra-vasated into the deeper parts of the palmar region beneath the flexor tendons of the fingers. Dupuytren quotes the case in his *Leçons orales*, 1834, t. iv. p. 183.

Rognetta quotes M. Flaubert (of Rouen) as having seen a similar case which had been treated as a simple contusion of the wrist-joint. The specimen was in the Anatomical Museum of the Hôtel-Dieu in Paris, and is also quoted by M. Malgaigne as having been treated for a simple dislocation of the wrist.

B. Anger figures (*Traité iconographique des maladies chirurgi-cales*, 1865, p. 197) the only specimen of separation of the lower end of the radius which he had been able to observe anato-mically. It was taken from a youth, a printer, whose hand had been caught in a machine. The lower epiphysis of the radius was separated, and from the backward projection of the lower end of the bone the deformity in every respect was similar to that of fracture of the lower end of the radius. From the figure it appears that the styloid process of the ulna was uninjured, that the periosteum in front is torn across at the level of the lower end of the diaphysis, and that scarcely any displacement had occurred.

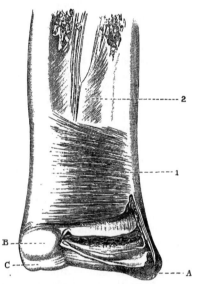

Fig. 140.—PURE SEPARATION OF LOWER EPIPHYSIS OF RADIUS WITH SLIGHT DISPLACEMENT BACKWARDS

A, styloid process of radius; B, head of ulna; C, styloid process of ulna; 1, pronator quadratus; 2, interosseous ligament. (ANGER)

The specimen in Guy's Hospital, described below, is also an example of separation without fracture of the diaphysis.

Athol A. Johnson, in a clinical lecture at the Hospital for Sick Children (*British Medical Journal*, January 21, 1860, p. 44), refers to a preparation with laceration of the inferior epiphysis of the radius, but the exact age of the patient is not known.

In Hartmann's case the separation on each side was perfectly clean and transverse, and without the slightest indication of an osseous particle.

St. Bartholomew's Hospital Museum (*Catalogue of Pathological Museum, St. Bartholomew's Hospital*, Addenda 1881-93, 1894, p. 44) contains a specimen, No. 758B, one half (posterior) of the lower end of the radius and ulna which have been sawn through longitudinally, showing, as the result of an accident, the separation of the lower epiphysis of the radius from the shaft. It was obtained from a boy, aged sixteen, who was brought dead to the hospital. The epiphysis of the right radius is seen to be displaced backwards almost completely off the diaphysis. The triangular fibro-cartilage and wrist-joint are intact, while the periosteum is stripped up on the dorsal aspect for one and a quarter inches. The styloid process of the ulna is broken off, but the bone is otherwise uninjured; its lower end is very prominent. There is no fracture of the diaphysis of the radius

One of the earliest cases of compound separation of this epiphysis is recorded by Mr. John Hilton (*Guy's Hospital Reports*, 3rd series, vol. xi. 1865, p. 338–44). There was compound separation of the carpal epiphyses of both radii from the shafts of the bones; tetanus ensued on the sixth day, and terminated in death the following day.

The patient (B. B.), aged fourteen, a bricklayer's labourer, was admitted into Cornelius Ward, under the care of Mr. Hilton, on December 13, 1864. He had fallen from a scaffolding half an hour previously, a distance of about forty feet, and had alighted on a heap of bricks with his face downwards, and both arms and hands stretched out after a kind of spreadeagle fashion. There was a contused lacerated wound of the forehead and concussion of the brain. The continuity of the right radius was destroyed at the junction of the lower epiphysis with the shaft, the distal portion being displaced backwards; the ulna of this side seemed to be entire. There were two transverse slits in the skin over the anterior surface of the same wrist, laying bare the flexor tendons, but not exposing the bone. Only one could have been caused by the protrusion of the broken radius; the other was probably produced by extreme flexion of the hand backwards, causing great tension of the skin in front, which then gave way. The hæmorrhage from these wounds was trifling. The displacement was readily reduced by extension, and was accompanied with a feeling of crepitus over the region of the fracture.

The left radius was fractured similarly to the right, with a corresponding displacement; only in this case the end of the diaphysis projected through a wound anteriorly, and there was more hæmorrhage. On feeling the exposed end of the bone it was noticed to be comparatively smooth, and suggested to the house surgeon a separation of the epiphysis from the shaft. The displaced extremity of the bone was fixed with considerable firmness in its abnormal position, and there was much difficulty in getting the fragments into good position. The projecting bone had passed between the closely grouped and tense tendons, indicating that great force had been expended in producing this separation of the epiphysis. The radial artery, but not the ulnar, could be distinctly felt. After 'the setting' of the fractures a pistol-shaped splint was put on the outer side of each forearm and hand.

As Mr. Hilton says : 'These splints were wrong and unnecessary, and were applied by the dresser, who thought he had two instances of Colles's fracture to deal with. The median nerve could scarcely have escaped injury at the time of the accident, lying, as it did, in the midst of the tendons through which the fractured bone protruded.

'On December 19, six days after the accident, the patient complained of a little soreness about the throat, and of stiff neck. On the 20th, 8 A.M., the corrugatores superciliorum were contracted, the lower jaw fixed, neck rigid, and abdomen hard ; at 3 P.M. he had a severe opisthotonic spasm, and his chest became rigid. The spasms became more severe, and recurred frequently till 5.35 P.M., when he died of tetanus, caused, Mr. Hilton thought, by injury to the median nerve. At the *autopsy* only the wrists were allowed to be examined. As soon as the splints were removed the displacements recurred. At the right wrist the radial epiphysis was found separated from the shaft of the bone, but the wrist-joint was uninjured. There was no suppuration about the fracture. On the left side a similar displacement was found, and also an oblique fracture of the ulna about an inch and a half above the wrist-joint. Suppuration existed about the fractured bones, which were bloodless and saturated with fetid pus. The periosteum of the shaft of the radius was stripped off to a considerable extent.'

Mr. Jonathan Hutchinson, in his report as chairman of the committee of the International Medical Congress Museum of 1881 (*Transactions of the International Medical Congress*, London 1881, vol. i. p. 116), says : 'An excellent specimen of separation of the carpal epiphysis of the radius was lent from the Dublin College of Surgeons, in which was shown the precise condition of parts in a complete separation, with complete dislocation of the epiphysis on the dorsal aspect of the radius. I was able to supplement this by a drawing from a precisely similar case, showing the appearance presented by the hand immediately after the accident. It is quite possible that specimen and drawing may each be unique, for this accident, with this degree of displacement, is certainly very rare, and I have never myself, until this occasion, had an opportunity of examining a preparation. Dr. Geoghegan's patient died of injuries received in a fall from a scaffolding ; in mine, reduction was found exceedingly difficult, and suppuration subsequently occurred, but the arm was saved.'

Körte mentions a specimen, alluded to later on, from a boy, aged eighteen years, in which the lower radial epiphysis was completely separated, although it was still connected with the diaphysis by means of the periosteum.

Displacement backwards with fracture of the diaphysis.—Many specimens in which dorsal displacement occurred show the existence of a slight fracture of the diaphysis. In the majority of cases some small osseous scales adhere to the posterior margin of the epiphysis. The fragment is almost always from the back of the diaphysis.

A specimen, No. 758A, in the museum of St. Bartholomew's Hospital (*St. Bartholomew's Hospital Reports*, 1887, vol. xiii. p. 367; *Catalogue of the Anatomical and Pathological Museum of St. Bartholomew's Hospital*, Addenda 1881–93, 1894, p. 43), a section of the lower end of the radius of a child, is described as an incomplete separation of the lower radial epiphysis, or separation combined with fracture of the diaphysis, the separation being complete along the radial border, but towards the ulnar side the line of injury running obliquely, and consequently the bone has been fractured above the epiphysis. On examining the specimen, however, it appears that this small shell of the shaft adhering to the epiphysis is on the dorsal aspect, towards which the epiphysis has been displaced two-thirds of the way off the diaphysis. The periosteum is torn through at the anterior aspect, and the diaphysis, which is quite devoid of cartilage, projects at this point.

The specimen was from a girl, aged three years, who fell from a height of thirty feet on to the pavement, and died two days after the injury.

Another specimen, No. 39A, in St. George's Hospital Museum (*Catalogue of Museum of St. George's Hospital*, 1882), is figured by Holmes (*Surgical Diseases of Children*, 1868, p. 255, figs. 42, 43), in which some displacement backwards of the epiphysis has taken place, and the diaphysis, in the description of the specimen, is stated to be displaced by the action of the pronator quadratus; but an examination of the specimen shows that the periosteum is torn off, together with the lower part of the pronator quadratus, from the anterior aspect of the lower end of the diaphysis, so that the bare end of the diaphysis protrudes. The separation is clean through the epiphysial junction, with the exception of the posterior margin of the end of the diaphysis, which is broken off as a rim of bone situated just a quarter of an inch above the epiphysial line and still adherent to the epiphysis. The symptoms during life are not recorded.

A similar specimen is in the London Hospital Museum, No. 404 (*London Hospital Museum Catalogue*, 1890, p. 96), and is figured and described by Mr. Hutchinson (*Pathological Society's Transactions*, vol. xiii. 1862, p. 182, fig. 1, plate xi.; and *London Hospital Reports*, vol. i. p. 89). It shows complete detachment of the carpal epiphysis of the radius, with the exception that, on its dorsal aspect at the inner side, a small portion of bone has been broken from the extremity of the shaft and carried along with the epiphysis. The lower extremity of the shaft presents no cartilaginous covering, but shows numerous rounded elevations which had fitted into corresponding depressions in the cartilage of the epiphysis. Its surface

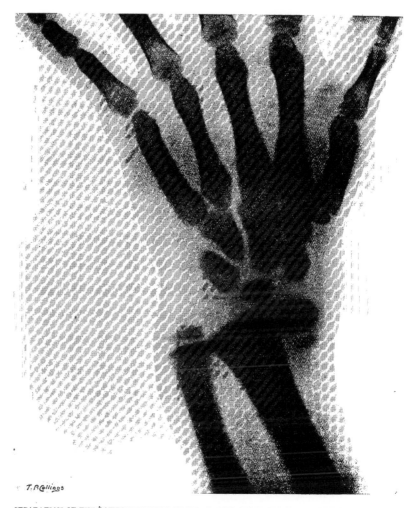

T. P. Collings

SEPARATION OF THE LOWER EPIPHYSIS OF THE RADIUS, WITH ALMOST COMPLETE DISPLACEMEN
BACKWARDS AND TO THE OUTER SIDE.

he backward displacement was well shown in another skiagram taken laterally. A flake is detached from the posterior as
of the diaphysis of the radius. The ulnar epiphysis appears to be uninjured. From a boy aged eleven years.
Another skiagram of the same case after reduction showed the epiphysis in exactly normal position.

Mr. THOMAS MOORE'S case.   Taken by Mr. THOMAS MOORE.

is entire and unbroken, excepting at the back, from which the small fragment of bone has been detached. The detached epiphysis is everywhere covered with cartilage, and is in normal relation with the carpal bones. None of the ligaments are injured. The head of the ulna having been removed, it was impossible to state whether or not the styloid process of that bone, or the triangular ligament connecting it with the radius, had been injured.

The specimen was taken from a boy aged sixteen years, who died a few days after admission from various severe injuries sustained in a fall. The symptoms of the epiphysial injury during life are unfortunately not given.

The same museum contains another preparation, No. 405 (*London Hospital Reports*, vol. iii. 1866, p. 401), consisting of the radius and ulna of a young subject, whose left arm was removed by primary amputation. The carpal epiphysis of the radius has been detached, and almost the whole of the epiphysial cartilage has gone with it; but two small patches remain on the extremity of the shaft. The end of the shaft at its margins is a little splintered, but there is no material fracture. On the palmar aspect, about a quarter of an inch from the outer border, is a linear fracture about an inch long, the upper end of which looks as if a tooth of some machine had entered the bone. This linear fracture does not involve the whole thickness of the bone, and consequently does not permit of motion; possibly it is only a scratch, and if so the epiphysis was probably pulled off by the tooth which inflicted it. Unfortunately, the carpal end of the bone has not been kept. The ulna presents a dentated, almost transverse, fracture an inch and a quarter from the extremity of the styloid process.

Mr. Jonathan Hutchinson junior's specimen in the Royal College of Surgeons Museum presents a traumatic separation of the lower radial epiphysis with great displacement and slight diaphysial fracture from a fall on the hand.

The patient was probably aged about sixteen years. The lower radial epiphysis has been displaced completely backwards, so that the anterior margin is about on a level with the diaphysial end and looking downwards, still adhering to the shaft by the periosteum.

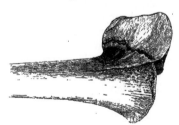

Fig. 141.—SHOWING EPIPHYSIS FROM OUTER SIDE DISPLACED BACKWARDS WITH PERIOSTEUM. SEEN FROM THE INNER SIDE THE DISPLACEMENT APPEARED MUCH GREATER

(Royal College of Surgeons Museum, No. 956c)

The separation has occurred exactly at the epiphysial line, except on the posterior aspect, where a small ridge of bone has been torn off the diaphysis. The top of the styloid process of the ulna is broken off, but the conjugal line is uninjured.

An interesting recent specimen in the Pathological Institute of the University of Turin is figured and described by Dr. De Paoli (*loc. cit. supra*). It was taken from a boy aged nine years, who had fallen from a great height, and died from fracture of the skull and visceral lesions (figs. 142 and 143).

A little above the radio-carpal articulation there was to be seen issuing through a transverse laceration of the anterior part of the periosteum and lower part of the pronator quadratus, the quadrangular lower end of the diaphysis of the radius, with its somewhat rounded corners. Its lower aspect was slightly granular, and showed here and there a scale of cartilaginous tissue; its anterior surface, especially towards the inner side, is deprived of its periosteum for a distance of seven to eight millimetres, but a little higher up it is covered by the periosteum and pronator quadratus. The small portion of the periosteum stripped from the diaphysis here in front is still adherent to the upper margin of the epiphysis, and covered by the lower part of the pronator quadratus. The upper aspect of the epiphysis was principally covered by the conjugal cartilage, although a thin scale or two of the osseous tissue of the diaphysis still clung to it.

Posteriorly, the periosteum remained intact, although stripped for a distance of about one and a half centimetres from the posterior and inner aspect of the diaphysis, a very thin strip of which remained adhering to it.

The displacement of the epiphysis was not completely off the epiphysis, but it could be readily accomplished, and reduction was then found to be almost impossible in the preparation. The ulna was partially displaced below and in front, and the internal lateral ligament and the posterior part of the articular capsule presented lacerations; that of the latter opened the radio-ulnar articulation.

There was also an incomplete fracture of the diaphysis of the radius about its middle, the periosteum and posterior half of the bone being involved. The bone was bent at an angle of about 120°.

De Paoli in 1877 dissected a similar specimen taken from the body of a mason's apprentice, aged fourteen, who had fallen from a third floor and died of severe abdominal lesions—lacerated kidneys, &c.

There was the usual projection in front of the forearm, about one centimetre above the radio-carpal articulation, and a corresponding depression behind. The hand was in a hyper-extended position and the styloid processes in their normal relations, and there was some effusion of blood on the palmar aspect of the forearm.

The radial epiphysis was found almost cleanly separated from the diaphysis, and covered with the conjugal cartilage; while posteriorly and internally the periosteum was stripped for a distance of about two centimetres off the outer surface of the diaphysis, many small particles of the compact substance of which adhered to it. Anteriorly the periosteum was lacerated, and remained adherent to the epiphysis. The diaphysis which protruded through this laceration had its anterior surface somewhat rotated backwards towards the inner side, and the epiphysis, on the other hand, was turned slightly outwards and backwards; which facts led De Paoli to suppose that the lesion had been produced by violent extension and supination of the radio-carpal articulation, such as would be produced by the boy falling on his outstretched hand with the forearm pronated. The radio-ulnar joint was intact.

M. Johnston describes (*Bullet. de la Soc. Anat.* 1839, p. 184) a specimen of perfect separation of this epiphysis, with the exception of a very small fractured fragment which had been detached from the posterior margin of the diaphysis, and still adhered to the

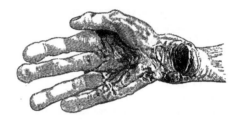

FIG. 142.—DISSECTION OF TRAUMATIC SEPARATION OF THE LOWER EPIPHYSIS OF THE RADIUS, AND DISLOCATION OF THE ULNA. (ANTERIOR VIEW)

(Specimen in the Pathological Institute, University of Turin)

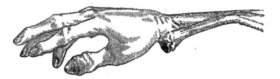

FIG. 143.—THE SAME. (LATERAL VIEW.) (DE PAOLI)

posterior border of the epiphysis. The periosteum was stripped up from the dorsal aspect of the diaphysis, was thickened and markedly injected, and completely torn through in front. The epiphysis was displaced backwards, and the diaphysial end projected forwards beneath the flexor tendons. There was said to be also a tendency to displacement outwards from the action of the radial muscles.

The articular ligaments uniting the ulna to the carpus were lacerated behind, and the head of the ulna projected strongly below through the inclination of the carpus outwards, but was not displaced off the carpus. On the opposite, the left, side there was a precisely similar, though less marked fracture.

During life the injury was thought to be a fracture of the lower end of the right radius, as all the signs of this injury were said to be present. There were several other bones fractured, including the femur. The lesions·resulted from a fall from a height of about thirty or forty feet.

The patient, a lad aged eighteen years, died, on the fifth day after the accident, from gangrene following laceration of the popliteal artery and vein.

J. Colignon describes (*Disjonction traumat. des épiph.*, Thèse de Paris, 1868, p. 72) an almost perfect separation of the lower radial epiphysis, to which adhered some osseous scales, broken from the posterior margin of the diaphysis. There was extensive separation of the periosteum from the diaphysis, and two fringe-like processes of the former remained adherent to the epiphysis. There was a little extravasated blood in the situation of the epiphysial cartilage; the ulna was intact.

The patient, a boy aged seven years, died from severe injuries to the head thirteen days after a fall from a second story, and was under the care of M. Marjolin at the Hôpital St. Eugénie in 1868.

During life the left forearm was much deformed, swollen, and somewhat shortened. The 'fork-back' deformity described by Velpeau in cases of fracture of the lower end of the radius was well marked. The styloid process of the radius was on the same level as that of the ulna, which projected more than in the natural condition. The hand appeared to be somewhat thrown towards the radial side ; the forearm consequently presented a slight incurvation at its lower part. The form of the projecting lower end of the diaphysis, with its abrupt ridge, could be easily made out, about a centimetre above the intra-articular interline. Mobility from before backwards was distinctly felt, and a smooth soft crepitus which did not permit of any doubt as to the true nature of the lesion. The pain was very great on the slightest movement, and the limb quite powerless. M. Marjolin readily reduced the fragments by means of extension and manipulation, but the deformity was almost immediately reproduced.

In Gripat's and in one of R. W. Smith's cases the separation was accompanied by a slight fracture of the diaphysis; this also existed in Bœckel's case.

Occasionally it is noted that fragments of the diaphysis are torn away from its anterior aspect, and it is probable, as De Paoli remarks, that the lesion has occurred nearly at the period of complete development and union of the epiphysis with the shaft. This view·is further supported in the recent specimen figured by De Paoli, by the fact that the ulnar epiphysis has almost completely ossified to the shaft, and that the measurements of the displaced portion of the radius are those of the fully formed epiphysis (being sixteen millimetres in depth at the styloid process).

The lower end of the ulna was fractured at the middle in an antero-posterior direction, detaching on the inner side the styloid process and a portion of the diaphysis, and on the outer side the head of the bone at the upper level of the epiphysis, together with a small portion of the diaphysis behind (see fig. 144).

The two portions detached from the compact layer of the lower end of the diaphysis of the radius were, posteriorly, nine millimetres in length, and remained attached to the upper margin of the epiphysis, while on the inner side of the anterior aspect some irregular pieces of the diaphysis, five to six centimetres in depth, also adhered to the epiphysis. The epiphysis was displaced backwards.

COMPLICATIONS. **Separation with fracture of the epiphysis.**—From the thinness of the epiphysis, especially about the middle, it might be supposed that fracture of the epiphysis in this position would be of frequent occurrence, but an examination of the records shows that this is not the case. Several museum specimens demonstrate its existence, however.

The epiphysis is more solid than the lower end of the bone of the adult, and by this means escapes the fracture, comminution, or even impaction which are so frequent in later life.

The specimen, No. 931, in the museum of St. Bartholomew's Hospital (*Catalogue of the Anatomical and Pathological Museum of St. Bartholomew's Hospital,* vol. i. p. 134) of separation of the lower epiphysis of the left radius is of considerable interest. The separation from the shaft has taken place almost quite cleanly at the epiphysial line, and a fracture extends vertically through the middle of the epiphysis into the wrist-joint. The periosteum with a small flake of the diaphysis is torn upwards for half an inch on the dorsal aspect, and the lower end of the ulna is fractured above the epiphysial line. The styloid process of the ulna is also broken off.

On the right side (specimen No. 932) the radius is fractured transversely an inch and a quarter from its articular surface. The shaft was driven into, and firmly impacted in, the cancellous tissue

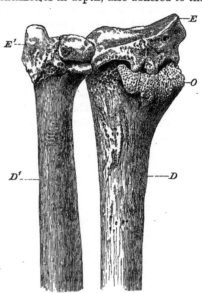

FIG. 144.—RECENT TRAUMATIC SEPARATION OF THE LOWER EPIPHYSIS OF THE RADIUS, AND SEPARATION WITH FRACTURE OF THE LOWER EPIPHYSIS OF THE ULNA. (DE PAOLI)

E, epiphysis of the radius; *O*, fragments of the compact tissue of the posterior part of the diaphysis adhering to the epiphysis; *D*, diaphysis of radius; *E'*, epiphysis of ulna; *D'*, diaphysis of ulna

of the lower extremity, which was displaced backwards, the epiphysial line below being intact. The epiphysis of the ulna is separated from the diaphysis and broken into several pieces. The intra-articular fibro-cartilage is still attached to one of the larger pieces comprising the head of the ulna on the inner side. The shaft of this bone is uninjured. Owing to the impaction, no crepitus could be felt, even after the removal of the surrounding soft parts. The specimens were taken from the body of a boy aged fourteen years, who fell from a window and died, a few hours after, from injuries to the head.

Callender ('Fractures injuring Joints,' *St. Bartholomew's Hospital Reports*, vol. i. 1865, p. 281) alludes to the same case in St. Bartholomew's Hospital museum. The right radius, he adds, was deformed through the projection of the lower end of the bone.:

The bone was broken transversely at a point one inch from its articular surface. The shaft was impacted and driven into the cancellous tissue of the carpal extremity, so that the latter was displaced backwards and fixed at an angle of 160 degrees with the shaft.

In 1884 Professor Annandale, of Edinburgh, showed the author an almost precisely similar specimen in his pathological collection in the Edinburgh Infirmary. The lesion had been a compound one. The lower epiphysis of the radius was displaced backwards halfway off the diaphysis, and there were one or more fissures extending through the epiphysis into the wrist-joint. Primary amputation of the forearm was performed, and the patient recovered.

In the Musée de la Société de Chirurgie de Paris (*Bullet. de la Soc. de Chirurg.* 1865, 1866, 2 Sér. vi. p. 524, and *Gazette des Hôpit.* 1865, pp. 145–147) there are specimens presented by M. Dolbeau of almost perfect separation of the lower epiphysis of the radius and ulna on the left side and of the radius alone on the right. On this side (the right) the aponeurosis of the forearm was torn, and the flexor muscles formed a kind of buttonhole, which was placed between the diaphysis and the epiphysis. The epiphysial cartilage still adhered to the right epiphysis together with a thin flake from the posterior margin of the diaphysis, and the separation on the left side was moreover complicated with a fracture of the epiphysis penetrating the wrist-joint; otherwise the wrist-joint on each side was intact. The specimens were taken from a child thirteen years old, who died nineteen days after from fracture of the skull, the result of a fall from a second story.

E. H. Bennett describes (*British Medical Journal*, vol. i. 1880, p. 759) casts and specimens taken from the limbs of a boy who died from injury to the skull a few days after a fall from a height. On the one side the displaced epiphysis was comminuted, with detachment of a small scale of bone from the diaphysis; on the other the separation was simple. There was to be noticed the contrast of deformity with Colles's fracture in the transverse features of their dorsal and palmar projections, the folding of the skin in the palmar depression, absence of abduction of the hand, easy reduction, and the facility of obtaining crepitus, as well as of keeping fragments in position.

In an article upon 'Clinical Observations on Disjunction of the Lower Epiphysis of the Radius' (*Dublin Hospital Gazette*, vol. vii. 1860, p. 49) and in his 'Address in Surgery' (*British Medical Journal*, vol. ii. August 17, 1867, p. 123; and in the *Proceedings of the Pathological Society of Dublin*, N.S. vol. i. 1862, p. 126), Professor R. W. Smith describes a case in which the diagnosis made during life was confirmed by an autopsy. The separation was bilateral, and on one side the epiphysis was comminuted.

A lad, under twenty years of age, was admitted into the Richmond Hospital, Dublin, having fallen from a considerable height. He sustained a very severe injury of the head, and in each forearm the radius was broken close to the wrist-joint. The external characters of the fracture were as nearly as possible alike upon each side. In the left forearm two projections were visible immediately above the radio-carpal articulation, one upon the dorsal, the other upon the palmar surface of the limb, the latter being the more distinctly circumscribed. Their outline was directed transversely, but neither of them extended across the entire breadth of the forearm. They were limited to the transverse extent of the radius, and were not placed directly opposite to each other, the lower boundary of the anterior corresponding to the superior margin of the posterior. Immediately below the abrupt termination of the anterior projection there was a deep transverse sulcus, in which the integuments presented a few transverse folds, as if relaxed. Upon the right side, although there existed a greater amount of deformity, the peculiar signs which characterise the injury under consideration were not so distinctly marked. Owing to the comminution of the lower fragment of the radius, the neighbourhood of the wrist here presented a combination of the signs of Colles's fracture with those of disjunction of the radial epiphysis, but the peculiar twisted appearance which forms so striking a feature in the former injury was entirely wanting. Upon both sides the antero-posterior diameter of the limb was increased, and the sharp margin of the superior fragment of the radius could be very distinctly felt. The diagnosis made was 'separation of the lower epiphysis of the radius upon each side.' The patient died from the injury to the head a few days after the accident, the symptoms having been those of compression of the brain.

The examination of the bones after death demonstrated the correctness of the opinion which had been formed as to the nature of the injuries sustained, the epiphysis being found separated from the shaft of the radius upon each side, and carried backwards along with the carpus to the extent of about three-eighths of an inch.

Upon the left side there was no other injury, but upon the right a thin scale of bone was detached along with the periosteum from the posterior surface of the shaft, and the epiphysis was broken into four pieces. There was no injury of the ulna upon either side.

Laceration of pronator quadratus, &c.—This small muscle can exert but little influence on the lower fragment or epiphysis, or cause any displacement inwards, for only a few fibres of this muscle are attached to the epiphysis, and these are usually torn across.

The action of this muscle would only tend to draw the shaft of the radius towards the ulna, but there is really no interosseous space in epiphysial separation into which the diaphysis may fall, and its displacement in this direction therefore becomes impossible.

In the Guy's Hospital specimen dissected by the author, the anterior margin of the diaphysis is seen protruding for three-eighths of an inch beyond the transverse laceration in the lower third of this muscle.

The same laceration of the pronator quadratus exists in both of the specimens in St. George's Hospital Museum and in that in the University of Turin.

In Johnston's case this muscle was found to be infiltrated with blood, and in the author's specimen the effusion of blood around the lacerated muscle in front of the diaphysis was a noticeable feature. This effusion has been remarked in many of the other specimens.

The interposition of the flexor tendon (profundus) of the middle finger prevented reduction in Hartmann's case.

Injury of wrist-joint.—The wrist-joint frequently escapes injury, and in this respect separation of the lower epiphysis of the radius differs very considerably from Colles's fracture in the adult.

In many instances, e.g. Bœckel's, it is distinctly stated that on dissection of the specimen the wrist-joint was uninjured.

Detachment &c. of periosteum.—In displacement backwards the periosteum is usually torn through at the anterior aspect, about on a level with the conjugal cartilage, and more or less extensively stripped up from the dorsal aspect of the diaphysis in the majority of the dissected specimens, but it is not usually lacerated in this latter direction.

De Paoli notes this laceration of the periosteum at the anterior part, with displacement of the diaphysis forwards, in ten out of his thirty-five cases, while in Bœckel's case a small strip of periosteum on the dorsal aspect was the only part remaining intact.

In the Guy's Hospital specimen the periosteum is torn off for a distance of three-quarters of an inch, and the space between it and the shaft is occupied by blood clot; in front it is lacerated in the usual way transversely across at the level of the anterior margin of the diaphysis. Precisely the same condition is described by Johnston (loc. cit. supra).

Dorsal detachment of the periosteum is also noted in one of

R. W. Smith's cases (*loc. cit. supra*), and also by other surgeons. In Colignon's case the separation of the periosteum from the diaphysis was described as extensive.

In one or two rare examples the periosteum has been found stripped from the front of the diaphysis. Thus in one of the specimens in St. George's Hospital the periosteum, together with the lower part of the pronator quadratus, was torn off the anterior aspect of the lower end of the diaphysis, and in the King's College Hospital specimen it is torn upwards for three-quarters of an inch from the front of the diaphysis.

Fracture of the styloid process of the ulna.—The frequency of fracture of the styloid process in Colles's fracture has been noted by Malgaigne, Cameron, Bennett, Lucas, and others, and the same lesion is not uncommonly found to exist in separation of the lower radial epiphysis.

At the Pathological Society in 1890 Mr. S. G. Shattock (*Transactions of the Pathological Society,* vol. xli. 1890, p. 236 ; St. Thomas's Hospital Museum, No. 115A) showed a specimen in which the lower epiphysis of the radius was clearly detached along its plane of junction with the shaft, and displaced backwards at an obtuse angle about a quarter of an inch off the diaphysis, precisely as the lower fragment commonly is in a Colles's fracture, rendering the head of the ulna very prominent. The styloid process of the ulna was also broken off. The injury probably resulted from the shock of the fall having been received by the outstretched hand. The boy, eight years of age, had fallen from a window a height of about twelve feet, and was supposed to have struck an anvil which was lying in the yard below. He sustained at the same time a rupture of the small intestine. For this a partial but unsuccessful enterectomy was performed on the day following the accident.

In a specimen in St. George's Hospital Museum, No. 3424 (114*b*) (*Catalogue of the Pathological Museum of St. George's Hospital,* 1882, p. 7), the lower radial epiphysis is displaced upwards and backwards almost off the diaphysis, and the apex of the styloid process is broken off. The ligaments of the left wrist were said to have been torn and the diaphyses of the bones uninjured.

In the description of the specimen it is stated that the lower end of the radial diaphysis may be seen protruding through the lacerated anterior ligament. If by this is meant the true anterior ligament of the wrist-joint, it is quite impossible to see how this could occur ; but, on the contrary, on examining the specimen it is clearly seen that the end of the diaphysis has lacerated the periosteum and lower part of the pronator quadratus, and protrudes in front through the fibres of this muscle. The patient, a boy aged fifteen, had fallen fifty-five feet, and fractured both his skull and his right clavicle.

In one of the specimens in St. Bartholomew's Hospital mentioned above, the styloid process was fractured, as well as the lower end of the ulna above the epiphysial line.

In 1883 the author made the following dissection of a case of separated lower epiphysis of the radius which simulated a Colles's fracture. The specimen is in the Guy's Hospital Museum, No. 1117⁴², and the specimen No. 956B in the Royal College of Surgeons museum is the inner portion of the same after vertical section. It is also figured by Mr. Bryant in his 'Practice of Surgery,' and by the author in 'Pediatrics,' New York and London, 1897, iv. p. 49.

The patient was a boy (Jas. H.), aged twelve, who, in sliding down the banisters of a warehouse, overbalanced and fell from the third story. Death ensued on the second day from fracture of the

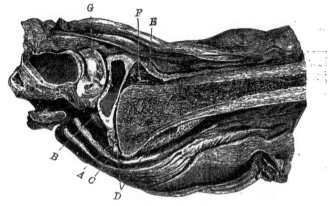

FIG. 145.—AUTHOR'S DISSECTION OF SPECIMEN IN GUY'S HOSPITAL MUSEUM. FROM A LAD AGED TWELVE YEARS

A, diaphysis of radius; *B*, carpal epiphysis of radius incompletely ossified; *C*, flexor tendons displaced forwards; *D*, pronator quadratus lacerated by anterior margin of end of radial diaphysis; *E*, periosteum stripped off dorsal aspect of diaphysis; *F*, blood clot filling space between periosteum and diaphysis; *G*, scaphoid

anterior fossa of the skull. The characteristic deformity of a Colles's fracture was still present after death, but crepitus was not felt.

The lower radial epiphysis was displaced more than halfway off, towards the dorsal aspect of the diaphysis, carrying with it the carpus and hand. It made an angle of forty-five degrees with the dorsal aspect of the shaft, the anterior third of its separated epiphysial surface being still in contact with the posterior or dorsal edge of the lower end of the diaphysis. The anterior margin of the latter had completely torn across the lower third of the pronator quadratus, and projected three-eighths of an inch beyond the lower portion of this muscle. This projecting margin of the diaphysis covered by the flexor tendons gave rise to the prominent convexity on the anterior aspect of the forearm above the wrist.

The periosteum was stripped off the dorsal aspect of the shaft to the extent of three-quarters of an inch upwards, and a triangular interval was thereby left between it and the diaphysis, which was occupied by firm blood clot. On the palmar aspect the periosteum binding the epiphysis to the diaphysis was entirely ruptured across.

The styloid process of the ulna was broken off, and together with the internal lateral ligament of the wrist-joint, which still remained connected with it, displaced for a distance of half an inch upwards and backwards. The lower end of the ulna, with its fractured styloid surface, projected prominently on the inner side of the wrist, but the dorsal branch of the ulnar nerve was uninjured, although the periosteum and ligamentous tissues were detached from the dorsal aspect of the ulna for a distance of three-quarters of an inch upwards. The triangular fibro-cartilage had its apex torn from the ulna, but a few fibres still remained attached to the root of the styloid process, and the cartilage was displaced backwards with it.[1]

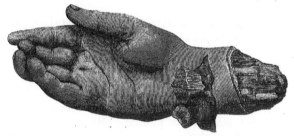

Fig. 146.—COMPOUND SEPARATION OF LOWER EPIPHYSIS OF RADIUS, WITH FRACTURE OF STYLOID PROCESS OF ULNA. (GUY'S HOSPITAL MUSEUM)

This inner portion of the wrist-joint (articulating with the cuneiform bone) was full of blood. The inferior radio-ulnar joint also contained some blood. The capsular ligament of the wrist-joint and the diaphyses of the bones of the forearm were uninjured.

The tendon of the extensor carpi ulnaris on the posterior aspect of the wrist was exceedingly tense, and on the outer side the supinator longus, still attached to the displaced epiphysis, was in a like condition. These, as well as the other extensor tendons passing through the thecal grooves at the back of the epiphysis, largely contributed by their action to the maintenance of the displaced condition of the fragment, and no doubt afforded considerable hindrance to the proper reduction of the deformity.

The accompanying drawing is from a case in Guy's Hospital Museum, No. 5⁸⁷, in which primary amputation was performed by Mr. Hilton in July 1865. There was a compound separation of the lower radial epiphysis, with great displacement backwards of the

---

[1] Differing from many instances of rupture of the fibro-cartilage in Colles's fracture, which takes place at its attachment to the inner margin of the radius.

carpus and hand. The styloid process was broken off, and the ends of the radius and ulna projected for some distance through the rent in the skin in front above the wrist-joint. The end of the radial diaphysis has the appearance as if it were fissured upwards about its centre.

This specimen is also figured by Bryant.

Separation of the lower epiphysis of the ulna.—The lower epiphysis or head of the ulna is but rarely detached. Its styloid process or its diaphysis, three-quarters of an inch above the lower end, gives way more frequently.

Barbarin mentions (*Les fract. chez les enfants*, Thèse de Paris, 1873, p. 34) the case of a youth, eighteen years of age, in whom amputation of the shoulder-joint was performed on account of gangrene. He had fallen from a tree, and there was found a very clean separation of the radial epiphysis, to which the conjugal cartilage still adhered. There was also on the same side a separation of the lower epiphysis of the ulna. The patient was under the care of M. Ollier.

Professor Annandale, of Edinburgh, informed the author in 1884 of a case in his practice of compound separation of the lower radial and ulnar epiphyses. A boy, aged about fifteen years, fell from some crags when bird-nesting. There was a lacerated transverse wound across the lower end of the forearm on the palmar aspect; the tendons were not torn, but the ends of the shafts of the radius and ulna protruded and were bruised and covered with dirt. The epiphyses remained in position. Mr. Annandale excised the protruding portions of the radius and ulna, and also removed the epiphyses. The result was a good recovery, with a movable wrist and fairly strong hand.

Dr. C. A. Sturrock records (*Edinburgh Hospital Reports*, vol. ii. 1894, p. 602) a case from Mr. Annandale's wards at the Royal Infirmary, Edinburgh. A boy of fourteen sustained a compound separation of the lower epiphyses of the radius and ulna, the result of a machinery accident. The shafts of both bones, which protruded and were partially stripped of periosteum, were tightly gripped by the flexor muscles of the fingers. It was found to be impossible to reduce the displacement, and accordingly Dr. R. J. A. Berry, after enlarging the wound, removed about three-quarters of an inch of the shafts of the radius and ulna, replaced the bones in position, and sewed up the wound. The patient made a rapid recovery, and when seen some fifteen months after the accident was found to have regained almost completely the movements at the wrist, and to suffer from little or no shortening.

In one of De Paoli's specimens figured above (fig. 144) there existed a separation and a fracture of the lower epiphysis of the ulna. He has noted the existence of separation of the ulnar epiphysis in three other instances.

Mr. E. Percy Paton (*Transactions of the Pathological Society,* vol. xlviii. 1897, p. 191) showed at the Pathological Society of London, on January 19, 1897, a specimen of fracture of the ulna and radius at the epiphysial lines.

Mr. Stonham kindly placed the specimen at the author's disposal for the purpose of the accompanying drawing.

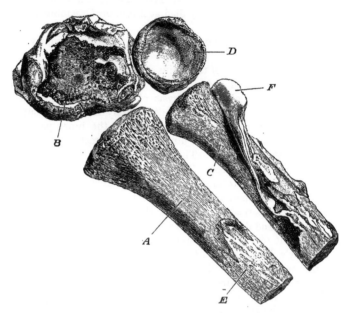

Fig. 147.—COMPOUND SEPARATION OF THE LOWER EPIPHYSES OF THE RADIUS AND ULNA. (WESTMINSTER HOSPITAL MUSEUM.) SUPPURATIVE PERIOSTITIS. THE EPI- PHYSES HAVE BEEN ROTATED IN ORDER TO SHOW THEIR DIAPHYSIAL SURFACES

A, diaphysis of radius bereft of periosteum ; *E*, new osseous deposit from peri- osteum ; *B*, epiphysis of radius with conjugal cartilage almost entirely destroyed by suppuration ; *C*, diaphysis of ulna ; *D*, epiphysis of ulna with conjugal cartilage intact ; *F*, periosteum stripped off the diaphysis of ulna

For the following notes of the case the author is indebted to Mr. Paton.

D. S., aged fourteen, plumber's mate, was admitted into West- minster Hospital under Mr. Stonham on December 11, 1896, having just fallen twenty feet from a ladder. He was found to have a transverse wound from two to three inches long on the flexor aspect of the right forearm just above the wrist-joint. It was begrimed with dirt, and from it protruded the lower end of the diaphyses of both radius and ulna. An anæsthetic was given, and the bones and wound were thoroughly cleansed by the house surgeon. The bones were then reduced without difficulty and the wound sutured, the hand and arm being put in a splint. The temperature rose somewhat during the next day or two and the wound suppurated, but not very extensively; all stitches were taken out and the hand transferred to an arm-bath, the deformity being still controlled by a splint. On December 18 signs of tetanus set in at 6 A.M. (trismus and some dorsal spasm). This was treated with large doses of chloral and bromide, scraping of the wound under an anæsthetic, irrigation with oxygen gas, and the injection of anti-tetano-toxin, obtained from the Institute of Preventive Medicine, in three doses to the amount of 35 c.c., but the boy died at 2 P.M. on December 19, in an acute spasm.

Nothing special was found at the autopsy but the injury shown in the specimen.

The carpal epiphyses of the radius and ulna were cleanly separated, with the exception of a few osseous granules from the posterior margin of the end of the diaphysis of the radius. The conjugal cartilage of this bone had been almost entirely destroyed by suppuration—a few flakes only remained attached to the inner part of the epiphysis—while that of the ulna was still intact, adhering in its entirety to the epiphysis. The styloid process of the ulna and wrist-joint were uninjured. The periosteum was stripped for two and a half inches from the whole circumference of the shaft. Above this, new periosteal deposit extended upwards for some distance. The periosteal sheath of the ulna was much thickened and inflamed, and detached for two and a half inches upwards from the outer half of the circumference of the shaft.

At Guy's Hospital in 1880 Mr. Cooper Forster had under his care the case of a boy (Henry T.), aged fourteen years, who had fallen through the stair-rails the height of the flight of stairs on to his hands. There was found compound separation of the lower epiphyses of the radius and the ulna, with displacement of the radial epiphysis. Mr. Forster resected half an inch of the lower end of the diaphysis of the radius by means of a saw, and reduced the displacement. This was followed by some necrosis of the diaphysis and by recovery. Dislocation of the elbow backwards was also present.

At the museum of the International Medical Congress, London, in 1881 (*Museum Catalogue of International Medical Congress*, London 1881, p. 52, No. 550) Dr. Geoghegan exhibited a specimen, from the Royal College of Surgeons, Ireland, of separation of the epiphyses of the radius and ulna. The subject from which this specimen was taken was a young man who died of injuries received in a fall from scaffolding.

M. Voillemier gives an example in a child aged fourteen years, who had fallen a height of eight feet on to the palm of the hand.

Besides the detachment of the lower epiphysis of the radius, there was a fracture of the ulna which involved two thirds of its thickness at the union of its lower epiphysis with the shaft. But this author makes no further allusion to the subject in his valuable memoir on fractures of the lower end of the radius.

Fracture of shaft of ulna.—Fracture of the ulna is of frequent occurrence towards its lower end.

In a child of about fifteen the weakest and smallest part of the diaphysis is three-quarters of an inch above the lower end.

In Roux's specimen the ulna was fractured in its lower fourth, but in this case the radial epiphysis was displaced forwards.

De Paoli, in four cases, found this separation accompanied by fracture of the ulnar diaphysis near its lower extremity.

In Hilton's case of compound separation of both radial epiphyses, on the left side there was also an oblique fracture of the ulna an inch and a half above the wrist-joint; on the right side the ulna was uninjured.

The ulna was fractured, in Bœckel's case, three centimetres above its lower end.

An interesting case of epiphysial separation of the lower end of each radius—compound on the right side, with fracture of the ulna a little above its lower end—is recorded at length by H. Hartmann (*Bulletins de la Société anatomique*, Paris, July 1883, p. 328). Fracture of the right femur, rupture of the left kidney, and multiple contusions complicated the injury and led to death on the thirty-fourth day from general infection and suppuration of all the seats of injury.

(C.), a boy, aged twelve years, was admitted on June 8, 1883 under the care of Dr. Terrier, into the Bichat Hôpital, having fallen that afternoon from the top of the ramparts while at play. There was a contused wound of the forehead and slight contusion of the nape of the neck, fracture of the lower part of the left forearm (with displacement backwards of the hand, which was easily reduced, and a posterior plaster splint applied), and fracture of the right thigh at the junction of the upper with the lower thirds (which was treated by continuous extension). At the inner and front aspect of the right forearm there was a wound, through which protruded the lower end of the radius, displaced forwards and inwards off the epiphysis. Its surface displayed a slightly mammillated appearance, without any trace of spongy tissue or osseous roughness, and was more like the articular end of the bone than a fractured one. The styloid process held its normal relations. The radius was irreducible on account of the interposition of the tendons and its embracement by the skin wound, and the urine was found to contain blood. The following day, under an anæsthetic, reduction was somewhat difficult, for the middle finger, which was kept flexed, could not be extended, whilst all the other fingers could be, with ease; this was caused by the tendon of the flexor profundus to the middle finger being interposed. After this had been drawn aside and disengaged the radius was placed in position. Lister's dressings were employed, and a posterior splint applied.

On June 10 an external splint was applied to the thigh. On

June 16 some sloughs began to separate from the wound of the forearm, and two days later a blackish slough the size of the palm of the hand formed on the right buttock, and hæmorrhage took place from the ulnar artery, which necessitated ligature of the two ends in the wound. On June 22 the patient, in his delirium, had a second time taken off the dressings, and there was noticed at the upper and inner part of the wrist a wound in which the end of the fractured ulna presented itself with an oblique (inward) division and very sharp end. There was also œdema of the abdominal wall and pain in the left flank. On June 27 a small purulent collection in nape of neck opened at the site of a contusion. The following day it was noted that the swelling of the right thigh had increased the last few days, and a puncture let out a quantity of gas and fœtid pus. On the 29th a small abscess opened at the level of the frontal wound. On the 30th an incision above the left crural arch evacuated a very large quantity of serous and brownish pus. T. 101°. On July 1 the right radius again became displaced, and projected between the muscles in front of the forearm. The slough of the right buttock was detached, leaving a vast wound. Emaciation increasing, tongue dry, eyes sunken, T. 101·4° F. Death ensued on July 12. Temperature rose gradually the last four days to 105·2° F. At the autopsy a large wound was seen on the anterior aspect of the *right forearm*, through which there protruded the lower part of the radius. It was directed obliquely downwards, forwards, and inwards, ending immediately above the pisiform bone. The whole mass of the flexor tendons was situate on its outer side, and prevented it being replaced in position. Its end presented a very abrupt, slightly mammillated, and black appearance. The bone was denuded for about three fingers' breadth, with a reddish, mottled, and slightly rough look. On dividing and removing the anterior tendons the radial epiphysis was seen to be in position, and the styloid process preserved its proper relations. The epiphysis had the appearance of a plate about a millimetre and a half thick, rising up at its outer part to constitute the styloid process. The cartilages were destroyed. The ulna presented a dentate fracture just above its lower end, passing obliquely downwards and inwards, so that the upper fragment was displaced in the same direction, overlapping the lower fragment (backwards and inwards), and was pointed at the inner side. The lower fragment occupied its normal position, while the upper was denuded for two centimetres in extent on its inner side, and projected through the integuments. No union was present, but suppuration was limited to the seat of fracture. The cartilages of the medio-carpal articulation and of the carpo-metacarpal articulation of the second and third metacarpal bones had disappeared, while the trapezo-metacarpal and two last metacarpal joints were healthy. At its upper part the synovial sheath of the flexor tendons was obliterated at the level of the wound by a greyish mass, the palmar portion presenting its normal pearly aspect. On the posterior aspect the extensor tendons in the whole of their extent were clear and shining. On *the left forearm* there was an extensive purulent collection extending between and separating the muscles, which did not appear to be very much altered. The bones were in their normal relations. The radial epiphysis was separated; the end of the upper fragment presented a general transversely divided and slightly mammillated appearance, while the lower fragment presented precisely the same appearance as that of the right side. The ulna was not fractured, and occupied its normal position; its small denuded head was surrounded by a deep furrow consequent on the partial destruction of the conjugal cartilage by the suppuration. The cartilages of the medio-carpal joint were destroyed. The synovial sheaths of the flexor and extensor tendons were intact.

On the *right thigh* there was a transversely dentate subtrochanteric fracture of the femur. The lower fragment was parallel to, but surmounted, the upper on its outer aspect for about three fingers' breadth. There was no trace of union between the ends, which were contained in a fairly large but limited collection of pus. Nephritic abscess and rupture of the left kidney. At the upper part of the left thigh, from four fingers' breadth below the crural arch, there was a large purulent collection extending upwards in the sheath of the psoas muscles into the abdominal cavity. The peritoneum was not opened. There was also a large lumbar abscess destroying the iliacus muscle, at the upper part of which the kidney was torn in two by a transverse rent at the level of the lower part of the hilus. The two parts were only held together by some tags at the posterior part, which appeared to be formed by some *débris* of the capsule. The lower part was surrounded by the abscess cavity. The whole of the hilus was completely torn through. The ureter was partially torn at the inner side. Interstitial nephritis, with foci of fatty granular degeneration, was present in the lower half of the lacerated kidney.

M. Hartmann draws attention to the slight displacement of the radius on the one side, while the upper fragment of the radius on the other side protruded through a wound, and to the difficulty of reduction and maintaining it in position after replacement, which he thought attributable to muscular action and to the absence of dentation, which permitted the easy reproduction of the displacement. He also remarks upon the suppuration of *all* the seats of injury and of these alone; he therefore considered the case a good example of those auto-inoculations so well described by Professor Verneuil.

Professor R. W. Smith (*Fractures and Dislocations*, Dublin, 1847, p. 164) figures and describes the condition of the forearm before and after dissection.

The patient, a young man, fell from a scaffold, and in addition to the fracture of the forearm, received other injuries, of which he

died in a few hours. No attempt was made to reduce the displacement consequent upon the fracture. When the limb was examined
after death the radius was found fractured transversely through the
line of its inferior epiphysis, and the lower fragment displaced
directly backwards, so far as to have very nearly cleared the
extremity of the upper fragment; the lower extremity of the ulna
was broken a short distance above the line of junction with its
epiphysis; this fracture was oblique from above and before downwards and backwards; the extremities of the two fragments formed
with each other an angle salient in front; the radio-carpal articulation

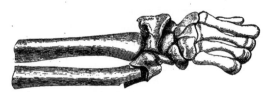

Fig. 148.—Separation of lower epiphysis of radius, with fracture of ulna.
(after r. w. smith.) appearance before dissection

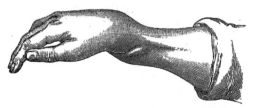

Fig. 149.—Separation of the lower epiphysis of the radius, with
fracture of the ulna. (r. w. smith)

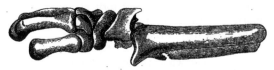

Fig. 150.—the same, outer side. (r. w. smith)

was uninjured, and the carpus accompanied the lower fragment of
the radius in its displacement backwards.

The same author describes (*Dublin Journal of Medical Science,*
vol. lvi. 1873, p. 424; *Proceedings of the Pathological Society of
Dublin,* N.S. vol. v. 1874, p. 245) the following case of compound
disjunction of the lower epiphysis of the radius accompanied with
fracture of the ulna. The patient, a boy aged twelve years, fell off
a parapet fifteen feet high, sustaining very extensive compound
fractures of the skull and laceration of the brain, from which he
died.

The lesion was situated in the immediate vicinity of the radio-carpal articulation ; a large lacerated wound existed here upon the palmar surface of the limb, through which rather more than half an inch of the radius protruded; it was disjointed from its epiphysis. The axis of the bone was directed forwards and considerably inwards towards the lower end of the ulna. The radial border of the forearm presented a very striking curve, the concavity of which (supposing the arm to hang by the side) was directed forwards, while along the ulnar margin was seen an equally remarkable convexity. The hand and carpus were in the position of extreme abduction. The dorsal surface of the limb presented equally remarkable features. It was curved to a great degree; the hollow of the curve (the limb being in the position mentioned above) was directed backwards. Above, it faded away insensibly, but below it ended abruptly at the margin of a tumour, which, extending from the radial to the ulnar border of the limb, constituted a most striking feature of the injury, and was, of itself, diagnostic of the nature of the injury

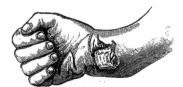 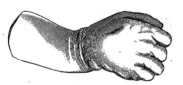

FIG. 151.—COMPOUND SEPARATION OF THE LOWER EPIPHYSIS OF THE RADIUS, WITH FRACTURE OF THE ULNA. PALMAR ASPECT (AFTER R. W. SMITH)

FIG. 152.—THE SAME, DORSAL ASPECT (R. W. SMITH)

which the bones had sustained. This tumour gave to the back of the hand an elongated appearance.

The condition of affairs disclosed by dissection was as follows : The radial epiphysis was found still connected with the scaphoid and lunar bones. The ulna was fractured directly above its epiphysis, and the lower fragment displaced backwards in such a manner as to form with the upper an angle salient in front. The dorsal tumour was thus constituted by the carpus, the radial epiphysis, and the lower fragment of the ulna, forming one system of parts, carried backwards, and giving to the hand its lengthened appearance and its resemblance to a luxation of the carpus in that direction. In the sulcus which marked the termination of the posterior curvature and the commencement of the dorsal tumour, the relaxed integument was thrown into transverse curved creases, whose concavities were directed downwards towards the hand. They closely resembled the crescentic folds seen above the displaced phalanx in many cases of Hey's luxation of the thumb.

In a case mentioned by E. H. Bennett the separated radial epiphysis was accompanied by a fracture of the ulna close above the epiphysial line, and a similar fracture is present in one of the specimens in St. Bartholomew's Hospital Museum.

In one of the specimens in the London Hospital Museum the fracture of the ulna was almost transverse, and an inch and a quarter from the extremity of the styloid process.

Labadie-Lagrave records (*Bull. de la Soc. Anat.* 1868, Paris 1874, p. 240) a case of compound separation in which the epiphysis was very cleanly and completely detached, with the exception of some small scales from the diaphysis adhering to the outer part of the circumference of this epiphysial fragment; the diaphysis protruded through a large lacerated wound of the skin on the anterior aspect of the forearm at the level of the upper articular crease. Its end appeared to be covered with a thin cartilaginous layer, which at first sight might have been mistaken for a compound dislocation of the wrist. The carpal ends of the radius and ulna preserved their normal relations with the carpus. The carpal ligaments were perfectly intact. The ulna was also transversely fractured at its neck, one centimetre above the articular surface. The injury occurred in a lad, aged six-teen years, who died in two hours in a comatose state from injuries to the head, the result of a fall from the fourth story of a house. He was under the care of M. Maisonneuve at the Hôtel-Dieu. Attempts by powerful traction were made, during life, to reduce the displaced fragments, but without success.

There was great increase in the antero-posterior diameter of the hand, with the usual characteristic 'fork back' deformity, and the hand, slightly flexed, inclined to the ulnar border at the same time that it appeared to be thrown (as a whole) towards the radial side, so that the hand made an angle with the forearm, which was open outwards. The forearm was in a position midway between pronation and supination.

Fracture of both bones of the forearm.—W. Körte junior, at the Berlin Medical Society (*Berliner klinische Woch.* Berlin 1880, No. 3, May 18, S. 263), showed a specimen of separated radial epiphysis and incomplete fracture of both bones of the forearm from a boy, aged eighteen. The separation of the lower end of the radius was perfect, but was not detected before dissection, although a careful examination had been made of the part. The boy had got his right arm caught between the barrel and the driving-strap of a machine, so that the limb was torn off at the middle of the humerus. Amputation at the shoulder was performed and terminated in recovery.

On examination the forearm was seen to be semipronate and bent like a bow with the concavity backwards; the hand was also bent backwards, but no fracture of the bones could be made out. Subsequently there was found to be a complete solution of continuity of the radius in the epiphysial line, although the epiphysis was still connected with the diaphysis by means of the

periosteum. The radius was incompletely fractured fifteen centimetres higher up, and also the ulna five centimetres above the
wrist-joint; in both, the dorsal fibres of the bones still held the
bones in position, although the anterior fibres were ruptured.

Dr. Körte thought that by the accident the hand was first of all
bent backwards and the epiphysis of the radius thereby separated,
which was analogous to a fall upon the hand bent backwards, and
that on further bending of the forearm the ulna yielded, and then the
radius, at their thinnest parts.

Dislocation of Ulna.—Professor E. M. Moore, of Rochester, U.S.A.,
mentioned in a letter to the author (September 1893) that he had in
his possession an excellent specimen of epiphysial fracture of the
lower end of the radius, accompanied with luxation of the lower
end of the ulna, from a boy, aged fifteen, who was killed by
machinery. Unfortunately no details were given.

Dislocation of the ulna was also present in De Paoli's case
described above.

Wounds.—These are much more frequent complications in
epiphysial separations than in the corresponding fractures in adults,
probably owing to the greater amount of force required in the former
case and to the thinness of the anterior edge of the projecting
diaphysis.

In the *Archives générales de Médecine* (1867, vol. ii. p. 228;
Gazette médicale de Strasbourg, No. 7, 10 Juin, 1867) Dr. E.
Bœckel gives the following description of a case of compound
separation followed by sloughing of the forearm.

A boy, aged twelve years, while endeavouring to climb a tree, fell
to the ground a height of about eight metres upon the outstretched
hands, producing a serious injury to the left wrist. The surgeon
who saw the case stated that the lower extremity of the radius had
passed through the integument of the anterior aspect of the forearm, and, finding this bone covered with a layer of cartilage, he
believed it to be a dislocation of the wrist. The displaced bone was
immediately reduced and kept in position by a suitable apparatus;
sloughing of the forearm, however, soon ensued, and only stopped at
the elbow. Dr. Bœckel performed amputation of the arm ten days
after the accident, and the patient recovered. On examining the
limb he found the following lesions: the lower epiphysis of the
radius, five millimetres thick, was separated, together with the
epiphysial cartilage, from the shaft of the bone; on its posterior
aspect it was surmounted by a fragment of the cortical layer of the
diaphysis, which had been torn off. A strip of the periosteum was
still intact on this side. The end of the diaphysis was eroded by the
pus, and on a fair way to necrosis. The ulna was divided by a
transverse dentate fracture, three centimetres above its lower
extremity, but the wrist-joint was not opened.

Gripat records (*Bull. de la Soc. Anat.* 1872, Paris, 1874,

p. 176) a case in which the lower epiphyses of both radii were separated.

On the right side the injury was compound, the end of the diaphysis protruding through the soft parts, and some fragments of bone were detached from the posterior margin of the diaphysis, but remained attached to the epiphysis. The diaphysial end presented some small particles of cartilage, and was stripped of its periosteum in front, but more especially behind. With this exception the epiphysial cartilage remained with the epiphysis. The specimen was obtained from a boy, aged thirteen and a half years, who died from the effects of a fall from a third story. There were other injuries present —viz. fracture of the skull and coronoid process of the ulna, with dislocation of the elbow-joint, as well as dislocation of the hip-joint.

Richet mentions (*Gaz. des Hôpit.* 1865, pp. 145–147, and *Bull. de la Soc. de Chirurg.* 1865, p. 528) the case under the care of M. Denonvilliers of a boy, aged fifteen years, who had fallen upon his hand. The end of the diaphysis of the radius projected between the flexor tendons through the skin in front of the forearm ; the projecting end was removed by a chain-saw, on account of the impossibility of reduction. The bone on removal was found to be covered with several thin lamellæ of the epiphysial cartilage, so that the separation was thought to have occurred through the epiphysial cartilage itself. Recovery took place.

M. Manquat records (*Les décollements épiphysaires traumatiques,* Thèse de Paris, 1877, p. 37) a precisely similar case observed by Péan. The projection of the diaphysis through the wound and the separated epiphysis bore the same characters. Resection of the diaphysis was followed by cure.

At Guy's Hospital in 1870 Mr. Cock had the case of John D., aged sixteen years, under his care. While at work in a sawmill his left hand became entangled in the band driving the machine, and was carried upwards several times, knocking his legs and arms against the beam above. A compound separation with displacement of the lower radial epiphysis was found, together with simple fracture of the lower third of the shaft of humerus and severe contusion of the right leg. Reduction could only be effected after the removal of half an inch of the end of the radial diaphysis by means of a saw. Recovery ensued after some suppuration and necrosis of the right tibia.

M. Curtillet describes (*Du décollement traumatique des épiphyses,* Lyon, 1891) a case of compound separation in a boy aged six years, who had fallen upon his hand. There was the usual deformity of displacement backwards of the epiphysis, and on the anterior aspect, just above the wrist, a transverse wound through which the end of the diaphysis, completely detached from the epiphysis and stripped of its periosteum, protruded with its characteristic uniform, flat, and somewhat granular surface, and mossy-looking rounded margins. There was no fracture of the ulna.

Under an anæsthetic, after the wound and bone had been carefully cleansed from dirt, pebbles, and other filth, and disinfected, it was found that reduction could not be effected ; the wound was therefore enlarged perpendicularly by an incision three centimetres in length. The end of the diaphysis was then easily and completely reduced. The articulations about the wrist were found to be intact. A strip of iodoform gauze was used for drainage, the wound closed by three sutures, and a plaster splint applied. The wound was dressed about the twentieth day, but there was no suppuration, and the patient left the hospital shortly afterwards.

When examined ten months after the accident there was no deformity of the wrist, with the exception of slight prominence of the lower end of the ulna, and the movements of the wrist, as well as those of pronation and supination of the forearm, were quite natural. The patient could then use his hand freely for writing and other purposes.

There was slight diminution in the length (half centimetre) of the radius, which was probably the result of slight transient disturbance of ossification, so frequently seen in many epiphysial detachments, and Dr. Curtillet did not think that it would be followed by any more serious disturbance of growth.

In all the other compound separations observed by R. W. Smith, Bennett, Hilton, Cock, Annandale, and Labadie-Lagrave, already mentioned, the wound was situated on the palmar aspect of the forearm in close proximity to, or just above, the wrist. In Hartmann's case it was on the inner side of the anterior aspect.

The cases of Messrs. Cooper Forster and Hilton at Guy's Hospital were also compound ; in the last-named primary amputation was performed.

In more than one case the end of the diaphysis of the radius has been mistaken for a compound dislocation of the radius—an error it is difficult to imagine, considering the presence of the articular cartilage covering the concave end of the bone in the latter form of injury.

In Hilton's case of compound separation of the carpal epiphyses of both radii, on the right side there were two wounds anteriorly, laying bare the flexor tendons, but not exposing the bone; one was thought to have been caused by the protrusion of the diaphysis, whilst the other was probably produced by severe flexion of the hand backwards, causing great tension of the skin in front, which then gave way. On the left side the smooth diaphysial end of the bone projected through a wound anteriorly, and was associated with an oblique fracture of the shaft of the ulna one and a half inches above the wrist-joint.

Bruns collected five cases of compound separation of this epiphysis.

J. Hutchinson junior found ten compound cases among fifty-four.

The author has collected fourteen cases.

Pressure upon the radial nerve from the displacement of the epiphysis has only been noted in one case, that of Brunner described below; but the occurrence of this may be easily brought about in cases of great displacement.

Pressure upon the median nerve by the displaced diaphysis in Hilton's case was thought to have been the cause of the tetanus from which the patient died on the seventh day.

Injury of radial artery.—Pressure upon the radial artery by the lower end of the diaphysis projecting in front has never occurred.

OTHER SEVERE LESIONS.—In most of the cases in which separation of the lower radial epiphysis has been found on dissection the injury is an insignificant one in comparison with the injury which proves fatal.

Fractured skull.—Of the twenty-one pathological specimens death was caused in eleven by a more or less extensive fracture of the base of the skull, after a fall from a height. It is probable that many more of these specimens were taken from patients after similar severe accidents, although it is not especially noted.

Among ten cases of compound separation death ensued in three, and in all of these from extensive fractures of the skull; in one after a fall from a parapet sixteen feet high; the second, after a fall from the third story; and the third after a fall from the fourth story of a house.

Severe abdominal lesion.—Laceration of the kidneys and intra- and extra-peritoneal hæmorrhage were the cause of death in the case from which one of De Paoli's specimens was taken. Complete rupture of the kidney and fracture of thigh and multiple contusion complicated Hartmann's case. Rupture of the small intestine occurred in Mr. Shattock's case after a fall of twelve feet from a window.

Dislocation of the forearm backwards.—In three cases De Paoli found the separation of the radial epiphysis accompanied by a dislocation backwards of the bones of the forearm.

Compound dislocation of forearm backwards.—Galand (Thèse de Paris, 1834, No. 196, p. 23) mentions the case of a youth under the care of M. Roux in 1834. The patient had fallen from a tree, and was thought by M. Roux to be the subject of two dislocations of the left arm—one being of the elbow, compound, and another of the wrist, both being backwards. M. Roux reduced the supposed dislocation of the wrist with difficulty, but it tended to be reproduced. At the time he had no doubt as to the correctness of his diagnosis. The patient died some days later, when, to the astonishment of M. Roux, a separation of the lower epiphysis of the radius was found on dissection.

Kramer (*Monatsschrift für Unfallheilkunde*, 1897, No. 4) relates a similar interesting but more successful example of compound separation of the lower radial epiphysis complicated with compound dislocation of the forearm backwards at the elbow. A boy, aged twelve years, whilst quickly running, fell, alighting first on the palm of the right hand, then on the ground with the weight of his whole body. The arm having lost its proper support through the solution of continuity of the radius, the whole weight of the body appeared to have been violently received upon the inner aspect of the flexed forearm, which slid to the ground; this, giving rise to forcible abduction and perhaps also to rotation of the forearm, led to laceration of the internal, lateral, and anterior ligaments, &c., of the elbow-joint, and ultimate perforation of the skin by the lower end of the humerus impinging against the flexure of the elbow. The lower radial diaphysis appeared through a wound on the volar side, while at the flexure of the right elbow there was an oblique wound through which a good deal of hæmorrhage occurred. The ulnar artery was crushed, the vein lacerated, and the median nerve torn through for a third of its distance. At the operation the dislocation was reduced, the nerve sutured, and the radial epiphysis replaced and secured by two silver sutures. Recovery took place without any untoward result. After six and a half weeks extension of the elbow-joint was almost complete, but flexion was only possible up to 100°. Pronation and supination were very restricted. The wrist and finger-joints were almost free in their movements. Later on functional restoration had considerably improved, yet the forearm appeared to have been somewhat retarded in its growth in length.

Incomplete fracture of the radius, &c.—De Paoli noted fracture of the coronoid process of the ulna in one case, and in another incomplete fracture of the radius in the middle, with dislocation forwards of the ulna at the hand.

LATER COMPLICATIONS. **Gangrene of hand and forearm.**—R. W. Smith mentions (*Treatise on Fractures and Dislocations*, Dublin, 1854, p. 170) the case of a boy, aged eighteen years, who had a fracture of the lower extremity of the radius, through the line of junction of the epiphysis with the diaphysis, caused by being thrown from a horse. A surgeon applied, within an hour, a narrow roller bandage tightly round the wrist. On the following day the limb was intensely painful, cold, and discoloured; still, the bandage was not removed, nor even slackened. On the fourth day he was admitted into the Richmond Hospital, when gangrene was found to have reached the forearm. Spontaneous separation of the soft parts finally occurred, and the bones were sawn through twenty-four days after the accident; afterwards ' everything proceeded favourably.'

Rognetta (*Gazette Médicale*, Paris, 1834, p. 514) records the case of a youth, aged fifteen years, who fell from a tree, dislocating his forearm backwards, and injuring the wrist of the same side. He was thought to have a dislocation of the wrist as well as the elbow. The parts were replaced somewhat in their natural position, and a retentive apparatus was applied; intense phlegmonous inflammation and gangrene ensued, followed by death. At the autopsy it was found that the supposed dislocation of the wrist was in reality a perfect separation of the lower end of the radius.

Gangrene of the arm also followed in Barbarin's case (see above) of separation of the lower epiphysis of radius and ulna, and gangenous cellulitis ensued in Dr. Bœckel's case of compound separation of the radius.

Suppuration of forearm or **phlegmonous inflammation** of limb has been noted in a few instances. In one instance of complete displacement of the epiphysis recorded by Hutchinson reduction was found exceedingly difficult, and suppuration subsequently occurred, but the arm was saved.

Suppuration is a not uncommon result in compound separations. Mr. Stonham's case of compound separation of the epiphyses of radius and ulna is a notable instance.

Necrosis of the diaphysis has been a not infrequent result in compound cases. In Bœckel's case the end of the diaphysis was infiltrated with pus and about to become necrosed.

Necrosis followed resection. in Mr. Cooper Forster's case of compound diastasis. .

Tetanus.—In Hilton's case tetanus occurred on the sixth day, after compound separation of the carpal epiphyses of both radii, and terminated in death the following day. This surgeon says: 'The median nerve could scarcely have escaped injury at the time of the accident, lying as it does in the midst of the tendons, through which the fractured bone protruded.'

The following remarkable case of traumatic tetanus is recorded by Brunner (*London Medical Record*, July 15, 1886, p. 298), in which compression of the radial nerve was caused by a separation of the lower radial epiphysis. Upon resection of the bulky callus and freeing of the radial nerve the symptoms disappeared.

A boy, fourteen years old, was admitted to Conrad Brunner's ward in Zürich for a fracture of the left radius which had occurred three weeks previously. The fourteenth day after the fracture the child found that he could not extend the fingers of the left hand, and his parents noticed that when he walked he was bent forward. The symptoms became gradually more marked, so that on his admission the symptoms of tetanus were evident—sardonic laugh, teeth firmly set, complete emprosthotonos, the head resting against the breast. There was evidence of a badly reduced fracture of the epiphysis of the radius, and bulky callus just below the articulation. It seemed evident that the tetanus resulted from pressure of the radial nerve by new formations connected with the callus, and this was proved by operation. The nerve was set free, the prominent portion of the radius being resected, and the symptoms of tetanus slowly disappeared. The patient was given morphine injections. Three weeks after the operation he was cured.

Articular inflammation is rarely met with, notwithstanding the proximity of the joint. It would ensue in fracture of the epiphysis into the joint, as has been found in one of the specimens in St. Bartholomew's Hospital.

Suppurative periostitis.—Suppurative periostitis was present in Hilton's case of compound separation of the epiphysis, and probably was associated with the death of the patient on the seventh day, although this was said to have taken place from tetanus. Both bones were removed after death with their epiphyses detached. The specimens from the left wrist were bloodless, saturated with fœtid pus, and dead. This resulted from the periosteum having been stripped off the bone at the time of the accident; the bone being thus deprived of its proper medium of nutrition, there resulted the death of bone and the purulent condition associated with it.

This serious complication may arise even in cases of simple separation.

A case of acute osteomyelitis following injury to the lower epiphysis of the radius is related by Mr. Page (*British Medical Journal*, July 20, 1889, p. 131).

On June 17, 1887, A. R., aged seventeen, a groom, was lifting a horse-collar down from its peg when, because of his insecure hold of it, the collar slipped back, and his right wrist was, as he thought, sprained. In about three hours his wrist began to be painful, but he continued at his work both on that and the next day. On the 21st he first noticed swelling of the wrist, and on the 23rd he came to St. Mary's Hospital. His temperature was 103·4° F., and there was some swelling on the flexor side of the wrist, which was also hot and tender. The next day an incision was made under most careful antisepsis, and a small quantity of clear serous fluid evacuated from the sheath of one of the tendons, but the periosteum was not opened. On the 26th examination of the wound led to the suspicion that he had acute inflammation of the radial epiphysis as the result of some injury sustained by it when the wrist was supposed to have been merely sprained. On June 30 fluctuation, redness, and swelling extended to the dorsum of the limb, and an incision was made on the back of the wrist and pus was let out from beneath both skin and fascia. It was then found that the whole lower end of the radial shaft was quite bare. Some improvement followed, but did not last long. The pus increased in amount, and soon began to burrow up the limb; next there was suppuration in the upper arm, then the elbow-joint became involved, so that amputation of the arm was performed in the middle third on July 19. Then he rapidly got well.

Examination showed that the periosteum had been stripped up from the shaft of the radius to a distance of five inches, but there was no inflammation of this part of the bone. The epiphysis, however, was quite detached, and what remained of it presented all the indications of having been affected by an acute destructive septic inflammation. It was soft, completely broken down, and infiltrated with pus. It was, indeed, abundantly clear that the beginning of the mischief had been in the epiphysis itself, that in all probability there had been some separation of it from the shaft, and that the unhealthy character of the boy's occupation had determined the virulent septicity of the inflammation which so speedily supervened. Whether at the time of the accident there had been likewise detachment of periosteum it is impossible to say with certainty.

Pyæmia has occurred in more than one case, and been followed by death.

Displacement forwards.—Forward displacement of the epiphysis is probably not so rare an occurrence as has been hitherto supposed.

In this injury the epiphysis is driven towards the anterior or flexor aspect of the wrist.

A case of M. Denonvilliers's is reported by Professor Richet (*Anatomie chirurgicale*, 4 éd. p. 90) of a child about eight years of age, in which the upper fragment or diaphysis protruded on the dorsal aspect of the forearm. The osseous projection was at first taken to be the lower end of the radius, but the irregularity of the surface of the fragment and the fact of its bristling with cartilaginous projections clearly showed that it was a true solution of continuity in the conjugal cartilage, and not a simple separation. Resection of the end was rendered necessary, and the patient completely recovered, without any untoward symptoms.

M. Péan observed a precisely similar case in the year 1856. This patient likewise recovered in a short time without the occurrence of any complications.

M. Roux (*La Presse Médicale*, July 12, 1837, vol. i.) describes the following case, in which there was disjunction of the lower epiphysis of the radius, of the styloid epiphysis of the ulna, of the upper epiphysis of the first phalanges of the thumb, and of the index and middle fingers of the left hand.

On July 22, 1821, the patient (M. A., a porter), when packing boxes, had his hand and forearm severely injured by an explosion of gunpowder. On his being taken at once to the hospital, it was found that the thumb and middle finger were held to the hand merely by the extensor tendons, the index finger had been completely blown off (this was found some days afterwards in a house near the scene of the accident), while the last two fingers were uninjured. The soft parts covering the carpus and metacarpus were severely contused, lacerated, and blackened by the powder. The forearm was also extensively injured. The ulna was fractured at its lower fourth. The lower end of the radius projected outwards through the skin and muscles on the dorsal aspect; it did not present the smooth polished appearance of the articular surface, but was more rough, and not so large in size. Amputation through the lower third of the forearm was the only treatment to be adopted, and was performed five or six hours after the accident. Rapid recovery took place. M. Roux subsequently made out the following lesions :—

(1) The pisiform bone had been carried away, as well as the index finger mentioned above. (2) The ulna was fractured in its lower fourth. (3) The shaft of the radius was separated from its lower epiphysis, as well as the styloid epiphysis of the ulna ; and the shafts of the first phalanges of the thumb, of the index and of the middle fingers were separated from their upper epiphyses, which remained connected with the bones of the metacarpus. Roux states that he sent the specimen to the Musée Dupuytren.

The following description of a dwarfed radius, with displacement forwards of its lower epiphysis (?), is given by the great surgeon Dupuytren (*Injuries and Diseases of the Bones*, translation, Sydenham Society, 1847, p. 129), and is worthy of being quoted in detail.

' The subject of this pathological condition was an adult female, respecting whom no history could be obtained. The forearm seemed shorter than natural. The lower extremities of the radius and ulna formed a considerable prominence beneath the skin, that of the radius, however, being less marked and not descending so low as that of the ulna. The upper extremity of the carpus was on a plane superior and anterior to that of the lower extremity of the bones of the forearm. The hand formed a right angle with the forearm, and was also inclined towards its radial side; and this inclination could be extended so as to bring their outer borders into contact. Extension was impracticable, but flexion could be carried much beyond a right angle. On dissection, M. Cruveilhier found that all the muscles of the arm were atrophied; but this condition principally affected the muscles acting on the wrist-joint and radio-ulnar articulations—viz. the radial and ulnar flexors and extensors, and the pronators and supinators. The tendons of the radial and common extensors were lodged in a deep groove which existed at the posterior surface of the lower extremity of the radius; to this osseous excavation they were firmly adherent. The extensor carpi ulnaris was reflected at a right angle from the ulna, to be inserted in the fifth metacarpal bone; the flexor carpi ulnaris was shrunken, and terminated as usual in the pisiform bone. The carpus presented a singular deformity. The upper row of bones, reduced to a rudimentary condition, had lost their form and their volume, being diminished to less than half of their normal size. The pisiform bone alone remained unchanged. The corresponding surfaces of the second row were likewise altered. There only existed trifling rudiments of the os magnum and unciform bone; and in like manner the upper half of the trapezium and trapezoid, which should articulate with the scaphoid, was contracted. The ulna, which was very little changed in form, was prolonged five or six lines below the extremity of the radius; but a little above its inferior extremity, at a height corresponding to the lower end of the radius, it presented a deep excavation to receive an articular apophysis of the latter bone. It was united to the cuneiform bone by means of an extremely long ligament, which permitted of very considerable abduction of the hand. The radius was shortened and deformed, and the latter defect was principally observable at its lower extremity, which was enlarged and presented an appearance as if it had been crushed. It was also deeply grooved posteriorly for the united extensor tendons.

'There was a sort of transposition of the articular facet of the radius, which occupied the outer side of this extremity, whilst a prominent apophysis on the inner side articulated with the ulna. Lastly, the shaft of the radius was more voluminous than in its natural state, and the lines and elevations marking the insertion of muscles were unusually prominent. Its upper extremity, instead of being excavated to receive the smaller head of the humerus, was convex, and its circumference appeared as if battered. This case is given by M. Cruveilhier as an instance of dislocation backwards of the forearm or the hand, or of the wrist forwards, but it is impossible to account for many of the appearances on the supposition of dislocation having existed. Thus, for example, in all dislocations the displacement of a bone on one side of an articulation always involves the inclination in an opposite direction of the lever which it represents, whereas here the hand is in front. But why is the articular surface found upon an apophysis above the joint? Why is the radius so much curtailed of its length, whilst the ulna, which was at least luxated with it and retained even less mobility, is half an inch longer below? On the supposition that there had been fracture or separation of the epiphysis, there is no difficulty in explaining and linking together all these phenomena. It is probable that the accident occurred in infancy, and thence atrophy of the carpal bones. It is further likely that the fracture was the consequence of a fall on the back of the hand, in which case the violence of the shock would have thrown the epiphysis of the radius forwards together with the hand. In this way one may conceive that the extensor muscles would have been but little stretched; for if the fragments were separated in respect of their thickness, they were approximated in point of length. On the contrary, if there had been dislocation, the amount of tension would have corresponded to the breadth of the articular surface of the radius, which would have been very great. Again, the separation of the epiphysis accounts for the unusual apophysis which supports the new articulation, and the dislocated ulna is, as it should be, longer than the broken radius. It may be further observed that atrophy of the bones would follow long disuse of the limb consequent on dislocation of the radio-carpal articulation, and motion would become impracticable, whereas in the present instance the joint could be flexed. We may therefore conclude that the case in question is one of dislocation of the ulna backwards, with fracture of the radius and displacement of the inferior fragment forwards—a very remarkable case, without doubt, but at the same time one which does not touch the disputed question of dislocations of the wrist.'

It has already been stated that J. B. Roberts (*Fracture of the Radius*, Philadelphia, 1897, p. 42) experimentally produced epiphysial separation with anterior displacement by extreme flexion of the wrist on the amputated arm of a boy aged fourteen years. He also (p. 26) gives a drawing of a specimen in the Mütter Museum of the College of Physicians, Philadelphia, in which it seems probable that the injury was an epiphysial fracture with moderate anterior displacement.

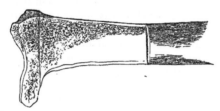

Fig. 153.—PROBABLE EPIPHYSIAL FRACTURE WITH MODERATE
DISPLACEMENT FORWARDS
Mütter Museum, Philadelphia. (After Roberts)

SYMPTOMS.—M. Colignon, in his thesis, 1860, has described at some length the signs of this lesion, and Manquat likewise made (1877) some attempt in the same direction.

Writing in 1884, Packard (*International Encyclopædia of Surgery*, vol. iv. 1884, p. 171) dismisses this important subject as follows: 'Epiphysial separations of the lower end of the radius have been spoken of by some authors; but they do not present any special features as compared with ordinary fractures in this region.'

SEPARATION OF THE LOWER RADIAL EPIPHYSIS WITHOUT DISPLACEMENT.—The lower epiphysis of the radius may be separated without any displacement, and the injury is usually looked upon as a sprain or severe contusion. These cases are of great importance from their liability to be overlooked and their tendency to be followed by arrest of growth of the shaft. Some authors believe that they are more common in the first few years of life than later, but this does not appear to be borne out by any clinical facts.

There will be **pain** about the wrist, especially on pressure over the epiphysial line of the radius, but there will be none over the line of the joint, provided no extravasation has taken place there.

Mobility of the epiphysis in the antero-posterior direction, but not laterally, is always present at the line just mentioned; it is more limited than when displacement is present. Care must be taken not to confuse this with the movement at the wrist-joint, for the conjugal cartilage is only five or six millimetres above the wrist.

Impaired active movement of the hand.—The hand may be more or less helpless; flexion may be performed fairly well, as well as extension, but pronation and supination are impaired to some extent, or even become quite impossible.

There is **no deformity**, but Colignon mentions that a slight depression at the seat of separation may be felt in certain cases during traction on the hand, when there is no considerable swelling. He does not appear, however, to have met with it in any case.

Muffled crepitus may be present or absent. Colignon thought it was not often present in this form of injury in very young subjects.

Some swelling will rapidly occur, especially towards the dorsal aspect of the forearm, from the detachment of the periosteum, and from extravasation of blood into it and the soft parts. Although it may extend over the lower part of the forearm, it will not, as a rule, be found to extend as far as the line of the wrist-joint, the cutaneous folds in this situation still remaining visible.

In other cases the swelling may be as marked on the palmar aspect, or even confined to it.

Colignon believed that this form of separation took place most frequently in the newly born and in early infancy, and that the pain was less acute and the swelling moderate; absence of deformity and presence of soft crepitus distinguished it from separation with displacement.

In seventeen cases which came under the observation of De Paoli, the majority were incomplete separations occurring after violence applied to the hand. They were characterised by very acute pain, localised to the line of the epiphysial cartilage, absence of distortion, loss of power of the forearm, especially in pronation and supination—all of which he had at one time believed to be merely the effect of some more simple injury, or of traumatic distension of the synovial sheaths, but now considered to be merely more or less extensive solutions of continuity of the epiphysis from the diaphysis, with slight extravasation of blood between their surfaces and under the periosteum, which is more or less widely separated.

SEPARATION OF LOWER EPIPHYSIS OF RADIUS AND ULNA WITHOUT DISPLACEMENT.—Ozenne (*L'Union Médicale*, Paris, 1887, 3rd series, xliii. January 4, pp. 13–15) describes a case of simultaneous traumatic separation of the lower epiphysis of the radius and ulna, with inter-epiphysiary separation, in a child aged ten.

The boy, while wrestling, was thrown on to his back, and in trying to disengage himself with his arms extended, his comrade fell with his entire weight on to the palm of his right hand, which underwent forcible extension. Great pain was experienced at the lower part of the forearm, and on examination six hours after the accident the axis of the hand was in a position midway between pronation and supination, but there was no lateral deviation from the axis of the forearm. The fingers were flexed to a right angle with the hand. There was no wound or discoloration of the skin, but slight swelling was evident on the antero-lateral aspect, scarcely any, however, on the posterior aspect of the lower part of the forearm. The styloid processes of the radius and ulna were in their normal relations, and there was no pain or pressure over them. No transverse prominence, abnormal projection, or prominence could be detected. No displacement had been effected, and the periosteal connections had probably not been destroyed; on slight pressure, however, by the index fingers pretty acute pain was produced, ten to twelve millimetres above the tip of the styloid process of the ulna, and twelve to fifteen millimetres above that of the radius. This pain existed throughout the whole circumference of the epiphysiary line of junction, less on the posterior aspect, not more intense at the sides, but especially acute on the anterior aspect. In fixing with one hand the lower part of the two bones and seizing the epiphyses with the other, slight abnormal mobility was made out from before backwards and from behind forwards, but no displacement in the lateral direction. Crepitus was absent. The two epiphyses could be taken separately and displaced from one another with slight mobility, due, no doubt, to some laceration of ligaments. The active movements of the hand were preserved in part, that of flexion being the most extensive, although incomplete; that of extension was more limited and painful. Pronation, but more especially supination, was very limited.

Although there was no reduction of the fragments to be made, a moulded splint was applied to the forearm and wrist. By the third day the swelling had disappeared and complete recovery took place, so that by the twentieth day there was perfect use of the limb.

Hamilton (*American Medical Times*, August 18, 1865, p. 116) also had under his care in 1860 a case of separation of the lower epiphyses of the radius and ulna in a boy aged nine, who had fallen and struck the back of his right hand and wrist. On the following day motion was detected in both epiphyses, accompanied with the peculiar crepitus belonging to epiphysial separations. Palmar and dorsal splints were employed, and after the lapse of three weeks union was complete without any ankylosis. The splints were then discontinued.

SEPARATION AND DISPLACEMENT OF THE EPIPHYSIS BACKWARDS.—As long ago as 1834, Rognetta pointed out some of the symptoms which he observed in a case under his care, in which, however, the displacement does not seem to have been very great (*Gaz. Médicale*, 1834, p. 514).

A child, aged five years, while at play had been dragged about the floor in a bowl by his elder brother, who held him forcibly by one hand. The child gave some piercing cries, and his parents, finding his wrist very painful, thought it had been 'put out of joint.' M. Rognetta saw·the child six hours after the accident, and was unable to make a diagnosis on account of the great tenderness, redness, swelling, and ecchymosis of the wrist. The fingers were semiflexed. But the following day, the swelling and pain having much diminished, separation of the lower radial epiphysis was easily recognised. While holding the forearm, there could be easily made out at the wrist antero-posterior and a little lateral movement, and even a certain degree of rotatory movement. During the backward movement, the displacement simulated a dislocation of the wrist backwards. During pronation and supination, a fragment with a thin border was felt to roll under the examining fingers. There was no crepitus during these movements. The styloid processes of the bones of the forearm were too little developed to allow M. Rognetta to make use of them for the purpose of diagnosis. Two small wooden splints were applied, and remained on the limb for thirteen days. The epiphysis then appeared to be consolidated, and slight movements of flexion and extension were therefore commenced. Recovery took place without deformity.

Dupuytren says (*On the Injuries and Diseases of Bones*, Sydenham Society's translation, 1846, p. 123) that in young subjects separation of this epiphysis is more likely to occur than fracture, as he had seen in many instances.

Malgaigne has observed that this injury is perhaps the most common of all epiphysial separations, but he has not described at any length its signs, or pointed out any of its peculiar features, or figured a specimen of it; however, he mentions one case of 'his own, and alludes to the cases mentioned by Roux, Cloquet, and Johnston.

Nélaton did not consider an accurate diagnosis of this injury to be possible, but it might be presumed to have occurred before the twentieth year.

M. Dolbeau, during the discussion at the Société de Chirurgie of Paris in 1865, pointed out the distinguishing characteristics of this lesion from fractures of the wrist, the form of the diaphysial fragment, the mechanism of the injury, its relative frequency, and its complications.

B. Anger, in his *Traité iconographique des fractures et luxations*, notes the similarity of the deformities to fracture of the lower end of the radius in a case of separation of the lower radial epiphysis with displacement backwards. The accident happened to a young man, a printer, whose arm had been caught in a machine.

Bruns considers it very probable that separations of the lower radial epiphysis occur more often than any; for although in his statistics of cases verified by an autopsy the radius only stood second in point of numbers, yet he thought that from the fact of their being very often uncomplicated and uniting well, they seldom afforded an opportunity for dissection.

Mr. Hutchinson also says it is not an uncommon accident, and occurs in children where Colles's fracture would occur in the adult.

In the same connection Professor E. H. Bennett, while enumerating the phenomena of this injury, and speaking of his case (*loc. cit. supra*), says : ' The casts in this case contrast, as many similar casts in our collection do, with the representations of the deformity in Colles's fracture, in the transverse features of the dorsal and palmar projections, and in the folding of the skin in the palmar depression, and, again, in the absence of abduction of the hand. If we add to all these the necessary reduction of the fracture and the facility of obtaining crepitus, and, still more remarkable, the facility of maintaining the reduced fracture in place, phenomena all long since pointed out by Smith—which, I may state, I have frequently observed and verified myself—there are, I think, ample grounds for questioning the recent statement of Professor Macleod that "there are no distinctive signs by which a separation of it (the radial epiphysis) can be differentiated from an ordinary Colles's fracture." '

Agnew dismisses this injury very hastily thus (*Surgery*, vol. i. 1878, p. 903) : ' When the line of fracture is transverse and near the articulating extremity, it may follow the junction of the epiphysis and shaft.' And Packard, writing in Ashhurst's *Encyclopædia*, 1884, vol. iv., does the same in a few words, which are quoted on p. 523. The above quotations are sufficient in themselves to demonstrate the great difference of opinion that exists among surgeons as to the occurrence of separation of the lower epiphysis of the radius.

Deformity.—In some cases there is extreme deformity, the hand together with the epiphysis or lower fragment being carried behind the axis of the forearm, while the upper fragment or diaphysis is projected prominently forwards.

As in Colles's fracture, the displacement is determined by the direction of the force, usually from a fall upon the palm of the hand.

The displacement of the epiphysis is very rarely sufficient to allow it to be completely displaced off the upper fragment on to the dorsal aspect, except in compound cases.

Mr. Jonathan Hutchinson believed that there was complete dorsal displacement in a case figured by him (*Archives of Surgery*, vol. i. No. 3, January 1890, p. 287), in which the amount of deformity certainly appears to have been very great.

Two prominences are ordinarily seen in this injury—one on the posterior or dorsal aspect and one on the anterior or palmar aspect ; and two distinct depressions—a dorsal one directly above the prominence, and a palmar one below the anterior projection.

Posterior Prominence.—This prominence is not so distinct as the palmar ; it is formed by the upper projection of the lower

.fragment together with the carpus and base of the metacarpus. It is directly continuous with the dorsal aspect of the hand. Like the palmar one, it is transverse in its direction, and almost as straight and regular.

The displacement appears to be more prominent on the radial than the ulnar side, on account of the greater width of the styloid process in this direction, and the displaced epiphysis may occasionally have a backward and slightly outward inclination.

In some cases where the injury has been seen directly after the accident, the lower fragment displaced backwards may be felt quite plainly to have the form of the epiphysis, with its well-known upper margin on the posterior aspect and the prominent middle thecal tubercle.

The posterior sulcus, just above the projection, is also transverse.

The abrupt angle on the dorsal aspect, formed by the separated radial epiphysis and the shaft, is soon obscured by the effusion of blood beneath the periosteum and into the extensor sheaths, and if the child be at all fat a transverse depression only is to be seen.

Anterior Prominence.—The prominence in front commences just above the anterior annular ligament and wrist-joint, extends upwards for about two inches, and gradually subsides into the anterior aspect of the forearm above, with which it is continuous.

It is formed by the lower end of the diaphysis, and by the skin and the soft parts, with the flexor tendons, pushed forwards by its anterior margin. This transverse anterior margin may sometimes be felt projecting across and between the flexor tendons. The palmar projection is abrupt and sharp, quite regular at its anterior margin, and is transverse like the dorsal prominence, but is much more evident than this. It is especially evident in cases examined before swelling has taken place. The angle it forms is more acute than the corresponding angle of Colles's fracture. A precisely opposite condition is therefore presented to that met with in the latter injury, in which the dorsal swelling is more marked than the palmar. The lower end of the diaphysis has an appearance very similar in shape to that of the lower end of the entire bone, and the projecting angle on the outer side may be mistaken for the styloid process. Goyrand was the first to draw attention to the straight and regular transverse anterior margin of the diaphysis and the similar posterior border of the epiphysis in those cases observed by him.

The sharpness and regularity of the diaphysial end is, however, soon obscured, as in the dorsal sulcus, by serous and bloody effusion into and between the sheaths of the flexor tendons.

In cases of more or less complete displacement backwards of the epiphysis the lower fibres of the pronator quadratus will be lacerated by the projecting diaphysis, and lead to still further effusion of blood.

Anterior Depression.—Directly below the palmar prominence there is a depression over the wrist-joint.

M. G. Goyrand, in his article ' De la Fracture, par contre-coup, de l'Extrémité inférieure du Radius ' (*Journal Hebdomadaire des Progrès des Sciences médicales*, 1836, T. i. p. 170), relates the case of a child, aged eleven, who had fallen from a height on to his hands. The right hand was carried backwards at the wrist, close to the articulation. The fingers were flexed. The upper end of the lower fragment presented, posteriorly, a horizontal angular edge, causing a projection on the dorsal aspect of the forearm—unlike the rounded end of the carpus—whilst the radius made an equally well marked transverse projection in front above the hand. The styloid process of the radius held its normal relations with the carpus.

The displacement was easily reduced, and the reduction being accompanied by soft crepitus like that met with in the reduction of the displaced articular surfaces, anterior and posterior splints were applied for twenty days, at the end of which time .the child had completely recovered.

The same surgeon published in 1848, in the *Revue Médico-Chirurgicale*, Paris, the following case of separation of the lower epiphysis of the radius, and quotes it again in his paper on separation of this epiphysis read before the Société de Chirurgie in 1860 (*Bulletin de la Société de Chirurgie*, 1861, 2me Série, t. i. p. 537; and *Gazette des Hôpitaux*, 1860, 124, p. 494).

A boy, aged fifteen and a half years, fell (August 20, 1846) with his two hands stretched forwards. There was great pain about the left wrist, and deformity, like a Colles's fracture, with impaction. The hand and wrist were carried backwards, so that the axes of the forearm, wrist, and hand made a Z. The tendons of the radial extensors on the outer side were prominent at the line of separation. The transverse and even projection of the lower end of the upper fragment in front was very marked; its margin could be distinguished through and between the flexor tendons. Behind, at the level of separation, there existed a transverse depression forming a retiring angle; the margin of the lower fragment was a little raised and displaced backwards towards the dorsal aspect of the upper fragment, but the projection was not so distinct as the anterior margin of the upper fragment. Movements backwards and forwards, which M. Goyrand made on the hand, were followed by the lower fragment; the latter therefore being displaced still more backwards or carried forwards with it. There was no crepitus. Reduction was easily and perfectly carried out by extension and manipulation of the fragment, and there was no attempt of the fragments to become displaced again. Anterior and posterior splints were applied to the hand and forearm, and perfect recovery ensued without any trace of injury on the twentieth day, when the splints were finally removed.

Buck in 1865 mentioned at the New York Pathological Society (*New York Medical Journal*, September 1865, p. 462) a case of separation of the lower epiphysis of the radius in a child twelve years old, which was diagnosed by the remarkable square shape of the surface presented by the end of the shaft, its transverse line, and its close proximity to the articular surface.

Mr. Durham, at Guy's Hospital, in August 1884 had the following case of Ed. Jas. P., aged twelve years, under his care. The boy fell out of a wagon on to some grass, and on admission there was great pain in the left forearm and great deformity of the wrist. Backward displacement of the hand was found on admission just above the wrist, and a palmar projection a little lower down than the dorsal one in the usual situation. The hand was somewhat dragged towards the ulnar side, and supination and pronation of the hand were lost. Crepitus was absent. Anterior and short posterior splints were applied, and two days later a plaster-of-Paris bandage from hand to elbow. Some deformity still remained a few weeks later.

Although there is no marked inclination either to the radial or ulnar side like that observed in fractures with impaction, Colignon has described a very apparent sloping of the hand in his case, which was under the care of M. Marjolin, and Piscart thought that the epiphysis was drawn somewhat outwards by the action of the radial muscles on the outer side.

Projection of the lower end of the ulna is noticeable beneath the skin on the inner side only when the displacement is great and the styloid process of the ulna broken off.

The hand is also slightly *supinated* in cases of great displacement.

Professor R. W. Smith (*Dublin Hospital Gazette*, vol. vii. 1860, February 15) contrasts this injury (separation of the radial epiphysis alone) with others which resemble it to a greater or less extent in their external characters—viz. Colles's fracture, disjunction of the epiphysis of the radius with fracture of the ulna, and luxation of the carpus backwards. It resembles, he says, Colles's fracture in the loss of the power of rotation, the existence of a palmar and dorsal tumour, and in the increase of the antero-posterior diameter of the forearm, but differs from it in the absence of that singularly distorted and twisted appearance which is so characteristic of Colles's fracture and is owing to the lower fragment of the radius being drawn towards the site of supination besides being displaced backwards. In the injury we are now considering the radial epiphysis passes directly backwards, without any tendency to supination ; nor is there any elevation of the styloid process, so that the radial border of the forearm does not present the curved outline so frequently seen in Colles's fracture. In the last-named injury the dorsal prominence is usually more evident than the palmar, and the sulcus or depression which limits it above generally passes in an oblique direction downwards and inwards towards the lower end of the ulna; but when the lesion of the bone traverses the line of junction of the epiphysis with the shaft, the palmar projection is by far the more striking, and both tumours are placed transversely, so that there is none of the appearance of obliquity which so many cases of Colles's fracture present.

Professor Smith continues : 'I have, more than once, seen separation of the radial epiphysis mistaken for Colles's fracture, but I do not think that any surgeon who has had moderate experience of injuries in the vicinity of the wrist-joint is likely to commit this error. It is, in my opinion, much more readily confounded with fracture of both bones of the forearm close to the wrist, or, to speak more correctly, disjunction of the epiphysis of the radius with fracture of the ulna immediately above its lower extremity, for the external characters of these two injuries present a most remarkable resemblance. There is in each case, occupying the same position and presenting very nearly the same form, an anterior and a posterior tumour; in both cases the hand, viewed posteriorly, presents an elongated appearance; there is the same increase in the antero-posterior diameter of the forearm, and a similar impairment of the functions of the limb.

'In the case of fracture of both bones, however, the deformity is greater, and at first sight might readily be confounded with that observed in cases of luxation of the carpus backwards, an injury to which the separation of the radial epiphysis bears but little resemblance.

'Moreover, the projections in front and behind occupy the entire breadth of the forearm, and the anterior presents none of the abruptness and sharpness of outline which forms so striking a feature when the injury is confined to the radius. An error in diagnosis is here, however, of little or no importance, as the treatment is to be conducted upon precisely the same principles, no matter whether one or both bones are broken.'

There is *no rotation or tilting of the epiphysis* on a transverse axis; therefore, there is no radial inclination or obliquity of the hand and none of that abducted and twisted appearance which is so striking a feature of Colles's fracture.

This is probably due to the unbroken condition of the inferior radio-ulnar and radio-carpal ligaments, which has been especially noted in some of the specimens mentioned above.

This rotation of the lower fragment in Colles's fracture cannot be due, at any rate to any large extent, as stated by Hamilton, to the laceration of the triangular fibro-cartilage or the internal lateral ligament, for laceration of the triangular fibro-cartilage was present in the specimen of separated lower epiphysis dissected by the author, and fracture of the styloid process has been found in several instances of epiphysial separation where such rotation does not occur, and consequently we find in epiphysial separation no curving of the radial border of the forearm, no tendency to supination, and no elevation of the styloid process.

The *styloid process of the radius* is thrown out of the axis of the forearm, but preserves its normal relations with the carpus, and moves with the carpus, so that on moving the hand backwards and forwards the displaced epiphysis moves with it; but in many instances of Colles's fracture the lower fragment does not move with the hand when any motion is imparted to it, the movement taking place at the wrist-joint from the impaction of one fragment in the other.

Fracture of the styloid process of the ulna.—In the more complete displacement of the radial epiphysis off the diaphysial end, the styloid process of the ulna will be lower than that of the radius. However, in these more severe injuries there is, as we have just stated, a fracture of the styloid process, and sometimes a rupture of the triangular fibro-cartilage, but the process always maintains its natural connection with the hand by means of the internal lateral ligament of the wrist.

Fracture of this process is seen in four out of nine specimens in the London Museum, fully described above, and was probably present in the following case described by Malgaigne (*Traité des fractures*, 1855, vol. ii. p. 692).

A boy, aged fourteen years, fell upon his hand, producing the deformity as of a dislocation. There was a large projection backwards which seemed to belong to the carpus, with a corresponding projection in front. The latter was formed on the inner side by the head of the ulna, and ended on the outer side by an osseous point simulating the styloid process of the radius; but this process was behind in contact with the posterior fragment. The radius was shortened, and the hand lengthened. The diagnosis made was separation of the epiphysis of the radius and projection of the ulna forwards. Reduction was effected with a very evident sound, and the wrist from that time assumed its proper shape and movements. There was no pain on pressure over the joint, but it existed over the level of the fracture of the radius. Malgaigne states that the displacement was similar to that of the fracture depicted in Plate XXV. figs. 2 and 3 of his work.

The author had recently under his care at the Miller Hospital a marked example of separation of the lower radial epiphysis with moderate displacement backwards and fracture of the apex of the styloid process of the ulna on the one side, while on the other there was separation of the radial epiphysis with little or no displacement, the characteristic 'silver fork' deformity of the opposite side being entirely absent, thus affording a comparison of the results of mild and severe forms of violence in this very common injury.

D. W., aged fourteen years, fell from off a roof about fifteen feet on October 27, 1897, alighting on his face and hands. The author saw him within half an hour of the accident, when the transverse ridge or angle, so characteristic of radial separation, was so marked that the forefinger of the surgeon could be placed on the front portion of the end of the diaphysis. It was therefore clear that the epiphysis was only about halfway displaced off the diaphysis (fig. 154).

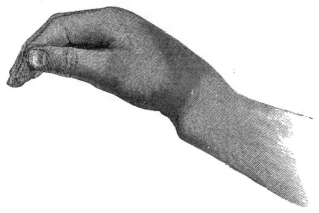

Fig. 154.—SEPARATION OF LOWER EPIPHYSIS OF RIGHT RADIUS WITH DISPLACEMENT BACKWARDS HALFWAY OFF THE DIAPHYSIS AND FRACTURE OF STYLOID PROCESS OF ULNA

From a photograph taken within half an hour of the accident, before any great swelling had taken place

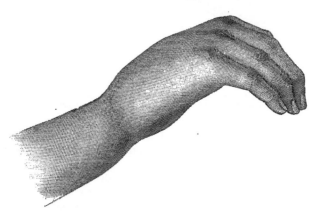

Fig. 155.—THE SAME CASE SEEN FROM ITS POSTERO-INTERNAL ASPECT

The slight obliquity of the hand towards the ulnar side is accurately represented

There was slight obliquity of the hand towards the ulnar side, which is seen in the accompanying drawings taken from photographs and in the annexed skiagraphs, due to slight displacement outwards as well as backwards from fracture of the apex of the styloid process. The apex of this process was displaced backwards, with the radial epiphysis behind the lower end of the ulna. Here there was some swelling and ecchymosis, but none existed in front to obscure the deformity (fig. 155). On the left side there was only a slight projection of the diaphysis in front on forcibly extending the wrist, which was accompanied by mobility. There was no fracture of the styloid process of the ulna, and only slight swelling on this side from extravasation of blood. Photographs were immediately taken of both hands, and skiagraphs the next day (fig. 156). Three days later the patient was kindly placed under the author's care by one of his colleagues, reduction of the displaced right radial epiphysis in the meantime having been partially effected by the house surgeon without an anæsthetic. The anæsthetic was now administered and the reduction completely effected; characteristic soft crepitus was

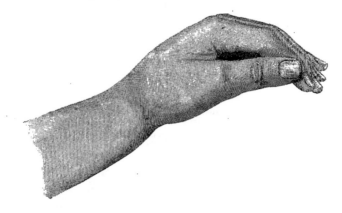

Fig. 156.– SEPARATION OF THE LOWER EPIPHYSIS OF THE LEFT RADIUS WITHOUT DISPLACEMENT

Slight swelling is seen in the region of the diaphysial end from effusion of blood into the soft tissues. From same case as the preceding

felt, and a wooden anterior and posterior splint applied, with pads over the epiphysis and diaphysis on the posterior and anterior aspects respectively. On the left side mobility and soft crepitus were now very evident on seizing the radial epiphysis and moving it in an antero-posterior direction, the end of the diaphysis becoming very prominent in front; in fact, with little more force the epiphysis could have been easily displaced backwards and the characteristic deformity produced. A short anterior wooden splint was applied to prevent mobility and any subsequent displacement. The skiagraph on the right side shows a small splinter of bone, very clearly delineated from the slight displacement of the epiphysis outwards, detached from the posterior aspect of the diaphysis.

The patient made a good recovery without any deformity of the wrists.

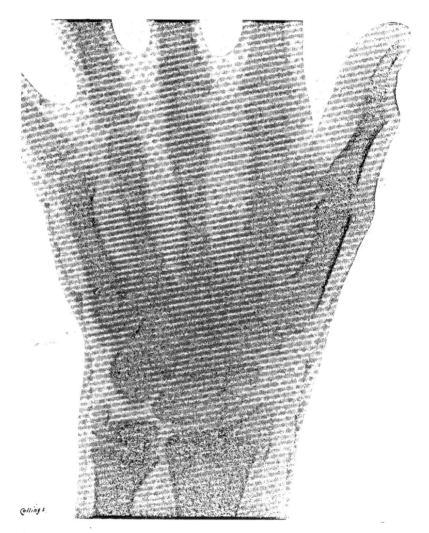

Collings

PARATION OF LOWER EPIPHYSIS OF RIGHT RADIUS. DISPLACEMENT BACKWARDS WITH A FLAKE
FROM POSTERIOR ASPECT OF DIAPHYSIS.

AUTHOR'S case.   Taken by Mr. THOMAS MOORE on day after injury.

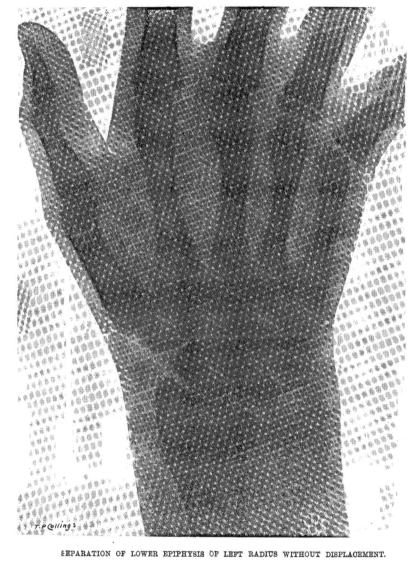

SEPARATION OF LOWER EPIPHYSIS OF LEFT RADIUS WITHOUT DISPLACEMENT.

AUTHOR'S case.   Taken by Mr. THOMAS MOORE on day after in;

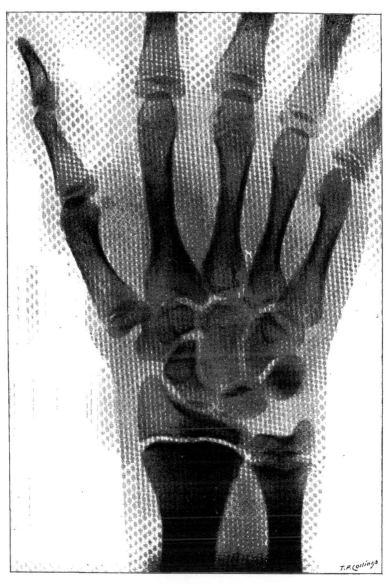

T.P.Collings

SEPARATION OF LOWER EPIPHYSIS OF RADIUS WITHOUT DISPLACEMENT.
Same case.   Left hand, palm downwards.   (Fourth week).

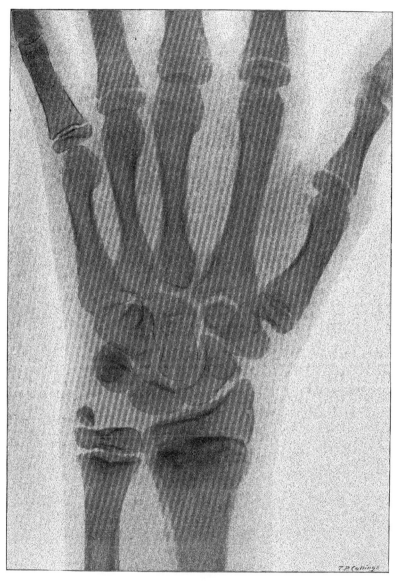

SKIAGRAM TAKEN IN THE FOURTH WEEK AFTER SEPARATION AND DISPLACEMENT BACKWARDS
OF LOWER EPIPHYSIS OF RADIUS, WITH FRACTURE OF STYLOID PROCESS OF ULNA. PERFECT
REDUCTION OF DISPLACEMENT.

Right hand, palm downwards. AUTHOR's case.

Skiagraphs of the wrists were again taken at the commencement of the fourth week. On the right side the epiphysis was in excellent position, with the slightest inclination towards the ulnar side, as revealed by the minute spicule of the diaphysis projecting on the outer side. New periosteal bone was represented as a faint shadow along the inner aspect of the radial diaphysis. The fracture of the apex of the styloid process of the ulna was also clearly displaced. The skiagraph showed the condition of affairs at the left wrist to be exactly normal, and although in this instance it proved most useful for comparison with the more serious lesion on the right side, it conclusively demonstrated that the employment of the Röntgen process in an epiphysial separation without displacement could give no affirmative assistance in the matter of diagnosis of such an injury.

Shortening of radius.—The radius appears to be shortened and the hand lengthened. However, in its actual length the radius is but little shortened—in displacement of the epiphysis halfway off the diaphysis, not more than an eighth of an inch.

It will only be shortened to any extent in the rare case of complete displacement of the epiphysis.

Although the styloid process may in these severe cases of displacement be found to be somewhat above its normal height, it will never be to the same degree as is met with in cases of fracture in older persons.

Mobility of epiphysis and site of lesion.—Mobility of the epiphysis with the carpus and hand takes place at its line of junction with the diaphysis ; this is situated less than a quarter of an inch from the articulation of the wrist-joint, and is thus nearer than the line of solution of continuity in fracture, which is usually three-quarters of an inch from the lower end. Manquat gives almost the same measurements—a centimetre and a half for fracture, and never more than six millimetres for epiphysial separation. The movement can only take place in simple cases in the antero-posterior direction, and very slightly or not at all laterally. It is due to the absence of impaction.

The separated epiphysis can be still further displaced towards the dorsal aspect by pushing the hand in this direction. Rognetta considered this a very distinguishing feature of the injury (*Gazette médicale*, 1834, p. 514), but he adds that the wrist may be displaced a little laterally, and even a rotatory movement may be effected. During the movements of pronation and supination a mass can be felt, according to this author, rolling under the finger, but with an absence of crepitus.

In certain rare cases this movement will be prevented by the fixation of the lower fragment by impaction, or only a hinge-like movement of the lower upon the upper fragment will be permitted ; but as a rule the bones of the forearm will not be moved when the

hand with the lower fragment or epiphysis is pushed backwards and
forwards, or even slightly supinated.

M. G. Goyrand erroneously thought that in separation the
abnormal mobility was much greater than in the case of fracture,
as in the latter the fragments were more or less impacted in one
another.

This surgeon related a case of separation of the lower epiphysis of the radius before the Société de Chirurgie in 1860 (*Bulletin
de la Société de Chirurgie*, Paris 1861, 2me Série, t. i. p. 534;
Gazette des Hôpitaux, 1860, 124, p. 494), giving the principal
features in detail.

Albert D., aged seventeen years, while exercising on a trapeze,
fell and alighted on his right hand. Acute pain and great deformity
were found at the wrist. The lesion on a superficial examination
might have been mistaken for a dislocation, for the hand was carried
behind the axis of the forearm, and there was a transverse projection of the radius in front above the displaced hand which
elevated considerably the skin and flexor tendons. The displacement, which was very close to the articulation, appeared to be more
extensive towards the radial than on the ulnar side. The ulna was
intact. The styloid process of the radius preserved its normal
relations with the hand, and although the fragment which surmounted the carpus had very little depth, M. Goyrand could, while
fixing it, impart to the wrist-joint movements which were easy and
painless. The mass formed by the hand and the lower extremity of
the radius was inclined towards the dorsal aspect of the limb, but
without being fixed, so that on pushing the hand backwards it could
be displaced more forcibly in this direction without producing any
crepitus. The solution of continuity was exactly transverse, and
much nearer the articulation than ever fracture is. Separation of
this epiphysis was diagnosed—in spite, M. Goyrand says, of the age
of the patient—from fracture, by the mobility of the fragment of the
radius surmounting the carpus and the absence of crepitus. In
the case of fracture, if it were not impacted, as is mostly the case,
it could not move on the upper fragment without crepitus being
felt. Reduction was effected without crepitus, and without any
tendency for the displacement to be reproduced. Anterior and
posterior splints were applied, and the patient recovered perfect use
of the limb. There was no trace of the injury five weeks later,
except a little wasting of the forearm and hand and slight numbness of the little finger.

Impaired movements.—The fingers of the hand are usually slightly
flexed, and the movements of pronation and supination impaired,
or even completely lost, the patient being unable to rotate the hand
in the least degree.

Ease of reduction.—Reduction is generally effected with great ease,
but in some cases only after the administration of an anæsthetic; for

not until the extensor muscles have been relaxed, which permits only of a hinge-like movement of the lower upon the upper fragment or posterior edge of the diaphysis, is it possible for the lower epiphysial fragment to pass across the face of the end of the diaphysis.

Hutchinson says that not unfrequently great difficulty is experienced in effecting complete reduction, and in afterwards retaining the two portions in accurate apposition.

Reduction will be difficult in the rare cases of impaction of the fragment, or only permitted to a certain degree.

On the other hand, Goyrand says that the natural shape of the parts is perfect after the reduction of a separation, whilst in the case of fracture if the extension (before the splint is applied) is relaxed the displacement is more or less reproduced. This cannot, however, be considered a distinguishing feature, when it is remembered that many cases of fracture unite rapidly without leaving any deformity.

M. Leroux, of Versailles, in 1865, observed a case of separation of the lower epiphysis of the radius of both forearms (Nélaton, *Pathologie chirurgicale*, 2nd edit. t. ii. p. 237). The prominent border of the diaphysial fragment stretched and threatened to lacerate the skin. The condition presented an absolute irreducibility. **Rigidity of supinator longus and other extensors** on the posterior aspect, which are raised up over the separated epiphysis.

Doubtless impaction of the fragments has occurred in a few cases and has prevented reduction, but is it muscular action alone that can maintain the deformity? This may be possible, as shown by the tense condition of the extensors on the dorsum and towards the radial side, which has been noted by several authors and was a marked feature in the specimen dissected by the author.

Through the attachment of the posterior annular ligament—which is only a transverse thickened portion of the fascia of the forearm—to the thecal ridges on the lower epiphysis of the radius, and, on the inner side, to the styloid process of the ulna and cuneiform and pisiform bones, the tendons of the extensor carpi radialis longior, the extensor carpi radialis brevior, the extensor communis digitorum, the extensor indicis, and the extensors of the thumb, are all held down in their grooves close to the epiphysis. All these muscles, aided by the supinator longus attached to the epiphysis, by their action tend to displace the separated epiphysis backwards. The flexor muscles, on the other hand, have no such influence on the epiphysis in front, for the anterior annular ligament (deep portion) is not attached to the radius, but to two of the carpal bones—the unciform and trapezium.

Muffled crepitus.—The characteristic muffled crepitus is sometimes detected during the reduction of the fragments, but more often it is entirely absent, whereas in fracture crepitus can frequently be detected when true impaction does not exist between the fragments, or when hinge-like movement of the lower upon the upper fragment is absent; at any rate, when the lower fragment can be moved to the extent that is possible in epiphysial separations.

Goyrand goes so far as to say that crepitus is not produced during the reduction of the separated epiphysis, and gives this as a distinguishing sign from fracture.

Manquat thought that as the separation is seldom pure, this sign is of little importance.

No tendency to reproduction of deformity after the epiphysial fragment has been reduced.

Subsequent malposition of the fragment is unlikely to occur from the more or less square condition of the separated surfaces in pure separations. In fracture, on the other hand, the displacement is often reproduced—at least, in part.

But M. Robert, in certain cases of fracture of the lower end of the radius, has not applied any apparatus after reduction, and with satisfactory results—results which he could not have obtained if there had remained any great tendency to displacement after the fracture had once been reduced. Such fractures are certainly met with in the case of children, without any tendency to reproduction of displacement, but they rarely occur.

Colignon thought that the epiphysis often returned to its displaced position after it had been reproduced.

Pain.—Pain is intense over the situation of the epiphysial lines, but not usually at the joint.

Swelling, although greater than in separation without displacement, is usually not very extensive.

COMPLICATIONS.—Out of seventeen cases alluded to by De Paoli, in one case the lesion was bilateral, in another there was, in addition, separation of the epiphysis of the ulna, and in a third a fracture of the diaphysis of this bone.

In Roux's case the lesion was double.

Separation of the lower epiphysis of the ulna.—Bertrandi is said to have reported that he had seen the epiphyses of the radius and ulna separated in a child who had been violently lifted by the hand from the ground.

The following case, which the author had the opportunity of observing, is a good example of separation of the lower epiphyses of the radius and ulna. On July 7, 1894, Hilda J., aged eleven, fell (whilst playing) off a wall seven feet high on to both her outstretched hands, but the right touched the ground first. The forearm was painful, and she was unable to move it; she kept it in the flexed position, supported by the other hand. Twenty minutes after the accident she came to the Miller Hospital holding the arm in this position. The forearm was also in a position midway between pronation and supination, and there was great pain on the slightest attempt at movement of the hand. On the dorsal aspect, just above the wrist, there was a very prominent and characteristic swelling projecting three-quarters of an inch beyond the posterior aspect of the forearm, with a depression above. Corresponding to the latter on the anterior surface was another prominence, which, on account of the small amount of swelling and bruising present, it was not difficult to make out as the lower ends of the radial and ulnar diaphyses. Soft crepitus was easily felt. The hand was not deflected either towards the inner or outer border of the forearm. Reduction was easily effected by extension and manipulation of the dorsal swelling (caused by the displaced epiphyses) into position. This was accompanied by soft crepitus, and there was no tendency for the displacement to recur. The forearm was then put up in splints. Through the courtesy of Dr. H. D. Coles the author saw the case eight days after the injury. There was then absolutely no deformity whatever, the fragments were in accurate position, and there was only the smallest amount of thickening about the lower ends of each bone; in fact, examining it at this early period, it would have been difficult to say that there had been any solution of continuity of the bones. As gentle movements of the wrist did not cause pain, passive motion was commenced. On the fourteenth day the splints were taken off, and the arm was carried in a sling. The patient now used her wrist for flexion and extension. Three days later there were no signs of any injury. Flexion and extension, and all movements of the wrist, were perfect. Eight months after the injury there was no appearance of shortening. There was the nearest approach in this instance to immediate union of separated epiphyses—if the author may so call it—that he has ever seen. But in other cases he has seen the union has not been so rapid or so good, doubtless on account of the incomplete reduction of the displaced epiphysis.

The following case (of H. H.), aged ten years, the author saw at the Miller Hospital, July 5, 1895, three weeks after the accident. The boy had fallen from a bar, eight to ten feet high, on to the palmar surface of his left outstretched hand; he was attended to at once, and the displacement, which was not very great, was reduced; this reduction was, however, imperfect, for at the time there was still some displacement of the diaphysis forwards, pressing the radial artery forwards. The epiphysis was somewhat mobile, showing that the new bone, which was pretty abundant, had not consolidated so firmly as in the instance just recorded. There was some thickening about the lower end of the ulna, but no displacement; this, together with the absence of any deflection of the hand, pointed to the probability of the lower epiphysis of the ulna having been separated, at any rate partially, without being displaced. The movements of the wrist were already good passively, but not actively.

Dr. C. A. Sturrock reports (*Edinburgh Hospital Reports*, vol. ii. 1894, p. 602) that Mr. Annandale has treated successfully several cases of separation of both epiphyses, in one of which, however, excision of the lower fragments was necessary. He also relates a good example of this injury.

N. F., a boy aged twelve, sought advice in Mr. Annandale's out-patient department at the Royal Infirmary, Edinburgh, for an injury which he had sustained by falling from a swing on to the dorsum of his hand. When seen within half an hour of the accident, the lower ends of the shafts of the radius and ulna were felt to be displaced forwards, while there was a prominence on the back of the wrist caused by the separated epiphyses; there was epiphysial crepitus, and only when traction was made on the hand, under an anæsthetic, could the bones be brought into position, the displacement recurring the moment extension was withdrawn. The arm, with the hand flexed, was put up in a temporary apparatus until next day, when anterior and posterior splints were applied and retained for a fortnight. Passive movements of the wrist and fingers were then commenced, and continued for fourteen days, when the boy ceased attending the Infirmary. Four months after the accident the movements at the wrist were slightly restricted, there was some thickening at the epiphysial line, and a fluctuating swelling extending one inch below and two inches above the anterior annular ligament, apparently in the flexor sheaths, which closely resembled a compound ganglion. A wristlet was worn for five months more, at the end of which time the swelling had gradually disappeared, movements at the wrist had become more extensive, no shortening could be detected, and there was only slight thickening at the epiphysial line.

Dr. J. F. Erdmann, of New York, quotes (*New York Medical Record*, October 26, 1895, p. 588) a case of epiphysial separation occurring in both bones of the wrist, and a separation of the lower epiphysis of the humerus. A girl (M. D.), four years of age, fell down a flight of fourteen steps. She complained of pain in the right wrist and elbow. Upon examination, a peculiar transverse deformity, sharply outlined, upon the posterior aspect of the forearm, about half an inch above the wrist-joint, was observed, while anteriorly there was a deformity continuous with the shafts of the bones. At the site of the deformity during manipulation a soft crepitation was apparent. At the elbow there were the characteristic evidences of an epiphysial separation of the lower end of the humerus. The separations were reduced, and the limb was placed on a long posterior splint extending down to the metacarpo-phalangeal joints. The patient was discharged in four weeks with a good result.

As stated above, these separations are often but insignificant lesions compared with those received at the time of the accident.

Fracture of the base of the skull is a frequent concomitant lesion.

In 1885 Mr. Davies-Colley had a case under his care at Guy's Hospital with the following lesions. James C., aged eight, fell about forty feet from a bridge on to a railway, and was picked up insensible. There were found, on his admission, separation of the lower epiphysis of each radius (with deformity similar to that of Colles's fracture) and of the right olecranon epiphysis, which was also vertically fractured, fracture of the shaft of the right femur, and fracture of the anterior fossa of the skull. The patient recovered, and left the hospital in about four weeks' time with half an inch shortening of the right leg, some impairment of flexion and extension of the forearm, and deformity of the limbs.

The following two cases at Guy's Hospital were also accompanied by fracture of the base of the skull.

In the first case, under the care of Mr. Cooper Forster in 1871, a youth (Daniel C.) fell out of a warehouse a distance of eight feet on to his chin and right arm. There was separation of the lower epiphysis of the radius and hæmorrhage from the right ear. The patient recovered, and was able to use his arm well. His age is not given.

In the second, under the care of Mr. Howse in 1887, the boy (Thos. W.), thirteen years old, fell from a balcony a distance of ten feet, and alighted upon his head. There was a separation of the lower epiphysis of the radius with backward displacement and fractured base of skull. Death ensued on the seventh day from meningitis due to extensive fracture of the anterior and middle fossæ of the skull.

Both the following cases of epiphysial separation of the lower end of the radius with other severe injuries were under the care of Mr. Howse at Guy's Hospital in 1883.

In the first instance the boy (William N.), aged seventeen, fell a distance of twenty feet from a second floor to the basement. There was the usual displacement of the lower fragment on to the dorsum, causing the projection with the hollow above and also the convexity on the palmar aspect. The forearm and wrist were much swollen, and there was a fracture of the internal condyle of the femur with much effusion into the joint. The injury to the radius was treated with a Carr's splint, and the patient recovered perfectly.

In the second instance the child (Herbert A.), three years old, fell down an area a distance of ten to twelve feet. The separated epiphysis of the radius was displaced backwards and the upper fragment forwards, the hand being in the extended position and extremely pronated. There was a comminuted fracture of the lower end of the humerus. An internal angular splint was applied after reduction, and subsequently an anterior rectangular one, with a posterior straight splint to forearm. Four weeks later he left the hospital, with both the elbow and wrist in good position. Movements of the elbow were excellent, only extreme flexion being a little painful, with some thickening about the lower end of the humerus. Pronation and supination and use of the wrist were perfect.

Injury to radial artery.—Mr. Hutchinson alludes to a case under his care in the London Hospital of separation of the radial epiphysis in which the displacement forwards of the diaphysis was so great that the lower end of the shaft was in front of the radial artery.

LATER COMPLICATIONS.—**Suppuration, necrosis, and osteomyelitis** are very uncommon complications in simple cases, although the periosteum is so often extensively stripped up.

Mr. Jonathan Hutchinson, however, records (*Illustrations of Clinical Surgery*, fascic. xix. pl. lxxi. fig. x.) and figures a case of simple separation of the carpal epiphysis of the radius in a boy, aged thirteen years, in which the first of these complications occurred. There was complete dislocation of the epiphysis on to the back of the end of the shaft, giving rise to extreme deformity. The styloid process of the radius was still in relation with the carpal bones. Reduction was found to be impracticable, and an abscess subsequently formed, probably in connection with great stripping of the periosteum from the shaft. Recovery took place with a much injured arm.

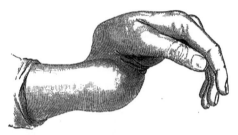

FIG. 157.—COMPLETE DORSAL DISPLACEMENT OF CARPAL EPIPHYSIS OF RADIUS

From a lad aged fourteen. Reduction could not be effected, although anæsthetics were given and much force used. Suppuration followed, and the arm was in the end much crippled. (Hutchinson)

The same surgeon gives (*Path. Soc. Transactions*, vol. xiii. 1862, p. 265) the following description of a case of detachment of the radial and ulnar (?) epiphysis, at the age of eight, in which suppuration occurred at the seat of injury, and was followed by ankylosis of the wrist and arrest of growth of the bones.

'J. P., aged twenty-three, came under my care, on account of a skin eruption, on November 19, 1860. I noticed that one of his wrists was deformed. The right hand was bent over to the radial border and firmly fixed by bony ankylosis at the wrist. There was not the slightest motion of the carpus on the radius. The wrist was thin and small, looking too small in proportion to the hand. It was considerably less in width than that of the other hand, but fully as thick, if not a little thicker. On his directing my attention to it, I noticed a small scar in front of the wrist. Being struck by the smallness of his wrist, I compared his arms, and found that both bones of the right forearm were an inch and a third shorter than those of the other side. The upper arms and the hands were of similar size. The diminution was in the lower parts of the bones of the forearm. The history of the case was that at the age of nine, in playing at leap-frog and "taking a seven-foot fly," he fell, and came with his hand violently on the ground. The wrist was supposed to be dislocated. It inflamed, an abscess formed, which a surgeon opened, and a piece of bone came out "about as large as his finger-nail." In two or three months it had soundly healed, and has remained quite well ever since. The hand is so useful to him that he is scarcely aware of any defect. It is his right hand, but he employs it as usual, and can write easily. Putting together the history of the accident, the supposed dislocation, the suppuration afterwards, the age of the boy at the time, and the subsequent arrest of growth of the bones, there can, I think, be little doubt but that the injury was a separation of the epiphysis. Very probably the radial epiphysis was fissured longitudinally, and the joint became involved in the inflammation which followed. In consequence of the abscess the nutrition of the epiphysis was, no doubt, greatly interfered with, and hence the arrest of growth of the bone.' ·

Gangrene of hand and forearm.—One instance is recorded by R. W. Smith (*loc. cit. supra*) in which gangrene of the forearm and hand was the result of tight bandaging.

In Rognetta's case (*loc. cit. supra*) death resulted from phlegmonous inflammation and gangrene of the arm, and a like result ensued in Barbarin's case.

Tetanus has been met with in two compound separations in both of which death ensued, and in a third in a simple separation, all described above. This fatal result occurred, it was thought, from pressure upon the median nerve in one of the first, and upon the radial nerve in the second case.

Pyæmia occurred in another compound case and death ensued.

DIFFERENTIAL DIAGNOSIS.—In former years a diagnosis of this injury was rarely made; indeed, in many of the earlier recorded cases, and in many in which the specimens were obtained and put up in museums, the nature of the injury was only discovered after death or amputation:

Dislocation of carpus backwards.—The error of mistaking separation for a dislocation of the wrist has been committed in former years by eminent surgeons.

Separation of the radial epiphysis alone does not bear so great a resemblance to dislocation as separation associated with fracture or separated epiphysis of the ulna.

In Bœckel's case the injury was mistaken for a dislocation, although the injury was compound. The diaphysial end, being covered with a layer of cartilage, was thought by the doctor who first ·saw the case to be the articular extremity, and reduction was effected.

M. Roüx (1834) had no doubt as to the correctness of his diagnosis during life in the case above recorded (p. 516). On death ensuing some days later he was astonished to find a fracture of the lower end of the radius with separation of its epiphysis.

In a child, a fall upon the palm of the hand, followed by deformity at the wrist, must nearly always suggest the occurrence of traumatic separation of the radial epiphysis.

Epiphysial separation is of frequent occurrence in youth, whilst dislocation of the wrist is almost unknown or extremely rare, though examples have been recorded by Guyon, Désormaux, Paret, and others.

Colignon, writing in 1868, says that since the death of Dupuytren, twenty years previously, dislocation of the wrist had only been noted three or four times (Marjolin, Thèse inaugurale ; Voillemier, *Archives de médecine*, Déc. 1839).

The specimen of displacement forwards of the radial epiphysis described by Dupuytren was taken from a patient who during life was considered by Cruveilhier to have had a dislocation of the wrist forwards.

Sir Astley Cooper has also recorded (*Fractures and Dislocations*, edited by Bransby Cooper, 1842, p. 485) an unusual case in a boy, aged thirteen years, in which both wrists were dislocated, one forwards and the other backwards.

Dr. H. Hollis records (*Lancet*, December 8, 1894, p. 1345) a rare case of backward dislocation of the wrist in a boy fourteen years of age. Half an hour previously he had fallen backwards from a ladder about twenty feet on to some sand. His hand was partly flexed at the wrist, and displaced slightly to the radial side ; the fingers were also flexed, and, including the thumb, could not be perfectly extended. There was no pain. On the posterior surface the upper end of the carpus with its convexity upwards and to the right was easily felt, the scaphoid lying higher than the other bones. Anteriorly there was a decided depression below the end of the radius, becoming less marked towards the ulnar side. The styloid processes were very easily felt below the skin. The dislocation was reduced by traction on the hand, but needed considerable force. Afterwards the boy could move the fingers and hand perfectly. There was some swelling of the wrist for a few days, but in a week the splint was removed and he resumed his occupation.

A similar case of dislocation of the carpus backwards was seen by Dr. T. H. Morton, of Sheffield (*British Medical Journal*, July 20, 1895, p. 131), and occurred in a boy, aged sixteen, who had fallen on his thumb with the arm backwards, the hand being probably pronated slightly and under him. On examination the radial and ulnar processes were in the normal plane. The carpus projected upwards and backwards, but not to any great extent. Reduction was effected easily by fixing the forearm, grasping the hand, and making forcible extension. A slight grating was felt. That no radial fracture existed was proved by the natural position being sustained when the patient moved the joint, and also by the satisfactory rotation of the radius without crepitus or displacement.

Mr. Jas. Hossack gives (*British Medical Journal,* December 7, 1895, p. 1424) another instance. J. B., aged sixteen, came to the Royal Infirmary, Edinburgh, on September 10, 1895. Twenty minutes previously he was riding on a lorry, and, in attempting to jump off when it was in motion, caught his foot against the edge and fell to the ground, landing on the flat of his hands. At first sight, to all appearances, it was a case of Colles's fracture, and, seen from the radial side, was a beautiful specimen of the 'silver fork' deformity seen in that fracture. The illustration shows the condition fairly well. On examination, however, the styloid processes of both the radius and ulna were in their usual positions, while the prominence on the back of the wrist was not limited to the radial side of the forearm, but was equally marked over the ulnar. On the palmar aspect the ends of both radius and ulna made an abrupt

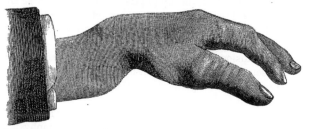

FIG. 158.—JAMES HOSSACK'S CASE OF BACKWARD DISLOCATION OF THE CARPUS

prominence, while the flexion lines there were especially well marked. Reduction was simple. The forearm was steadied and slight extension made on the hand. Suddenly the carpus slipped back with a distinct 'click.' There was no fracture present; this was definitely ascertained after reduction. No crepitus could be felt when rotating the radius. The whole bone rotated in one piece, and no prominence or deformity was to be made out along the course of either bone. There was no suspicion of return of the condition. It was put up in anterior and posterior splints, and resort was early had to passive movement. The wrist, three weeks after, was perfectly well; the boy, however, complained of its being weak and stiff.

R. W. Smith says: 'Nothing but extreme ignorance or extreme carelessness can lead to the injury under consideration being confounded with dislocation of the carpus backwards, for the means of diagnosis are simple and sufficient. In fracture or separation of the epiphysis the styloid processes of the radius and ulna hold their natural relations to the carpus, and follow any motion imparted to the hand; the reverse obtains in the case of luxation. Again, the distance from the upper edge of the dorsal tumour to the end of the middle finger is, in the case of fracture, greater than that between the corresponding point of the hand and the upper edge of the carpus of the sound limb; but in the case of luxation of the wrist backwards this measurement will give the same results upon each side.'

To this normal relationship of the styloid processes, and the fact that they move with the carpus when any motion is imparted to the hand, may be added movement at the wrist-joint when the lower fragment is fixed. Although this epiphysis which surmounts the carpus is of small size, it can be seized with the fingers and thumb and fixed, and movement made at the wrist-joint without pain. Again, in this injury the styloid process deviates from the axis of the radius, whereas in dislocation it still remains in a line with it. In dislocation the displaced hand remains almost fixed, whilst in epiphysial separation antero-posterior movement of the hand with the epiphysis upon the forearm can, as a rule, be effected. The radius in separation of the epiphysis will be found to be shortened to a greater or less extent when measured on the outer side from the styloid process; in dislocation this shortening does not take place.

Finally, a dislocation, when reduced, does not tend to be reproduced like some cases of separation of this epiphysis.

Colles's fracture.—Separation of the radial epiphysis resembles to a great extent Colles's fracture in the existence of a palmar and dorsal swelling, and loss of power of rotation. The deformity is, however, very different, for in disjunction of the epiphysis the displacement is directly backwards, and there is none of the rotation, obliquity, or curved outline of the radial border, characteristic of Colles's fracture. Moreover, in the latter injury the dorsal projection is usually more distinct than the palmar, the anterior projection being therefore not so abrupt. It forms a much more obtuse angle than in epiphysial separation. The dorsal groove is oblique, but in separation of the epiphysis it is transverse. The palmar swelling is therefore, in epiphysial separation, more evident than the dorsal, and there is no third prominence, as in Colles's fracture, from the projection of the styloid process.

The margins of the anterior and posterior projections, if they can be felt, are irregular in Colles's fracture.

The age and crepitus assist but little; for as to the former point, fracture of the lower end of the radius occurs in children, although but rarely, and as to the latter, the characteristic muffled crepitus is often absent in separation of this epiphysis as well as in fracture. If characteristic dry crepitus is present, a true fracture suggests itself, but even here the presence of a fracture of the diaphysis complicating the separation must not be lost sight of.

The mobility is greater, as a rule, in epiphysial separation, due to the gliding of one fragment upon the other; in fracture it is often of a see-saw movement only. Mr. D'Arcy Power says : 'It may be distinguished by observing that the outline of the wrist is angular, whilst in fractures it is curved. The projection, too, upon the palmar surface is more obvious after epiphysial separation than after fracture.'

Goyrand believed that crepitus was always absent in separation of the epiphysis, and therefore considered this a distinguishing sign from fracture, when mobility could be obtained.

In Johnston's case, related above, the injury was mistaken for a fracture during life.

In one of the interesting specimens in St. Bartholomew's Hospital, Nos. 931 and 932, on the left side there was a separation of the epiphysis, and on the right a fracture of the diaphysis one inch and a quarter from the articular surface, with impaction of the shaft into the lower end ; in the latter instance, with an absence of crepitus during life. The boy, aged fourteen, had fallen from a window, and he died from injuries of the head.

A comparison of the two injuries in this case during life would have afforded an important clinical study.

The following case of **fracture of the lower end of the radius** just above the conjugal line, closely resembling separation of the epiphysis, is one of many which have come under the author's care at the Miller Hospital.

H. S., aged eight years, fell, September 29, 1894, from a dustbin a distance of three feet, on to his hand. He came to the hospital within an hour, his mother having seen that his forearm was not of the right shape. He complained of great pain from the time of the accident. On examination the forearm was midway between pronation and supination, with loss of power, so that he was obliged to support it with the other hand. The dorsal aspect of the wrist presented a marked prominence with a concavity above, while the palmar aspect showed a corresponding depression and elevation. Pronation and supination of the hand produced no movement of the head of the radius. There was mobility in an antero-posterior direction just above the level of the lower epiphysis of the radius. The ulna was uninjured. The dry crepitus of fracture was very noticeable during reduction. An immovable apparatus was applied for a week, when union was found to have taken place ; the slightest thickening of the radius above the epiphysial line was the only discernible feature. Passive movement was commenced on the tenth day; no pain then on moving the wrist. At the end of three weeks the movements of the wrist and forearm were perfect, and there was no deformity. A photograph of this case was taken directly on admission to the hospital, but was not very successful.

De Paoli draws attention to this form of fracture, and illustrates it with the accompanying drawing (fig. 159).

Professor J. B. Roberts, in his excellent monograph (*A Clinical, Pathological, and Experimental Study of Fracture of the Lower End of the Radius with Displacement of the Carpal Fragment towards the Flexor or Anterior Surface of the Wrist*, Philadephia, 1897, p. 11), gives six instances observed clinically of fracture of the lower end of the radius, with displacement *forwards* of the carpal fragment, in children from ten to fourteen years of age. For a detailed description of the symptoms of this injury the reader must be referred to that work. It corresponds to 'Smith's fracture '—that is, fracture in adults with displacement forwards of the lower fragment, first described by R. W. Smith.

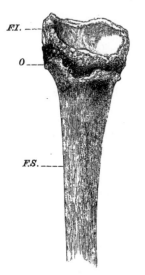

Separation of the lower radial epiphysis, with fracture of the ulna above the epiphysial line, will be discussed in the following section.

Fracture of both bones of the forearm near to the wrist will simulate radial separation, with fracture of the ulna, very closely, by the presence of the same palmar and *dorsal* swelling, giving rise to increase in the anteroposterior thickness of the forearm and loss of power over the forearm.

FIG. 159.—FRACTURE OF THE LOWER END OF THE RADIUS IN THE VICINITY OF THE CONJUGAL CARTILAGE, WHICH HAS ALREADY DISAPPEARED

F. I. lower fragment; *F. S.* upper fragment; *O*, fragments of compact tissue of upper fragment adhering to the lower. (De Paoli)

This is a rare form of injury in the child, the shafts of both bones usually giving way higher up.

In both these varieties of fracture of the shaft, however, the deformity is, as a rule, greater than in separation of the radial epiphysis alone, and in fracture of both bones the crepitus is of a drier character.

The following case of fracture of the ulna and radius just above the epiphysial line came under the author's care.

H. W., aged fourteen, on November 6, 1894, while playing football, slipped and fell on his hand, which he put out to save himself. On getting up he experienced great pain, and noticed that his wrist was bent. When he was seen at the Miller Hospital soon afterwards there was a dorsal projection of the whole wrist, the whole hand and width of the wrist being displaced backwards. The fingers of the hand were slightly flexed. There was a solution of continuity

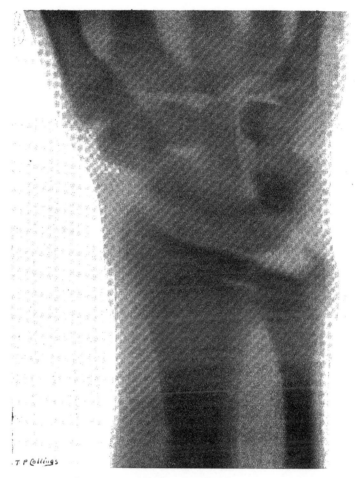

. T P Collings

EARLY RÖNTGEN PICTURE OF DISPLACEMENT OF LOWER EPIPHYSIS OF RADIUS.

The image of the bones is magnified on account of the close proximity of the tube to the patient's wrist.
The restlessness of the patient has produced double shadows. The apex of the styloid process of ulna appears
to be bent outwards or incompletely fractured.

Mr. CHARLES COPPINGER's case.　　　　Short exposure.　　　　Taken May 21, 1896, by Mr. CHARLES COPPINGER.

of the shafts of radius and ulna above the level of the epiphyses, with mobility. On moving the hand with the lower fragments, hard crepitus, as of ordinary fracture, was felt.

Reduction was easy, and the forearm and wrist were put up in straight anterior and posterior splints. By the eleventh day the bones had united and there was no pain, only some thickening of the lower end of the ulna, and three days later the splints were removed. On the eighteenth day passive movement, which had been carried out daily, resulted in perfect movement of the hand and forearm. At the end of three weeks there was perfect consolidation, without any deformity, and all movements were restored.

The method of photographing by means of Röntgen's rays will prove of the greatest assistance in the diagnosis of all these injuries to the bones of the forearm at the wrist, as in diagnosis of other forms of epiphysial separation in other parts of the body.

Mr. Charles Coppinger gives (*British Medical Journal*, June 6, 1896, p. 1411) a brief record of a case in which he found this process of use in the diagnosis of an epiphysial separation of the radius.

J. R., aged twelve, was admitted to the Mater Misericordiæ Hospital on May 21 with an injury to his right wrist, caused about an hour before by a fall from the horizontal bar at a gymnasium. The boy had fallen to the ground palm downward, and the existence of a fracture was at once apparent. The deformity was great and unmistakable, the dorsal and palmar elevations producing the usual appearance of undulation at the wrist. There was, however, no appearance of rotation, the displacement of the carpus being directly backwards, so that the deformity resembled that caused by a dislocation of the wrist in that direction. The absence, moreover, of the curved outline of the radial border of the arm characteristic of Colles's fracture was noticed.

A Röntgen photograph of the wrist was taken without delay, but with some difficulty on account of the patient's restlessness. The negative, though not fully exposed, showed, when compared with a radiograph of the normal wrist, that the injury was really a displacement at the epiphysial line, and not the well-known fracture of Colles, or the far more rare dislocation of the wrist backwards. The facility with which the deformity was subsequently reduced by simple traction, and the absence of bony crepitus during its reduction, confirmed the diagnosis.

Mr. Coppinger purposed taking another skiagraph of the boy's wrist at an early date for comparison.

SEPARATION OF THE RADIAL EPIPHYSIS WITH FRACTURE OF THE ULNA.—Separation of the radial epiphysis with fracture of the lower end of the shaft of the ulna will present the same symptoms as separation of the epiphyses of both bones.

Although simultaneous separation of both lower epiphyses of the forearm is not a rare event, yet the more common accident is for the shaft of the ulna to give way at its weakest point just above the epiphysial line.

R. W. Smith believes that both of these resemble more a dislocation of the carpus backwards than does a simple separation of the radial epiphysis. ' Moreover, in the latter injury,' he says, ' the anterior tumour does not extend completely across the entire breadth of the forearm, being limited to the transverse extent of the radius; but the opposite is the case when the lesion implicates both bones.'

Deformity.—Professor R. W. Smith, as long ago as 1847 (*Fractures and Dislocations*, Dublin, 1847, p. 164), described the deformity in separation of the inferior epiphysis of the radius with fracture of the lower extremity of the ulna.

' When the limb is viewed posteriorly it is found to present two planes, one extending from the elbow to the seat of fracture, i.e. from half to three-quarters of an inch above the wrist-joint; the other, which is placed more inferiorly, begins at the situation of the fracture and reaches to the fingers; where these two planes join there is a deep and abrupt depression, succeeded by a solid tumour placed above the carpus, but on a level with the dorsum of the hand; the latter presents an elongated appearance. Viewed anteriorly, the forearm presents an unnatural convexity, commencing immediately above the annular ligament of the carpus, and fading gradually as it ascends; the tendons of the extensors of the thumb, where they cross the hollow above the posterior tumour, are elevated and thrown into relief, and the antero-posterior diameter of the forearm is considerably increased at the seat of the injury. The injury consists in a fracture, usually transverse, of the lower extremities of both radius and ulna, close to the wrist-joint, or through the line of their epiphyses; the lower fragments are displaced directly backwards, and the superior consequently project in front.'

The deformity is greater than in separation of the radial epiphysis alone, and is more like that of dislocation of the wrist backwards.

The dorsal swelling is transverse, and also broader than in separation of the radial epiphysis alone, so that the anterior and posterior projections occupy the entire breadth of the forearm.

As in the case of separation of the radial epiphysis, the projection on the palmar surface is more pronounced than those on the dorsal aspect, the opposite condition to that found in Colles's fracture. The twisted appearance of this fracture also is absent; and the anterior margin of the diaphysis may be distinctly felt.

There is no abduction of the forearm, and both the ulnar and radial borders of the forearm are somewhat shortened.

Besides the palmar and dorsal prominences, a third is visible on the inner side due to the projection of the lower end of the ulna.

Muffled crepitus is more easy of production than in separation of the radial epiphysis alone, but is likely to be obscured by the crepitus associated with the fracture of the ulna.

Reduction is easy, but there is more difficulty in keeping the fragments in position than in the case of separation of the radial epiphysis alone.

Numbness of the little finger may be present, and is due to injury to the dorsal branch of the ulnar nerve, caused by the stretching or displacement of the nerve in fracture of the ulna, or in separation of its lower epiphysis.

The symptoms in a case of compound separation with fracture of the ulna are described by R. W. Smith (*loc. cit. supra*).

Loss of power over the forearm, especially rotation, will be present in this as in other forms of fracture of the lower ends of the bones of the forearm.

The following case came under the author's observation at the Miller Hospital in 1890.

John M., aged eleven years, fell and pitched on the palm of his outstretched hand. The arm was quite useless, and the patient unable to support it in the slightest degree. The hand, with the lower part of the forearm, was freely movable on the rest of the limb. There were the usual prominences above the carpus on the dorsal and palmar aspects, as well as the hollow characteristic of a Colles's fracture on the palmar aspect of the wrist. The hand was slightly abducted, and crepitus was easily felt along the line of fracture, which involved both bones. The deformity was easily reduced by extension, and the limb put up in anterior and posterior splints. It quickly and firmly united, with some thickening both on the dorsal and palmar surfaces.

Diagnosis.—Professor R. W. Smith says: ' This accident is very liable to be mistaken for dislocation of the wrist backwards, but cannot be confounded with the ordinary fracture of the radius ; the dorsal tumour is transverse, and the limb presents none of the peculiar deformity arising from the displacement of the lower fragment of the radius towards the side of supination which distinguishes Colles's fracture. Although this injury assumes very much the appearance of dislocation of the carpus backwards, it may yet be distinguished from it without any considerable difficulty, more especially should we be fortunate enough to see it before the occurrence of tumefaction has obscured the diagnostic signs. The styloid processes of the radius and ulna can be felt still holding their normal relations to the carpus, and, as has been remarked by Boyer, these processes move with the hand when any motion is imparted to the latter. If the distance between the superior margin of the dorsal tumour and the extremity of the middle finger of the injured limb be measured and compared with that between the corresponding point of the hand and the upper edge of the carpus of the sound limb, the former measurement will be found to exceed the latter by at least half an inch; sometimes the difference is greater, but if the case should be one of dislocation of the wrist backwards this measurement will give the same results upon each side, and the styloid processes will be found to remain at rest when the hand is moved; if we add crepitation, the easy reduction of the deformity by extension, and its liability to recur when the extending power is removed, we are at once furnished with a group of symptoms quite sufficient to enable us to distinguish this injury from that very rare accident, luxation of the wrist.'

DISPLACEMENT FORWARDS OF THE EPIPHYSIS.—Displacement of the lower radial fragment or epiphysis, anterior to the upper, is rare compared with the dorsal displacement. Several instances have already been quoted in which this position of the fragments was found by direct examination. It does not appear absolutely essential that forward displacement must be caused by a fall upon the back of the hand, although this is the usual manner in which the force is applied. In the case related below—Mr. F. Le Gros Clark's—it was produced in exactly the same manner as in the dorsal displacement by a fall on the outstretched hand.

Experimentally it has been produced by forcible flexion, placing the dorsal aspect of the hand on the ground and letting a weight fall on the upper part of the forearm placed in a vertical position. M. Curtillet found that separation thus produced occurred at the posterior half of cartilage, and was associated with a fracture in the rest of the thickness of the bone.

Mr. F. Le Gros Clark describes (*Medical Times and Gazette*, vol. ii. 1860, p. 27; *St. Thomas's Hospital Reports*, new series, vol. xvii. 1887, p. 2) a case in which the separated radial epiphysis was displaced forwards, and mistaken at first for a dislocation of the carpus.

The patient, a lad aged fifteen years, had fallen with violence upon his outstretched hand. The supposed dislocation had been reduced, but immediately the support was removed from the wrist the hand fell, and the radius projected on the back of the carpus. A brief examination showed that the case was one of separation of the epiphysis of the radius, which was thus carried *forwards* in company with the hand, the base of the bone being felt, deprived of its articular extremity, projecting on the back of the wrist. The source of the error in diagnosis was the similarity in the form of the base of the radius, minus the epiphysis, to that of the perfect bone. Le Gros Clark says: 'The diagnostic difference is in the interval between the base of the middle metacarpal bone and the projecting extremity of the radius, which is of course greater when the epiphysis accompanies the carpus; but more especially in the noticeable fact that the styloid process of the radius is identified with the carpus in its movements, and distinctly isolated from the radius. Moreover, if this joint can be, or ever is, dislocated, it would surely not be so

readily reducible as in the form of injury I am speaking of. I have
had an opportunity of dissecting a precisely parallel case to this,
and I believe the preparation is in our museum of St. Thomas's
Hospital.'

The treatment in this case consisted in confining the hand and
wrist in gutta-percha splints, moulded to the entire palm and the
lower part of the forearm, both before and behind. Passive motion
was commenced at the end of three weeks, and the boy recovered
a useful limb, there being free motion in every direction, and
scarcely perceptible deformity.

PROGNOSIS AND RESULTS.—There are no cases on record of
non-union.

Union without deformity.—In simple cases without complications,
without much displacement, without laceration of the periosteum
or fracture of the diaphysis, or in which the deformity has been
reduced, the union is very rapid and good from the thirteenth to
the twentieth day. The use of the limb under these circumstances
is perfectly unimpaired (see author's case from the Miller Hospital
already described).

All complications—such as wounds, fracture of the epiphysis or
of the diaphysis of the radius or ulna, and other rare lesions—affect
the progress, union, and ultimate result very considerably. The author
has, however, recorded a case of separation of the lower epiphyses
of the radius and ulna in which the most perfect union without
deformity took place within a fortnight of the injury.

Malgaigne treated separation of the lower epiphyses of both
radii in a child six years old, and consolidation ensued in the usual
time and without deformity.

M. Roux has recorded (*La Presse Médicale*, No. 55, July 15,
1837, vol. i.) a similar case of disjunction of the carpal end of both
radii which he had seen in consultation. B., a labourer, aged
seventeen years, fell from a building a distance of fifteen feet on
his face and on the palms of his hands, which were carried
forwards. The double lesion of the forearms was easily made out by
the peculiar character of the crepitus produced by rubbing together
the cartilaginous surfaces, by the uniformity of the solution of
continuity, and by the height at which it had taken place on the
two sides. The displacement was slight, although the pain was
acute. The apparatus applied to each forearm consisted of two
splints and a bandage. The treatment only lasted about twenty
days, when remarkably firm union had taken place. Such firm
union, M. Roux says, could not have been expected in the same
space of time in the case of a fracture, even if the fracture had
occurred in a subject of the same age.

Deformity.—Deformity from non-reduction of the displaced
epiphysis.

Consolidation in a vicious position should never be allowed to take place, yet even where the reduction of the displacement has not been effected the resulting deformity is slight, and in the course of a few years this will be completely effaced. There need not, therefore, be any fear that permanent deformity will result.

There is usually none of that persistent distortion on the dorsal and palmar aspect so characteristic of Colles's fracture.

Mr. Hutchinson describes (*Lancet*, August 24, 1861, p. 184; *New Sydenham Society's Retrospect*, 1862, p. 270) the case of a boy, aged eight, who was admitted into the London Hospital, having fallen from a tree upon his outstretched hands and afterwards struck his head. He sustained concussion of the brain and detachment of the epiphysis of the radius in both forearms. The deformity of the right wrist was more marked than that of the left, but exactly similar. It was so great in the right that the case looked like a dislocated wrist. No crepitus was felt. All deformity was removed by extension, and both forearms were put up in splints in the usual manner. Three weeks after the accident the epiphyses were firmly united to the shafts, with, however, a large amount of thickening and some displacement backwards.

Mr. Hutchinson says : 'Even in cases in which perfect reduction was not effected, the patients usually recovered with very useful arms, and in course of years all trace of deformity might be expected to be removed.'

When the reduction is effected early and completely, and the fragments are maintained in position carefully, the separation is very rapidly repaired.

In 1888 the author saw a young man, who was about to enter the army as an officer, aged eighteen and a half years, who had fallen on some grass with his right hand outstretched. When seen in the first instance by Dr. Creed, of Greenwich, there was dorsal displacement of the hand and lower end of radius, which he easily reduced and retained in position by anterior and posterior splints. Recovery took place without any deformity.

In the following case of probable injury to the lower epiphysis of the radius the state of the parts twenty months afterwards is given by E. H. Bennett (*British Medical Journal*, vol. i. 1880, p. 759). A little girl, aged four years, fell on her hand, and was brought to him twenty months afterwards. A separation of the carpal epiphysis of the radius had been diagnosed, and treated with plaster of Paris and a hinged splint. Pronation and supination were quite free, and the patient could use the arm for almost all purposes, except that the elbow-joint could not be flexed beyond 45°.

Roux records (*La Presse Médicale*, July 12, 1837) a case of separation of the carpal epiphysis on both sides, in which the deformity partially destroyed the symmetrical shape and the power of both upper extremities. He gives no description of the appearance of the limbs, but merely remarks that there was a 'shocking' deformity above the wrists. The patient, a girl, aged twenty-two years, had been under his care for a short time with some strumous affection. During infancy she had met with a double disjunction of the lower epiphysis of the radius, the cause of which she did not remember. This disjunction had doubtless been overlooked, and had not been treated.

MM. Bauby and Bardier (*Le Midi Médical*, Toulouse, 8 Octobre 1893), in their article, 'Considérations sur le Traitement des Fractures épiphysaires,' upon the immediate treatment by massage, quote the following two cases as examples of the evil result of fixation of epiphysial fractures of the lower end of the radius.

CASE I.—A healthy youth (P. B.), aged twenty, slipped on a waxed floor and fell backwards on to the palm of his outstretched hand. There was pain at the wrist, loss of power in the hand, and the characteristic 'fork back' deformity. The hand was inclined towards the radial border as well as strongly extended on the forearm. A doctor who saw the case immediately after the accident, before swelling occurred, attempted reduction by means of traction, and placed graduated compresses with wooden splints in front and behind in the interosseous space. Ten days later this apparatus was re-applied in a tighter manner. At the end of twenty-five days the fracture was united, with the hand bent towards the radial border, so that at its lower third the forearm presented a concavity postero-externally and a bony projection in front. Movements were very restricted and muscular atrophy very marked. Four years after the accident the bony deformity, from union in the bad position, was very marked, and although the joint had almost completely regained its power of action there still remained a certain hindrance to free movements together with muscular atrophy.

CASE II.—A youth (J. E.), aged sixteen years, came under care for operative treatment to free his right hand, which could scarcely be moved. At the lower extremity of the radius there was a cicatrix corresponding to an old injury, and the tendons on the dorsal aspect appeared to be bound together with cicatrised tissue. The fingers were almost completely fixed in the extended position, and there was scarcely any movement at the wrist. He said that ten years previously he fractured his wrist, and was treated by a bone-setter at Toulouse, who applied an immovable apparatus for twenty-three days. When this came to be taken off the fracture was found to be united, but in the bad position with which he presented himself. The forearm and hand were much atrophied.

The operation had not been carried out at the time of the report, but the fingers could be used more freely after the use of massage.

De Paoli relates a case of double separation of the lower

epiphysis of the radius of a month's duration, in which consolidation had taken place in a false position. The subject was a youth, aged nineteen, who had fallen from a tree on to the palms of his hands, and the deformity was practically identical on the two sides and had not been corrected at the time of the accident. The transverse form of the upper fragment in front and the lower fragment behind were easily recognised now that the swelling had subsided. The forearms were semi-pronated and semi-supinated, and the end of the radius and hand were forcibly supinated.

Pronation and supination were almost impossible, flexion being also very limited, and the patient was almost powerless to make any use of his hands. Dr. Margary, under whose care he was (September 1879) at the Hospital of S. Giovanni, broke down the osseous union between the fragments by forcible hyperflexion and pronation while the patient was under chloroform, and completely corrected the deformity. A short palmar and long dorsal splint were then applied and twenty-six days later removed, when it was found that pronation and supination had been in great measure restored. Nine days later the patient returned home, making careful use of his hands. When seen three years afterwards he could work perfectly, using his arms in fatiguing occupations.

The following case, under the care of Mr. T. Bryant at Guy's Hospital in January 1885, was probably one of separation of this epiphysis with dorsal displacement. Florence D., aged ten years, three weeks previously, while walking slipped and fell forwards on to her hands, especially the left; the latter became very painful and swollen, and she was unable to use it. The wrist was bandaged up, and arnica applied. Lately she had regained some use in the left hand.

On admission there was considerable deformity, some swelling over the dorsum of the carpus, and immediately above it a hollow about one inch above the lower end of the radius; on the anterior aspect, just above the wrist, another considerable swelling; the styloid process of the ulna was lower than that of the radius. The articulation was free from pain, and movable. Although the fragments had to a large extent united, Mr. Bryant attempted reduction under the influence of chloroform, and succeeded in diminishing the amount of deformity by bringing the styloid process of the radius on to a level with that of the ulna.

De Paoli figures a specimen preserved in the Riberi Pathological Museum which illustrates a separation of the epiphysis consolidated in an abnormal position.

The diaphysis is much enlarged, especially at the posterior and inner part, where it presents a somewhat rough surface, terminated by a clean edge, which, commencing below at the outer margin, ascends obliquely upwards, reaching to a height of three centimetres on the diaphysis, and terminates on the inner margin at the line of insertion of the interosseous ligament. The anterior surface of the diaphysis is turned outwards. Its lower extremity has left the upper surface of the epiphysis almost completely on the inner side, less so towards the outer side, and is flat and smooth owing to a thin strip of compact tissue which covers it. The epiphysis, the upper edge of which is throughout very distinct and does not show any considerable alteration from its normal shape, has been displaced backwards, and its articular surface looks downwards and backwards in such a way that the direction of its outer lateral edge, instead of following that of the lateral edge of the diaphysis, makes an angle of about 45° with its prolongation below.

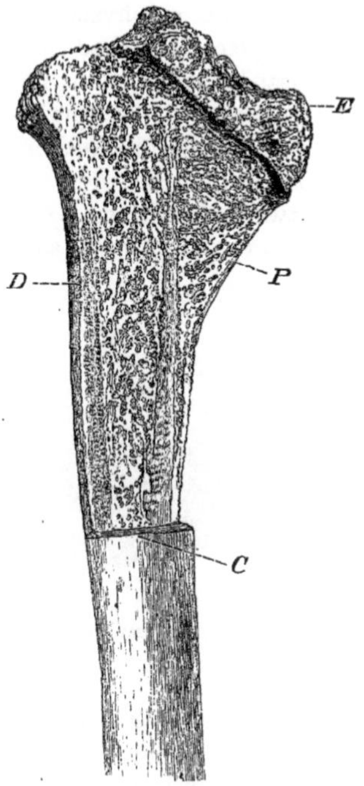

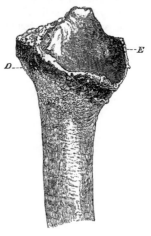

FIG. 161.—THE SAME VIEWED LATERALLY

FIG. 160.—TRAUMATIC SEPARATION OF THE LOWER EPIPHYSIS OF THE RADIUS UNITED IN BAD POSITION. SAGITTAL SECTION. (DE PAOLI)

Specimen in the Riberi Pathological Museum. D, diaphysis; E, epiphysis; P, newly formed osseous tissue from the periosteum; C, compact tissue of diaphysis.

An antero-posterior section of the specimen gives a clearer idea of what has taken place. It can be seen that the epiphysis is only in contact with the posterior part of the diaphysis for a distance of two millimetres; elsewhere it is completely separated from it, so that its upper margin makes an angle of 45° with the posterior surface of the diaphysis. About forty-five millimetres from the lower end of the diaphysis a thin compact layer covers the diaphysis for a short distance, gradually thinning upwards, and passes abruptly downwards and backwards to join the posterior margin of the epiphysis. The normal compact tissue of the posterior aspect of the diaphysis may be traced as far as its lower end. The irregular triangular interval thus left is filled up with new osseous tissue, which has its cellular spaces much smaller than those of the lower end of the diaphysis, and constitutes the posterior enlargement of the diaphysial end, and is the principal bond of union of the separated bones. The epiphysis was fifteen millimetres in width (height) at its styloid process, four at its middle, and five at its inner margin. The radio-carpal articulation was in a permanent condition of hyper-extension. The epiphysis of the ulna had united to the shaft, and the preparation was believed to have been taken from a woman, aged twenty, who had the lower epiphysis separated some years prior to her death. The displacement had not been corrected, and the epiphysis had consolidated in this vicious position.

A case of marked deformity after separation of the epiphyses of the lower ends of the radius and ulna came under the author's care at the City Orthopædic Hospital on October 12, 1894.

The accident had taken place between five and six weeks previously, and the author was asked to give an opinion as to the damaged condition of the limb.

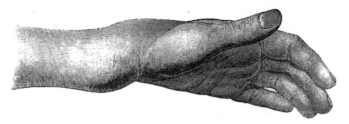

FIG. 162.—DEFORMITY FOLLOWING SEPARATION OF LOWER RADIAL EPIPHYSIS
(From a cast taken six weeks after the injury)

Fred P., aged ten years, on September 5, fell at school, whilst jumping, a height of five feet, and put out his left hand to save himself. He immediately experienced great pain in the wrist, which was much displaced, the deformity being of the same character as when he came under observation, only it was much more marked. He was taken immediately to one of the large hospitals in the north of London. The bones were there replaced in position, and anterior and posterior splints applied and retained for a month. At the end of this time the splints were removed, and the bones found to be displaced again in the same position as when he came for treatment. When the author saw him there was the typical 'silver fork deformity' indicating displacement backwards of the lower epiphyses of the radius and ulna, with the wrist and hand, although the epiphysis of the ulna did not appear to be so much displaced in this direction as the radius; the hand was not deflected to one side or the other. The styloid processes of the bones were in normal relation with the wrist and hand. The fragments were very firmly consolidated, and there was some thickening of the shafts of the bones to be felt on the dorsal aspect, extending upwards from the diaphysio-epiphysial line. The radial artery was pushed very prominently forwards by the displaced lower end of the diaphysis in front. The flexor tendons also were very prominent, and around them a ganglionic swelling had developed. The fingers were kept slightly flexed, and complete active extension was not possible; with this exception, all movements of the wrist and hand were good.

A leather moulded wristlet was worn for five months, and massage employed. At the end of this time the ganglionic swelling was much reduced, the flexor tendons were less prominent, and the diaphysial end of the radius rounding off and less distinct. The movements of the fingers were perfect.

When seen at the end of June 1895 there was little deformity left and no swelling about the flexor tendons, and in October 1896 there was no distinguishable deviation from the natural condition.

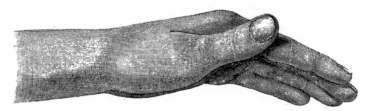

Fig. 163.—THE SAME CASE, SHOWING NEARLY COMPLETE ABSENCE OF DEFORMITY, TWO YEARS AFTER THE ACCIDENT

Professor L. Freeman, of Denver, U.S.A. ('Some Fractures of the Lower End of the Radius as seen by the Röntgen Rays,' *Annals of Surgery*, April 1897, No. 52, p. 471), describes the following case of deformity after epiphysial separation, which he attributed to stimulated growth of part of the epiphysial cartilage. The evidence he adduces is not by any means conclusive that the abnormal position was caused in this way. However, the case is quoted on his authority :

'A boy, about ten years of age, fell from a height on to his hands and fractured the lower extremity of each radius. There was marked "silver fork" deformity, with flexion of the fingers and inclination of the hands to the radial side. A diagnosis of probable epiphysial separation was made. Complete reduction was easily accomplished by dorsal flexion of the hands upon the wrists and pressure applied to the distal fragments. The forearms could then be shaken until the hands jerked to and fro with considerable violence without reproducing displacement of the fragments. A dorsal splint was employed, reaching to the tips of the fingers and padded at its extremity so as to maintain volar flexion at the wrist. The apparatus was purposely made large and clumsy, in order, as far as possible, to prevent the boy from using his hands. Following reduction there was no pain and little tenderness.

'The wrists were examined every day or two in order to note any tendency towards displacement. In about a week a slight deformity was seen upon the

right side, which was attributed to swelling of the soft parts. In a few days this
had increased to a considerable extent. Chloroform was administered and reduction
of the deformity attempted without success, although much force was employed in
combination with extension, dorsal flexion, and direct pressure. After several
days, the deformity in the meantime having increased, a second attempt at its
correction was made, likewise without result. It was found impossible to even
rebreak the bone with the amount of force which could be applied by the hands
alone.

'The little patient ultimately recovered, however, with a functionally perfect
right wrist, although with moderate deformity. It is impossible to detect that the
left wrist has been broken.

'During treatment, the boy, in spite of repeated warnings, insisted on using
his hands when he imagined himself free from observation. On several occasions
he reached backward from his bed and pulled open a drawer with his right hand.
At the time this was thought to account for the redislocation of the fragments. It
was difficult to understand, however, why the bones could not be replaced, or, in
fact, moved at all; and besides this, when closely questioned the patient said that
at no time had he felt any pain or been conscious of anything slipping.

'About fourteen weeks after the injury two skiagraphs of the wrists were taken,
one in the prone and one in the semiprone position. Cartilage being easily
penetrated by the Röntgen rays, the epiphysial lines of the bones of the forearm
were clearly shown, as were also those of the metacarpal bones and the phalanges.
The incomplete ossification of the bones of the carpus was also indicated.

'In the prone position of the forearms the epiphysial line of each radius was of
the same width throughout, one bone being apparently as perfect as the other. In
the semiprone position, however, the anterior half of the right epiphysial line was
obscured by a dark shadow, representing, undoubtedly, a growth of new bone, and
the anterior border of the epiphysis was tilted downward from the shaft.

'It may be that the injury alone was responsible for this excessive growth and
premature ossification of the epiphysial cartilage; or it is possible that the extent
to which the boy insisted upon using his hand may have had something to do
with it.

'The skiagraphs made it at once clear why no amount of force or method of
manipulation would cause the disappearance of the deformity; and why the boy,
in spite of an apparent redislocation of the fragments, had been free from pain and
tenderness.'

Professor Freeman adds: 'In several treatises upon surgery,
brief mention is made of the fact that subsequent deformity may
appear after separation of the epiphysis of the lower end of the
radius; but in most text-books the question is entirely ignored,
although its importance in prognosis is certainly considerable. The
only deformity mentioned, however, is that produced by cessation of
growth on the part of the radius, due to premature ossification of
the epiphysial line, while the ulna continues to elongate, thus
twisting the hand to the radial side. This is entirely different from
the case reported above, in which the abnormal position of the bones
is due to stimulated growth and not to inhibited growth, although
the latter may take place later.

'I know of no way in which this misfortune can be prevented
unless something may be accomplished by keeping the broken bone
absolutely at rest. It is perhaps possible that a marked deformity
could be lessened by stimulating the bone-producing power of the
remainder of the epiphysial line through injection of Lannelongue's

ten-per-cent. solution of chloride of zinc; but this is theoretical only, and more harm than good might be done. Seeing that the epiphysial line seems to be at least partially ossified upon its anterior surface, it may be that the remainder which is unaltered will cause a more rapid growth of the posterior half of the bone, thus tilting the epiphysis back into its normal position. The efficacy of re-breaking the bone would be, to say the least, doubtful, while operative interference might so damage the cartilage as to stop all growth. In case of great deformity an osteotomy might be made higher up.'

Impaired movements.—There is never seen in young subjects any of that almost permanent stiffness of the wrist, fingers, or hand which occurs in adults—lasting, e.g., for months or even years in the case of Colles's fracture; although some little embarrassment in the more severe cases is noticeable for some time. The effusion into the synovial sheaths of the numerous tendons passing over the wrist is rapidly absorbed, and but little fear need be apprehended of adhesions forming, provided passive motion has been properly carried out and commenced early.

In the case related by Dr. Sturrock, four months after the accident the movements of the wrist were slightly restricted, and a ganglion-like swelling extended one inch below and two inches above the anterior annular ligament, apparently in the flexor sheaths. But at the end of nine months this had disappeared, movements were more extensive, there was no shortening, and only slight thickening at the epiphysial line.

A similar swelling existed in the author's own case just mentioned.

In Professor Annandale's case, recorded by Dr. Sturrock, the patient when seen some fifteen months after the injury (compound separation of radial and ulnar epiphyses) had almost completely regained the movements of the wrist, and little or no shortening had occurred, although three-quarters of an inch of the shafts of the radius and ulna had been removed by operation.

Ankylosis of the wrist is not produced by extension of the inflammation to the joint, but may ensue in those rare instances where the separation is associated with a splitting or fracture of the epiphysis into the joint, or in compound separation.

Wasting of forearm and hand is never severe; if movements and massage have been properly carried, out it is slight and of a transient nature.

Non-union.—Although non-union and the formation of a false joint, from the separation being overlooked or badly reduced and the fragments allowed to move one upon another, have been alluded to by some writers as very uncommon, their occurrence is open to great doubt. No authentic case has ever been recorded.

Union may be retarded by these movements, but they appear never to produce non-union.

Arrest of growth and subsequent deformity.—In the forearm, as in the case of other bones which lie parallel, shortening of one bone from arrest of growth is usually accompanied with marked deformity.

Although the radius lengthens principally by its lower extremity, it is less dependent for its growth on the lower epiphysis than is the ulna, and hence the deformity after epiphysial separation is not usually so great in the former as in the latter. The hand is in a valgus position. The transverse diameter of the wrist is increased, the hand often a little atrophied and inclined to the radial side, making with that of the forearm a greater or less angle. The ulna appears to be displaced downwards and outwards, the end of the bone being very prominent. But the free mobility of the articulation is unaltered.

Ozenne thinks that arrest of growth is slight in separation without displacement on account of the union being rapid and consequently ossification of the cartilage less interfered with. But from some of the published examples of arrest of growth it is quite clear that there has been little or no displacement at the time of injury, which has been looked upon as a sprain.

De Paoli did not find any arrest of growth in seventeen cases, principally incomplete separations, observed by him, even after the lapse of two years. However, he agrees with some authors in thinking that arrest of growth usually occurs in cases of great or complete displacement of the epiphysis, for he says not only is there no longer any connection between the diaphysis and the epiphysis, but the latter is, in addition, united to some higher part of the former by means of an exceedingly dense osseous tissue, while it is only connected in a very remote degree with the nutritive artery of the diaphysis, and is therefore henceforth practically incapable of performing its function in promoting the increase in length of the lower end of the radius.

M. Goyrand, in referring to his two cases described above, states that there was no arrest of growth of the injured radius in either when he examined the upper extremities some years after the accident. There did not exist any difference in the corresponding arms, but both had grown well. He moreover says (1861): ' I can now, therefore, confidently say that separation of the radial epiphysis is an accident without serious consequences when it is simple, that union is accomplished in a very short time, and that no trace is left of the injury. Fracture, on the contrary, leaves some stiffness at the wrist for some time, even in infants, and after recovery it is possible to distinguish, even throughout the whole of life, the fractured limb. I will go still further: from many cases I have observed, two of which were published in my paper in 1848, it appears that in cases where the radius has been fractured before osseous union has taken place between the epiphysis and the diaphysis, the end of the bone has ceased to grow regularly, and when the patient has attained his full height the radius has been found to be perceptibly shorter and its carpal extremity atrophied. This condition apparently results from the ossification of the cartilage, and is produced during the formation of the reparative callus. This ossification will be found to occur more especially in comminuted fractures of the lower end, which involve the extremity of the diaphysis as well as the epiphysis. Separation of the epiphysis is therefore a much simpler and milder injury than fracture of the extremity of the bone.'

Goyrand mentions also the case of a girl (a member of his family), aged seven or eight years, who had separated her lower radial epiphysis, the result of a fall at the age of three years. The injured arm developed like the other in every respect.

In the author's own five cases of separated lower radial epiphysis there was no arrest of growth in any, nor did any arrest of growth occur in the several cases under his care of fracture of the radius immediately above the epiphysial line, which closely resembled epiphysial disjunction. This might have been expected, as fractures have in some instances, in the case of other bones, led to this result.

J. Hutchinson junior' has followed up six cases of undoubted separation of the lower epiphysis of the radius for a considerable time after the accident; in only one (in which some backward tilting persisted) was there decided shortening.

The deformity and attendant inconveniences from arrest of growth increase in proportion to the age of the patient and the time which has elapsed from the date of the accident.

The three following cases quoted by Curtillet as mentioned by Wilhelm Stehr (Th. inaug. Tübingen, 1889 ; Curtillet, *Du décollement traumatique des épiphyses*, Lyon, 1891) are good examples of the truth of this.

CASE I.—A boy (R. R.), aged sixteen years, fell from the second story of a house at the age of twelve. It was noticed that there was a lesion of the right wrist, but it was unimportant compared with the other lesions, which attracted more attention. He remained insensible for a long time after the accident. It was not until two years later that the patient perceived that he could not use his hand so well at his employment of hairdresser, and that it inclined to the outer side, whilst there was some projection of the styloid process of the ulna. When examined the hand was found to be in the position of extreme abduction, the axis of the hand making with that of the forearm an angle of 150 degrees. The right radius measured 18 centimetres, the left 22 centimetres ; the right ulna 23·3 centimetres, the left ulna 24 centimetres. Freedom of movement of the wrist-joint appeared to be normal. It was subsequently ascertained that the patient had been obliged to give up his work as hairdresser and had taken to work with a corn merchant, which did not appear to aggravate his condition, although there was no improvement in it.

Case II.—A lad (Bernard S.), at the age of fourteen years, in 1876 fell from a tree and produced an injury to the wrist, which was diagnosed at the time as a fracture. In 1885, when twenty-three years old, he complained of pain in the arm on military service, and in the following year the left hand was found to be in a position of extreme adduction, with great prominence of the head of the ulna. The left radius measured 19 centimetres, the right 24·5 centimetres; the left ulna 26·4 centimetres, the right 27·4 centimetres. The radius presented an osseous outgrowth at its articular margin, and a kind of depression about its epiphysial line.

Case III.—A lad (G. W.), aged eighteen years, was seen on February 14, 1889. In March 1884 he had fallen from a height of five metres upon a cemented surface. The left hip was contused, and he experienced very acute pain above the left wrist; he also asserted that he had noticed a very marked depression on the dorsal aspect of the forearm, whilst on the palmar aspect there was a bony prominence. The doctor, however, treated the injury by cold applications, &c., and made the patient carry the arm in a sling without attempting any reduction. At the end of four to five weeks he said he could very freely use his hand, and rotation was but little diminished. Since 1885 the patient had worked in a spinning factory, then as a locksmith, and could easily perform his work till the autumn of 1888, when he found that after he had been at work 'screwing' for some time and was obliged to use his left hand, it gave him slight pain; he also noticed that the hand inclined more to the radial side than before. On examination the left forearm was a little thinner than the right (the former being 23·2 centimetres in circumference, the latter 24·5 centimetres), while the left arm was normal. During the state of rest the left hand was bent to the radial side to an angle of 170 degrees, and the styloid process of the ulna projected very prominently. About the epiphysial line the left radius was somewhat thickened; it was also 4·7 centimetres shorter than the right. The left ulna was 1·7 centimetres shorter than the right.

Mr. Augustus Clay exhibited a boy, aged fourteen, at the Midland Medical Society in 1888 (*Lancet*, April 7, 1888) who had injured his forearm six years previously by falling off a cart. The injury had been treated then as a sprain, and after three weeks was apparently well. Three weeks previous to his appearance before the society he again hurt his arm, and the shortening was discovered. The wrist was much wider than the other, and the hand was pushed over to the radial side by the increased length of the ulna, which bone was exceptionally prominent and slightly bowed.

Museum specimens.—Several specimens in the museums of the London hospitals show great dwarfing of the radius and deformity of the forearm after what was probably an epiphysial separation.

The specimen, No. 956A, in the museum of the Royal College of Surgeons (*Catalogue of the Museum of the Royal College of Surgeons*, vol. ii. p. 129; *Trans. Patholog. Soc.* vol. xvii. 1866, p. 223, with fig.; and *London Hospital Reports*, vol. ii. 1865, p. 351, with fig.) shows arrested development of the radius, forearm, and hand after an injury in childhood. The following account is mostly taken from Mr. Hutchinson's description—both the long bones are unusually slender; the radius is relatively much shorter than the ulna. The radius measures five inches from the middle of its articular surface at the wrist to the articular surface of its head, and the ulna is eight and a quarter inches from the styloid process to the tip of the olecranon. Measured from the tip of the styloid process of the ulna to the inner side of the articular surface of the radius the latter is one and one-eighth inches higher than the former.

The carpal bones are drawn upwards with the radius, and the side of the ulna is consequently in apposition with the inner side of the cuneiform. The cartilage covering the articular surfaces of the bones at the wrist-joint is irregularly thinned at various places, especially that covering the extremity of the radius, and two or three bands of adhesions pass between them.

The lower articular extremity of the radius is widened, the articular surface is directed somewhat forwards, and upon the palmar surface is a prominent 'lip,' caused by the abrupt inclination forwards of the lower extremity of the bone. Near the posterior margin of the articular surface is a ridge with a prominent central spine, nearly corresponding to the concavity on the palmar aspect of the shaft. The grooves for the tendons on the dorsal aspect are well marked.

The articular facet for the lower end of the ulna is only faintly indicated; that of the head of the radius is very limited. It is placed obliquely, starting from within outwards and downwards, and at its outer side the cartilage is deficient over a patch, as if from attrition. From its appearance it would seem that pronation and supination must have been confined within narrow limits.

The bicipital tubercle of the radius is so far rotated outwards that it is directed upwards.

About the middle of the shaft the outer margin bulges considerably, but there is not the slightest indication of fracture of the shaft at any part. A longitudinal section of the radius shows no interruption of the continuity of the medullary canal or of the compact wall, even at the lower extremity. The ulna, except in the adaptation of its articular facets to the shortened radius, presents no unusual feature; its styloid process projected considerably. The carpal bones were displaced slightly forwards, being in apposition with the anterior portion of the articular surface of the radius. The remodelling of the parts has been perfect.

The specimen was removed by Mr. Hutchinson from a woman, aged twenty-five years, who died in the London Hospital of tetanus consequent on a burn. The patient stated that when five years old she had 'her wrist put out by a fall on the hand.' Her right forearm was less developed in all respects than the left, and the bones were much shorter; the right wrist-joint was considerably deformed, and the hand was inclined to the radial side. The hand itself was slightly smaller than the other one. From the condition of the bones it was conjectured that the lower epiphysis of the radius had been injured in early life. Although both the ulna and the radius were less developed than those of the opposite limb, and even the hand was somewhat smaller, yet the dwarfing of the radius was out of all proportion to that of the other bones. It seemed even probable that the retarded development of the rest of the forearm was secondary to that of the radius.

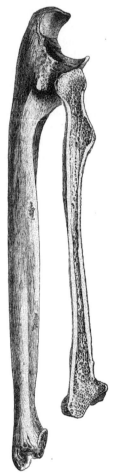

FIG. 164.—ARREST OF GROWTH OF RADIUS
(Royal College of Surgeons Museum)

The specimen in the London Hospital Museum, No. 400 (*Catalogue of the London Hospital Museum*, 1890, p. 95), is described and figured by Mr. Hutchinson in the *Path. Soc. Trans.* vol. xvii. 1866, p. 237, and is almost a counterpart of the one just related. Mr. Hutchinson obtained it from the forearm of a man between forty and fifty years of age at the time of his death.

The injury to the epiphysis had occurred in boyhood. The injured hand had been very useful; there was free motion at the wrist, and no defect whatever at the elbow. The ulna projected considerably, and the hand was pushed over to the radial side. A vertical section has been made through the carpal bones and the lower third of the ulna and the radius. The ulna is about three-quarters of an inch longer than the radius, and articulates with the side of the cuneiform bone, the triangular fibro-cartilage intervening. This cartilage is very much elongated. The styloid process of the ulna is short and ill-marked. Part of the articular surface of the ulna is devoid of cartilage, but there are no adhesions; at the other parts the cartilage is of normal thickness, and the edge is quite smooth and bevelled off where it has been removed. The carpal end of the radius is shaped exactly like that of the specimen described above. It has a strong lip anteriorly, projecting towards the palmar aspect, and occasioning a deep hollow on the front of the bone just above it. Against this lip the carpal bones chiefly rest; the cartilage of the radius is deficient or much thinned on that part of the bone nearest the ulna, and there are some strong bands of adhesion between it and the scaphoid and semilunar bones. There is free motion at the joint. There is nothing in the section of the bone to indicate the line of fracture, reparation having been complete and the alteration in form being the chief remaining peculiarity. The increased thickness of the compact tissue on the ulnar border of the radius is deceptive, and results from the section having passed close to its surface.

Mr. Hutchinson's belief respecting this and the preceding specimen is that they illustrate the results of displacement of the carpal epiphysis of the radius at a very early period of life, when the remodelling power was great. Probably the epiphysis was, he says, as is usual, displaced backwards, carrying with it, of course, the carpus. The bones of the carpus thus placed would probably tend to glide forwards, and hence the formation of a strong lip of bone in front to support them.

By the displacement backwards, the great depth of all the grooves for the tendons on the dorsum may also be explained, as these would have to play over a ridge, and would gradually deepen their channels. The evidence of absorption of cartilage in both specimens, and of strong bands crossing the articulation, is difficult to deal with, but it does not materially militate against the hypothesis of epiphysial detachment. In both cases, and in several other examples of similar deformity which Mr. Hutchinson had seen in living patients, there was the clear history of an accident in childhood—a supposed ' dislocation of the wrist.'

A specimen, No. 95, in St. Mary's Hospital Museum is figured and described by Mr. Hutchinson in the *Path. Soc. Trans.* vol. xiii. 1862; p. 264, plate xi. fig. 2; *London Hospital Reports*, vol. i. 1864, p. 95; *Catalogue of the Pathological Museum of St. Mary's Hospital*, 1891, p. 10, as an arrest of growth of the radius probably consequent on separation of its epiphysis. The specimen was obtained in the dissecting room of St. Mary's Hospital from the body of an adult man, of whom no history could be procured. The radius is about one inch shorter than the ulna, and articulates with a facet, on the side of the shaft of the latter bone, considerably below its head. The relative position, &c., of the bones, and the shape of the extremity of the radius, are well shown. On the outer aspect of the extremity of the ulna is seen a new facet, smooth and polished, but not covered with cartilage. With this facet the cuneiform bone was in apposition during life. The supposition as to the cause of the arrest of growth on the part of the radius is that the epiphysis of the latter was detached at an early period of life, and that the reunion was interfered with, either by inflammation or otherwise.

Dupuytren's specimen of dwarfed radius has already been fully described (see page 521).

Professor Nicoladoni figures (*Wiener medizin. Jahrbücher*, 1886, S. 264) a specimen of displacement of the hand into the valgus position from a male subject in the dissecting room of Innsbruck (see page 115).

This deformity had been brought about by the abnormal shortness of the radius, whose carpal surface was placed obliquely to its long axis (at an angle of 135°, open towards the ulnar side).

Above the obliquely placed radial epiphysis there was a rough edge on the volar and dorsal aspect. The head of the ulna projected three centimetres beyond the styloid process of the radius, while on the radial side of the lower end of the ulna there was a longish facet articulating in part with the radius, and in part with the inner border of the carpus. The articular surface of the head of the radius was placed obliquely, and sloped off towards the outer side; the lesser sigmoid cavity of the ulna had also an oblique direction, so that the elbow-joint must have assumed a considerable valgus position.

Clinical cases.—Mr. W. H. Brown figures and describes (*Lancet*, March 17, 1888) a case of arrest of development of the radius following injury, with resulting luxation of the head of the ulna.

A. W., a boy aged ten years, was admitted in June 1880 into the Leeds General Infirmary, having fallen from a two-storied house upon his face and right arm. He was unconscious. There were several severe wounds upon the face; the right wrist was swollen, but there was no displacement of bones and no fracture. He was discharged well after two weeks, being able to move his wrist freely and without pain. There was no alteration in the shape of the wrist at that time. Two years later his mother first noticed a 'lump' on the wrist, but as the boy had no pain she did not consult any one. The deformity gradually increased, and on February 6, 1888, she brought him to the infirmary. On examination the head of the ulna of the right side was found to be dislocated inwards and somewhat backwards; the movements of the joint were but little interfered with; the radius was in its normal position, and practically unchanged in contour. On measurement, the radius of the affected side was found to be one inch shorter than its fellow, whilst the length of the ulna on the two sides corresponded. Mr. Brown remarked that he had met with but one other instance where the radius almost entirely disappeared after a blow, leaving but the upper and lower epiphyses.

The injury in the present case was a very severe one, and it would seem probable that the lower epiphysis of the radius was impacted, and that as a result ossification followed, whilst the ulna continued to grow in the ordinary way.

Goyrand (*Revue Méd. chir. de Paris*, 1848, p. 25) observed an arrest of growth of the radius in two cases after separation of its lower epiphysis. One of the cases was that of a lady, aged twenty-seven years, who had received a lesion at the wrist which was treated as a fracture of the lower end of the radius when she was ten years old, and which had united without any deformity. It was only during the subsequent growth of the body that a corresponding and increasing

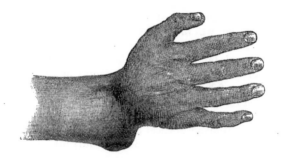

FIG. 165.—DEFORMITY OF HAND AND FOREARM FROM ARREST OF GROWTH OF RADIUS DUE TO EPIPHYSIAL INJURY. MR. W. H. BROWN'S CASE

deformity began to appear in the neighbourhood of the wrist. Examination disclosed a very striking shortening of the radius and abnormal projection of the lower end of the ulna. The outline of the radius, which was smaller than that of the opposite side, was quite regular, showing that there had been no overlapping of the fragments.

The other case was precisely similar in a man aged twenty-seven, who had met with the injury in very early childhood; the radius was slender and shortened by two centimetres, and its lower end displaced towards the dorsal aspect. In both cases there was abnormal projection of the styloid process of the ulna on the inner side.

Goyrand some years afterwards modified his opinions as to the frequent occurrence of arrest of growth after this injury, when reporting a few new cases which have already been described.

A. Poncet describes (Barbarin, *Des fractures chez les enfants*, Thèse de Paris, 1873, No. 206, pp. 57, 58; *Lyon Médical,* 1872) two cases of adults in which there existed marked deformity in the neighbourhood of the wrist, from the pushing of the hand towards the radial side and displacement of the lower end of the ulna downwards and outwards. In both there was an arrest of growth of the radius following a separation of the lower epiphysis in childhood, which was diagnosed and afterwards verified by dissection. The transverse diameter of the wrist was notably increased. In the one case the shortening of the radius followed a fracture at the age of ten to twelve years, and amounted to five centimetres, and in the other, in which the injury occurred at the age of sixteen, it was only three centimetres. In the former at the time of the accident no marked deformity was noticed.

Both had been carefully treated in the first instance with splints ; the latter was, moreover, treated as an in-patient at the Hôtel-Dieu de Paris.

In the former, although the limb was a very useful one, it was weaker than its fellow, and in the latter pronation, flexion, and extension were easily effected ; the lateral movement inwards of the hand, in addition, was limited by the ulnar projection.

At the Bradford Medico-Chirurgical Society in 1889 (*British Medical Journal*, January 19, 1889) Mr. J. Appleyard showed a child in whom an arrest of growth of the radius at its lower epiphysis occurred after a fall eleven months before. The lower epiphyses of the ulna and radius were connected with the bone above by fibroid tissue.

Before the Midland Medical Society, November 28, 1888 (*British Medical Journal*, December 22, 1888, p. 1397) Mr. Haslam exhibited a girl, aged seventeen, who three years before had sustained a fracture at the lower end of the radius. This had arrested the growth of the bone, and the hand was being gradually fixed to the radial side by the increase in length of the ulna.

Holmes (*Surgical Treatment of Diseases of Children*, 1869, p. 239) also mentions that he had observed several instances of loss of growth after fracture in the neighbourhood of the wrist.

G. A. Wright, of Manchester, figures (Ashby and Wright, *Diseases of Children*, 3rd edition, 1896, p. 754) another instance of an arrest of growth of the radius from separation of the lower epiphysis many years before.

A very interesting example of dwarfing of the radius after injury to its carpal epiphysis came under Mr. Hutchinson's notice (*Archives of Surgery*, October 1892, vol. iv. No. 14, p. 171) in the wrist of a medical friend. During a consultation he noticed that the ulna of his right wrist projected greatly, and, having asked permission to examine it, Mr. Hutchinson found the ulna at least three-quarters of an inch longer than the radius. There was not so much obliquity as is usual in these cases. The wrist was simply placed at the distance named above the end of the

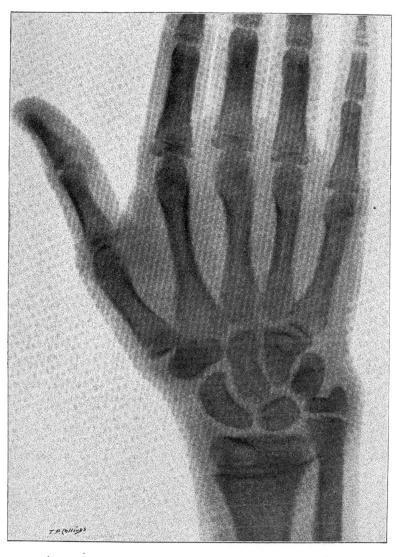

SKIAGRÁM OF WRIST OF A GIRL AGED TWELVE YEARS, SHOWING CONSIDERABLE DEFORMITY
AND ARREST OF GROWTH OF LEFT RADIUS.

Twelve months after a fall on hand, which was treated as a sprain. The ulna projects about half an inch
lower than its proper relation to radius ; the epiphysial cartilage of the radius is obliterated,
but that of the ulna is quite normal.

Mr. WM. THOMAS's case.

TABLE OF SHORTENING OF THE RADIUS AFTER EPIPHYSIAL INJURY

	Amount of shortening	Age of patient	Date of injury	Sex	Remarks
St. Mary's Hosp. Mus.	Radius about 1 in. above ulna	An adult man	No history obtainable	Male	
London Hosp. Mus.	About ¾ in. above ulna	40-50 years of age	In boyhood	Male	
Roy. Coll. Surg. Mus. Eng.	1⅛ in. above styloid process of ulna	25 years of age	Fall on hand at 5 years of age and wrist 'put out'	Female	Displacement forwards of epiphysis
Dupuytren	5 or 6 lines above the ulna	An adult	No history obtainable	Female	
Poncet	5 centimetres	Not stated	At 10-12 years of age	Not stated	
Poncet	3 centimetres	Not stated	At 16 years of age	Not stated	
Goyrand	Not stated	27 years of age	At 10 years of age	Female	No deformity at time of injury
Goyrand	2 centimetres	27 years of age	In very early childhood	Male	
Hutchinson	Radius and ulna both 1⅛ in. shorter than opposite side	23 years of age	Fall on hand at age of 9 years	Male	Abscess and necrosis followed the injury
Brown (W. H.)	1 in. shorter than its fellow	18 years of age	At age of 10 fall from second story	Male	No deformity at time of injury. (?) impaction
Clay (Augustus)	Not stated	14 years of age	Fall off cart at 8 years of age	Male	
Appleyard (J.)	Not stated	A child	Fall 11 months previously	Not stated	
Stehr (Wilhelm)	4 centimetres	16 years	At 12 years	Male	Other serious lesions
"	5·5 centimetres	23 years	At 14 years	Male	Diagnosed as a fracture
"	4·7 centimetres	18 years	At 18 years	Male	Displacement at time not diagnosed
Hutchinson	At least ¾ in. above ulna	Not stated	At 4 years	Male	Hand straight; little obliquity
Annandale	Little or none	14 years	15 months	Male	Compound separation of both epiphyses
G. A. Wright	?	?	Many years before	?	

ulna, the lower part of the forearm and hand being nearly straight. Mr. Hutchinson was told that the condition had resulted from an accident which occurred at the age of four.

Arrest of growth was attributed by Colignon to premature ossification of the conjugal cartilage leading to union of the epiphysis with the diaphysis, produced during the formation of callus in separations which were not simple but accompanied by pre-epiphysial or juxta-epiphysial fracture, or by a splintered fracture of the diaphysis. For the several views on this subject the author must refer the reader to the commencing chapters on epiphysial injuries in general (Part I., Chapters II. and VIII.).

Arrest of growth after suppuration and necrosis in epiphysial separation of the radius and ulna is noted in a case described by Mr. Hutchinson.

Gangrene, as a result of the improper use of splints, has already been alluded to.

It is usually due to the tight application of the splint impinging upon the two principal arteries of the forearm, which occupy a superficial position in the lower part of their course. Where the violence has been great and is followed by great inflammatory swelling, should the apparatus not allow of its being loosened as the swelling increases, this disastrous occurrence may result. However, we must not be too ready to attribute it entirely to the negligence of the surgeon. In cases of severe violence the hand and forearm should be carefully examined day by day, and in this respect the patient or his parents are often too ignorant or careless.

Again, the severe nature of the original violence, the extensive extravasation of blood, and the pressure of the diaphysial end upon one of the main vessels, are sometimes sufficient, especially in a feeble constitution, to produce such a result.

TREATMENT.—There is a very marked contrast in the rapid union of separations in comparison with that of fractures in older patients. In epiphysial SEPARATIONS WITHOUT DISPLACEMENT, and in the simpler forms of displacement when reduction has been effected, the most simple retentive apparatus is sufficient to keep the fragments in position—a moulded plastic splint to the forearm, wrist, or palm, or Gamgee tissue soaked in silicate of potash, or cardboard splints. Absolute rest for a few days in these instances is sufficient to remove all traces of the lesion.

The splint should, however, in most cases be applied for eighteen to twenty days, and the hand supported in a sling on account of the tendency to inflammation of the periosteum and bone. In a few instances the splint may be removed as early as the fifteenth day.

In these cases there is no tendency for the deformity to be reproduced on account of the broad and transverse surfaces of the epiphysis and diaphysis. A very different condition is present in fracture, where the greatest care is necessary to prevent a recurrence of the deformity. The majority of such cases do not unite without some deformity. Satisfactory results such as this can only occur, as a rule, in epiphysial separations.

In more or less COMPLETE DISPLACEMENTS reduction should in the *first* place be effected by means of extension and manipulation, and approximation of the displaced parts. It can always be accomplished easily and completely. In more complicated cases some periosteal tags may intervene between the diaphysis and displaced epiphysis and prevent complete reduction. The extension should be carried out with the hand in the supinated position. The thumb or fingers of the surgeon's hand will also help to press the epiphysis directly into its normal position. As a rule there is but little tendency to reproduction of the displacement.

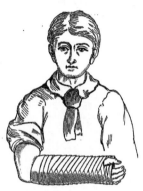

FIG. 166.—METHOD OF APPLYING ANTERIOR WOODEN SPLINT TO FOREARM AND HAND

The *second point* is to retain the epiphysis in position by means of Gordon's, or two straight wooden, splints, one on the anterior and the other on the posterior aspect of the forearm. The dorsal splint may be longer than the palmar (Nélaton's plan).

Nélaton's splint, or any other form of pistol-shaped splint, is unnecessary, and, as a rule, in simple cases of separation of the radial epiphysis alone, no inclination of the hand towards the ulnar side is necessary, as the fracture is transverse and not oblique. Indeed, a pistol-shaped splint is actually harmful, as it tends to separate the epiphysis from its diaphysis.

Dr. R. W. Smith says (*Dublin Hospital Gazette*, 1860, p. 49) : ' Compared with Colles's fracture there is but little difficulty in the treatment of this accident, nor need any apprehension be entertained of permanent deformity resulting, or of any lasting impairment of the functions of the limb. The pistol-shaped splint, usually employed in the common fracture of the lower end of the radius, is not required ; when the fragments have been brought into opposition by extension, a cushion, thickest opposite the disjointed epiphysis, is to be placed along the posterior surface of the limb, and a second along the front of the forearm, its thickest part corresponding to the lower end of the upper fragment ; two straight splints are then applied, reaching from the elbow to the metacarpophalangeal articulations at least, and secured either by a continued roller or by tapes ; the latter mode of securing them facilitates the use of evaporating lotions, and favours the early detection of any amount of swelling.'

Levis's metallic splint for the palmar aspect of the forearm and hand is a good one, provided an accurately fitting one can be obtained. Usually a special one has to be made for the particular case.

A moulded splint of gutta percha, plaster of Paris, or other material may be accurately moulded to the palmar aspect in a few minutes.

The forearm and hand should be enveloped as far as the metacarpo-phalangeal articulation in the plaster dressing; in separation of both lower epiphyses of the forearm the hand should be slightly inclined to the ulnar side after the fragments have been replaced in position. The dressing, if made of plaster of Paris in the form of palmar and dorsal splints, may easily be cut up along the inner or outer borders to examine the condition of the bones, and as readily re-applied. Great caution should be exercised in avoiding any tightness of the bandage applied to the retentive apparatus, especially in the more severe cases, on account of the great amount of extravasation of blood present.

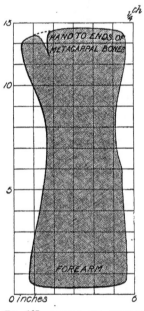

FIG. 167.—PATTERN FOR ANTERIOR AND POSTERIOR PIECES OF ANTERO-POSTERIOR SPLINTS (CROFT'S), FOR THE HAND AND WRIST AND FOREARM OF A BOY OF FIFTEEN YEARS

Reduced to one-quarter size on scale of inches

No graduated compress between the bones of the forearm is necessary, inasmuch as the lower end of the diaphysis of the radius is almost the same shape as the articular end, and hence the interosseous space has no tendency to become obliterated.

Great care must be exercised in applying the splints, on account of the not infrequent accident of gangrene from tight bandaging. A bandage should never be applied to the limb before the splints are fixed.

Professor Roux was the first to lay stress upon the frequency with which gangrene occurred in fracture of the forearm from retardation of the circulation, in severe injuries from pressure of effused blood upon the vessels.

The arm and hand should be examined frequently. Once a day at least the surgeon should carefully examine the condition of the limb. It would be far better to apply no splints at all than to allow them to be on the limb with the danger of increasing the inflammatory swelling.

J. Hutchinson junior says that out of fourteen cases, nine of which were under his own observation, of simple detachment of this epiphysis, most of them with very marked displacement, reduction was in every case effected, and a very good result obtained by treatment.

Passive motion must be commenced early; after the tenth day the fingers, at any rate, should be freely moved.

The splints should be finally removed on the fifteenth to the twentieth day in cases of separation without displacement; but

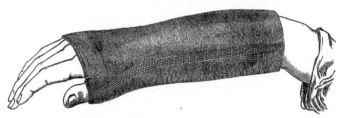

FIG. 168.—CROFT'S ANTERO-POSTERIOR SPLINTS OF PLASTER OF PARIS APPLIED TO THE RIGHT FOREARM AND HAND

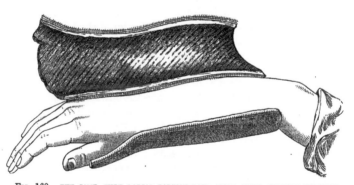

FIG. 169.—THE SAME, WITH DORSAL PORTION LAID ASIDE AFTER CUTTING THROUGH THE MUSLIN ALONG GAP ON OUTER SIDE

where displacement has been present they should be removed on the eighteenth to twenty-fifth day, or even a few days later if thought to be necessary.

After removal of the splint when union has taken place, the movements of the wrist-joint are soon regained, the swelling of the forearm rapidly disappears, and supination and pronation soon become normal; whereas in the corresponding fractures in older persons great stiffness of the wrist-joint and tendon-sheaths and wasting of the muscles of the forearm are a frequent result from the penetrating fracture of the joint, the feebler circulation, &c.

An injury at the lower end of the radius in a boy, described by John Ashhurst junior (*International Clinics*, 2nd series, 1892, vol. i.

p. 200) as an ordinary fracture a short distance above the joint, was probably a separation of the epiphysis produced by a fall upon the hand, which sustained the weight of the body. The deformity was well marked, being the ordinary 'silver-fork' deformity, and mobility, though not crepitus, existed at the seat of fracture.

He recommends two compresses, which should be large enough to effect the desired purpose. The upper compress is applied over the lower end of the upper fragment, on the palmar surface, and the other is applied on the dorsal surface over the lower fragment. When the compresses are brought together, the bones are necessarily pushed into position. Even if this cannot be accomplished at once, it will be found, he says, that by careful dressing the deformity will in a few days disappear. The hand should be put in the supine position and a Bond's splint applied.

Dr. Thomas S. K. Morton recently advocated (*New York Medical Journal*, July 7, 1894, p. 26) a new method for reduction of fractures of the lower end of the radius, which had proved satisfactory in his hands during the previous few years. By this manipulation a separated epiphysis of the lower end of the radius was easily reducible. The method was as follows :

'The surgeon stood in front of the patient and interlaced his fingers beneath the supinated wrist and palm of the injured member, so that his two index fingers lay parallel crosswise beneath the lower end of the upper fragment of the radius. The palms of the surgeon's hands were then closed in upon the thenar and hypothenar portions of the patient's hand respectively, while the surgeon's thumbs rested parallel lengthwise upon the upwardly displaced lower fragment of the radius. The parts were thus firmly grasped by the surgeon while the following movements were made : The patient's wrist was excessively extended by carrying his hand upward. When superextension had thus been secured, the surgeon made powerful traction upon the wrist in the line of superextension. While this traction was maintained the hand was suddenly carried into full flexion, and at the same time powerful downward pressure upon the upwardly displaced lower fragment of the radius was made by the surgeon's thumbs opposed by the interlaced index fingers beneath the lower end of the upper fragment. The excessive extension of the first portion of the movement had always, so far in my experience, loosened or disentangled the displaced lower fragment, while the subsequent traction, flexion, and direct thumb pressure had not yet failed to accurately force the lower fragment into its proper position. Anæsthesia was unnecessary for making a single effort at reduction by this method, but was necessary for a second attempt.'

The immediate treatment by massage without the use of retentive splints, lately recommended by French surgeons, has been adopted by M. Bauby and M. Bardier (*Le Midi Médical*, Toulouse, 8 Octobre,

1893, p. 473, 'Considérations sur le traitement des fractures épi-physaires') in this as in other forms of epiphysial fracture.

The reduction of the fragments is said to be slower and surer by this method.

The author quotes the following case mentioned by them in order to strongly deprecate their procedure—at any rate, if it be carried out to its fullest extent in children, as it is in adults.

A patient (M. B.), aged twelve, fell from a trestle upon his hands. A fracture occurred at the level of the lower epiphysis of the right radius, and was easily diagnosed by the characteristic deformity. A compression-bandage was applied for twelve hours and then taken off, and massage commenced at the seat of the fracture. There was discoloration and swelling of the wrist, with great pain on pressure, and all movement was impossible.

Massage was carried out daily for five minutes, the pressure being progressively increased. At the end of fifteen days consolidation took place, and there was neither pain, swelling, nor deformity. During the intervals of the massage a very light dressing was applied, but not sufficient to fix the part, the arm being in a sling.

At the time of the report (four months later) recovery was said to be perfect, without any articular stiffness and without the slightest untoward sign.

COMPOUND SEPARATION.—An attempt should always be made to save the limb, even though it be so severely damaged as to apparently preclude recovery.

The wound must, of course, be carefully and thoroughly cleansed from all dirt and grime; for this purpose it may be found necessary to remove the superficial parts of the soiled soft tissue of muscle, cellular tissue, &c. If the subject be very young, soiled portions

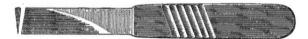

FIG. 170.—STOUT KNIFE EMPLOYED BY AUTHOR (MAY ALSO BE USED AS A CHISEL WITH A MALLET) FOR REMOVING FOILED PORTIONS OF THE DIAPHYSIS IN COMPOUND EPIPHYSIAL SEPARATIONS

of the diaphysial end may be cut away with a stout knife; and in older subjects the careful use of a saw may be found advantageous for the same purpose. The wound and bone should then be dis-infected by means of a suitable antiseptic solution, such as carbolic acid (1 in 30), hyd. perchlor. (1 in 1,000).

The wound may require to be enlarged before the diaphysis can be replaced in its normal position through the rent in the periosteum. In some of the recorded cases this reduction appears to have been very incompletely carried out.

Resection of the diaphysial end may be necessary to effect the reduction of the fragments. This irreducibility of the diaphysis is

P P

mainly due to its particular shape—viz. its marked enlargement in its lower fifth from above downwards—and to the shrinking of the skin, which has lost its proper circumference, and the buttonhole condition of the aponeurosis and flexor muscles.

Resection was performed in the cases of Denonvilliers, Péan, Richet, Annandale, and others with a successful result.

Antiseptic dressings and great care are required to prevent subsequent inflammatory complications.

In two cases of compound separation in children, both aged thirteen years, one recorded by M. Péan in 1856 and the other by M. Richet in 1859, M. Denonvilliers, under whose care they were placed, resected the protruding end of the diaphysis, rather than incise the skin, to effect reduction.   Both patients recovered in a short time, and without any unfavourable occurrence.

J. Hutchinson junior found ten compound cases among fifty-four otherwise uncomplicated cases ; in four it was found necessary to resect the end of the protruding diaphysis before it could be reduced.   In all these good recovery ensued ; in the other six this course was not followed, but more or less imperfect reduction was obtained.   Two patients died, both with suppuration, tetanus being responsible in the one case, pyæmia in the other ; one case recovered with a crippled wrist-joint after tedious suppuration ; three underwent amputation on account of gangrene.   Two deaths and three cases of loss of limb occurred out of six, nearly all being comparatively recent cases.

Secondary amputation may be required, from sloughing or gangrene of the forearm.

Dr. Bœckel performed amputation on the tenth day after compound separation for sloughing of the forearm, and the patient recovered.

Resection of whole or part of the epiphysis may be expedient in some few exceptional cases of comminuted fracture of the epiphysis (see Professor Annandale's case, described above), and in cases where ankylosis of the wrist appears to be inevitable.

Replacement by operation in old cases.—L. von Lesser, of Leipzig, has drawn attention (*Centralblatt für Chirurgie*, No. 15, April 9, 1887, S. 265) to the operative treatment of badly united fractures of the radio-carpal epiphysis, and mentions the case of a boy, aged thirteen years, in which the lower end of the radius, which had been displaced towards the dorsum, was detached by means of a chisel.   Other complications in this case—ankylosis of the meta-carpo-phalangeal joint of the thumb, matting together of the flexor tendons, and marked atrophy of the muscles of the hand—had rendered operative interference necessary.

Conjugal chondrectomy, or excision of the conjugal cartilage of the ulna, may be performed to produce its arrest of growth in deformity arising from cessation of growth of the radius after epiphysial separation. This may be especially desirable when there is a considerable period of time to elapse before the bone reaches its limit of increase in length.

The distances given by Ollier (through the skin) from the conjugal cartilages to the top of the styloid processes are as follows :

Radius : at four years of age, eleven to twelve millimetres ; at fifteen years of age, fifteen to sixteen millimetres.

Ulna : At four years of age, eight to nine millimetres ; at fifteen years of age, eleven to thirteen millimetres.

The deformity of the wrist caused by shortening of the radius after fracture in an adult has been successfully treated by Dr. Gill (U.S.A.) by the removal of a portion of the shaft of the ulna (*New York Medical Record*, January 6, 1894, p. 9). The portion of the ulna removed was five-eighths of an inch in length, and was taken from just above the attachment of the pronator quadratus.

Correction of deformity by osteotomy.—Dr. McBurney operated on a boy of about sixteen years for the relief of deformity and impaired function caused by a Colles's fracture of the radius, one and a half inches from the lower extremity. Perfect union had resulted after the fracture, with well-marked silver-fork deformity, loss of power of flexion at the wrist, partial loss of flexion of the fingers, and a good deal of pain on motion. He did not think he could with propriety attempt refracture without cutting down upon the bone. He therefore divided this as nearly as he could in the line of the fracture, which ran somewhat obliquely. He was then able to put the parts up in proper position and retain them with a plaster-of-Paris splint. Subsequently there was very little deformity left, and the restoration of function was extremely satisfactory (*New York Medical Record*, April 3, 1897, p. 495).

However, the author cannot consider this an example of Colles's fracture, inasmuch as the fracture occurred one and a half inches above the wrist.

CHAPTER XIII

SEPARATION OF THE LOWER EPIPHYSIS OF THE ULNA

ANATOMY.—Up to three years the lower end of the shaft of the ulna keeps its cylindrical form, and it is the lower epiphysis which chiefly gives the shape to this end of the bone.

About the fourth, fifth, or sixth year the chief nuclei of the carpal extremity appear towards the centre of the head and base of the styloid process. These lie close together, and soon blend, forming an osseous plate which extends downwards on the inner side into the styloid process. This process is formed principally from this centre, but an additional centre is sometimes seen at the summit, appearing about the twelfth year, and joining the rest of the osseous epiphysis three or four years later.

Béclard described two centres, one for the articular end and the other for the styloid process, appearing soon after birth.

This epiphysis joins the shaft at twenty years of age, often a little later.

The fully formed epiphysis comprises the whole of the articular surface of the head on the outer aspect, for the radius, as well as on the inferior aspect towards the inarticular fibro-cartilage ; it also includes the styloid process projecting downwards on the inner side, which is grooved behind for the tendon of the extensor carpi ulnaris. Its upper aspect is concave and mammillated, and fits the corresponding convexity of the diaphysis.

The level of the epiphysial line of the lower end of the ulna is very slightly above the level of that of the radius, about $\frac{1}{16}$th of an inch. The cartilaginous disc is twelve millimetres vertically above the apex of the styloid process in the fully formed epiphysis, and seven millimetres at fourteen years of age. On the inner side or head it is eight millimetres vertically above the lower articular surface, and at fourteen years of age five millimetres. Where the head joins the styloid process on the outer side the thickness (vertically) of the mature epiphysis is only five millimetres, at fourteen years three millimetres.

The head of the ulna is covered by the synovial membrane of the inferior radio-ulnar articulation, and rotates within the sigmoid cavity of the radius and on the surface of the triangular fibro-cartilage.

This epiphysis is held to the lower epiphysis of the radius in front and behind by the anterior and posterior inferior radio-ulnar ligaments, and also by means of the triangular fibro-cartilage, which is attached by its apex to the root of the styloid process, and by its thin base to the lunar margin of the radius. To the carpus it is held by the numerous anterior and posterior fibres of the capsular ligament of the wrist.

The apex of the styloid process affords attachment to the internal lateral ligament of the wrist.

The synovial membrane of the inferior radio-ulnar articulation is especially loose in front, where it slightly overlaps the epiphysial margin of the ulna; on the outer side it extends upwards between the radius and ulna, and overlaps the epiphysial line at this point. This *cul-de-sac* is not necessarily opened in epiphysial detachment, on account of its being firmly attached to the epiphysis and but loosely to the diaphysis, from which it is readily separated.

PATHOLOGICAL ANATOMY. SIMPLE SEPARATION.—This is an exceedingly rare injury. The author knows of no specimen where simple detachment of this epiphysis has taken place without some accompanying serious injury to the neighbouring bones or soft parts.

SEPARATION WITH OTHER LESIONS.—In separation of the lower epiphysis of the radius it is surprising to see how very infrequent is an accompanying separation of the lower end of the ulna. In radial separation the styloid process of the ulna is mostly broken off, or, as we have seen above in R. W. Smith's and several other instances, the diaphysis of the ulna is broken at its smallest part—namely, three-quarters of an inch above the lower extremity (considered at fifteen years of age).

In Bruns's 100 cases of epiphysial separation, of which the anatomical details were given, only two were of the lower end of the ulna.

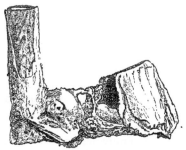

FIG. 171.—SEPARATION OF LOWER EPIPHYSIS OF ULNA, AND FRACTURE OF RADIUS

Specimen, Royal College of Surgeons Museum, No. 956D.

Mr. Jonathan Hutchinson junior's specimen in the Royal College of Surgeons Museum shows this lesion, amongst others, caused by direct crushing violence. It consists of the lower ends of the right radius and ulna taken from a lad, aged fourteen, whose forearm had been caught in a jute-tearing machine, rendering primary amputation necessary. The lower epiphysis of the ulna (the head and styloid process), cleanly detached, is displaced outwards, so as to be firmly wedged between the shaft and the lower end of

the radius, which is extensively fractured. The membrana sacci-
formis and wrist are uninjured; the former has been cut open in
order to expose the epiphysis.

The fracture of the radius occurs on the inner side, rather more
than a quarter of the width of the diaphysis being broken away;
the rest of the conjugal line is uninjured (see fig. 171).

Incomplete detachment, with greenstick fracture of the shaft.—In
the Charing Cross Hospital Museum there is a specimen, No. 355
(*Catalogue of Museum of Charing Cross Hospital*, 1888, p. 33;
Lancet, January 8, 1859), showing incomplete separation of this
carpal epiphysis, associated with a greenstick fracture of the shaft.
The detachment of the epiphysis has been effected only on the
outer and anterior aspects; the posterior and inner are still connected with the diaphysis by means of the periosteum, so that there
is no displacement, and only a slight gap between the epiphysis and
the shaft on the outer side. The latter presents a greenstick
fracture one and a half inches above the lower end for three-quarters
of an inch of its thickness, with bowing (convexity) outwards of the
remaining portion of the bone. The lower epiphysis of the radius
is completely separated.

The patient was a boy, aged fourteen, who received a lacerated
wound of the outer side of the arm in a printing machine. The
forearm was amputated by Mr. Canton.

Comminution of epiphysis with fracture of shaft of radius.—In a
specimen, No. 932, in the Museum of St. Bartholomew's Hospital
(*Catalogue of Museum of St. Bartholomew's Hospital*, vol. i. p. 134).
the lower epiphysis of the ulna is separated from the diaphysis
and broken into several pieces. The largest piece of the epiphysis
with the triangular fibro-cartilage is displaced outwards off the
diaphysis towards the radius, and the periosteum still attached to it
is stripped upwards from the shaft for nearly half an inch. The
diaphysis is displaced somewhat inwards off the comminuted
epiphysis. The radius is fractured transversely one and a quarter
inches from its articular surface and above the epiphysial line. The
shaft is firmly impacted in the cancellous tissue of the lower end,
which is displaced backwards. No history is appended to the case.

Separation of the epiphysis with that of the radius.—Instances
have been recorded in which separation of this epiphysis was
associated with that of the radius, and have already been alluded to
in the previous chapter.

It occurred in Voillemier's, Geoghegan's and other cases already
described.

Dolbeau (*Bullet. de la Soc. de Chirur.* 1865; *Gazette des
Hôpitaux*, 1865) mentions a separation of the carpal epiphyses of
both bones of the forearm and of the opposite radius in a child,
aged thirteen years, who fell from a second story and died nineteen
days later from fracture of the skull.

Barbarin relates (*Les fract. chez les enfants*, Thèse de Paris, 1873, p. 34) a similar case of separation of the carpal epiphyses of the radius and ulna on the same side in a boy, aged eighteen years, who fell from a height. Amputation was performed at the shoulder-joint for gangrene.

In Roux's specimen of separation of the radial epiphysis the styloid epiphysis of the ulna, as well as the epiphyses of the first phalanges of the thumb, index, and middle fingers, were detached by an explosion of gunpowder.

ETIOLOGY.—Severe direct violence appears to be the usual cause in the published examples.

Bertrandi said he had seen in a child 'the epiphyses of the radius and ulna separated by its being violently raised by its hand from the ground.'

AGE.—Of the eleven cases recorded six are *pathological specimens* and five *simple cases of arrest of growth*. Of the former the age is stated in four: one at eighteen, two at fourteen, and one at thirteen years. Of the latter the injury is said to have occurred: two at five, one at two, one at eleven, and one in a little boy.

SYMPTOMS.—No instance has been published, apart from those accompanied by other severe injuries to the wrist, in which the injured lower ulnar epiphysis formed an insignificant part, while more than one was caused by direct crushing violence as just stated.

It is possible that a less degree of violence does not unfrequently cause a partial separation, which is then overlooked; the signs of these partial separations cannot differ materially from those of other bones. (See Part I. Chapter VII.)

PROGNOSIS. Suppurative periostitis.—Mr. Cock had a case under his care at Guy's Hospital (*Lancet*, 1850, vol. ii. p. 652) of a child, aged three and a half years, with acute periostitis and necrosis of the entire ulna from suppuration extending upwards beneath the periosteum. Three months previously the child had received a severe blow with a stick on the inner side of the arm just above the wrist. Mr. Cock considered the acute periostitis to be the result of the original injury—viz. a fracture or separation of the epiphysis just above the styloid process. The end of the ulna, which projected through a large ulcerated opening immediately above the wrist, was seized, and the entire ulna, with olecranon and coronoid processes complete, was drawn out through the opening. Thickened soft tissues only remained, as no new shell of bone had been formed round it. Four months later the use of the arm was completely restored, but with entire deficiency of the ulna and the absence of any attempt at restoration by the deposition of new bone.

Arrest of growth.—The ulna depends almost entirely upon the integrity of the lower epiphysis for growth in length; the upper epiphysis being of comparatively little importance in this respect. From the examples of arrest of growth now recorded it would appear probable that injury to the lower epiphysis of the ulna is not so rare as has been supposed. At any rate a partial separation without displacement or juxta-epiphysial sprain appears to be not uncommon.

Arrest of growth from injury to the lower end of the ulna, as in the case of the other parallel bones (the radius, tibia, and fibula), is usually seen to give rise to much lateral displacement or adduction of the hand, from the continued growth of the second bone (radius). The hand is thereby thrust over into the varus position.

Mr. Jonathan Hutchinson figures (*Illustrated Medical News*, November 17, 1888) the peculiar deformity of the forearm which followed an injury to (detachment of) the carpal epiphysis of the ulna in early life. The hand seemed to be pushed over to one side. It was the radius which had grown in excess of the ulna.

The patient was a young man of about eighteen, who had received an injury to his wrist when a little boy. No history of the precise diagnosis at the time of the accident was forthcoming, and although separation of the carpal epiphysis of the ulna is very rare, yet it had in all probability occurred in this instance and occasioned the arrest of growth. Mr. Hutchinson continues: ' I do not know that I have ever seen a recent example of detachment of this epiphysis, and the present is, I think, the only case in which I have seen dwarfing of the ulna of the kind which suggested its occurrence.'

The following notes by the same author (*Pathological Society's Transactions*, vol. xvii. 1866, p. 251) appear to be of the same case, shown by this surgeon at the Pathological Society in 1866.

Mr. Hutchinson says: 'The young gentleman, aged seventeen, was sent to me on account of an unusual condition of his right arm. The hand was bent over to the ulnar border. The extremity of the ulna was hidden. The styloid process of the radius projected, and the lower fourth was bowed outwards. It was clear, from the thickening and bend, that the radius had been fractured between two and three inches above the wrist. I could not find any evidence of former fracture of the ulna, but the whole of the lower half of this bone was very thin, and so buried amongst other muscles that it was not easy to examine it. The ulna of the left arm measured from the olecranon to the styloid process nine and three-quarter inches; the ulna of the right arm, eight inches; the radius of left arm, nine and a half; the right, nine inches; the girth of the left forearm at thickest part, nine and three-quarters; and the right, nine inches. The accident occurred at the age of five, from a kick from a horse; it was said to be a fracture at the time, and the skin was not lacerated. The deformity has gradually increased as the lad grew. He complains that the right arm is much weaker than the other, but still he can use it for most things. The right hand is not smaller than the left to any perceptible degree. There is no deformity at the elbow. My diagnosis was that there had been a fracture of the radius in its lower third, and probably at the same time detachment of the epiphysis of the ulna, and that thus the growth of the ulna had been arrested.'

Mr. Edmund Owen showed before the Medical Society of London, March 26, 1888 (*British Medical Journal*, vol. i. 1888; *Medical Society's Proceedings*, vol. xi. 1888, p. 353; *Lancet*, October 3, 1891, p. 767), the following case of arrested growth after injury to the lower epiphysis of the ulna. The girl, aged eighteen, had been under his care sixteen years previously at St. Mary's Hospital for an incised wound of the left wrist. The blade of a chaff machine had passed through the ulna, just above its articulation with the lesser sigmoid cavity; that joint was not opened, but the lesser sigmoid cavity was sliced from the radius, and the wrist-joint was laid widely open. The tendon of the flexor carpi ulnaris, the ulnar nerve and artery, and some of the adjacent flexor tendons were cleanly severed. Circulation and cutaneous sensibility were ultimately restored along the inner side of the hand, and though inflammation attacked the surrounding tissues and an abscess formed on the back of the hand, the power of movement became in due course as free as ever. Indeed, the child was left-handed; as she grew up she easily used her knife in that hand. Ultimately she became a useful domestic servant. But when the ulna had ceased to be developed, it played the part of a bowstring, bending the radius over to that side, so that the hand was greatly adducted. In September 1887 the girl fell upon the inner side of the damaged wrist, and immediately afterwards (according to her account) sensation became diminished along the inner side of the hand, and the member became useless. How far the case might be influenced by hysteria Mr. Owen could not say, but it was evident that the ball of the little finger and the web of the thumb were wasted; probably the nerve was injured. The chief interest consisted in the apparent overgrowth of the radius; actually, however, that bone was half an inch shorter than the opposite one, whilst it was bowed in its lower two-thirds towards the ulna, which latter bone was three inches and a half shorter than its fellow on the right side. Mr. Owen excised one inch of the lower third of the shaft of the radius, with the result that the hand and forearm became much straighter, and their usefulness was increased. See cast specimen No. 96 in St. Mary's Hospital Museum (*Catalogue of the Pathological Museum*, St. Mary's Hospital, 1891, p. 10).

The figure in Part I. Chapter VIII. p. 118 is of a case described by Curtillet (*Du Décollement traumatique des épiphyses*, Lyon, 1891) from the clinique of M. Poncet, in which a compound traumatic separation of the lower epiphysis of the ulna was followed by suppuration and necrosis of the epiphysis, and subsequently by arrest of growth and considerable deviation of the hand.

The youth (V. P.), aged 22, was admitted into the Hôtel-Dieu in November 1890. At the age of eleven he had fallen from a trapeze about two metres in height, causing a wound at the lower part of the left forearm through which the ulna projected for about six centimetres. The patient stated that the end of the bone was smooth and regular. It was reduced by a bone-setter. Profuse suppuration occurred through several openings which were found on the inner side of the forearm, and extended over four months. Three or four months after the accident the patient perceived a movable piece of bone in the wound, which he removed with his fingers. The fragment was

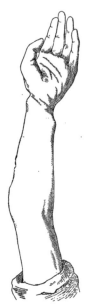

cylindrical, about two centimetres in length, with a flat surface at each end. The wound completely healed shortly afterwards. The deformity seen was considerable. The radius, although normal at its upper end, was bent like a bow at its lower end, being thrust over to the ulnar side. The axis of the hand made with that of the forearm an angle of 130 degrees. The ulna was likewise normal at its upper end, as well as at the superior radio-ulnar and humero-ulnar joints; its lower end, however, terminated abruptly, thereby leaving a hollow one and a half centimetres in length, which corresponded precisely with the fragment which had been removed. The forearm was somewhat atrophied, but pronation, supination, and flexion were effected naturally, whereas extension was slightly less than normal.

Fig. 172.—Varus position of hand and elbow the result of arrest of growth of ulna following injury (Nicoladoni)

The right radius measured from the epicondyle to the styloid process 24·5 centimetres; the left, 22·5 centimetres; the right ulna from the olecranon to the styloid process, 24·5 centimetres; the left, 17·5.

The length of the humerus was the same on the two sides, and there was no difference between the two clavicles.

Professor Nicoladoni, of Innsbruck, noticed (*Wiener medizin. Jahrbücher*, 1886, S. 264) a striking example of this varus position of the hand complicated with deformity at the elbow-joint, following arrest of growth of the ulna in a boy aged eleven years.

The left hand (fig. 172) in complete supination of the forearm was placed in a very marked varus position—that is, inclined to the ulnar side. The line of the wrist passed obliquely from the styloid

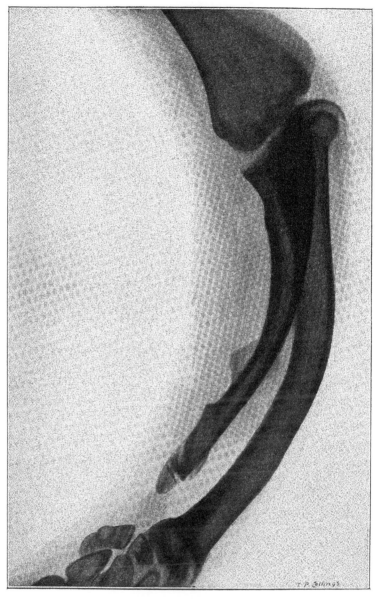

CURVATURE OF RADIUS, DUE TO ARRESTED DEVELOPMENT OF THE ULNA
AT ITS DISTAL EPIPHYSIS.

Prof. J. W. WHITE's case.

process of the radius upwards and inwards towards the head of the ulna, which was represented by a spindle-shaped projection. The elbow-joint, when extended, was likewise in a varus position, the axis of the humerus forming with that of the forearm an angle inwards of 165 degrees. The head of the radius projected on the outer side of the elbow-joint, and the epitrochlea stood more than a centimetre higher than the (outer) epicondyle. The right ulna measured twenty-two centimetres and the left sixteen, while the right and left radius were of equal length. The extremity was otherwise well developed, and the movements of the wrist and elbow-joints were free. The boy was said to have had a fall when five years old, and to have injured his left hand. The injury, however, appeared to his relatives to be so slight that no medical assistance was called in. Dr. Nicoladoni thought that the thickening of the lower end of the ulna indicated a disjunction of the lower epiphysis at the time of the injury, and that this had led to arrest of growth and consequent deformity. The deformity had perceptibly increased (1886) since the time it had been first observed (1884).

J. Hutchinson junior records (*British Medical Journal*, March 31, 1894, p. 669) another case, of a student aged twenty-four, which came under his own observation. When five years old he had been kicked by a horse on the right wrist. There was no wound and no subsequent suppuration. The radius gradually became curved, and the ulna was ultimately nearly two inches shorter than that on the other side. The forearm muscles were not so well developed as on the left side, but the patient had very good use of the hand.

A skiagraph produced by Professor A. W. Goodspeed (*The American Journal of the Medical Sciences*, August 1896) shows very well the condition and appearance of the forearm produced by curvature of the radius due to arrested development of the ulna at its distal epiphysis. E. A., aged fifteen years, came to the University Hospital of Pennsylvania, under Professor J. W. White, in January 1896. The affection began in the seventh or eighth year, when a little lump was noticed on the arm and the patient complained of pain located at that point. There was no sign of curvature at that time; it had come on gradually since, while the pain had been inconstant and rheumatic in character, seemingly after a slight cold at each attack. As the patient had fair use of the hand, and could write with it and do almost everything useful, no operation was advised.

TREATMENT.—The general rules of treatment are the same as in other epiphysial separations.

CHAPTER XIV

Separation of the Epiphysis of the Metacarpal Bone of the Thumb—
Separation of the Epiphyses of the True Metacarpal Bones—Separation of the Epiphyses of the Phalanges of the Digits

SEPARATION OF THE EPIPHYSIS OF THE METACARPAL BONE OF THE THUMB

ANATOMY.—The first metacarpal bone, or metacarpal bone of the thumb, is developed like one of the phalanges, the epiphysis being situated at its proximal end. In the four inner or true metacarpals the epiphysis is placed at the lower extremity. Both morphologically and developmentally this bone should be regarded as a phalanx.

The epiphysis begins to ossify about the third year, and unites with the shaft about the twentieth year.

The epiphysis is at fourteen years of age five millimetres thick vertically at the posterior border, and four millimetres anteriorly; in width, laterally, eleven millimetres. The epiphysis is at eighteen years of age six and a half millimetres thick vertically at the posterior border, and seven millimetres anteriorly; in width, eighteen millimetres.

To the margin of this epiphysis is attached the capsular ligament of the carpo-metacarpal joint, which is stronger behind and on the outer side than in front.

The synovial membrane of the carpo-metacarpal joint of the thumb, although loose, does not extend downwards so far as to overlap the epiphysial cartilage.

Traces of a distal epiphysis in this metacarpal bone are usually to be seen, and in some instances a distinct epiphysis (as in the seal and some other animals) is visible at the age of seven or eight years.

The nutrient artery of this bone is situated on the ulnar aspect and runs downwards.

ETIOLOGY.—Indirect as frequently as direct violence is the cause of separation of this epiphysis.

Indirect injury, such as a fall upon the thumb, or a blow with the fist in pugilistic encounters.

Direct violence, such as a blow from a stick or cricket-ball.

AGE.—There are only two simple cases recorded; one at eighteen, one at sixteen years of age.

PATHOLOGICAL ANATOMY.—There is no specimen of this lesion in the London hospitals or elsewhere, and no case has been verified by immediate dissection.

SYMPTOMS.—Pain is experienced on pressing the thumb towards the carpo-metacarpal articulation.

Deformity arises from the displacement of the base of the diaphysis more or less completely off the epiphysis, giving rise to a projection on the dorsal or palmar aspect, together with shortening of the thumb.

Displacement backwards.— The only case which has been diagnosed during life is one recorded by Mr. R. Clement Lucas (*Lancet*, October 31, 1885, p. 801), in which he was able to determine the exact character of the lesion by examination under chloroform.

C. W., aged sixteen, came to Guy's Hospital on March 6, 1885. He had fallen with his hand bent under him, the weight of the body being received upon the outer side of the left thumb; this was bruised and painful, and he was unable to move it without great pain. There was a projection outwards and backwards. at the base of the metacarpal bone which at first sight appeared to

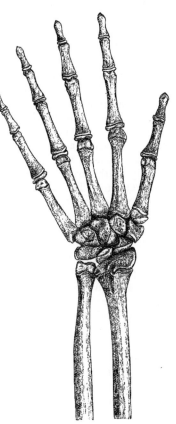

FIG. 173.—EPIPHYSES OF THE METACARPUS AND PHALANGES AT THE AGE OF FIFTEEN AND A HALF YEARS. $\frac{1}{2}$ NATURAL SIZE

be caused by a dislocation of the carpo-metacarpal joint. The dresser attempted a reduction and failed. Under chloroform Mr. Lucas traced the metacarpal bone down towards its base, where it terminated in a projection situated on the outer and posterior aspect of the thenar eminence. It could be easily pressed into its place, but showed a tendency to recur to its unusual position. There was no true bony crepitus. The seat of abnormal movement was too inferior to be in the joint between the metacarpal bone and the trapezium, and the symptoms present were considered sufficient to distinguish it from dislocation of the metacarpal bone. Reduction was effected by pressure and extension, and a well-padded splint was applied from the wrist to the end of the thumb on its dorsal aspect. Complete recovery without deformity took place in three weeks.

Abnormal mobility between the fragments is difficult of detection by reason of the smallness of the epiphysis and the difficulty experienced in grasping it. If this can be accomplished by the finger and thumb, mobility may be felt during attempt at flexion of the metacarpus.

Crepitus of the characteristic soft kind may be found during reduction; it will be slight on account of the small size of the separated surfaces.

Dr. C. A. Sturrock (*Edinburgh Hospital Reports*, vol. ii. 1894, p. 603) has seen 'one case in which separation of the head of the first metacarpal as an epiphysis was diagnosed by an eminent surgeon, though the epiphysis for the extremity of this bone is usually at the base; in many instances there is also one for the head (Quain). The accident referred to occurred in a patient aged eighteen, and now, fourteen years after the accident, there is very slight stiffness of the joint, with some thickening, but no shortening.'

J. Hutchinson junior alludes to a case in which the proximal epiphysis of the first metacarpal bone was separated during an attempt (fortunately successful) to reduce a dislocation of that bone.

COMPLICATIONS.—Inflammation of the carpo-metacarpal joint may follow epiphysial separation.

DIAGNOSIS.—Separation of the epiphysis of the metacarpal bone of the thumb might be mistaken for a **dislocation**, which it closely resembles either in its forward or backward displacement.

Shortening of the thumb and *mobility* may be present in both injuries, although in separation of the epiphysis the latter may be detected somewhat lower down than the joint.

Tendency to re-displacement after reduction may exist in dislocation, as well as in separation of the epiphysis.

Muffled crepitus is the only trustworthy sign; it may be absent from the small size of the separated surfaces.

TREATMENT.—The treatment of separated epiphysis is much the same as that for dislocation of the metacarpal bone backwards or forwards. The reduction will readily be accomplished by employing extension and making direct pressure upon the displaced end of the diaphysis.

A moulded splint of gutta-percha, or other material well padded, should then be applied, and the hand kept in a sling.

Operative treatment by open incision may be necessary if the displacement of the base of the diaphysis be completely off the epiphysial plate, and reduction cannot be accomplished by more simple means.

COMPOUND SEPARATIONS should be carefully dissected down upon, freely exposed, and the fragments placed in their normal position and fixed together by sutures.

Amputation should perhaps never be performed, although the diaphysis may be comminuted and apparently crushed in an almost hopeless manner.

SEPARATION OF THE EPIPHYSIS OF EITHER OF THE TRUE (FOUR INNER) METACARPAL BONES

ANATOMY.—In the four inner or true metacarpal bones the epiphysis is developed at the distal extremity. The osseous nucleus appears about the centre of the cartilaginous end from two and a half to five years of age, commencing in that of the index finger.

The epiphysis unites with the shaft about the twentieth year. The proximal end in each metacarpal bone is formed by the shaft.

In the second metacarpal bone the nutrient artery runs upwards on the ulnar side; in the other three it runs upwards on the radial side.

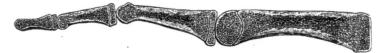

FIG. 174.—EPIPHYSES OF THE PHALANGES AND METACARPAL BONE AT SIXTEENTH YEAR (AFTER RAMBAUD AND RENAULT)

Mr. Allan Thompson states that there are traces of a proximal epiphysis to be seen in the second metacarpal bone.

The fully formed epiphysis constitutes the whole of the condyloid head, and has the lateral ligaments attached to the tubercles and hollows on each lateral aspect.

The length of the epiphysis (of the index finger) vertically from the epiphysial line is nine millimetres posteriorly and seven millimetres anteriorly. The width from side to side is at fourteen years, ten millimetres; at eighteen years, twelve millimetres; the width anteroposteriorly at fourteen years, twelve millimetres; at eighteen years, fifteen millimetres.

The synovial membrane is firmly fixed to the epiphysis laterally below the attachment of the lateral ligaments, but in front and behind it overlaps the epiphysial cartilage. Even here the membrane springs from the epiphysis, and is but loosely attached to the diaphysis.

ETIOLOGY.—**Indirect violence.**—Falls upon the hand with the fist closed, in such a manner that the lower end of the metacarpal bone strikes against the ground, whilst the upper end receives more or less the weight of the body. The natural curve of the bone is thereby increased, and the epiphysis thrown forwards.

By reason of their greater length, on receiving the violence in a fall upon the closed fist, the epiphyses of the first and second metacarpal bones are more likely to be separated than those of the other metacarpal bones of the fingers.

Striking with the fist closed or a fall on the palm or heads of the metatarsal bones when the fingers are in the over-extended position may produce displacement of the epiphysis backwards.

Direct violence.—Direct blows upon the knuckles are more likely to separate one or more epiphyses, while indirect violence is more likely to separate single bones.

AGE.—There are seven clinical cases recorded : two at ten, one each at fourteen and a half, twelve, nine, eight, and six years respectively.

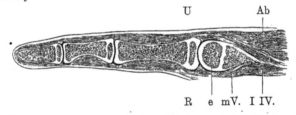

Fig. 175.—FRONTAL SECTION OF THE LITTLE FINGER OF THE LEFT HAND OF A BOY AGED EIGHT YEARS, SHOWING RELATION OF SYNOVIAL MEMBRANES TO THE EPI-PHYSIAL LINES

Posterior sectional surface: U, ulnar, and R, radial side ; mV, fifth metacarpus ; e, its epiphysis ; Ab, abductor of little finger ; I IV, fourth interosseous muscle: The section has been made a little obliquely, so that the synovial membrane of the metacarpo-phalangeal joint appears to be higher on the outer than on the inner side. (V. Brunn)

PATHOLOGICAL ANATOMY.—No example has been verified anatomically.

SYMPTOMS.—It is exceedingly probable that many examples diagnosed as fracture of the head of these bones were really cases of separation of the epiphysis.

From its more exposed position the epiphysis of the metacarpal bone of the index finger is more likely to be separated than that of the other metacarpal bones.

DISPLACEMENT OF THE EPIPHYSIS FORWARDS.— From the direction of the violence and the anatomical connections of these bones, it will be found that displacement forwards of the epiphysis is the most frequent, the epiphysis being driven forwards into the palm.

Deformity.—Besides the projection of the epiphysis in the palm of the hand beyond the level of the neighbouring bones, there is an angular projection of the diaphysial end on the dorsum. It is quite

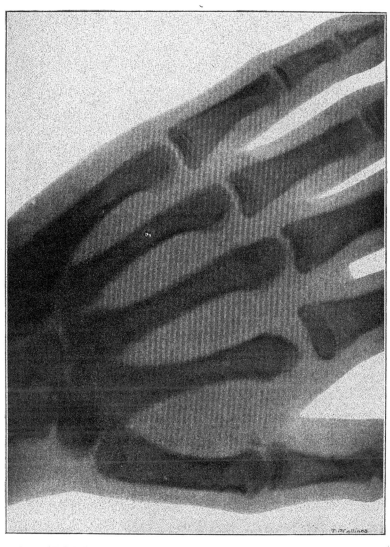

DISPLACEMENT FORWARDS OF EPIPHYSIS OF METACARPAL BONE OF INDEX FINGER.

AUTHOR'S case.   Taken by Mr. SYDNEY ROWLAND in March 1896.

possible that the concavity on the upper aspect of the epiphysis may be felt in the palm.

After the deformity has been reduced there is a great tendency for it to recur, due in part to the smallness of the separated surfaces, in part to the action of the powerful flexors, aided by the interossei.

The finger is shortened from the overlapping of the diaphysis by the epiphysis.

Hamilton (*Fractures and Dislocations*, London, 1884, 7th edit., p. 393) relates the following case, in which the metacarpal bone was probably separated at the epiphysis.

Thomas R., aged eight, fell down a flight of steps, September 11, 1855, breaking the metacarpal bone of the index finger of the right hand near its lower extremity, and apparently at the junction of the epiphysis with the diaphysis. The lad was seen sixteen hours after the accident. The lower fragment, projecting abruptly into the palm of the hand, could be easily replaced, or with only moderate effort, yet immediately when the support was removed it would become displaced. There was no crepitus. It was dressed very carefully with a splint and compress; but, notwithstanding continued efforts to keep the fragments in place, the epiphysis united considerably depressed towards the palm.

M. Polaillon quotes another case from a thesis by Pichon in a child aged twelve years.

The following interesting case was sent to the author by Dr. Atkins of Sutton. The patient (W. F. C.), aged fourteen and a half, the son of a well-known medical man, injured his right hand on April 17, 1893, by falling with a stick twisted in between his fingers. Separation of the epiphysial head of the metacarpal bone of the first finger, with displacement forwards, was diagnosed at the time. Under chloroform the epiphysis was readily replaced backwards into its normal position, but on account of some deformity recurring the author was asked to see the case. There was still some tendency for the epiphysis to ride forwards towards the palm, and also some displacement outwards. Beyond this there was subluxation of the first phalanx. Chloroform was again administered, and the finger placed in a good position. In spite, however, of repeated and careful application of plaster-of-Paris and other splints, the epiphysis again became a little displaced forwards, but all lateral displacement was entirely corrected. In this position it finally united to the diaphysis. As a result, at the present time (March 1896) the head of the metacarpal bone is still prominent in the palm, as seen by the photograph (see fig. 176). The power of flexion at the metacarpo-phalangeal joint is a good deal restricted and the finger shorter than its fellow, but its usefulness is scarcely impaired.

In March 1896 Mr. Sydney Rowland kindly took a skiagraph (*British Medical Journal* of March 1896, p. 620) of the hand, which confirmed absolutely the diagnosis of separation of this epiphysis. The space noticeable between the first phalanx and the displaced posterior margin of the epiphysis and the diaphysial end is probably occupied by fibroid tissue, forming some portion of the new articular surface between the bones. The epiphysial discs of the other metacarpals, as well as of the phalanges, are clearly seen.

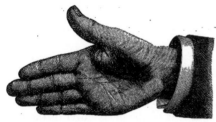

Fig. 176.—Separation of the head of the meta-carpal bone of the index finger, with displacement forwards. a somewhat prominent knob is seen in the palm. the finger is slightly shorter than its fellow

. **Crepitus** of the usual muffled character is often absent. M. Mirault detected it in his case.

There will be **acute pain** in the hand, and a crackling sensation at the time of the accident; also pain at a point opposite to the epiphysial junction, more marked than in dislocation.

Swelling or ecchymosis will be chiefly noticeable on the dorsal aspect, and but seldom on the palmar.

There will be some **loss of power** of moving the finger, it is somewhat bent up towards the palm, and the patient is unable to extend it.

In cases of great displacement, the extensor tendon may be pushed to one or other side of the dorsal projection.

Mobility may be obtained in forcibly flexing the finger and pressing with the finger or thumb in the palm opposite to the level of the epiphysial junction. In the metacarpal bone of the index finger about the fifteenth year the line is about a quarter of an inch above the articulation, but great care must be exercised on account of the natural mobility of the lower ends of the metacarpal bones and the smallness of their epiphyses.

DISPLACEMENT BACKWARDS.—Guéretin describes (*La Presse Médicale*, 1837) a case of separated epiphysis of the metacarpal bone of the index finger observed by M. Mirault, surgeon to the Hôtel-Dieu d'Angers, in a child aged ten years. The child, whilst lying on his back at play, June 2, 1836, was said to have received his brother (who rushed at him from a distance) on his hands and feet, so that the fingers of his left hand were turned forcibly backwards. Acute pain and deformity of the index finger immediately took place. A dislocation of the first phalanx of the index finger from the metacarpal bone was supposed to have occurred, and numerous ineffectual attempts were made by the doctor who first saw the case to reduce it. The finger was fixed, the second phalanx flexed almost at a right angle upon the first, whilst the latter was in extreme extension upon the metacarpus, so as to form with it an obtuse angle. The

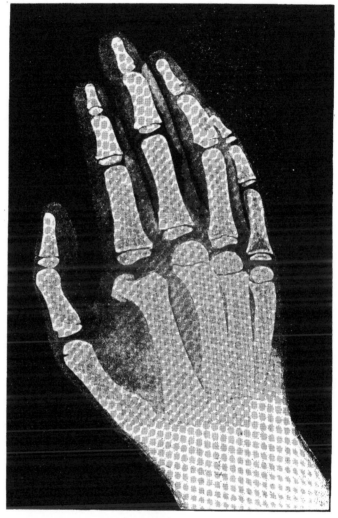

DISPLACEMENT OUTWARDS OF EPIPHYSIS OF METACARPAL BONE OF
INDEX FINGER.

Dr. E. KEY. HERRING'S case

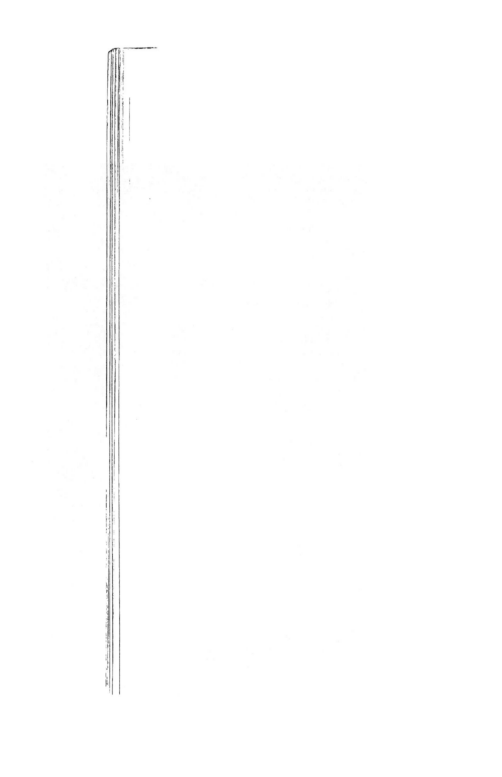

whole finger was placed on a plane posterior to the direction of the metacarpal bone, and the metacarpal phalangeal joint appeared to be much thicker than normal. But neither towards the dorsal nor palmar aspect of the hand was there an abrupt projection such as is usually met with in dislocation. Flexion and extension of the first phalanx could be effected; these movements, however, did not take place at the metacarpo-phalangeal joint, but about four lines higher up. It was at this spot that an abrupt solution of continuity perpendicular to the long axis of the metacarpal bone was recognised. M. Mirault thought he could distinctly detect a rough friction sensation, which was somewhat less harsh than that of two irregular osseous surfaces. The solution of continuity of the metacarpus was therefore clearly made out, and the lower end of the upper fragment of the bone distinctly felt towards the palm of the hand. The lower fragment was displaced obliquely upwards and backwards between the metacarpus and phalanx. It was the latter which gave the thickened appearance to the joint, and the finger was no longer in the same plane as the metacarpus.

This oblique position of the fragment had also produced a shortening of about two lines in the length of the index finger, whilst the measurement of the index finger itself from the seat of separation appeared to be longer than that of the opposite side. The epiphysis, intimately attached to the end of the phalanx, followed it in all its movements. Unfortunately, the mode of reduction, the retentive apparatus used, and the length of time to effect union are not mentioned.

M. Guéretin adds that, from the symptoms enumerated by Mirault, the case had probably been seen a short time after the accident, and that there did not appear to have been any swelling to obscure the diagnosis.

DISPLACEMENT OUTWARDS.—Dr. E. K. Herring of Ballarat (*Intercolonial Medical Journal of Australasia*, March 20, 1897, vol. ii. No. 3, p. 144) publishes the notes of a case of dislocation outwards of the epiphysis of the metacarpal bone of the index finger, and gives a skiagraph of the hand.

O. W., aged ten, was brought by his mother on account of a lump in his hand. He had fallen from a tree six or seven weeks previously, and says he fell on his outstretched hand. He complained of pain in the hand next morning, and the mother says the lump was there then. On examination of the palmar surface of the right hand, just over the neck of the second metacarpal bone, there was found a small, rounded, hard, and firm nodule, about the size of a pea, not movable from the metacarpal bone, which otherwise appeared normal. Flexion and extension were free, and there was no pain on pressure. On closing the fist, the knuckle was not quite so prominent as the others. The injury was diagnosed by several medical men as an exostosis, but the skiagraph revealed a detachment of the epiphysis. By a tenotome, separation and replacement were effected, but the nodule could not be kept in position, and had finally to be removed.

DIAGNOSIS. Dislocation of first phalanx of finger forwards.—Dislocation is rare, and is not accompanied by cartilaginous crepitus during reduction. The finger is more fixed than in separated epiphysis except in the case of the index finger, while the dorsal projection has a less sharp edge, is less painful to the touch, and is on a level with the heads of the other metacarpal bones.

In dislocation there is less tendency for the deformity to be reproduced after reduction.

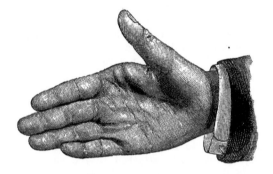

Fig. 177.—DISLOCATION AT METACARPO-PHALANGEAL JOINT WITH SLIGHT FRACTURE OF THE HEAD OF METACARPAL BONE. THE PALMAR PROJECTION IS SEEN TO BE LOWER DOWN THAN IN THE CASE OF SEPARATION OF THE EPIPHYSIS. MR. THOMAS MOORE'S CASE

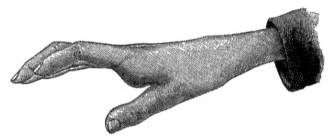

Fig. 178.—THE SAME, LATERAL VIEW

Dislocation at metacarpo-phalangeal joint backwards.—Guéretin notes the similarity of the symptoms met with in Mirault's case to dislocation backwards, but the signs given in this case were too precise to admit any doubts as to epiphysial separation.

Fracture.—Polaillon only found (*loc. cit. infra*) two examples of fracture of the metacarpus in children. One of them is the case alluded to below.

In fracture the dorsal prominence is pointed, and in separation

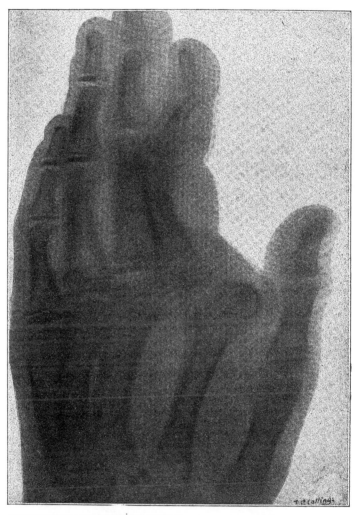

DISLOCATION OF METACARPO-PHALANGEAL JOINT, WITH FRACTURE OF EPIPHYSIS
OF METACARPAL BONE OF INDEX FINGER.

Mr. THOMAS MOORE's case.   Taken by Mr. THOMAS MOORE.

of the epiphysis angular, while in both the distance from the tip of the finger is greater than in dislocation, and in them it may be possible to detect some movement of the metacarpo-phalangeal joint.

Simple contusion.—It is doubtless true that many cases of epiphysial separation are masked by the pain and swelling, especially cases of but little displacement. In the progress of these, when the swelling and pain have subsided, the diagnosis will be made clear. A separation, in these difficult cases, may be presumed to have occurred if the patient has experienced a crackling sensation at the time of the accident, and pain persists at a certain point with some loss of power in the finger.

PROGNOSIS AND RESULTS.—**Non-union** is not likely to occur; the epiphysis quickly rejoins the diaphysis without any deformity in two to three weeks.

There was failure of union, however, in the following case, although there was no loss of function thirteen years after the injury.

M. Polaillon describes (art. ' Main,' *Dict. Encycl. des Sciences Médicales*, 2e Section, vol. iv. 1870–71, p. 51) this case, which Malgaigne considered to be one of epiphysial disjunction resulting in non-union. The patient (E. H.), aged twenty-two years, had had a fall at the age of nine years which gave rise to a fracture of the fourth left metacarpal bone, and resulted in a false articulation. The head of the bone was deformed and movable, and appeared to have a concave surface. When the patient flexed her fingers the head sank down towards the palm of the hand, and the upper fragment made a marked projection backwards. This projection became so marked that at the same time the extensor tendon slipped to the outer side of the bone by the side of the middle finger. During extension this projection diminished, but did not entirely disappear, and then on the palmar aspect, opposite to the head of the bone, the flexor tendon could be felt thickened and enlarged, and appeared to contain a cartilaginous or osseous nodule. All movements could be carried out freely and to their natural extent. As Polaillon states, it is very difficult to form a precise opinion on the nature of a lesion observed thirteen years after the accident, but he gives his opinion that epiphysial separation was more probable than a fracture in this case.

M. Renault, however, thought that if there had been a separation this was probably owing to its having been predisposed to it by rachitic enlargement of the epiphysial cartilage.

Even in those instances where great difficulty has been experienced in retaining the epiphysis in position, and some *deformity* has been the inevitable result, the utility of the hand will not be seriously affected.

Some *synovitis* of the metacarpo-phalangeal joint may prolong the diminished power of moving the finger, and even delay the union.

An instance of deformity of the hand from epiphysial injury to the metacarpal bone of the third finger is reported by Dr. J. H. Sequeira (*Hunterian Society Trans.* 1897, p. 109). The patient, a healthy girl aged nine years, presented a remarkable shortening of the ring finger of the left hand—in fact, it was but slightly longer than the little finger. The shortening was in the metacarpal bone, and amounted to three-eighths of an inch. It was well seen when the finger was strongly flexed into the palm, the absence of the prominent head, the fourth metacarpal, being marked by a hollow in the line of the knuckles. Three years previously the patient injured that hand, and there seemed little doubt that the metacarpal epiphysis had been injured, and in consequence there had been failure of growth; but it was probable also that part of the shortening arose from the displacement forwards of the metacarpal head into the palm of the hand.

TREATMENT.—If the separation is **without displacement**, the simpler the form of apparatus the better, and the hand and forearm should be kept at rest for fourteen days in the elevated position. Evaporating lotions should be applied to the dorsal aspect to allay any inflammation.

Displacements.—Reduction should be effected by means of moderate extension on the finger, and pressure on the epiphysis, either on the palmar or dorsal surface, towards the end of the metarcarpal bone, and counter-extension made on the forearm by an assistant.

A moulded gutta-percha or poroplastic splint should then be applied to the whole of the palmar and dorsal surfaces of the hand and fingers. In some cases of displacement *forwards* it may be found advisable to insert a thick pad of lint or tow in the palm before applying the splint. Notwithstanding all efforts, in others the fragments are not easily retained in position. The hand should be worn in a sling and carefully examined each day.

Passive motion should be commenced on the tenth day.

In *displacement backwards* the fingers of the hand should be kept in the extended position with a flat dorsal splint or moulded gutta-percha splint, including the fingers.

Malgaigne's method of treatment of fractures in the adult will be found of service in certain instances. A thick compress is placed on the dorsal projection and another on the palmar surface over the head of the bone, which is pushed backwards. Two large splints are then placed across—one on the palm, the other on the dorsum, of the hand, and their ends brought near to one another and fixed by bandages or plaster. By this means the fingers are left quite free.

SEPARATION OF THE EPIPHYSES OF THE PHALANGES OF THE DIGITS

ANATOMY.—In all the three rows of phalanges of the fingers, and in the two rows of the thumb, the epiphysis is placed at the proximal end. The lower ends are developed from the shafts.

There is commonly one osseous centre, but M. Serrès describes two centres appearing in the middle of the cartilaginous epiphysis side by side, which rapidly unite and form one osseous plate.

The same writer states that three centres are sometimes seen in the epiphysis of the first phalanx of the thumb.

Ossification takes place successively from the first phalanges to the second, and lastly in the third ; in the first row from the third to the fourth year, and in the second and third row from the fourth to the fifth year.

The epiphyses unite to their respective shafts about the nineteenth year.

The nutrient canal runs upwards in each phalanx.

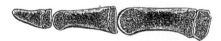

FIG. 179.—EPIPHYSES OF THE PHALANGES AT THE SIXTEENTH YEAR (AFTER RAMBAUD AND RENAULT)

It should be noted that the ungual phalanges of the fingers commence the ossification of their shafts at the distal end instead of in the middle like all the other long bones.

The proximity of the sheath of the flexor tendons on the palmar aspect of the epiphyses should be remembered.

The flat disc-like epiphyses (of the first row) are in depth, vertically, at fourteen years, at the sides four millimetres, posteriorly two millimetres, anteriorly three millimetres at eighteen years, at the sides six millimetres, posteriorly two and a half millimetres, anteriorly four and a half millimetres.

In width across, laterally, they are at fourteen years thirteen millimetres, at eighteen years seventeen millimetres.

ETIOLOGY.—**Direct violence,** as a blow from a bat or cricket-ball, and **indirect violence,** as from a fall upon the fingers, or by the fingers being caught in a hole or between two rigid bodies and wrenched, have been described as the cause in the published examples.

AGE.—In M. Roux's specimen of separation of the epiphyses of the index and middle fingers by direct violence the age is not stated, but in Hamilton's clinical example the lad was aged four years ; Macdonnell's was also in a lad.

PATHOLOGICAL ANATOMY.—The only specimen recorded is that by M. Roux in 1822, in which an explosion of gunpowder produced separation of the lower radial epiphysis, as well as of the shafts of the first phalanges of the thumb and of the index and middle fingers from their upper epiphyses.

The upper epiphyses of these three phalanges remained connected with the corresponding metacarpal bones (see Part II. chap. xii.).

SYMPTOMS.—Epiphysial separation of the phalanges is extremely rare.

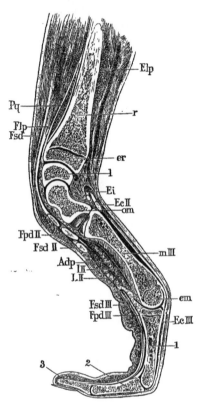

Fig. 180.—SAGITTAL SECTION THROUGH MIDDLE FINGER—ULNAR SURFACE OF SECTION, SHOWING RELATION OF SYNOVIAL MEMBRANES TO THE VARIOUS EPIPHYSES

r, radius; er, epiphysis of radius; l, semilunar bone; Ei, extensor indicis tendon; Ec II and Ec III, tendons of extensor communis digitorum; om, os magnum; mIII, third metacarpal bone; em, its epiphysis; 1, 2, 3, phalanges; Fpd II, flexor profundus digitorum tendon to index finger; Fpd III, the tendon of same muscle to second phalanx of middle finger; Fsd, flexor sublimis digitorum; Fsd II and III, the same tendons of flexor sublimis digitorum; Adp, adductor pollicis cut obliquely; III, second dorsal interosseous muscle; LII, second lumbricalis muscle; Pq, pronator quadratus; Elp, extensor longus pollicis. In none of the joints in this section does the synovial membrane come in immediate relation with the epiphysial discs. (After Brunn)

Mobility at the epiphysial line, which is almost immediately below the upper end of the bone, will be the most constant sign.

Deformity.—Displacement may occur in any direction, viz. *forwards*, most frequently from the powerful flexor tendons, *laterally* to one side or the other, or the epiphysis may be *rotated* on its vertical axis.

Muffled crepitus may be readily detected, but *swelling* is not very great, the thin covering of skin over the phalanges usually permitting a close examination.

J. Macdonnell says (*Cyclopædia of Practical Surgery*, vol. ii. p. 331, art. ' Fracture ') that he had once seen, in a lad, the epiphysis of the upper end of the first phalanx of the forefinger detached from the shaft.

In the following case recorded by Hamilton (*Fractures and Dislocations*, 1884, 7th edit. p. 395) there was probably an epiphysial disjunction.

A lad, four years old, was admitted to the Buffalo Hospital of the Sisters of Charity, December 24, 1849, with a simple fracture of the first phalanx of the ring finger of the left hand; the fracture being at the proximal end of the bone, and at the junction of the epiphysis with the shaft. The finger was so much swollen at first that no dressings were applied until the fifth day, at which time a gutta-percha splint was moulded to it carefully. It resulted in a perfect cure.

DIAGNOSIS. Dislocation.—The first phalanx is usually dislocated backwards. It may be distinguished by the fixation before reduction, and by the less tendency to displacement after reduction.

PROGNOSIS.—Deformity should be guarded against, especially in the case of girls, where any deformity is an unsightly disfigurement.

Non-union must be of rare occurrence.

Suppuration of the flexor sheath is not likely to occur unless the injury be a compound one, yet osteomyelitis, terminating in **necrosis of the epiphysis or shaft**, may result from contusion at the time of the injury.

Probably many of the examples of acute inflammation of the finger and whitlow, accompanied by necrosis of the epiphysis, which is situated at the proximal end of the phalanges, are the result of epiphysial sprain or separation. In one case, of a girl aged seven years, in which the author removed the necrosed epiphysis of the first phalanx, the finger had been injured by being caught between two pieces of wood whilst the girl was at play.

The author has seen a similar portion of bone removed on two occasions, on opening acute suppuration of the finger.

TREATMENT.—Reduction of displacement should be effected by gentle extension and manipulation of the epiphysis.

A moulded splint of gutta-percha (or small straight wooden

splint) should be carefully applied to the dorsal or palmar aspect of the finger.

In some cases it will be found convenient to apply the splint to two or more fingers.

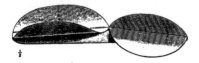

FIG. 181.—TIN FINGER SPLINT.   ONE HALF SIZE.

The finger should be examined daily.

Passive motion should be commenced early during the second week, as union occurs rapidly.

PART III

SEPARATION OF THE EPIPHYSES OF THE LOWER EXTREMITY

———◦—◦———

CHAPTER I

SEPARATION OF THE EPIPHYSES OF THE OS INNOMINATUM

Separation of the Epiphysial Parts of the Acetabulum

Anatomy.—Seen at the second year of life, the three, already well developed, primary pieces of the os innominatum—viz. the ilium, ischium, and pubes—are received into the hollows of the intervening cartilage, usually designated the Y-shaped cartilage; at this period this cartilage comprises the ilio-pectineal eminence, the anterior inferior spine of the ilium, the spine of the ischium, and the bottom of the acetabulum. The pubes and ischium are also separated by a wide cartilaginous interval.

In the acetabulum at the ninth year the ilium, pubes, and ischium are still separated by the Y-shaped cartilaginous interval, which is intimately connected with the cartilage covering the articular surface.

About this period—ninth to tenth year, some anatomists say as early as the sixth year—this cartilage begins to ossify in two or more pieces, usually commencing at the ilio-pectineal eminence. When ossification has advanced, it is seen that the largest and most constant piece of bone is of a triangular shape, and placed towards the fore and upper part of the acetabulum, of which it forms the whole of the pubic portion. It is called the *cotyloid* or *acetabular bone*. Its upper surface is placed between the ilium and pubes, and assists in forming the ilio-pectineal eminence; its external surface, also triangular, corresponds to the articular head of the femur, is slightly concave, and forms a part of the cavity as well as the inner lip of the same.

Between the ilium and ischium there are some irregular nodules of bone, which appear about the thirteenth year and form a somewhat thick mass. Occasionally some thin osseous plates are developed in addition over the iliac and ischial portions of the articular surface.

The ossific centre at the bottom of the acetabulum may be Y-shaped like the cartilage in which it arises, but the limb between the ilium and ischium is said to be usually the thickest in the male subject, and that between the pubes and the ilium in the female. The part between the ischium and pubes is generally absent or very thin. This unites at fourteen years of age with the ilium and ischium, and at about fifteen with the pubes.

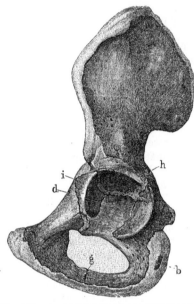

FIG. 182.—OS INNOMINATUM AT THE TWELFTH YEAR (Rambaud and Renault.) ½-size.

h, line of cartilage between the ilium and ischium (which are blended about the thirteenth year) extending to the interior of the acetabular cavity; *i,* narrow line of junction of the pubes and ilium (which unite a little later than the last two primary pieces); *g,* the junction between the ischium and pubes is indicated by a small line: it is often consolidated a few years earlier (eighth year); *b,* osseous centre of tuberosity of ischium has just commenced to appear as a small nucleus in the thick cartilaginous mass which forms this portion of the bone; *d,* cotyloid or acetabular bone placed between ilium and pubes towards the upper border of the acetabular cavity, and forming nearly the whole of the pubic portion of this cavity.

The several portions of the acetabulum are completely united at the seventeenth to nineteenth year.

From the twelfth to the thirteenth year, or even a little later, the ischium has reached the ilium and joins with it, at first on the inner surface, and later externally; the convex line of junction persists here throughout life, but on the acetabular aspect these two portions of the bone are still separated by a thin layer of cartilage. The union of the pubes and ilium is a little later, but up to this time they are still separated in the acetabulum by a narrow cartilaginous line containing osseous deposit.

The ischial and pubic rami unite at eight years of age—according to Béclard at the sixth year; but in some instances this union may be delayed up to twelve or fourteen years of age.

The synovial membrane covers all the epiphysial lines in the acetabulum, and no separation of one of the three primary pieces of the os innominatum from the other two can be effected in the acetabulum fossa without the articular cavity being involved. It is possible, however, for a separation to occur between the pubic and ischial portions without the joint being directly involved, on account of the synovial membrane being protected by the fat and soft structures filling in the acetabular fossa, provided, of course, in this case that no displacement of either the ischial or pubic portions has occurred.

Pathological anatomy.—A few specimens exist in museums which show the possibility of partial or complete separation of the epiphysial ends of the pubes, ischium, and ilium at the hip-joint.

These lesions will necessarily be accompanied by a more or less complete detachment of the acetabular bone developed in the Y-shaped cartilage.

Dupuytren speaks of a case in which the bones forming the cotyloid cavity had been forced in, and the head of the femur had passed completely into the cavity of the pelvis.

In St. George's Hospital Museum (*Catalogue of St. George's Hospital Museum*, 1866, p. 40, No. 121) there is a specimen of separation of the epiphysial ends of the pubes and ischium in the hip-joint accompanied by fracture of the pelvis; it is also recorded by Holmes in the *Pathological Society's Transactions*, vol. xiii. p. 187. It occurred in a girl aged ten, who was run over by a carriage and lived three months after the injury. In the specimen a fracture traverses the hip-joint at the junction of the ischium and pubes, another passes through the horizontal ramus of the pubes near the former, and a third through the ascending ramus of the ischium.

Mr. T. Wilkinson King mentions (*Cyclopædia of Practical Surgery*, vol. ii. art. on 'Fracture, Special,' p. 356) the fact that fracture of the acetabulum may occur as a kind of diastasis, but that other attendant injuries are

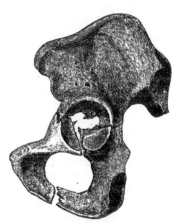

FIG. 183.—SEPARATION OF THE OS INNOMINATUM INTO ITS ORIGINAL PARTS

(Drawing from Guy's Hospital Museum, Mr. King's case)

to be expected. He gives an illustration of separation of the os innominatum into its original parts in a young person.

Sir William Stokes, of Dublin, showed at the International Medical Congress, London, 1881 (*Catalogue of Museum, International Medical Congress, London* 1891, p. 83, No. 775, Series A, No. 6), a specimen of epiphysial fracture of the acetabulum from the Museum of the Richmond Hospital, Dublin.

The author has been unable to obtain any history or details of this case of epiphysial separation, but in a letter to him in 1884 Sir William Stokes spoke of the specimen as being a most beautiful and rare one.

Separations in the acetabular cavity, with the exception of that of the cotyloid bone, should properly be classified under fractures of the pelvis.

Separation of the Epiphysis of the Iliac Crest and Anterior and Posterior Superior Iliac Spines

Anatomy.—Béclard fixes the commencement of osseous development of the iliac crest at the sixteenth year.

Some osseous granules, which show themselves in the cartilaginous margin of the iliac crest, congregating especially at two points —in the front and back parts to form the anterior and posterior spinous processes—are often seen at the fifteenth year.

At the nineteenth to twentieth year two thick and broad epiphyses are seen, the anterior one forming the anterior superior iliac spine and the anterior three-quarters of the iliac crest, the posterior one the posterior superior iliac spine and contiguous part of the crest. The point of interruption between the two is at the posterior flexion of the letter S, which represents the outline of the iliac crest.

More often these two parts are united into one long epiphysis capping the iliac crest.

This epiphysis does not join the body of the ilium till the twentieth to twenty-fifth year, usually at the twenty-first year.

The anterior superior spine has attached to it numerous muscles—the sartorius, tensor vaginæ femoris, external oblique, internal oblique, and transversalis and iliacus on the inner aspect, besides the fascia lata and Poupart's ligament.

To the posterior superior spine are attached a few fibres of the gluteus maximus (externally), the oblique portion of the posterior sacro-sciatic ligaments, and a few fibres of the multifidus spinæ (internally), while the intermediate portion of the iliac crest, which is thinnest about the middle, affords attachment to the fascia lata, tensor vaginæ femoris, obliquus externus, latissimus dorsi, internal oblique, transversalis, quadratus lumborum, and erector spinæ muscles, and iliac fascia.

Etiology.—The anterior superior iliac spine being developed as part of the iliac crest, a much greater amount of muscular violence will be necessary to effect its separation than in the case of the anterior inferior iliac spine, which develops from an isolated centre, while direct violence, such as in a fall against some hard surface, or by a severe blow, or by the patient being run over by the wheel of a vehicle, may not be an uncommon mode of separation.

Fracture of the anterior superior iliac spine, as a consequence of direct injury, is not uncommon in the adult.

A case of fracture of the anterior superior spine of the ilium by muscular action is recorded by Nickerson (*Deutsche medicinische Wochenschrift*, Leipzig, March 6, 1890). It was the case of a lad, aged seventeen years, who felt something give way while running, and was unable to walk; the symptoms were tenderness, crepitus, and mobility on pressure.

Nickerson adds abstracts of four other reported cases.

Dr. C. Haig Brown relates (*British Medical Journal*, August 16, 1884, p. 320) the case of a lad, aged seventeen, who separated the anterior superior iliac spine by muscular action. At some sports he was commencing to jump, after having finished his run (or, in technical language, 'taking off'), when he felt a sudden snap on the right side of the pelvis, and fell, being in considerable pain. In jumping from his right leg the boy had called into sudden and violent action the external oblique, internal oblique, and transversalis muscles (all of which are, in front, attached to the anterior superior iliac spine), and had separated the spine from the body of the bone. On examination, fifteen minutes after the accident, it was found that he could not stand, and though each hip-joint moved naturally, movements at the right hip-joint caused pain in the lower part of the abdomen on that side. Coughing and passing water also caused pain in the same place. The right anterior superior spine was not to be felt in its place, but was represented by a rough piece of bone. All round this was a considerable hæmatoma, while the spine itself was distinctly felt displaced upwards and a little inwards. With the abdominal muscles relaxed it could be brought back to its proper position, and the characteristic soft but marked crepitus was elicited. The boy was kept in bed on his back for ten days with a stout spica bandage round the right hip-joint and a pad to keep the displaced fragment in position. Movement was allowed at the end of a fortnight, and at the end of eight weeks he was able to walk about as well as ever, although crepitus was still present over the seat of injury. The whole epiphysis was not separated—i.e. the whole iliac crest—but only a small portion of it, which has no separate centre of ossification from the rest of the iliac crest. The iliac crest in this case—the age being seventeen—was in an unossified condition.

A case of fracture of the anterior superior iliac spine by the action of the sartorius muscle is recorded by C. E. Corlette (*Australasian Med. Gazette*, March 15, 1895, p. 99). S. D., aged seventeen years and eight months, was admitted into Sydney Hospital, August 24, 1894. As he was getting down behind from the top of an omnibus the omnibus suddenly went forward, causing him to slip and lose his footing. He came down with his whole weight on the right foot, and immediately felt a pain in the region of the anterior superior iliac spine. He fell forward and could not rise. On being assisted up he could not stand on the left leg, and could bear very little weight on the right, the attempt causing pain. On examination when standing, he stood bent forward, with the right hip and knee partly flexed, the toes touching the ground and turned slightly inwards. When he lay down passive movement of the hip and knee could be done freely without causing pain, so long as the hip was not extended beyond a certain point. There was an evident loss of prominence over the right anterior spine as compared with the opposite side, with pain at this site, but absent elsewhere. Manipulation caused great pain; closely localised and distinct crepitus was obtained. The treatment adopted was flexion of the hip by a high pillow beneath the knee. A considerable amount of callus subsequently formed. He was discharged September 24, 1894.

Age.—A separation of the true osseous epiphysis can only occur from the fifteenth year, the time of its formation, to the twenty-fifth year, its union with the body of the bone.

Pathological anatomy.—Separation of the anterior and inferior iliac spines was found (*Bull. de la Soc. Anatomique*, 1867, p. 283) in Bousseau's case of separation of the head of the femur quoted in the next chapter. The anterior superior spine was still held to the ilium by a small portion of cartilage and periosteum ; the inferior spine was completely detached. There were other severe lesions of the soft parts in this case produced by the passage of a wagon-wheel over the left hip.

M. Gosselin has reported (*Gazette Médicale de Paris*, 1879, 6, s. I. p. 129) a case in which the whole marginal cartilaginous crest of the ilium and the cartilaginous apex of the inferior iliac spine were both detached in a boy aged fourteen.

Gosselin thought that this was due to the suppurative inflammation extending from the fractured pelvis and fractured thigh (complicated with an extensive wound) rather than to the primary injury at the time of the accident. The child had been knocked down in the street and run over by the wheel of an omnibus.

Symptoms.—Although a rare accident, a separation of the iliac crest should always suggest itself to the surgeon's mind when a child has been knocked down in the street and its pelvis run over, although there may be no external evidence of contusion. Local pain, soft crepitus, and mobility are the chief signs.

The following case related by Bransby B. Cooper (*Lectures on the Principles and Practice of Surgery*, 1851, p. 251) was probably one of epiphysial separation. A sailor boy, aged fourteen, was admitted into Guy's Hospital. He had fallen from the rigging of a ship and alighted on his hip. When brought to the hospital he appeared to suffer severe pain, particularly when the abdominal muscles were called into action. A fracture was discovered separating the superior spinous process and about a fourth of the crista ilii from the rest of the bone. A bandage was placed round the pelvis and upper part of the right thigh. The lad was soon able to get out of bed, and could stand very well, although he walked rather lame. Shortly afterwards he was discharged as perfectly cured, the pain having entirely, and the lameness almost, disappeared.

Mr. Davies-Colley had under his care at Guy's Hospital in July 1885 a girl (Ellen D.), aged eight years, who was run over by an omnibus, which separated a portion of the cartilaginous iliac crest. Dull crepitus was detected over the right iliac crest, and a long ridge of bone was felt at the anterior part of the crest. This was accompanied by an obscure abdominal injury, from which she slowly recovered.

Treatment.—Rest in bed, with the legs flexed and knees tied together, and a stout broad bandage round the pelvis and hips, combined with a pad above and in front of the epiphysis to keep it in position, are the best indications for treatment. Or a firm spica bandage may be applied round the pelvis and hip of the injured side.

Some unimportant deformity about the region of the iliac spine and crest may result.

Separation of the Epiphysis of the Anterior Inferior Spine of the Ilium

Anatomy.—The epiphysis for the anterior inferior spine of the ilium is not always present, but is more frequent in the male than in the female subject.

It appears from the eighteenth to the twentieth year, often as early as the sixteenth year, and joins the body of the bone from the nineteenth to the twenty-first year, or as late as the twenty-fifth year.

It is of a largish size, prominent, and rounded in outline, having attached to it the straight head of the rectus femoris muscle, and a few fibres of the ilio-femoral ligament at its lower part. On the inner side a few fibres of the iliacus muscle are attached.

According to Sir George Humphry (*The Human Skeleton*, 1858, p. 458), the anterior inferior spine is peculiar to the human pelvis. It serves to give a slight leverage to the rectus femoris, making some amends to that muscle for the unfavourable position in which it is placed by the erect position.

Etiology.—The iliac or straight head of the rectus is exceedingly strong in muscular subjects.

Of the two heads the acetabular is the primary, the other (the

R R

straight) develops early in the third month of fœtal life as a secondary thickening of the sheath, owing to the change of axis of the limb consequent on the assumption of the capacity of full extension of the hip and knee. The muscle acts chiefly from its

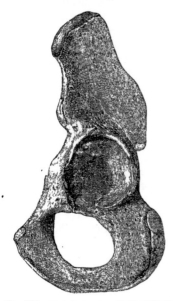

straight head when the hip is extended, but from its curved head when it extends the knee during flexion of the hip (Macalister). Thus in the position which was described in the case of Dr. Whitelocke's two patients as obtaining prior to starting in running—viz. that of flexion of the hip and semiflexion of the knee—the posterior head would fix the rectus above; but in the first bound of the start, when the knee- and hip-joints were suddenly, rapidly, and forcibly extended, the direct or straight head would come into action.

The flexed position of the fœtal extremities necessitates only the acetabular head, which in this position of the hip-joint is in a direct line of action.

FIG. 184.—OS INNOMINATUM AT THE END OF THE EIGHTEENTH YEAR. THE EPIPHYSIS OF THE ANTERIOR INFERIOR SPINE HAS COMMENCED TO JOIN TO THE ILIUM

Mr. Roger Williams states (*Journal of Anatomy and Physiology*, vol. xiii. 1879, p. 204) that only at about the sixth month of fœtal life can this head be distinguished. The iliac head cannot be discriminated from the fascia of the part. At full term the acetabular head is as large as the main tendon, of which it is obviously the direct continuation, whilst the iliac head, though plainly visible, is relatively insignificant. The size of the straight head is proportional to the muscularity of the subject, but the reflected head does not undergo a corresponding variation. Hence the difference between the heads is most marked in women. The histological structure of the two heads is different, the straight head containing many elastic fibres, and partaking more of the nature of a ligament than a tendon.

Mr. Maunder observed (*Lancet*, May 6, 1876, p. 668) at the London Hospital a case of separation of the epiphysis of the anterior inferior spinous process of the ilium by muscular action in a boy (W. G.) aged eighteen years. The patient stated that while running in a flat race he thought it necessary to 'put on a spurt,' and whilst doing so suddenly felt a sharp snap, followed by acute pain in the right groin, and accompanied by a sensation of 'something being out of its place.' He found it impossible to stand upright without great pain in the right groin, which was somewhat relieved by resuming the stooping posture. On examination he lay flat on his back with the thighs extended and the right foot slightly everted. He could rotate the right thigh inwards or outwards, but with slight pain. There was total inability to flex the thigh upon the pelvis, and the attempt caused great pain in the groin. A little fulness was evident in the position of the spinous processes, and the inferior spinous process (the attachment of the straight tendon of the rectus femoris muscle) was found to be detached and freely movable. Cartilaginous crepitus was very distinctly felt, both by the patient and the surgeon. This, together with the age of the patient, led to the diagnosis of separation of the epiphysis. The treatment adopted was rest in bed with the thigh flexed by a pillow beneath the knees to relax the rectus femoris muscle. At the end of three weeks firm union had taken place, and the patient could walk with ease and flex the thigh without discomfort.

In Dr. Whitelocke's two cases, and in that of Mr. Symonds, of Oxford, the injury was the result of running in a race. It appears from these examples to occur not uncommonly from sudden strain in young athletic men of good muscular development with powerful recti muscles.

Treves, in his *Surgical Applied Anatomy*, p. 370, says: ' In one case the anterior inferior spinous process was torn off by the rectus muscle during the act of running a race.'

The anterior inferior spine is so well protected from *direct violence* on all sides by muscles that separation from this cause is extremely improbable.

Symptoms.—Loss of power or difficulty of flexing thigh, accompanied by pain, flexion of hip, and crepitus, are the chief signs. The latter may not easily be detected on account of the deep position of the parts, especially in a muscular limb, although the posterior head of the muscle will not allow very great displacement of the epiphysis.

Ecchymosis, swelling, and pain will not be very great.

From the close association of the ilio-femoral ligament with the anterior inferior spinous epiphysis it is not unlikely that the hip-joint may be affected when this process is separated.

Dr. R. H. A. Whitelocke describes (*Lancet*, November 25, 1893, p. 1302) two instances of detachment of the epiphysis of the anterior inferior spinous process of the ilium through enforced muscular action. The respective ages of the patients were eighteen and nineteen years. The clinical histories, causation, and symptoms of the two cases were nearly identical. In February 1891 an under-graduate, in starting to run in a race of a hundred yards length, while practising for his college sports, 'seemed to have scarcely travelled ten yards when he had suddenly to stop, as he felt

something snap, and at the same time his limb became powerless.'
There was then some pain, but it was 'by no means severe,'
although he 'became faint and felt sick.' There was little to be
seen excepting that the injured limb assumed the position of semiflexion and was in advance of its fellow, which, being fully extended,
was sustaining the whole weight of the patient. On attempting to
straighten the injured limb by extending the hip- and knee-joints,
he felt increased pain, and he had extreme difficulty in extending
the knee-joint. The chief complaint was an unpleasant feeling of
numbness and tingling perceived all down the extensor surface of
the thigh. There was very little discoloration, accompanied by an
inconsiderable swelling situated for the most part beneath and to
the outer side of the middle of Poupart's ligament. After carefully
comparing the two sides and palpating, a distinct crepitation could
be elicited on deep pressure at that point, and this could be
even more distinctly made out when, while the pressure was made,
the patient made an effort to bring the rectus muscle into action.
The movable piece of bone gave a feeling on palpation not unlike
that of a loose cartilage in a joint. A pad with a temporary spica
bandage was applied. Another undergraduate gave an almost
similar history. He had been starting to run 'a quarter mile.' In
the very act of starting—in the first bound, as it were—he 'felt
something give, and became powerless to proceed.' With Dr.
Whitelocke's experience of the former case it was not difficult to
discover what was the matter. In this case a mere scale of bone, as
far as could be elicited, came away with the straight head of the
rectus, and crepitus was with difficulty made out at first. The
tingling sensation and other symptoms described in the former
case were also evident.

Each patient had started with his left limb somewhat flexed
both at the hip- and knee-joints, and in advance of the right, the
body being bent forwards and, as it were, poised upon and supported by it. In the sudden act of starting, the limb behind was
used to give the spring, and in the first bound the body and the
advanced and flexed limb were suddenly and quickly straightened
together, and the rectus muscle, already contracting and fixed at its
lower attachment to support the weight of the body on the semiflexed knee, being forcibly put upon the stretch during the sudden
extension of the hip-joint, tore away the unossified epiphysis of the
anterior inferior spinous process of the ilium.

The treatment in both cases was immobilisation of the flexed hip
in a plaster spica bandage for four weeks, and then a simple spica
was substituted. Recovery was complete in both. The 'tingling and
feeling of cold water' were the most persistent symptoms in one
case, and in this one a considerable amount of callus was thrown
out.

Dr. Whitelocke mentions a similar case with a satisfactory

result under the treatment of Mr. Symonds of Oxford, and believes that this accident is probably not so rare as at first would seem to be the case.

Separation of the Epiphysis of the Symphysis Pubis

Anatomy.—The angle of the pubes has an epiphysial plate appearing towards the end of puberty—i.e. about the sixteenth or seventeenth year—and consisting of two parts or branches, one extending on the horizontal ramus of the pubes, the other on the inner side of the symphysis to the descending ramus, downwards, in some cases, as far as the anterior end of the epiphysis for the tuberosity of the ischium. To the epiphysis the fibro-cartilage of the symphysis is firmly attached.

This epiphysis joins about the twentieth or twenty-first year to the body of the bone.

Although it is said that the crest of the pubes may be torn off by the action of the abdominal muscles (rectus abdominis, pyramidalis, conjoined tendon, &c.) in the adult, yet this epiphysis in its entirety in children can only be detached by severe crushing violence.

Many examples that have been recorded as separations of the symphysis pubis, especially those in patients of two years of age and thereabouts, were separations of the pubic articulation associated with fracture of one or other ramus. Holmes's case of separation of the symphysis pubis occurred, as is common enough in severe pelvic injuries, between the cartilaginous articular surfaces.

Traumatic separation of the osseous epiphysis is only possible from the sixteenth to the twentieth or twenty-first year; before this it is a question of detachment of the cartilaginous margin.

The proximity of the bladder to the epiphysis must always be a source of danger after severe direct violence—e.g. being run over by a cart, or crushing between two opposing forces.

Hæmaturia associated with dull crepitus, mobility at the symphysis, or with a depression at this spot, will suggest to the surgeon's mind a separation of the epiphysis.

Separation of the Epiphysis of the Spine of the Pubes

At times a distinct epiphysis forms at this point about the sixteenth year or a little later. It is usually of a lenticular or irregular shape, and more often present in females than males. It is analogous to the marsupial bone of the didelphidæ (Béclard).

This epiphysis, when present, unites with the epiphysis of the symphysis pubis first, and later with the body of the bone itself about the twentieth year.

The abdominal muscles acting upon the pubic spine by means of Poupart's ligament may tear it off, but no instance of separation has as yet been recorded.

Separation of the Epiphysis of the Sciatic Spine

Sometimes the sciatic or ischial spine has a distinct epiphysis of small size which appears about the sixteenth to seventeenth year, and joins the body of the bone at the eighteenth year.

To the apex of the ischial spine is attached the lesser sacro-sciatic ligament—the gemellus superior to its outer aspect, and the coccygeus and posterior fibres of the levator ani to its inner aspect. No case of separation has been recorded.

Separation of the Epiphysis of the Tuber Ischii

This epiphysis is a wide and thick plate, wider and thicker than any of the other epiphyses of the hip bone. It extends from the lesser sacro-sciatic notch to the upper end of the ascending ramus of the ischium, reaching occasionally on to the descending ramus of the pubes.

The centre of ossification appears about the fourteenth year.

This epiphysis consolidates with the body of the ischium at the twentieth year.

Considering the powerful hamstring and other muscles, adductor magnus, &c., and the great sacro-sciatic ligament attached to this epiphysis, it would appear that detachment of this epiphysis might readily occur from muscular action.

Mr. R. W. Parker has observed a separation of the epiphysis of the tuber ischii with suppuration following a kick, and the author has seen a similar example, the result also of direct violence.

CHAPTER II

SEPARATION OF THE EPIPHYSIAL HEAD OF THE FEMUR

ANATOMY.—The epiphysis of the head of the femur is developed from a single ossific centre appearing just about its centre—that is, above and somewhat behind the attachment of the round ligament—from the tenth to twelfth month after birth. This centre is often

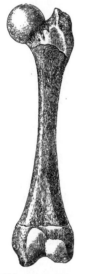

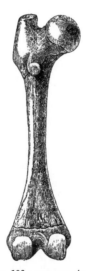

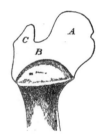

FIG. 187.—CORONAL SEC-
TION THROUGH UPPER
END OF FEMUR BEFORE
BIRTH, CARRIED THROUGH
THE LIG. TERES AND TRO-
CHANTER MAJOR

A, the head ; *B*, neck of thigh bone ; *C*, trochanter major. (Küstner)

FIG. 185.—UPPER AND LOWER
ENDS OF THE FEMUR A
FEW WEEKS BEFORE BIRTH.
NATURAL SIZE. (ANTERIOR
VIEW.) (AFTER RAMBAUD
AND RENAULT)

FIG. 186.—THE SAME (POS-
TERIOR VIEW). NATURAL
SIZE. (AFTER RAMBAUD
AND RENAULT)

surrounded by a number of small osseous granules, especially at its upper part. The cartilaginous head is still connected at this period with the great trochanter by a thick layer or mass of cartilage. This layer or strip at the end of the second year is thin and hollowed out, and presents many small depressions caused by the upward extension and increase in size of the osseous shaft to form the neck of the bone. It is all that remains now of the original cartilaginous upper end of the femur, from which the head and great and lesser trochanters are developed. These are gradually separated away from each other by the growing neck, and subse. quently increase in size quite independently of each other. The head passes upwards and inwards from the growth of the neck

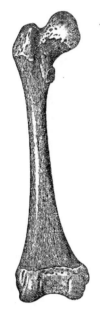

Fig. 188.—FEMUR AT THE END OF THE SECOND YEAR

The head is connected with the great tro- chanter by means of a thin cartila- ginous strip which appears as if riddled with holes. At the bottom of these the osseous tissue is seen, indicating that the connecting strip has already been invaded by osseous material. The lesser trochanter is now separated from the great trochanter by the elongation of the neck, so that the upper end is divided into two parts, one of which comprises the head and great trochanter and the other the lesser trochanter. (After Rambaud and Renault, ½-size.)

in that direction, whilst the great trochanter continues in the direc- tion of the shaft. At this time, the end of the second year, the cartilaginous lesser trochanter is already widely separated from the other two cartilaginous epiphyses. By the end of the fourth year nearly the whole of the epiphysis of the head is osseous, and sepa- rated from the great trochanter. At this time the thin dentate car- tilaginous epiphysial line between it and the shaft is visible, and by the sixth year is seen to almost exactly correspond to the articular surface. The epiphysial head is of a hollow hemispherical shape, and caps the mammillated end of the projecting neck. In many cases the upper surface of the neck is encroached upon by a thin irregu- lar rim extending outwards from the upper part of the head, and assists in transmitting the weight from the head above to the calcar femorale or vertical plane of com- pact bony tissue projecting upwards into the cancellous tissue of the neck and the great trochanter from the lower part of the neck (Macalister). On the other hand, the lower aspect of the epiphysial rim is exceedingly thin, and the last portion of the epiphysis which becomes entirely osseous. The epiphysial line is now still better marked. At the seventeenth year the epiphysis is entirely ossified, and appears about to join to the neck, but this is not finally accomplished until the nineteenth to twentieth year. A line of separation at its circumference, especially at its lower part, often persists, although it may be firmly joined in the centre.

On section, a line of dense bony tissue may be seen remaining for some years, traversing the cancellous tissue of the head and neck, and indicating the cartilaginous line of union.

With the exception of the first few years of infancy, the neck of the femur is therefore a prolongation of the shaft, not a part of the superior epiphysis.

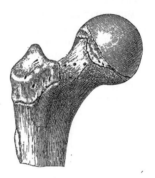

FIG. 189.—ANTERIOR VIEW OF UPPER END OF FEMUR, SHOWING THE EPIPHYSES OF HEAD AND GREAT TROCHANTER AT SEVENTEEN AND A HALF YEARS

($\frac{1}{2}$-size)

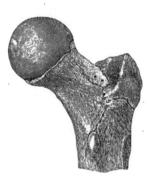

FIG. 190.—POSTERIOR VIEW OF THE UPPER END OF FEMUR. THE EPIPHYSES OF THE HEAD, GREAT AND LESSER TROCHANTERS, BETWEEN THE SEVENTEENTH AND EIGHTEENTH YEARS

($\frac{1}{2}$-size)

The femoral neck beyond the epiphysial line is covered in the whole of its circumference by the synovial membrane of the hip-joint. At thirteen years of age, on its inferior aspect it is covered by the membrane for nearly two centimetres, and above for nearly one centimetre (Sésary).

Although this epiphysis is situated entirely within the capsule and is completely surrounded by the synovial membrane, yet it might in some instances be detached without opening the joint, by reason of the easy detachment and stripping up of the synovial membrane and capsule from the neck of the bone right up to the head, thereby leaving the joint intact. The extent to which the synovial membrane covers the head and neck of the bone may be seen from the diagram.

Of course the joint would be unopened if separation of the upper end of the bone occurred before the fourth year. Not only is the cartilaginous head at this early age still connected with the great trochanter by the thick cartilaginous layer along the upper surface of the neck, but the synovial membrane on the under surface of the neck is more readily detached than later on.

De Paoli gives the following table of measurements of the height of the upper epiphysis of the femur in a frontal section.

AGE		HEIGHT		BREADTH
And periods of development		At the middle of the articular head	From the apex of the great trochanter to the lower edge	From the lower surface
—	Before birth	13 mm.	15 mm.	20 mm.
As shown from the osseous nucleus to the summit	1	12 ,,	19 ,,	29 ,,
—	4	14 ,,	23 ,,	42 ,,
—	5	13 ,,	24 ,,	45 ,,
As shown from the osseous nucleus to the trochanter	6	14 ,,	22 ,,	49 ,,
	7	16 ,,	22 ,,	51 ,,
Separation of the epiphysis	8	{ 16 ,,	{ 22 ,,	{ 52 ,,
		{ 19 ,,	{ 32 ,,	{ 52 ,,
	9	17 ,,	30 ,,	51 ,,
—	13	19 ,,	31 ,,	—
	14	17 ,,	35 ,,	—
—	15	20 ,,	36 ,,	—
As shown from the osseous nucleus to the small trochanter	16	17 ,,	35 ,,	—
Line dividing the epiphysis from the diaphysis	17	18 ,,	36 ,,	—
To the end of development	—	{ 18 ,,	{ 44 ,,	—
		{ 17 ,,	{ 40 ,,	

AGE.—From the condition of the upper end of the femur it is evident that a pure detachment of the head cannot take place—until the fourth year, at least—the head not being a separate epiphysis from the upper part of the neck and great trochanter, although a fracture may take place through the cartilage of the neck anywhere between the head and the great trochanter. After this period the possibility of its occurrence is rendered more certain by the growth of the neck of the bone, which by this time will have attained sufficient length and

strength to afford a very powerful arm of a lever. At the age of
two it is only three-quarters of an inch long. The whole epiphysis
of the head at the fourth year is almost entirely osseous. Therefore
epiphysial separations described as occurring under the age of four
cannot be regarded as simple detachments of the head, and would
more correctly be placed under separations of the upper end of the
femur, and their symptoms must differ very considerably. Salmon
readily separated the upper end of the bone in experiments on
the bodies of infants, but this author could not record any case
in which this lesion was diagnosed during life. Out of thirty-three

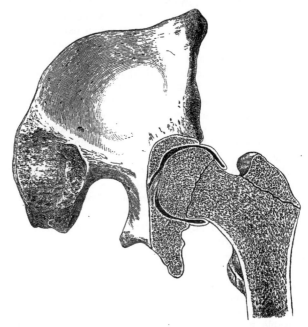

FIG. 191.—FRONTAL SECTION OF LEFT HIP-JOINT OF A LAD AGED SEVENTEEN AND A HALF
YEARS. RELATION OF SYNOVIAL MEMBRANE TO EPIPHYSIAL LINES

cases described in this chapter (two of these being simple cases, two
operative cases, and three pathological specimens) recorded as separations of this epiphysis—excluding the five below two years of age
(three at 2, one at 1 year, and one in infancy), and two in which the
age is not stated—fourteen were between the ages of 14 and 18 years
(thus two at 18, three at 17, two at 16, three at 15, four at 14) and
five between 6 and 11. Of the rest, two were at 19 years, one each
at 10, 5, 4½, 4, and 3 years.

Hutchinson says that it is probably the length and inclination
of the neck which save the epiphysial line by throwing the force upon
other parts; and that as both of them are less pronounced in early

life, we may reasonably suppose the risk of detachment to be greater then than later. This is not borne out by other recorded cases, nor by experiments upon the dead subject.

Below the fourth year and during the earliest periods of infancy it is only a question of separation of the upper cartilaginous end of the femur, whilst later on it is a matter of separation of · the different epiphyses formed from this—viz. the head, the greater and the lesser trochanters.

Separation of the whole upper end of the femur has only been proved by anatomical observation, and it is probable that ' separations of the upper epiphysis' of the femur produced during the first few years of life, or during delivery of infants, were of this nature. The author has produced it on many occasions in experiments on the bodies of recently born infants. In Sayre's case the accident occurred at the age of two years, and was probably due to separation of the epiphysis of the head, accompanied by fracture of the upper carti- laginous end uniting the head to the great trochanter.

Of the two other cases verified by direct examination, one occurred at the age of six years and one at fifteen years.

In two instances in which the lesion was discovered at the time of operation, the age of the patient was fourteen years in one, and in the other the age is not stated.

ETIOLOGY.—In the recorded cases many were caused by direct violence applied to the front or outer side of the hip, such as the passage of a cart-wheel, or the heavy blow from a falling boiler, or in jumping and alighting on the feet, &c., and some few were said to have been caused principally by sudden muscular action, as in slipping, or in the patient trying to save himself from falling.

Indirect violence.—Dr. Post (*New York Medical Journal*, vol. iii. p. 190, July 1840) related a case in a girl, aged sixteen, who, when carrying a child in her arms, made a false movement in stepping, and, feeling something give way, was obliged to lean against a wall. The next day the limb was found to be shortened one inch, but movable with the foot erected. There was no swelling, but slight pain at the upper part of the thigh. The great trochanter moved with the shaft, and crepitus was felt. From the age of the patient and the slight amount of violence producing the injury a separation of the epiphysis of the head was diagnosed. Extension was applied, and recovery took place with a quarter to half an inch shortening of the limb.

Dr. G. Stetter, in a paper on the etiology of fractures of the neck of the femur (*Centralblatt für Chirurg.* Sept. 8, 1877, No. 36), related a case in a boy, aged fourteen, who slipped on a smooth floor, and in trying to keep on his legs threw himself violently backwards and fell on his left side. Great pain was felt in the right hip; and he was unable to stand. The right limb was shortened three centi- metres and very strongly everted, with slight flexion of the knee.

There was inability to move the limb, and passive movement caused intense pain in the neighbourhood of the hip-joint. There was slight swelling about the great trochanter, which was painful on pressure. The left hip-joint was normal.

Dr. Stetter believes that the separation in his case was brought about by the powerful ilio-femoral ligament, which plays much the same *rôle* in this injury as in dislocations of the hip-joint.

In Dr. C. A. Sturrock's case the boy fell and twisted his hip.

In experiments the author has made in the post-mortem room, it was found that separation of the femoral head was most easily accomplished by means of extreme extension of the thigh, especially if accompanied by slight abduction.

Longaker, in relating a case of this injury (*loc. cit. infra*), draws attention to the mode of action of extreme extension of the limb. He says : ' The explanation of the accident was that as the patient fell prone the left leg was carried to a point of extreme extension, and possibly at the same time it was abducted. Great force was thus brought to bear upon the epiphysial junction, which, being the weakest part, yielded. We can easily appreciate the action of the powerful lever : the force is applied at the knee ; extension can be carried only to a certain point, when it is resisted by the tension of the strong ilio-femoral ligament ; this becomes the fulcrum, the weight is the point upon which the short arm of the lever is brought to bear, viz. the anterior margin of the acetabulum and the ligamentum teres and cotyloideum.'

This is probably the explanation of Dr. Stetter's case, in which the lesion is said to have been caused by muscular action, for it is exceedingly doubtful whether in a healthy subject the action alone of the muscles can be powerful enough to cause complete separation with displacement. That it is sufficient to cause a partial or incomplete separation without displacement we have abundant evidence to prove in cases of acute disease of the hip, accompanied by necrosis of either the whole of the head or some part of the neck of the bone, the result of slight injury.

Boerhaave's celebrated commentator, Van Swieten, was, the author believes, the first to observe that this was the most frequent cause of certain of these detachments.

Charles Bell believed that separation of this epiphysis was produced by children, while being carried in the arms of a nurse, violently throwing themselves backwards in a passion, whereby the full weight of the trunk is thrown on to the upper end or neck of the femur.

Bruns merely quotes as the etiology of this lesion the experiments of Colignon—viz. in using forcible abduction and rotation.

In proof of the statement as to the ligamentous character of the periosteum being often its strongest bond of union between the diaphysis and the epiphysis, it has been shown, according to

Dr. R. H. Harte (*Trans. Amer. Surg. Association*, 1897, vol. xv. p. 216) in the small epiphysis of the head of the femur, where the periosteum was divided circularly, that one-fifth of the amount of force will suffice to detach the epiphysis which would be required under other circumstances.

From the history of some cases it would appear that the violence was applied to the knee or outer side of the thigh while in the slightly adducted position, or to the foot or knee while the limb was in the extended and slightly adducted position.

In both these conditions the force acts from below upwards, backwards, and outwards, in a direction almost perpendicular to the axis of the neck.

Speaking of separations produced in the foetus, Küstner (*Die typischen Verletzungen der Extremitätknochen des Kindes durch den Geburtshelfer*, Halle, 1877, S. 45) is quoted by Simpson (*Edinburgh Medical Journal*, June 1880) as follows : 'As regards the recorded cases of epiphysis separation, Henke, indeed, notes the possibility that " the upper cartilaginous epiphysis may be detached from the femur by strong traction on the foot," but he records no case. Thudichum (*Illustr. med. Zeitung*, 1855) knows a case of separation of the upper epiphysis (Bertrandi) ; Ruge has none ; to myself also no case is known. Yet my experiments show that hyperabduction of the leg is very likely to produce this kind of injury ; the leg may get into this situation during version, perhaps also during extraction.'

Incomplete separation of the whole cartilaginous upper end of the bone—or, as Ollier terms it, juxta-epiphysial separation—is often brought about in young children by violent abduction or adduction of the limb, more especially the former, as when a child falls, slipping with its legs apart.

Ollier (*Traité des résections*, tom. iii. 1891, p. 70) gives a representation of the lesions produced at the upper end of the femur by violent abduction—viz. commencing separation of the diaphysis on the inner side—so that there is a gap left of about a centimetre and a half between the diaphysis and epiphysis, while on the outer side below the trochanter the spongy tissue of the diaphysis is somewhat crushed up. (See Part I. Chapter VI. fig. 5.)

Such an injury is often the starting-point of tuberculous disease of the hip-joint.

Dr. J. D. Rushmore relates (*Trans. Amer. Surg. Association*, 1895, vol. xiii. p. 502) a remarkable instance of separation of the femoral head, probably the result of unsuccessful attempts to reduce a supposed recurrent dislocation of the hip. Male, aged sixteen years, admitted to Brooklyn Hospital May 12, 1890, with a pubic dislocation of the right femur. The inability to use the limb was developed suddenly while walking, but the patient had been in the habit of separating his legs as wide apart as possible for several months, and had gradually acquired the ability to bring the buttocks into contact with the floor with the knee-joints extended. The hip-joint was opened and the dislocation reduced with some difficulty, and healing was complete by June 15. Subsequently, under the care of one of Dr. Rushmore's colleagues, the limb was thought to be shortened and the head of the bone displaced. Efforts were made unsuccessfully to reduce the dislocation; the joint was then opened and the head of the bone found in place, but separated from the neck. The loose bone was removed, the neck sawn off, and the limb placed in a plaster-of-Paris splint. Suppuration with marked loss of flesh and strength followed, but when seen on December 1 the wound had been healed for several weeks and the patient's general condition was much improved. The knee, however, without having been originally injured and without having subsequently shown any evidence of inflammatory trouble, was found, on removal of the plaster splint, to be stiff from extra-articular adhesions. On commencing to break up the adhesions the tibia was fractured just below the tubercle. The leg was put up in a plaster splint, and united at the end of a month. In February 1891 the patient left the hospital with the limb one and a half inches shorter than the opposite limb, the hip- and knee-joint becoming more and more useful under gentle passive motion. At the time of the report, more than four years afterwards, he had all the movements of the hip and complete use of the knee-joint. Except for the one and a half inch shortening, the limb was as good, but not so well developed, as its fellow.

Direct violence.—As the age of the child advances, the epiphysial junction of the head of the femur gains in width and strength, while the neck of the bone becomes the weaker point. Epiphysial separation is at this period commonly the result of great violence applied directly to the upper end of the bone, but nevertheless the neck of the bone is more likely to be fractured under these circumstances.

The author found that separation was most easily produced by a direct blow on the outer side of the thigh below the great trochanter while the limb was adducted and semiflexed, and in this case it was found that it was sometimes accompanied by some splintering of the neck of the bone.

Separations brought about by direct violence during life are recorded by several writers. Mr. J. F. South mentions (*Chelius's System of Surgery*, vol. i. 1847, p. 565, note to German translation), a case in a boy, aged ten years, who had fallen out of a first-floor window upon his left hip. The foot was slightly turned out, and scarcely any difference in the length of the limbs could be observed. The thigh could be readily moved in any direction and without much pain, but on bending the knee and rotating the limb outwards a very distinct dummy sensation was very frequently felt, as it seemed, within the hip-joint, as if one articular surface had slipped off another.   Mr. South and Mr. Green came to the conclusion that it was a case of separation of the head within the capsule.   The boy suffered such little inconvenience that he had two or three times got out of bed and walked about for a short distance.   He was put upon a double inclined plane.

A fall on the side has been noted in a few instances, e.g. in the cases of Sabatier and Fabrice de Hilden quoted by Rognetta, both of which were mistaken for fracture of the neck of the femur by these surgeons, while in both those recently recorded by Professor Kocher it is important to note that the cause of the epiphysial separation is expressly stated as a fall on the great trochanter. Both were instances of removal of the head by operation.

Mr. Mayo Robson (*Lancet*, vol. ii. August 21, 1886) has reported and given a drawing of the case of a child, aged five, who was brought to the Leeds General Infirmary on account of lameness, due to shortening of the left lower extremity, with the history of having, four years previously, been thrown up by her uncle, who, failing to catch her, let her fall heavily on the left side.   Beyond rest no treatment had been followed out, and the mother was unaware of any other accident having happened to the child, but she had noticed the limp to become more marked during the previous few months.

On examination the signs were as follows : marked limping on walking, the patient leaning to the left ; well-marked eversion of the foot, which could, however, be brought parallel with the right without giving pain ; ability to completely flex and extend the thigh.   Shortening of limb three-quarters of an inch.   Left great trochanter raised three-quarters of an inch, as shown by Nélaton's line.   Folds of the buttocks well marked.   On flexing and rotating the left femur inwards the fingers could clearly feel the neck of the femur as far as the head, but the prominent part of the caput femoris was apparently in the acetabulum, and was not attached to the cervix.

The muscles of the limb were well developed, and a thickened sole on the left boot almost abolished the limp.

From the anatomical condition of the upper end of the femur at the early age at which the accident occurred—viz. one year—it appears to the author that a true separation of the head alone in this case was impossible, but the history and symptoms would rather lead to the supposition that it was a fracture through the neck and cartilaginous band uniting the head to the great trochanter.

Packard thinks that there is 'an important difference between this injury and fracture of the neck of the bone close to the head, as appears from the recorded cases—viz. the much greater violence generally assigned as the cause of the epiphysial disjunction.'

PATHOLOGICAL ANATOMY.—Fabrice de Hilden, about the middle of the seventeenth century, and Verduc, at the end of the same century, J. L. Petit (*Maladies des os ; Description exacte des os*, Leyden, 1709), and G. J. Duverney (*Maladies des os*, 1751, translated by G. S. Ingham, 1762) all allude to epiphysial separation in speaking of fracture of the neck of the femur. Writing in 1837 Guéretin considered this injury as a very rare one, and mentions the cases of Bertrandi and Reichel as having been confirmed by an autopsy.

Dupuytren alluded to the possibility of its occurrence, but has not recorded any example of it.

Liston supposed, and many others since his day have asserted, that epiphysial separations of the head of the femur may occasionally take place.

Gurlt also, in 1862, although admitting the possibility of this lesion, had no knowledge of any case.

Holmes says (*Surgical Diseases of Children*, 1869, p. 258) 'that fractures of the neck of the femur are hardly known in childhood, and the upper epiphysis is so small, and lies so completely within the hip-joint, that its disjunction is unknown, except perhaps in the fœtus.'

Hamilton was very doubtful as to its occurrence.

Henry Morris, in his article ' On Injuries of the Lower Extremity,' in the last edition (1883) of Holmes's *System of Surgery*, states that ' several supposed examples of this accident have been recorded, but I agree with Mr. Holmes in thinking that they are not conclusive as to the real existence of the lesion.'

It is true that this epiphysis, including only, as a rule, the cartilaginous articular surface, accurately fits into the acetabulum, and rather more than fills it in youthful subjects. This fact, together with the deep situation of the part, renders the detection of its separation difficult, yet such a disposition of the head of the bone and the mechanical disadvantage arising from the length of the neck must favour separation to a considerable extent.

The real existence of this separation has been established by direct examination in eight instances. The first case is described and figured by Bousseau (*Bull. de la Soc. anatomique*, 1867, p. 283, Plate) in a boy, aged fifteen, who was severely injured by the passage of a wagon-wheel over his left hip and arm. The left lumbar and hypogastric regions and upper part of the thigh were considerably swollen and contused. There was inability to move the limb, which was shortened, slightly flexed, and completely rotated outwards, the left heel being in contact with the right internal malleolus, and the limb lying upon its outer side. The thigh was also slightly abducted. Death ensued in a few hours. Severe laceration of the muscles and soft parts of the thigh was found, together with extensive hæmorrhage in the thigh, the iliac fossa, and around the pelvic viscera (sub-peritoneal), although all the large vessels of the thigh were intact. A complete separation of the femoral head at the epiphysial line appeared, as though a section had been made of the femoral head perpendicular to the neck at the level of the brim of the cotyloid cavity. A small strip of cartilaginous and periosteal tissue still clung to the upper third of the neck on the outside. The periosteum was extensively detached from the neck all round, excepting on its outer side and above, as just mentioned, but it still remained attached to the epiphysis. The strip, which alone bound the two fragments together, was two millimetres wide. A vertical laceration existed on its inner side and extended downwards to the lesser trochanter. The capsule of the joint was also lacerated extensively at its inner part, through which the margin of the femoral head could be seen. Separations of the anterior superior, and inferior iliac spines were also found, the former still holding to the ilium by a small portion of cartilage and periosteum, the latter completely detached, with the exception of a small tag of periosteum uniting it to the superior spine. The rectus tendon remained attached to it. The iliac fossa was full of blood (sub-peritoneal). Each spinous process presented a thin osseous layer in the centre of the cartilaginous separated surface. There was also a transverse fracture of the lower end of the humerus.

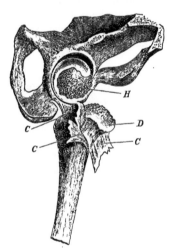

Fig. 192.—Traumatic separation of the epiphysial head of the femur. (after Bousseau)

H, head of the femur; *D*, end of diaphysis; *C*, detached periosteum and capsule

The convex end of the femoral diaphysis was wavy in outline, and had scattered over its greyish-looking surface small projections and excavations, two or three of the latter really forming holes. Under the microscope the surface of bone was seen to present osteoblasts, which were incompletely formed, and a considerable number of cartilage cells in various stages of transformation.

The surface of the epiphysis was deeply excavated, especially on the inner side, and also presented some less marked elevations and depressions scattered over it. Under the microscope little else than cartilage was seen, although some calcareous groups and unformed osteoblasts could be detected.

The separation had taken place between the chondroid and spongy layers.

The second remarkable case is recorded by Lewis Sayre ('On Diastasis of the Head of the Femur,' *American Practitioner and London Medical Record*, 1873, p. 393) of a child, aged ten, who died of cholera eight years after the occurrence of the accident. The acetabulum was found to be of small size and irregular shape, and was filled by the remnants of the head of the femur; a new acetabulum had been formed on the dorsum of the ilium, the upper part of which was attached to. the great trochanter by a firm dense ligament, the lower portion being polished and eburnated, and corresponding to a similar eburnation of the part of the neck of the femur fitting against it.

This case cannot be regarded as a true separation of the head alone at the time of the accident, when the child was only two years old. The fibrous band alluded to by Professor Sayre was probably the remains of the upper part of the epiphysis uniting the head to the great trochanter. A section through the upper end of the shaft and trochanter would have thrown much light upon this interesting specimen.

Longaker (*Medical and Surgical Reporter*, Philadelphia, 1883, xlix. pp. 228–231) relates the case of a male child, aged six years, who had up to that time good health and no.tendency to inherited disease. Nine weeks previously a heavy boiler fell against him, causing a large wound at the back of the upper part of the right leg. One week after the accident there was high fever with chills. Rapid emaciation and swelling of the upper part of the front of the left thigh increased steadily and rapidly to the time when he was seen. There was a cicatrix three-quarters of an inch in width and two inches long running obliquely across the .right leg. The patient lay on his right side with thigh flexed upon pelvis and leg on thigh. Pain on movement of left leg. Enormous fluctuating swelling of thigh extending upwards as far as the crest of the ilium. Any attempt at extension caused great pain. There was aching of the lumbar vertebræ, and the pelvis moved with the femur. Occasional diarrhœa. An incision was made behind the trochanter and a quantity of pus evacuated. The hip-joint was found to be opened and the head of the femur detached, and only adherent by the ligamentum teres. The upper end of the shaft presented a distinct sharp edge, from which the periosteum was not separated, but normal. .The part of the line which was separated was grasped by an ordinary dressing forceps, and with little difficulty removed from its attachment. There was no erosion of the articular cartilage of the removed fragment; it was normal in appearance. Carbolic acid was injected and a drainage tube inserted. On the sixth day the thigh was extended with considerable force, and some adhesions were felt to give way. A moulded splint was then applied to the anterior and outer aspect of the left side. Death occurred three days later from exhaustion.

At the post-mortem examination of the thigh the body was found in a state of great emaciation. Bands of adhesions had formed between the neck of the femur and the innominate bone, some of them being ruptured, and the others effectually preventing complete extension. The upper extremity of the bone presented an almost even surface with no necrosis.   There was no periostitis or ostitis.   Tissues about the joint had evidently suffered from violence.

Mr. Davies-Colley refers (*loc. cit. infra*) to a case he had seen under one of his colleagues at Guy's Hospital.   Excision of the head and neck of the femur was performed, and it was found that there was a separation of the epiphysis which had united by bone after the gliding upwards of the shaft.   He inferred that separation of the upper epiphysis had occurred from the shortening of the limb accompanied by great projection of the trochanter.

Professor Theo. Kocher (*Beiträge zur Kenntniss einiger praktisch wichtiger Fracturformen*, Leipzig, 1896, S. 238) describes in every clinical detail, and gives semi-diagrammatic drawings of, two interesting cases of traumatic separation of the epiphysial head of the femur,

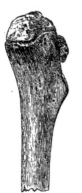

FIG. 193.—PURE SEPARATION OF HEAD OF FEMUR. A PORTION ONLY OF THE EPIPHYSIAL END OF THE NECK APPEARS IN THE DRAWING
(McGill College Museum, Montreal)

both caused by a fall upon the trochanter major, and both subjected to an exact diagnosis before operation.

In the first case, of a girl aged sixteen years, the head of the femur was removed by a posterior incision in February 1889, about three weeks after the accident.

In the second the operation was undertaken in a girl, aged fourteen, four years after the accident, when the diagnosis was made.

In the latter the neck of the bone appeared to have a very oblique downward direction, was tuberculated, and seemed as if it had formed a new head, while the epiphysial head itself was attenuated.

König has also performed resection in two cases of epiphysial separation of the head of the femur.

Amongst the photographs of specimens which Professor J. G. Adami, of McGill University, Montreal, generously handed to the author, was one of separation of the epiphysial head of the femur.   The specimen is so valuable that it is reproduced here, though the drawing shows but little of the part involved in the injury.   Dr. Adami supplied the author with the following note—viz. 'that it was taken from a child and was a fracture of the epiphysis of the head; it was photographed to show the trochanteric imperfect union.   In this specimen the head has been broken off sharply along the epiphysial line.   Unfortunately the head is missing' (see fig. 193).

The following case of epiphysial separation in a lad, aged twelve years, came under the author's observation at the City Orthopædic Hospital on July 20, 1894, two years after the accident.   S. S., aged twelve years, was admitted under the author's care for deformity of the left hip, with the history that on August 30, 1892, he had been knocked down in Rosebery Avenue and run over by a hansom cab. He was taken to a hospital, where 'traumatic dislocation of the hip was diagnosed and easily reduced'—so the author was informed by a letter from the registrar of the hospital. After seventeen days he left the hospital with a plaster-of-Paris dressing and crutches. The plaster casing was removed after a month, but at the end of three months he was only able to walk with a 'limp.' This got worse, and in April 1894 he again slightly injured the hip whilst at play, and at the end of May, six weeks later, he was taken into the same hospital for a week on account of the stiffness. Under an anæsthetic some adhesions were found and broken down. The stiffness recurring, the patient was brought to the City Orthopædic Hospital. He was a muscular boy for his age. The left leg was everted, so that the inner side of the foot looked forwards and inwards and the patella outwards. The muscles of the thigh were wasted, and there was rather more than a quarter of an inch shortening. The great trochanter was very prominent, with great thickening both in front and behind, especially in front towards the neck of the bone, so that this process felt almost twice as thick as on the opposite side; it was half an inch

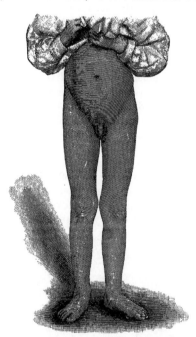

FIG. 194.—TRAUMATIC SEPARATION OF THE EPIPHYSIAL HEAD OF THE FEMUR. APPEARANCE OF THE LIMB TWO YEARS AFTER THE ACCIDENT (AUTHOR'S CASE)

nearer the iliac crest than that on the right side. The gluteal fold was lost on this side. The leg was neither adducted nor abducted, and the patient was quite unable to raise it from the bed. Passive flexion of the thigh was only permitted through an angle of forty degrees from the extended position, whilst rotation was almost lost; the slight amount of rotation inwards that was possible produced some pain.

On October 30 forcible flexion of the hip-joint was carried out up to an angle of seventy degrees with the trunk, and was accompanied by some 'crackling.' Forcible rotatory movements were also effected. For six weeks the patient was kept in bed, gentle movements of the hip-joint being carried out from time to time, and a month later he was discharged from the hospital, able to walk well without any limping. Flexion could be effected up to an angle of sixty degrees without causing any pain. The trochanter appeared less prominent, but this was no doubt partly due to the improved condition of the muscles, although the thigh was still considerably smaller than the opposite one. There still remained a good deal of thickening of the front of the neck of the bone. Two years later the patient was again under the author's treatment at the Miller Hospital, the deformity having greatly increased.

The eversion of the limb was so great that the outer malleolus rested on the bed ; its shortening amounted to nearly half an inch. The bony prominence in front of the hip was now very marked, owing probably to the wasting of the muscles, the continued displacement forwards of the end of the neck, and the rotation of the epiphysial head in the acetabulum. The position was very like that of a dislocation forwards of the head of the femur.

Active and passive movements of flexion of the hip-joint were almost absent. From the extended position the thigh could only be flexed about ten degrees. The great trochanter was in its normal position as regards Nélaton's line.

On November 19, 1896, by an anterior incision along the border of the tensor vaginæ femoris, the author excised, by means of a chisel, the end of the neck of the femur which was rotated forwards, so that its epiphysial surface presented in front and formed the

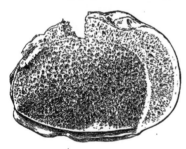

mass noticed previously. A small portion of the front margin of the head of the bone appeared to have been broken off and displaced forwards and outwards with the neck ; the rest of the head of the bone had undergone some rotation in the acetabulum. The articular cartilage was undergoing fibroid degeneration, and slight adhesions existed in the joint. No traces of the ligamentum teres could be found ; it had

FIG. 195.—PORTION OF HEAD AND NECK OF FEMUR EXCISED FOR DISPLACEMENT FORWARDS OF THE LATTER FOLLOWING EPIPHYSIAL SEPARATION. POSTERIOR VIEW OF DIVIDED SURFACES. (AUTHOR'S CASE)

evidently been ruptured. The neck of the bone was firmly united to the epiphysis. The parts were removed in several pieces, since it was desirable to leave as much of the posterior part of the neck as possible in contact with the back of the acetabulum to form a new joint with it. The great trochanter was uninjured, and therefore left intact.

After the operation the eversion was entirely corrected, and the limb could be freely flexed. No drainage. The patient made a good recovery, but the precise condition of the limb could not be ascertained at the time of this report, after he had left the hospital.

There is no specimen of this injury in any of the London hospital museums.

Although specimens are so rare, the author believes the accident to be by no means an uncommon one.

Several specimens from the lower animals have been obtained by Mr. Hutchinson, all resulting from violence in attempts at sexual connection. He believes that 'in almost all instances the injury is partly a fracture as well.'

Separation with fracture of a portion of the diaphysial neck.—It is probable in some cases that the separation does not follow exactly the line of conjugal cartilage, but that some small splinters of the neck may be detached, as in other epiphysial separations.

At the same time it must be remembered that the epiphysis of the head extends somewhat over the neck, especially on the upper and anterior aspects.

Incomplete separation.—Incomplete separation of the diaphysis is a very common origin of acute suppurative hip disease, the primary lesion being often overlooked.

It has been stated above that Ollier has recently drawn attention to these injuries under the name of juxta-epiphysial sprain.

Professor De Paoli, of Perugia, describes and figures (*Comunicazioni della clinica chirurgica propedeutica*, Perugia, 1891) a typical case of this kind in which he performed excision of the hip in a boy aged seventeen years. The injury (caused by jumping a ditch) had produced a partial separation or fracture of the epiphysis at its upper and anterior margin, and led to inflammatory softening of the conjugal cartilage.

This produced separation of the upper epiphysis with backward displacement of the diaphysis and acute suppurative inflammation of the hip-joint.

De Paoli believed that in this case there was added some pyæmic infection from a 'boil' which had been in existence on the back of the hand for some days previous to the injury. The ordinary micro-organisms of suppuration, and especially streptococci, were found in the pus on cultivation.

Most surgeons have seen various conditions of acute hip disease, succeeded by similar detachments, many of which have not been detected before the operation of excision of this joint.

SYMPTOMS.—In his memoir in 1834 M. Rognetta states that after a careful investigation he was persuaded that separation of the epiphysial head of the femur happens more frequently than was thought, and that it was often not detected.

Duverney thought that this lesion could only occur as the result of disease (*Maladies des os*, 1751, t. i. p. 354).

J. L. Petit, writing in 1837, at the end of a chapter on fracture of the neck of the femur, makes the following remarks, but it does not appear that he had ever met with a case:

'Il s'agit, pour finir cette matière, de dire un mot du décollement ou de la séparation du col d'avec l'épiphyse qui forme la tête. Cette épiphyse ou cette tête est unie, comme on sait, au corps de l'os par un cartilage qui se trouve entre eux et qui, comme une colle, fait la jonction de ces parties. On conçoit par là que le décollement ne peut arriver que dans les jeunes sujets en qui le cartilage qui joint l'épiphyse n'est point ossifié : car dans ceux en qui l'ossification est parfaite, le cou et l'épiphyse ne faisant qu'un, s'il arrive que la tête se sépare, ce sera par fracture et non par simple décollement. . . . Pour déterminer si ce décollement est simple ou s'il est causé par une fracture, il faut donc avoir égard à l'âge. . . . Après tout, il ne sert pas beaucoup, pour la guérison, de distinguer le décollement de l'épiphyse d'avec la fracture du col, puisque l'opération est la même et que les moyens de maintenir les os, quand ils sont réduits, ne diffèrent point.'

Although M. Colignon was able to collect ten cases of this injury, many of them cannot be accepted as trustworthy on account of the insufficient data given by their authors at a very remote period.

MM. Cruveilhier, Récamier, and Marjolin diagnosed a probable separation of this epiphysis in a child aged three years, who presented all the characters of a fracture of the neck of the femur.

Boyer, in his *Traité des maladies chirurgicales*, says that separation of the head does not differ at all from fracture of the neck, that the symptoms are the same for both, and that consolidation takes place as readily as after fracture. He quotes Paré as having described the symptoms of this lesion and alluded to the possibility of mistaking it for a dislocation.

Chelius says that the symptoms of this injury can in no respect be distinguished from those of fracture within the capsule.

One of the earliest cases recorded is related by E. Spillmann (*Dict. Encycl. des Sci. Med.* vol. xxiv. p. 238), as observed by Sabatier in a boy aged eleven, but he gives no account of the case. Spillmann also refers to another seen by Verduc.

The late Mr. John Hilton of Guy's Hospital made a diagnosis of this injury in two cases, and Mr. G. A. Wright, of the General Hospital for Sick Children, Manchester (*Hip Disease in Childhood*), has once met with diastasis of the upper femoral epiphysis. Mr. Hutchinson (*Medical Times and Gazette*, vol. i. 1866, p. 195), in speaking of separations of this epiphysis, maintained that 'at best a plausible guess is all that is possible.' However, the same surgeon in a recent article (*Archives of Surgery*, April 1892) upon detachment of the epiphysial head of the femur, speaks of the diagnosis of this injury in more certain terms. Also, Hamilton states that 'we have as yet no means of determining absolutely the symptoms of epiphysial separations.'

The numerous cases which have now been published should enable us to make an accurate diagnosis.

SEPARATION WITH DISPLACEMENT.—The symptoms of complete separation with displacement resemble mostly those of fracture of the neck of the femur within the capsule in adults, to which some of the signs of dislocation are often added.

Many examples of fracture of the neck of the femur in children have been verified by anatomical examination; a few only of these need be quoted here to show their existence.

Mr. Henry Morris (Holmes and Hulke's *System of Surgery*, 3rd edit. vol. i. p. 998) points out that occasionally undoubted intracapsular fractures occur in the young, and quotes cases recorded by Morgagni, Stanley, and others, while he gives a drawing from a specimen in the Middlesex Hospital taken from a person under seventeen years of age. In Guy's Hospital Museum there is a specimen of a similar fracture united by so large an amount of callus, obscuring the upper end of the bone, that it is probable that a more extensive fracture of this portion of the bone had existed.

Hamilton reported another case (F. H. Hamilton and Stephen Smith, *Fractures and Dislocations*, 1891, p. 369). A girl, aged sixteen, was caught between the wheels of two carriages, the blow being received directly upon the trochanter major of the right side. The symptoms which presented themselves showed conclusively that there was a fracture—viz. shortening, loss of voluntary motion, eversion, and well-marked crepitus. At the end of three years she died of acute disease, and it was found that there had been a transverse fracture of the bone just at the junction of the head and neck, and not an epiphysial separation. The head of the bone was still attached to the acetabulum by the ligamentum teres.

Schultz records another case of fracture of the neck of the femur under the care of Dr. Hoffa (*Zeitschrift für orthopädische Chirurgie*, i. S. 49), who removed the head of the femur in a girl of fourteen for ununited fracture six weeks after the injury from a fall.

Epiphysial separations cannot, therefore, be judged simply from the age; the narrowest portion of the neck of the femur is below the epiphysial line of junction of the head, and would therefore appear to be more liable to fracture than the broader epiphysial head to be separated above; but the subject will be alluded to again more fully under the head of diagnosis.

Shortening is the most marked sign; it is noted in eighteen out of twenty cases, and may be considerable, ranging from three-quarters to one and a half or two inches; in others it may be slight, and unrecognisable unless careful measurements be taken. On the other hand, it may be absent at the time of the accident, only being evident subsequently when the femur has become displaced in walking or by muscular action.

It may therefore be said to be dependent upon the extent of the displacement of the neck of the bone. Extension of the lower extremity readily reduces slight displacement, consequently short- ening may be overlooked.

In Hamilton's case there was three-quarters of an inch shorten- ing, in Post's one inch, Hutchinson's one inch, and in Maunder's half to three-quarters of an inch.

De Morgan has recorded (*Med. Times and Gazette*, 1859, vol. i. p. 137) the case of a young man, aged nineteen years, as a fracture of the neck of the femur; whilst standing on some movable steps, they slipped from under him, and he was thrown four feet on to the flags below, striking the back of his hip with great violence against the edge of some railings. The symptoms were eversion of the foot; the outer surface of the trochanter looked backwards; there was one and a half inch real shortening (which was readily reduced and as easily recurred). The trochanter, less prominent than on the opposite side, rotated with the shaft; there was obscure crepitus. He recovered with bony union.

A separation of the epiphysis probably occurred in this case.

Mr. Noble Smith (*Lancet*, March 20, 1886, vol. i.) records and figures an instance in a young lady, aged seventeen, who nearly fell while walking on wet boards, the right leg slipping outwards and forwards. She recovered herself, but felt pain, chiefly in the knee, but also in the region of the hip-joint. No shortening of the limb could be detected, but the toes inclined outwards at about 30° from the vertical.

The case was diagnosed as 'severe strain' of the femoral muscles from violent external rotation of the limb, with probably some rupture of the capsular ligament. She rested in bed for three weeks, and then endeavoured to get up, but found the leg useless. Five weeks before the accident the patient strained the right knee in walking, and this, although apparently recovered from, had probably contributed to the second severe accident. When seen by Mr. Smith eleven weeks after the accident, there was one and a quarter inch shortening of the limb. The trochanter was somewhat prominent laterally. The foot was rotated outwards to the extent of 50°; whilst in the recumbent position she could flex the thigh to an angle of 45° with the straight line of the body, without moving the pelvis. Limb utterly useless for standing. When placed on her side the patient could extend the thigh almost completely. The toes could be rotated inwards one inch towards the vertical without causing the slightest pain in the hip. Mr. Smith further states: ' The first slight accident caused a sprain of the muscles surrounding the hip- joint, leaving them somewhat weak, and favouring injury to the joint. At the time of the second accident, when the patient stumbled, the leg slipped outwards and forwards. Upon this latter occasion I believe the epiphysis was separated from ·the shaft, but was kept in position by the capsule, as occurs in intracapsular fracture, and subsequently the bone became displaced by muscular action. It will not, I think, be doubted that the head of the bone was separated from the shaft. The trochanter being an inch and a quarter higher than that of the opposite limb, and the two trochanters on the same level with the front of the body, although the right one was rotated out while the left was held with the foot vertical, indicated one of two conditions : either the head of the femur must have been dislocated from the acetabulum, or, if it remained in its place, it must have been separated from the shaft. If it had been dislocated, the head must have been discovered in the displaced position. In rotation outwards of a thigh the trochanter is naturally carried backwards ; but here the trochanter was level with the other, and therefore the head of the bone would have been very prominent had there been dislocation. There was no sign of it. Assuming that the head of the bone was separated from the shaft, its production by disease of the joint was contraindicated by the history, the symptoms, and the result of treatment. Under ether, the thigh could be flexed upon the body nearly to a right angle. The movement of the joint in all directions was more free than before. While in a flexed position traction was applied .to the thigh, rotation inwards, and the limb brought down to a straight line with the body by very moderate force. A cartilaginous grating was felt in the joint. The deformity was completely reduced with the exception of less than a quarter of an inch. Liston's long splint was applied for six weeks ; the patient then moved about on crutches for twenty-five days. Since then she has walked about comfortably with the assistance of a mechanical support. Firm union took place, but the movements of the joint were very restricted.'

Dr. Harvey (*Brit. Med. Journal*, February 19, 1887, p. 396) mentions the case of a child in whom there was **lengthening** of the limb by three-quarters of an inch after injury, reduced when in the recumbent position, but returning on standing, the result of separation of the upper epiphysis of the femur. A long splint was applied, and recovery took place.

The facts given in this case are unfortunately insufficient to explain this unusual symptom of lengthening.

Eversion of the limb is a most frequent symptom ; it appears to have been a more or less marked feature in eighteen out of twenty cases. As in intracapsular fracture, it is chiefly owing to the weight of the limb, and may be accompanied by slight flexion, abduction, or adduction of the limb.

In Bousseau's case the limb was completely everted, lying upon its outer side, the heel touching the internal malleolus of the opposite limb.

It is less marked in younger children, where muscular action comes less into play.

Inversion of the limb.—Inversion of the limb was present in one case mentioned by Mr. Hutchinson (*Archives of Surgery*, April 1892) under his care at the London Hospital in 1873. It was that of a boy (Herbert B.), aged four and a half years, who had fallen out of a high bed. There was at least an inch of shortening with inversion, and a distinct cartilaginous crepitus was detected when the limb was drawn into position. The deformity was reproduced immediately that extension was remitted. Mr. Hutchinson says : ' We did our best to keep the bone in position, but I am not sure that we obtained union.'

Like the rare cases of intracapsular fracture of the neck in the adult with inversion, the internal rotation must be due, as R. W. Smith thinks, to the relative position of the fragments—the lower being placed in front of the upper—rather than to the influence of muscular action, which must only act secondarily. The limb at the time of the accident is probably in the inverted position. In this relation of the fragments he is of opinion that the pectineus and the upper portion of the adductor magnus would then act as internal rotators, and the position of the fragments would mechanically hinder eversion.

One or two of those rare cases in the adult, described by Stanley, Spence, Dupuytren, Hamilton, Cruveilbier, Guthrie, Smith, &c., have been mistaken for dislocation on to the dorsum of the ilium, or into the ischiatic notch.

Crepitus is of the usual muffled or dull character. Mention is made of it in nearly one half of the recorded cases.

The following are the particulars of the only instance of epiphysial detachment of the head of the femur which up to 1866 had been under Mr. Hutchinson's care (' On Separation of the Upper Epiphysis of the Femur,' *Med. Times and Gazette*, vol. i. February 24, 1866, p. 195). He was sent for one night to the London Hospital to see a patient with a supposed dislocation of the femur. The house surgeon believed that he had reduced it more than once, but it had slipped again. The patient was a lad of eighteen, who had been violently knocked backwards by an explosion of gunpowder. His left limb was slightly everted, and shortened to the extent of about an inch. The great trochanter moved with the shaft. The limb could be drawn down, but it slipped up again as soon as the traction was remitted. No distinct bony crepitus could be elicited, but a somewhat rough grating could be easily produced. Chloroform was given to facilitate accurate coaptation. When the muscles were fully relaxed the limb was very forcibly extended, and then carefully secured at full length on a straight splint with perineal band. The splint was re-adjusted at the end of a fortnight, and taken off at the end of six weeks, when the union was found to be tolerably firm ; but as a precaution it was retained for three weeks longer. The result was perfect, the limb being of the same length as the other, and the union quite firm.'

Hamilton (*op. cit.* p. 424) describes a case reported by Dr. H. Wardner, of Cairo, Illinois, as one 'of intracapsular fracture of the neck of the femur,' which he regarded, from the 'dull crepitation' and other symptoms, as really epiphysial.

A boy, aged fourteen, hurt himself by jumping and alighting upon his feet, this being followed by a lameness in the hip-joint and some difficulty in walking. Twenty-four hours later, on attempting to get out of bed, one foot became entangled in the bedclothing, and this led him to exert forcibly the adductor muscles, when he suddenly cried out with pain, saying his hip had gone out of place and he found himself unable to rise. Under chloroform, reduction was attempted unsuccessfully. The following day the limb was found to be shortened one or two inches, and was lying nearly parallel with the other limb, with the toes rotated. Dull crepitus was detected. Extension was applied for several weeks, and at the end of thirteen months there was one inch shortening, and the motions of the hip-joint were limited to about one half the normal extent, the muscles, leg, &c., of that side of the pelvis being considerably shrunken. The patient walked a little lame, and complained of weakness of the limb.

The same author quotes a more decided case under his own care at Bellevue Hospital. Andrew L., aged fifteen, fell from the fourth story of a house; the following morning he was admitted into Professor Hamilton's wards at Bellevue Hospital. The right thigh was found to be shortened three-quarters of an inch, and slightly abducted; toes everted. Under chloroform feeble crepitus was felt in the vicinity of the joint, unlike the crepitus of broken bone. The shortening was entirely overcome with fifteen pounds of extension, the limb put in position, and maintained with Buck's apparatus. At the end of two weeks there was still half an inch shortening. The ultimate condition of the limb could not be ascertained.

Cartilaginous crepitus was determined in one case by Dr. Elder between the head of the femur and trochanter.

Dr. E. H. Bradford, of Boston, U.S.A. (*Boston Medical and Surgical Journal*, 1892, vol. cxxvi. No. 9, p. 212), records a case of the separation of the epiphysis at the head of the femur, in which the diagnosis was clear.

A boy, seventeen years old, fell from a window, striking upon a shed of the story below. He was brought to the hospital with symptoms suggesting a fracture of the right limb. On examination, however, no fracture was found of the leg or the thigh. The limb was held in a position of eversion and was slightly shortened, but no injury was discovered below the trochanter, which rotated on twisting the leg. On examination under an anæsthetic, abnormal mobility and a cartilaginous crepitus were determined between the head of the femur and the trochanter. The trochanter was higher on the affected than on the other side.

Mr. W. H. Battle, in a short paper on ‘Traumatic Separation of the Upper End of the Femur in Early Life,’ gives (*St. Thomas's Hospital Reports*, N.S. vol. xxii. 1894, p. 22) an account of two cases in which soft crepitus and some of the other usual signs were present, and the diagnosis established.

Case I.   J. P., aged eight years, was admitted under the care of Mr. A. O. MacKellar into St. Thomas's Hospital on July 7 and discharged August 19, 1887.   Whilst climbing a stack of timber (twenty feet high) he fell on his right side, and a plank struck him on his left hip and forehead.   He was unable afterwards to stand, or to put the left leg to the ground.   On admission he complained of slight pain over the left hip and down the front of the thigh.   There was no eversion of the limb, no apparent shortening, and he could flex the thigh on the abdomen.   On firmly grasping the thigh with one hand, and placing the other over the hip-joint, the movements of rotation were not diminished; crepitus was not obtainable, neither was it on pressing the bone firmly upwards towards the acetabulum, and the pain during these manipulations was slight, being felt in the upper part of the thigh.   On firmly grasping the great trochanter, pressing inwards whilst extension was made on the thigh, and then gently moving it backwards and forwards, fine crepitus could be felt.   Under an anæsthetic, the great trochanter was found to be half an inch above Nélaton's line; the femur could be rotated to a greater extent than normal, and grating was distinct.   After this examination the shortening was three-quarters of an inch, and eversion became evident.   There was no marked crepitus, but the sensation was undoubtedly that conveyed in cases of separation of epiphysis in other parts of the body.

The shortening could be done away with on extension of the limb.   Extension and weight of four pounds, with plaster and long outside splint, were applied.   On July 16 the splint was taken off and a quarter of an inch shortening found.   The splint was then re-applied.

Case II. was that of a boy, aged seven, who was admitted under the care of Sir W. MacCormac on May 15, and left on June 26, 1882.   He was running along when he caught his left foot against the pavement, felt a crick in his hip, and fell down on the opposite limb; he did not strike the injured side at all.   On admission there was well-marked eversion and one inch shortening, but crepitus could not be felt until the boy had been placed under ether.   He made a good recovery, but no note was made as to the ultimate result as regards shortening.   No doubt was entertained of the nature of the injury in this case, but in a third case described by Mr. Battle the epiphysial separation rather pointed to disease.

The *absence of crepitus* in Sturrock's case formed (it is said) one of the signs in making a diagnosis.

Deformity.—The chief noticeable alteration of the natural shape of the hip is the result of the *displaced position of the great trochanter.*

This displacement is usually detected in fractures of the neck of the femur by Nélaton's line, by Morris's bi-trochanteric or transverse measurement (*System of Surgery*, 3rd edit. vol. i. p. 1003), or by Bryant's test line (*Lancet*, vol. i. p. 119, 1876).

Mayo Robson's method of measuring the shortening at the neck of the femur is a very exact one with the patient in the dorsal decubitus. The method consists (*Lancet*, December 14, 1895, p. 1506) in drawing a transverse line from the tip of the great trochanter forwards and inwards across the front of the thigh on each side, and dropping a vertical line to meet this from the tips of the anterior superior spines; the latter constitute the measuring lines.

The trochanter generally will be seen to be unaltered in shape, but more prominent and placed higher, and to be nearer the anterior superior spine of the ilium than that of the sound side.

There is a great tendency for the deformity to recur when the reducing force is relaxed, while there may be an absence of tenderness about this process.

In others some fulness or swelling may be noticed at the upper part of Scarpa's triangle.

J. M. Barton, in a paper (*Medical News*, Philadelphia, 1883, xliii. p. 43) on separation of the epiphysis of the head of the femur, relates a case in which he had taken careful measurements of this displacement. John L., aged fifteen years, while crossing a yard a few days previously, carrying a bundle, was pushed; the bundle fell, but he saved himself from falling by resting his hands on it. While thus leaning forwards a second push was received, and he came to the ground seated, supporting his weight by his hands. His hip came but lightly, if at all, in contact with the ground.

On examination there was one inch shortening and eversion of the foot, so that its outer margin was at an angle of twenty degrees with the bed. Knee and back in contact with bed. Fascia lata relaxed. Great trochanter higher, more prominent, and nearer anterior superior spine than on the opposite side. No spasm of muscles of hip. Buttock flattened, gluteo-femoral fold not well marked.

Under chloroform the limb could be as readily and fully rotated as its fellow, the trochanter describing a large arc of a small circle, or, in other words, rotating on its own centre, and not increasing its distance from the median line of the body. On extension the limb readily acquired its full length, and all deformity disappeared; both shortening and prominence of the trochanter immediately re-appeared on relaxing extension. Crepitation as of large surfaces of denuded bone was felt. By placing the patient on his side the knee of the injured side could be made to pass three inches further posteriorly than its fellow. The boy had slightly limped for some weeks before the accident, and had had pain on the inner side of the knee, but was able to work and play football, even kick the ball with his leg.

Sandbags with extension were applied for five weeks, when there was less than half an inch shortening.

In taking the distance of the great trochanter from the middle line, Barton recommends the patient to be placed on the back with a book against each trochanter; the legs to be then rotated, and the distance measured of the book from the middle line.

An interesting case of unusual displacement has been recorded by Mr. Maunder (*Lancet*, 1870, vol. i. p. 192). A lad, aged fourteen, received a blow upon the front of his thigh, and fell upon his hip. He walked home, some hundred yards, leaning on the shoulder of a comrade. On examination the limb was much rotated outwards and shortened to the extent of from half to three-quarters of an inch, but it had not the thoroughly helpless appearance of fractured neck of femur. Manipulation of the upper part of the limb caused great pain. There was a firm resisting bony swelling in the groin, under the line of the rectus muscle, which moved with the thigh and seemed to increase the antero-posterior width of the upper end of this bone. The patient could rotate the limb very slightly inwards. The following day, neither swelling nor ecchymosis existing, chloroform was administered, and the limb drawn down to its normal length. A soft crepitus was felt about the head of the bone. Mr. Hutchinson, who saw the case, also regarded it as one of epiphysial separation, notwithstanding the boy could flex the thigh slightly on the pelvis.

At the Clinical Society, on February 26, 1892 (*Clinical Society's Transactions*, vol. xxv. 1892, p. 288), Mr. Davies-Colley showed the following interesting case, which will be given in his own words : ' E. C., æt. fifteen, while playing at football about the end of November 1891, fell with another boy on the top of him, and hurt his left hip. He was able to walk home, and there he remained almost entirely in bed for a fortnight, but occasionally he got up and hobbled about in much pain. At the end of that time he was admitted under my care into Guy's Hospital. There was pain and tenderness about the hip, and some fulness of Scarpa's triangle with slight eversion of the foot. The most remarkable symptom was great prominence of the trochanter major, which was of natural shape and hardly at all tender. This prominence at once suggested dislocation of the hip, but the head of the femur could not be felt in any abnormal position. At first no shortening was detected. There was no active movement of the hip, but passive movement, though painful, was almost complete. The next day, December 10, I examined him under ether. A rubbing sensation, or very slight crepitus, could be felt when the thigh was rotated outwards. There was some limitation to the movement of abduction, while adduction and the other movements of the hip were free. I made a careful measurement, and found that the injured limb was a quarter of an inch shorter than the other. The injury was unlike a fracture of the cervix on account of the prominence of the great trochanter. Moreover, if, as is usual in so young a patient, the fracture had been extracapsular, I should have expected to find the great trochanter altered in shape and very tender.

'The diagnosis of dislocation was excluded by the fact that the head seemed to be in the acetabulum. I could find no other explanation of the symptoms than that a separation of the epiphysis of the head had occurred, and that the upper surface of the shaft had glided upwards and outwards upon the obliquely placed plane of the epiphysial line, so as to produce a slight shortening, together with the marked projection of the great trochanter. Probably some fibres of the periosteum had remained untorn, so as to prevent the two surfaces from becoming completely free of one another. This would also account for the fact that the boy had been able to walk about a little. The rubbing sensation felt when the limb was moved about under ether was also confirmatory of the diagnosis of separated epiphysis.

'The subsequent progress of the patient was satisfactory. He was kept in bed about four weeks with a long outside splint and perineal bandage on, and two weeks afterwards he went out nearly well. The shortening had increased to half an inch. When shown at the meeting he could move his leg about as freely as the other. There was no pain, but the great trochanter was as prominent as ever, and distinctly nearer to the crest of the ilium than upon the uninjured side.'

The amount of displacement at first present in separation of the femoral head, as in other epiphysial separations, will be found in great measure to vary with the violence which has been applied to the hip. Yet the diaphysis is very prone to even great displacement if the lesion be undetected and the patient be allowed the use of the limb.

The relaxed condition of the fascia lata between the crest of the ilium and the great trochanter, and of the ilio-tibial band on the injured side, to which Dr. Allis has drawn particular attention in the case of adults, may assist in young muscular subjects in forming a diagnosis.

Active movement of the lower extremity is almost entirely absent where the fragments are separated to any extent.

In others, where the head is still held to the neck by the tough fibrous periosteum and but little displacement has taken place, a considerable amount of active movement may still be retained, and mislead the surgeon into the supposition that no serious lesion has occurred.

Inability to move the limb or bear the least weight on it may be present, but on the other hand it has been found that the limb can sometimes be slightly moved, for the patient can raise the limb somewhat, flex the thigh, or even rotate it inwards to some extent, though with a little pain.

Pain more or less severe in character is experienced at the time of the accident. The subsequent pain is often no more than in cases of a severe sprain to the hip-joint.

When the patient is resting in bed but little pain or tenderness is felt at the hip, and it is only when pressure is made and the limb is rotated or moved during manipulation that it becomes noticeable, but even then it may be almost entirely absent. Dr. R. H. Harte is of opinion that, as a rule, the pain is distinctly less than in fracture, when two bony surfaces are drawn past each other, as in the attempt to elicit crepitus.

Abnormal mobility of the great trochanter, in describing a smaller circle, although a larger segment than on the sound side, is not such a trustworthy sign as in fracture of the neck, and has only been noticed in a few instances. This may be accounted for by the fact of the neck still being attached to the shaft of the femur. Dr. Harte says that the movements of the hip-joint in which the ligamentum teres is made tense—e.g. external rotation and adduction—are exaggerated.

In all cases of recent injury the use of an anæsthetic is necessary to establish the diagnosis accurately.

DIFFERENTIAL DIAGNOSIS.—As Hutchinson says : 'We may probably venture to assume that of the three accidents, fracture of the neck, dislocation, and separation of the neck from the head at the acetabular edge, the latter is by far the most likely injury to occur in young persons.'

But it is quite impracticable to agree with him that it would be next to impossible to establish a diagnosis during the patient's life, and that fractures of the neck as distinct from detachments of the head are perhaps unknown, or that not improbably all cases in which they have been suspected were really examples of the. latter.

Dislocation.—Rognetta states that Ambrose Paré and J. L. Petit both mistook a separation of this epiphysis for dislocation, and F. de Hilden one for a fracture of the neck.

E. Spillmann also mentions that Verduc was once called in consultation by J. L. Petit for an injury to the hip which was mistaken for a dislocation, but which was afterwards recognised as a separation of the femoral epiphysis (*Dictionnaire Encyclopédique,* art. 'Cuisse,' p. 238).

Although infrequent in an extreme degree, many cases of dislocation in young children from a few months to seven or eight years of age have now been recorded—the majority on to the dorsum ilii— the almost constant and well-marked inversion and fixation of the limb being sufficient to distinguish them—and a few into the thyroid foramen, giving rise to apparent lengthening of the limb. It must. be remembered, however, that in a few rare examples of separation inversion of the limb occurs, and the injury will then simulate dislocation more closely.

In all dislocations the head of the femur may be felt in its abnormal position, whereas in separation it appears still to occupy the acetabular cavity ; in the latter case, also, the end of the bone is found very difficult to retain in position after reduction. It usually slips out again immediately.

Sir Astley Cooper has recorded a case of dislocation of the femur upwards on to the dorsum ilii in a girl aged seven years, and Mr. Arnallt Jones, of Aberavon, mentions (*British Medical Journal*, May 31, 1890) a typical case of this dislocation on to the dorsum ilii ; the thigh was flexed and the limb adducted and rotated inwards, and there was shortening to the extent of an inch and a half. See also recent examples in *British Medical Journal*, March 28, 1896 (in a boy aged four years), *Lancet*, October 12, November 2 (in a child of six), November 9, 1889 (in a child of seven and a half), and others.

Fracture of the neck.—The signs that will assist in distinguishing complete separations with displacement from fracture of the neck are the age of the patient and the absence of bony crepitus. However, it must be remembered that, as Mr. Morris has pointed out (*loc. cit. supra*), true fracture may occur before the epiphysis has united. Still, it becomes extremely improbable in the younger periods of age, when separation is frequently met with, no doubt from the short and undeveloped condition of the neck of the bone. From the reported cases it would seem that the violence causing the separation is much greater, as a rule, than that producing fracture of the neck of the bone.

The signs are similar in both—viz. eversion, usually slight shortening, pain, and inability to raise the limb, and swelling about the trochanter—except that in fracture the crepitus is more distinct and rough, while in epiphysial separation it is more indistinct, muffled, and soft.

Besides the cases of fracture of the neck of the femur in children mentioned above as verified by direct examination, Stanley describes (*Med. Chir. Trans.* vol. xviii. 1833, p. 256) the case of a lad, aged eighteen years, who fell from the top of a loaded cart upon his right hip. He was unable to move the limb ; it was bent to a right angle with the pelvis, could not be extended, and abduction was difficult ; an attempt at passive motion caused pain. There was eversion, but no shortening or crepitus. He died three months afterwards of small pox. The capsule was a little thickened, the ligamentum teres uninjured; a line of fracture extended obliquely through the neck entirely within the capsule; the neck was shortened, and its head approximated to the trochanter. The fractured surfaces were in the closest apposition, and united nearly in their whole extent by bone. There was an irregular deposit of bone beneath the periosteum and the synovial membrane along the line of the fracture. Stanley believed that this was the only recorded case of this injury.

John Johnson relates (*New York Journal of Medicine*, 1857, p. 303) an instance of an intracapsular fracture. The patient was a young lady, aged sixteen years, who had been caught between the wheels of two carriages. Her symptoms showed conclusively that there was a fracture; crepitus was well marked. The fracture failed to unite, and at her death, three years later, of an acute disease, the head and neck were found very soft and partly absorbed. The head was soft and spongy. The fracture was transverse at the junction of the head and neck.

The following remarkable instance of fracture of the neck of the thigh bone was placed under the author's care at the Miller Hospital, through the courtesy of Dr. John Mackern, of Blackheath, in December 1897. The lad (A. J. B.), aged twenty-one, had, ten months previously, fallen off a ladder to the ground, a distance of eight or nine feet, on to his right side. At the time of the accident the pain in the hip was rather severe and he felt ' shaken,' but after a few minutes both these symptoms passed off and he could walk without lameness. No treatment was employed. Four months later the patient noticed that ' the side of his hip was growing out,' and he began to limp. The limb appeared to be getting short and continued so up to the time of admission, while pain was only experienced on a sudden jerk to the limb or after walking five or six miles. On examination there was lameness in walking, and the right limb was greatly everted, and adducted so that the knee was placed in front of the opposite limb when the pelvis was straightened. There consequently existed very considerable apparent shortening and tilting of the pelvis, and compensatory bending of the vertebral column (see fig. 196) when the lad placed both feet on the ground. Real shortening of the limb scarcely amounted to one-eighth of an inch. The great trochanter was very prominent, and projected further backwards than on the left side, but was not placed above Nélaton's line. The hip joint was almost completely fixed, the slightest flexion being the only movement permitted. The adductors of the thigh were tense and contracted. In front of the hip-joint an irregular mass of osteophytic growth could be felt; this fact, taken in connection with the signs just enumerated, determined the diagnosis of detachment of the head of the femur from gradual displacement at the neck of the bone the result of the injury. Several skiagraphs were now taken, which confirmed absolutely the diagnosis, and an operation upon the neck of the femur was undertaken to remedy the crippling condition. Under

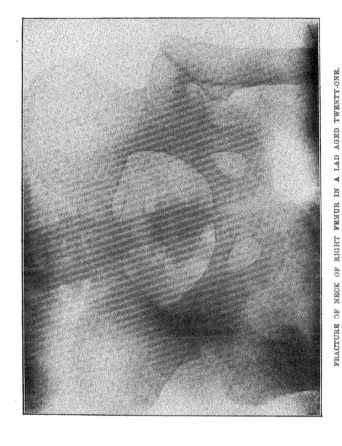

FRACTURE OF NECK OF RIGHT FEMUR IN A LAD AGED TWENTY-ONE.

Pubic and iliac portions of os innominatum still separate. Epiphyses of ilium were well displayed in the original.

AUTHOR'S case.   Reduced one-third size.

Taken by Messrs. ALLEN & HANBURY.

chloroform the adductor tendons were first divided, and the joint forcibly moved in all directions; but although flexion and extension were carried out almost to their furthest limit the eversion was in no way lessened. An anterior incision was therefore made, the distended joint incised, letting out about two ounces of dark bloody fluid. The neck of the bone was divided, and the head of the femur removed from the cotyloid cavity. The end of the neck was replaced in position. The ligamentum teres was found to be ruptured, the head

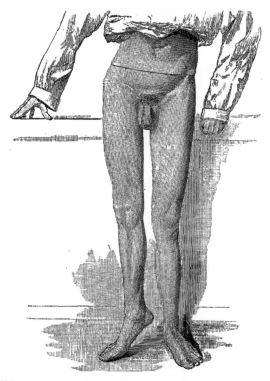

Fig. 196.—FRACTURE OF NECK OF FEMUR CLOSE TO EPIPHYSIAL JUNCTION OF HEAD. GREAT EVERSION AND ADDUCTION OF LIMB

becoming atrophied with its articular cartilage in a shrunken and crumpled condition. The fracture had been firmly united, though the end of the diaphysial fragment projected forwards into the osteophytic mass, probably the result of the atrophied and rotated condition of the epiphysis. On section of the portion removed the neck of the femur was found to have been divided nearly three-quarters of an inch from the remains of the conjugal line of cartilage, traces of which were still visible, the cancellous tissue of the epiphysis becoming rarefied. The patient was making an uninterrupted recovery with the limb in good position at the time of this report.

Prof. Jeannel (*Archives Médicales de Toulouse*, 1ᵉʳ Juin 1897, p. 236) relates the case of a young soldier, aged 22, who had fallen from a height of about eight metres. The patient did not know upon what part of his body he had fallen, but the injury was regarded at first as a contusion of the left hip. Ten months later he came under Dr. Jeannel's care, who found the limb wasted, the thigh slightly flexed and rotated outwards, but without abduction or adduction. The limb was also shortened three and a half centimetres, and the great trochanter above Nélaton's line. In spite of the external rotation, a diagnosis of irreducible iliac dislocation of an exceptional character was determined upon, and reduction attempted under chloroform. This having failed, a posterior incision was made, the detached head of the femur removed from the acetabulum, and the neck placed in the cavity. The result was perfect, the patient walking with scarcely a limp.

A case, probably of the same nature, is reported by Mr. Adams (*Med. Times and Gazette*, vol. i. 1859, p. 137) of a sailor aged seventeen. He had just before fallen into the hold of a ship, a distance of about sixteen feet. He did not know on what precise part he had been struck. He was unable to raise the right leg, and had pain in the hip. There was one inch shortening, eversion of the foot, and crepitus was distinctly felt on the great trochanter. An ordinary straight thigh splint was applied, but owing to the restless condition of the patient it had to be frequently re-applied. At the end of six weeks the fracture was found to be ununited, the splint was re-applied, and firm union eventually took place after some months. It was thought at the time that separation had occurred at the epiphysis, where it was not wholly cartilaginous, but contained some bony spiculæ.

Dr. Royal Whitman records (*New York Medical Record*, February 7, 1891, p. 165) a case of fracture of the neck of the femur, probably impacted, in a boy, aged eight, who had fallen eighteen feet. The symptoms upon which the diagnosis was made, six months after the injury, were half an inch shortening, elevation of the trochanter and its approximation to the middle line, while the movements of the joint were free, painless, and practically unimpaired.

Whitman thinks that under normal conditions the epiphysial junction of the head of the femur is not a weak point in the continuity of the bone; that, as a result of violence, fracture may occur above, below, and through the line of cartilage, and says (*New York Medical Record*, February 25, 1893, p. 230): 'Such fractures or displacements are of especial importance, because of the vicinity of the joint; because of the difficulty in keeping the fragments in apposition, and because cessation or diminution of growth or non-union may result.'

The same surgeon read a paper before the New York Academy of Medicine in December 1892 (*New York Medical Record*, January 14, 1893, p. 59) on 'Observations on Fractures of the Neck of the Femur in Childhood, with especial reference to Treatment and Differential Diagnosis from Separation of the Epiphysis.' The number of patients· shown in illustration of fracture of the neck of the femur in childhood was five, all of whom had been brought to the Hospital for the Ruptured and Crippled with a different diagnosis, usually that of hip-joint disease. He had seen none of the cases during the earlier stage, or not until the fourth week to the sixth month. Most of the children had fallen a distance of fourteen feet or more. In all the cases there was perfect or nearly perfect motion of the limb. The degree of shortening was usually from

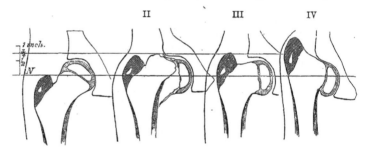

Fig. 197.—DIAGRAMS OF INJURIES TO THE NECK OF THE FEMUR (ROYAL WHITMAN)

I. The upper extremity of the femur, at the age of five years, drawn from a specimen in the Museum of the Hospital for Ruptured and Crippled, showing the epiphysis of the head and trochanter and the relation of the trochanter to Nélaton's line, N. The shaded area in the head and trochanter represents the cartilages.

II. A diagram to illustrate epiphysial disjunction, showing the separation of fragments necessary to account for upward displacement of the trochanter to the extent of three-fourths of an inch.

III. A diagram to illustrate fracture and depression of the neck of the femur and consequent elevation of the trochanter, also the limitation of the range of abduction of the limb that must result.

IV. A diagram to illustrate further depression of the neck and its effect in causing permanent abduction of the thigh.

three-fourths of an inch to one inch. There was in all an elevation of the trochanter which constituted a projection; in walking there was a dragging of the foot and eversion. The pain in most of the cases had disappeared. From the return of mobility in all directions, there could be no doubt but that the head of the femur rested in the acetabulum; there must have been a fracture between the head and the neck which changed the angle from an obtuse to almost a right angle. It was this alteration which caused the projection of the trochanter and the immediate shortening of the limb. The shortening had increased subsequently.

Dr. Whitman said that this accident in childhood had not been admitted as true heretofore. He did not deny that separation of the epiphysis might take place, but insisted that such was not the case in the patients presented, and expressed the belief that fracture was by far the more common accident in early life. The treatment employed by him consisted in obtaining immobility by the modified double Thomas splint.

Dr. Whitman (*Annals of Surgery*, June 1897, p. 673) has recently made some further observations on this fracture in childhood, and added five more cases. He also presents two skiagraphs showing the consequent deformity of the bone at the seat of injury, and he draws especial attention to this peculiarity—viz. that although the immediate results are extremely favourable even without treatment, yet the final outcome is likely to be a disability even more noticeable than after fracture in adult life. He also holds that it would be rather extreme violence followed by non-union of the fragments and subsequent disability that would favour the diagnosis of separation of the epiphysis. The less the violence and the less the immediate disability, the greater would be the probability of fracture when signs of fracture are present.

Mr. W. H. Battle, in a short paper on 'Traumatic Separation of the Upper End of the Femur in Early Life' (*St. Thomas's Hospital Reports*, N.S. vol. xxii. 1894, p. 19), has found four cases of intra-capsular fracture of the neck of the bone, below twenty years of age, from an analysis of the statistical reports of this hospital for ten years—viz. 1881 to 1890 inclusive—three males, aged seven, eight, and fifteen, and one female aged thirteen years, out of a total of 106 fractures of the neck. One, in the girl aged thirteen, was probably an intracapsular fracture, for the crepitus was rather more distinct than would be expected after epiphysial separation. Another, in the boy aged fifteen, was an example of separation the result of disease of the hip. The other two, aged eight and seven respectively, were epiphysial detachments.

Hip disease.—If a diagnosis has not been made at the time of the accident, it is easy to understand how, at a later period during the stage of recovery, it may be mistaken for hip disease. The subsequent halting walk of the patient, the pain and restricted movements of the hip-joint, the shortening and deformity of the limb, the pain in the knee (occasionally present) may be erroneously interpreted as symptoms of disease. The differences between the two are, however, well marked. The history of more or less severe injury, immediately followed by severe signs, is unlike the insidious nature of tuberculous disease following slight injury. The amount of deformity, also, caused by the former injury would, if it were the result of disease, be due to great disorganisation of the joint, and would be necessarily accompanied by other local phenomena of disease.

R. W. Parker (Heath's *Dict. of Practical Surgery*, vol. ii. 1887, p. 414) says that he has seen a case which simulated hip-joint disease.

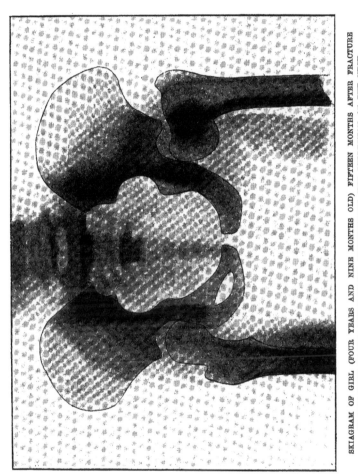

SKIAGRAM OF GIRL (FOUR YEARS AND NINE MONTHS OLD) FIFTEEN MONTHS AFTER FRACTURE
OF THE NECK OF THE RIGHT FEMUR, ILLUSTRATING THE DEPRESSION OF THE NECK.

Outlines traced on skiagram.   (ROYAL WHITMAN.)

In the *International Clinics* (4th series, vol. ii. p. 187) Dr. R. H. Sayre alludes to a case of diastasis of the left femur in a girl, and contrasts the manner of walking after union with that met with in hip disease, with which it might be confounded.

Congenital dislocation of the hip may be at once excluded by the absence of history of injury, its chronic and painless condition, and by the fact of the femoral head being felt in the gluteal region.

Simple contusion of the hip.—In contusion the normal relations between the anterior superior spine and great trochanter are preserved.

The shortening of the neck or of the limb, though often small in amount in epiphysial separation with displacement, apart from other signs, should at once remove all doubt as to its correct nature.

Incomplete separations without displacement the author believes to be far from uncommon. Unfortunately, a conjecture is all that can be made from the age, pain in the region of the head of the bone, and the history of injury, which may be slight. A much smaller amount of violence is required in these than in complete separations— e.g. a slight over-extension of the joint.

PROGNOSIS.—It is probable that good *bony union* will usually result, provided the limb be brought down and maintained in good position.

The ultimate result is also often good, although the union may only be a fibrous one.

In Mr. Davies-Colley's case of traumatic separation of this epiphysis repair had taken place, leaving considerable range of movement, but with marked projection of the great trochanter.

A similar good result, both as regards union and function of the limb, is recorded by Mr. A. E. Maylard (*British Medical Journal*, April 2, 1892, p. 709) in the following case under his care at the Victoria Infirmary at Glasgow.

'A boy, aged seventeen, was admitted on November 15, 1891. He had stumbled over a plank and fallen into a pit about eighteen feet deep. He had no power to raise the left leg from the bed; the foot was everted and there was slight shortening. On measuring from the anterior superior spine of the ilium to the great trochanter, the distance on the left side was increased by one inch. The left trochanter was, in appearance, more prominent than the right, and was on a higher level. Passive movement of the limb caused a corresponding movement of the trochanter, accompanied with the sensation of " cartilaginous " crepitus at the seat of fracture. He suffered very little pain. After about two months' residence in the infirmary he left, with neither appreciable shortening of the limb nor impairment of its function.'

In the two cases mentioned by Mr. Hutchinson (*Med. Times and Gazette*, vol. i. 1859, p. 162) undoubted true bony union occurred, although in one there was some doubt as to its being a real fracture of the neck of the femur; he also thinks that this tends to support the opinion that among the most efficient factors in non-union after fracture of the neck of the thigh bone in elderly persons is the age of the patient. Writing in 1866 (*Med. Times and Gazette*, February 24, 1866, page 195) he said he had seen two cases under the care of other surgeons in which this accident was diagnosed. In each the patient was between seventeen and twenty. In one union was delayed for several months, but in both it was eventually completed.

Dr. E. H. Bradford, of Boston, U.S.A., records (*loc. cit. supra*) the result in two cases which had been diagnosed as epiphysial separation.

CASE I.   A healthy boy, sixteen years of age, reported himself for examination with the following history: He had been perfectly well, and had not been lame. On attempting to milk a cow, seated on an ordinary milking-stool, he was kicked at by the cow and turned quickly to avoid a blow, suffering a sensation of sudden pain. Immediately after this he was unable to step and was taken to the house, being obliged to remain in bed several weeks.

He was etherised, and the limb, which was flexed, painful, and useless, was put into position, and made a recovery, but he was able to walk about only with crutches for some time. At the time of examination, three months later, he walked with crutches and could do so without them, but with marked lameness. He suffered no pain. An examination showed that the affected limb was shorter by an inch than the fellow. The trochanter was above the Nélaton line to that extent. The motions at the hip-joint were perfectly free, with the exception of inversion, which was not possible beyond the right angle. It was entirely free on the other side.

CASE II.   A child, seven years old, of fairly good health, sustained a fall from the window in the first story. The patient was taken up, placed in bed, and complained of great pain; but no injury of the limb was determined at the time. The child was of a nervous type, and it was thought that her symptoms were due to fright rather than to any injury to the bone. She remained in bed for several weeks, finally was able to get up, and after a while to walk, though she still limped. Upon examination, four months after the accident, it was found that the head of the trochanter was half an inch higher on the right, the affected side, than normal. The head of the trochanter was also placed more posteriorly than is normal, and the foot was everted. The motions at the hip-joint were free, with the exception of the inversion, which was not possible beyond the vertical. The patient was free from pain and able to walk. A rotation of the thorax had taken place in the four months, and the ribs on the right side projected.

Where no treatment has been adopted, the limb has been found permanently shortened and everted, but the patient had more or less complete use of it; this was the condition in Mr. Robson's case (*loc. cit. supra*). In this connection Dr. E. H. Bradford mentions two cases of deformity after separation of the epiphysis of the head of the femur which were brought to the Children's Hospital, Boston, U.S.A. (*Medical and Surgical Report of the Children's Hospital*, 1869–94, Boston, U.S.A., 1895, p. 292), with a history of a fall, followed by severe pain for three or four weeks, and lameness subsequent to ·this. In neither of the cases had the lesion been recognised. In one there was shortening of an inch, in the other of half an inch. In one there was marked inversion (? eversion) ; in the other there was but little. In the first, a girl of twelve, osteotomy of the neck of the femur was performed, and the limb brought into a normal position and treated by traction for several weeks. The result was satisfactory, but the shortening of an inch was not entirely overcome. Perfect motion at the joint was re-established six months after the operation. The eversion of the foot, which constituted a disfiguring deformity, was entirely corrected.

In the second case, a boy of four, there was no noticeable eversion, and no operation was attempted.

Dr. R. H. Harte (*Trans. Amer. Surg. Association*, vol. xv. 1897, p. 222) reports the following example of epiphysial separation of the head of the femur, in which the recent condition after injury is described as well as the appearance of the limb four months later. There was about one inch of shortening.

R. C., aged fifteen years, of fair physical development but of impaired mental condition, was admitted to the Episcopal Hospital on December 28, 1896, several days after the injury. He had slipped on the ice when walking, striking his hip, and was carried home, being unable to walk. On admission there was inability to stand or bear weight on the injured limb, and some tenderness over the hip. In the dorsal position with the legs together and moderate extension, the shortening disappeared so completely that at first Dr. Harte was disposed to consider it simply as a contusion of the hip ; moreover, all movements could be performed almost without pain, and with little restriction of motion. On the following day there was again marked deformity, with about one inch shortening, and some prominence of the trochanter ; there was no eversion of the foot, although this could be effected with pressure on the inner side of the foot. Inversion of the foot was equally carried out ; in fact, under ether all the normal movements of the joint could be exaggerated. The trochanter could be rotated more than on the uninjured side, but without any apparent diminution in its arc. No distinct crepitus could be elicited, although some slight rubbing sensation was detected, as though two rough cartilaginous surfaces were brought in contact. A skiagraph was taken with an indifferent result. The patient was treated in bed with extension by means of weight and sandbags for lateral support. The extension was removed on February 9 with apparently good union, and measurements showed no difference ·in the length of the limbs. The patient was soon permitted to leave his bed, but owing to his mental condition he acquired the art of walking slowly, and left the hospital soon at the request of his parents. On examination, four months after the injury, there was a slight limp on walking and a shortening of about one inch. The movements of the injured limb were slightly embarrassed, apparently unaccompanied with pain; no eversion of foot, although it could be everted beyond normal; it could be equally inverted; the thigh could be flexed, without tilting the pelvis, to about forty-five degrees, no roughening on moving the joint, the articular functions being performed without friction; fair abduction without tilting of the pelvis, of about two and a half feet from the median line; the upper margin of the trochanter being slightly above Nélaton's line, and the prominence of the trochanter being increased about three-quarters of an inch, with distinct depression behind it. There was some flattening of the gluteal muscles and disappearance of the rima-natium. The muscles of the injured limb were equally nourished with the opposite side. Another attempt to skiagraph the joint proved unsatisfactory. Dr. Harte also saw another example under Dr. Barton at the Philadelphia Hospital in which the most pronounced remaining symptoms were the undue prominence of the trochanter, with one and a half inches shortening, impairment of motion, which appeared to be intensified by a number of osteophytes or periosteal new growths round the joint, and a distinct limp on walking.

Non-union.—The grave prognosis—the lameness and atrophy of the limb—which are said by so many of the older writers to be the inevitable consequences of separation of this epiphysis, may be traced to Van Swieten, who quotes Boerhaave as giving a grave prognosis in this as in epiphysial separation in general.

Reichel relates (*loc. cit. supra*) a case seen by Ludwig of a young man, aged twenty, who had had from infancy a separation of the femoral head. There was no union, and a false joint developed, which allowed the man to turn the limb in all directions and to carry his foot easily up to his head. The limb was twelve inches shorter than the other.

Mayo Robson's case also appears to be one of non-union.

Mr. Jonathan Hutchinson says: ' In the later stage of confirmed non-union, which according to my experience is that which most frequently comes under notice, the symptoms are those of unreduced dislocation upon the dorsum, but with very free mobility and with inability to find the rounded head of the bone. The femur can generally be rotated with unusual ease, and in some instances pushed upwards and pulled downwards with considerable freedom.' He then gives the following three cases (' On Detachment of the Epiphysial Head of the Femur,' *Archives of Surgery*, vol. iii. No. 12, April 1892) as examples of this condition of things, in conjunction with a history entirely negative as regards disease.

The following note, he states, is only an unverified fragment, but all that bears upon detachment of the upper epiphysis of the femur is so valuable that he did not like to wholly neglect it. A very intelligent man told him that one of his brothers had been obliged all his life to wear a high-heeled boot because 'one hip had been dislocated' in a fall from his rocking-horse when a child. The 'dislocation' had not been recognised or reduced, and hence permanent shortening of the limb. The diagnosis of dislocation was based upon opinions given by consultants long after the accident. Looking at the age of the patient, and also at the fact that the early diagnosis was missed, it is far more likely to have been a detached epiphysis than a real dislocation. Mr. Hutchinson never saw the patient.

His next case is a more detailed one. A little girl presented conditions which were very suggestive of an ununited separation of the epiphysis. She was four years of age, very active, said to be always in motion, and never complaining of pain. She had never been laid up by any illness. There was a history of two accidents in infancy, one at the age of one month, and the other at the age of six months; but after neither of them had there been any special treatment. Her condition when brought to Mr. Hutchinson was that the right limb was one inch shorter than the other, the shortening being apparently at the hip. There was neither inversion nor eversion, but the limb was simply shorter and too movable at the hip. The great trochanter was much nearer the crest of the ilium on that side than on the other; and the distance between these points could be considerably altered by pulling the limb up and down. Eversion and inversion were also much too free. The examination did not cause the child the slightest pain. A diagnosis of infantile paralysis had formerly been given by a distinguished physician. Any indications in support of this opinion could not, however, be found. The limb was well nourished, just as useful as the other, and not liable to become cold. The two calves were of the same girth; nor was there any wasting to be observed about the thigh or buttock. The diagnosis seemed to rest between an ununited separation of the head and disease of the hip-joint with absorption of the head of the bone; or possibly a pathological detachment of the epiphysis. With the exception of a rumour that the child used at one time to complain of pain in the knee, there was no history of any symptoms pointing to inflammation of the joint. The child had never been laid up, nor had she ever worn an apparatus.

The preceding case came under notice seven or eight years previously, and Mr. Hutchinson had recently seen its exact counterpart. Indeed, he found it hard to believe that it was not the same patient who was again brought to him, for it was the same limb, and the advance in age fitted exactly. Miss G., a little slim active girl, aged twelve, was wearing a boot with two inches of additional heel, and her right limb measured exactly two inches shorter than the other. Yet she could scarcely be considered lame, and he was told that she would run and play as freely as other girls. There was no history of any disease. She had never had any illness, and had never at any time complained of pain in the hip. The monthly nurse, who was a careful person, observed nothing peculiar in her limbs at birth. It was not until she was several months old that it was discovered that there was something amiss with her right hip, and in the interval (her mother having died) she had been in the sole charge of a nurse girl, who had on one occasion, it was rumoured, in a passion thrown the crying baby from one end of the bed to the other. This was the only history of injury which could be obtained. From the time of the first discovery of deformity to the present date, the shortening of the affected limb had been steadily increasing, and it has been needful to make the heel thicker and thicker. With the exception of this, there has been no inconvenience. On examining the limb, its nutrition was perfect. There was, as above stated, two inches of real shortening. The hip was very obviously prominent, and the great trochanter was not more than an inch and a half below the middle of the crest of the ilium. The foot was usually pointed straight, but it could be inverted or everted very easily. It was not easy to push the great trochanter upwards or downwards, but its freedom of rotation was remarkable. The buttock being very thin, it was quite easy to feel a prominence of bone slanting obliquely upwards from the trochanter. This might be the head or only the decapitated neck of the bone. Mr. Hutchinson was inclined to believe that it was the latter, for the following reasons. Firstly, the rounded head could not be felt; secondly, it was shorter than usual in dislocations; thirdly, it was very freely movable; and fourthly, it might be rotated to such an extent that it could be felt now behind and now in front of the shaft. It cannot be possible that this last-named alteration of position could be effected in a case of dislocation of the entire bone. These conditions made it, he thought, quite certain that in this case the femur had lost its articular head. The diagnosis lay between a detachment of the epiphysis by violence, a congenital dislocation of a deformed bone, and absorption or detachment of the head by disease. He inclined to the first-named. There was not a tittle of evidence in favour of disease; nor, if the conditions were pathological, could it be believed that the freedom of motion would be what it was.

The cases which he recorded in this paper clearly proved that there are conditions occasionally met with which are most easily explained on the supposition that the cartilaginous head of the bone has been left in the acetabulum, wholly detached from the neck, as the result of violence in very early infancy. They must not, he says, be held to do more, however, than to establish a certain amount of probability. That they constitute a very interesting group of cases which has as yet received very little attention will be readily admitted.

The views of the author on this subject of epiphysial separations of the upper femoral epiphysis in infants have already been given.

Mr. D. Wallace, of Edinburgh (*Lancet*, August 20, 1892, p. 421), gives the following account of a case he saw in April 1892 which was supposed to have been an old-standing dislocation of the hip-joint. On examination he concluded that it was probably a diastasis through the neck of the femur, not a dislocation.

M. B., aged eleven years, a girl of good build, tall and strong for her age, was said by her mother to have been a well-nourished child, who walked before she was nine months old. When arrived at this age she fell out of her cot, and the mother believes that when falling the right foot caught between the bars, so that the leg was severely twisted. The child cried, and refused to stand up or allow the leg to be moved. There were pain and swelling in the neighbourhood of the hip. Hot fomentations were applied during the first few days, but in the course of two or three weeks (?) a doctor was called in, who said the hip-joint was dislocated, and attempted to reduce it, but failed to do so. Two or three years later the child walked with a distinct halt, and the hip was prominent. At this time the mother showed the girl to a 'bone-setter,' who tried 'to put the bone in,' but also failed. The swelling and lameness persisted until the time of examination, but the girl walked, ran, and jumped usually without any pain, although after much romping she now and then complained of pain at the hip. No other injury had been sustained, and there was no history of joint or chest disease in the patient or in other members of the family. The patient complained of no pain or discomfort, but said she was lame and that the 'leg comes out at the haunch.' She walked with a distinct limp, and when she stood the right foot was observed to be a little more everted than the left, while there were marked drooping and rotation forwards of the right anterior superior iliac spine. The right limb was evidently shorter than the left.

The measurements were : From anterior superior iliac spine to internal malleolus : right, 27 inches ; left, 29¾ inches. From anterior superior iliac spine to tip of patella : right, 14 inches ; left, 16 inches. From tip of trochanter major to external condyle : right, 13¾ inches ; left, 14¼ inches. Nélaton's line on the right side passed 1½ inches below the tip of the trochanter ; on the left side it was normal. The right thigh could be flexed on the abdomen, but not quite so fully as the left. Rotation of the right was greater than the left. Abduction was equal on the two sides. When the right leg was flexed on the thigh and the thigh on the abdomen the trochanter major was felt as a distinct prominence midway between the anterior superior spine of the ilium and the ischial tuberosity, and moved through a much wider radius than the left. No rounded prominence corresponding to the head of the femur could be felt, but there was a distinct mass of bone projecting internally to the trochanter, which moved with the trochanter. When rotary movements were carried out, a rough grating was felt deeply seated. The right leg was thinner than the left, but was muscular and showed no sign of malnutrition.

From a consideration of the above points in this case Mr. Wallace concluded that it was a diastasis of the neck of the femur, because of (1) a history of injury at an early age, but subsequent to the child walking; (2) no history or appearance of tuberculous disease; (3) marked displacement of the trochanter major upwards, associated with very free movement and eversion of the foot; and (4) a slight degree of shortening of the femur.

The author cannot think that *non-union* is the rule after epiphysial separation of the head of the bone, provided the lesion has been diagnosed; an examination of the result of cases in which a diagnosis was made soon after the accident points in quite an opposite direction—a firm and good union.

Non-union occurs in exceptional cases where the displacement of the neck is very great, and the periosteum of the neck extensively lacerated; such a condition must be quite exceptional, and associated with great violence and severe injury to the soft parts. We must remember the great strength and toughness of the periosteal covering of the femoral neck.

The cases which the author has quoted as described by Hutchinson, Wallace, and others were, as these surgeons suggest, in all probability separations of the head or of the cartilaginous upper end of the bone in infancy, but it is most likely that there was but little displacement at the time. From the fact of no immediate diagnosis being made and from the fact that no treatment was adopted, the child being allowed to move or walk about, it is more than probable that displacement took place gradually, thereby effectually preventing any union taking place between the diaphysis and the head of the bone. In many of these instances the violence causing the injury was by no means severe.

Sayre, in addition to the case quoted above (*loc. cit. supra*) as having a new acetabulum formed, mentions another which was still under his treatment. Both cases presented marked similarity in history and symptoms. The injury occurred to each patient at the age of two years, and when seen two years later the symptoms in both instances were: flexion of the thigh to a right angle; slight adduction; extreme rotation outwards; almost complete fixation of the limb in this position; and, with these, the total absence of pain, tenderness, suppuration, or interference with health, such as are the usual evidences of carious disease of the articulation. The treatment in both cases consisted in subcutaneous section of the adductor longus, gracilis, and tensor vaginæ femoris muscles; reposition of the limb in the extended state; breaking up the existing adhesions; and the subsequent employment of this author's wire breeches and extension splint.

Rigidity of joint and limb.—Subsequent mobility of the joint is usually good. However, in some instances new periosteal deposit or osteophytic processes round the neck of the bone, especially in front, may greatly hamper or even annihilate the function of the hip-joint.

Suppuration may ensue from periostitis or ostitis, or may be due simply to the injury to the epiphysial cartilage line.

Hamilton quotes a case recorded by Dr. Parker of New York (*Amer. Med. Gazette*, November 30, 1850, vol. i. p. 342). A girl, aged eighteen, had been injured by a fall upon a curb-stone when eleven years old. The accident was followed by suppuration and a fistulous discharge, from which, however, she finally recovered, but with the foot everted and a shortening of one inch and a half. ' Flexion and rotation of the joint occasioned no inconvenience.' This latter circumstance alone was thought sufficient to distinguish it from hip disease, in which ankylosis is the termination.

Suppuration and necrosis of any extensive portion of the diaphysis are not, however, common results of separation of this epiphysis, judging by the recorded cases.

Acute hip disease. with rapid necrosis of the head or some small part of the neck, is more commonly the effect of epiphysial detachment, mostly of the incomplete form, rather than the cause of displacement at this epiphysis.

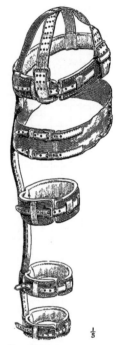

Fig. 198.—THOMAS'S HIP SPLINT, WITH BROAD PELVIC BAND

Death from pyæmia may even result under certain circumstances.

Arrest of growth of the femur does not occur to any appreciable extent after injury to this epiphysis, for very little of the growth of the femur takes place at this end of the bone.

TREATMENT. SEPARATION WITHOUT DISPLACEMENT.—Any of the forms of plastic splint about to be mentioned below should be carefully and firmly applied wherever a partial separation is supposed to have occurred. Careful padding with cotton wool should be used wherever necessary. In the milder forms of separation without displacement a Thomas's hip splint may be

U U

preferred with or without extension. A very guarded prognosis should be given, on account of the possible subsequent affection of the hip-joint.

SEPARATION WITH DISPLACEMENT.—In all cases of displacement the end of the femur should be brought down by gentle steady traction into as accurate apposition with the head as possible. No circumduction or severe manipulation is permissible, on account of the risk of further stripping the periosteum from the neck of the bone. The limb should be maintained in position by

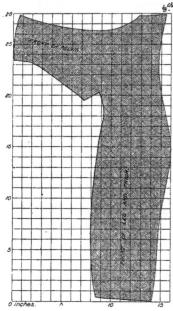

FIG. 199.—PATTERN IN HOUSE-FLANNEL OF PLASTER-OF-PARIS SPLINT FOR HIP, ENCIRCLING PELVIS AND LOWER EXTREMITY. FOR A CHILD OF EIGHT YEARS

Reduced to one-eighth size on scale of inches

means of an immovable apparatus, with extension, for three to four weeks. Bryant's double outside splint with interruptions and the long thigh splint with perineal band and extension are suitable, or a plaster-of-Paris splint round the pelvis and whole of thigh may be immediately applied during extension, under an anæsthetic. At the end of the month the pelvis and thigh should be surrounded by a plaster-of-Paris, poroplastic, starch, laminated plaster, or Hide's splinting, and the patient allowed to move about on crutches, or the plaster-of-Paris splint may be applied from the commencement. Good union may be anticipated in these cases, but it is not so rapid as in other separations on account of the probable contact of synovial secretion with the fractured surfaces.

'Far more,' says Packard, 'may be expected from treatment, in a lesion of this kind, than in the fractures which affect the same region in advanced life. Such shortening as exists may be corrected by extension with the weight and pulley, and the joint may be immobilised by means of a well-applied plaster-of-Paris bandage round the pelvis and thigh. This confinement may be continued, with sandbags on either side of the limb, and the extension kept up, for two or three weeks in the case of a child; a longer confinement would be advantageous in patients beyond the age of puberty. Cautious experiments should be made at first in allowing flexion of the hip-joint, but if they are productive of no pain or irritation more and more freedom may be accorded to the patient until he can move the limb without hindrance, after which, with equal caution, he may be encouraged to put the foot to the ground and bear his weight upon it.'

A number of years ago Packard had (Ashhurst, *Encyclopædia of Surgery*, vol. iv. 1884, p. 198) a case which he believed was really a separation of the epiphysis. A boy, nineteen years of age, by a fall from a very high wagon-seat, had sustained a fracture of the cervix femoris, the existence of which was verified under ether. He was treated in the manner above mentioned, and in six weeks was

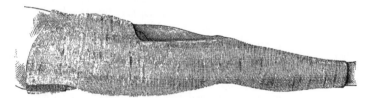

Fig. 200.—Plaster-of-Paris splint applied to right hip, pelvis, and lower extremity

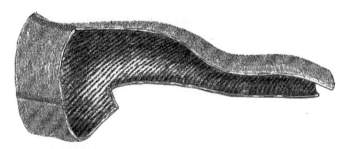

Fig. 201.—Plaster-of-Paris hip splint removed

driving his wagon again, with scarcely any perceptible lameness in walking.

Passive flexion and massage should be carefully carried out at the hip-joint and daily repeated more and more freely. It should be commenced at the end of the third week, and at the beginning of the fifth week the child will be able to bear some weight upon the leg.

Excision of the epiphysial head.—Should it be found impossible to replace the diaphysis in its normal position after severe displacements, excision of the detached head is to be recommended.

Notwithstanding that there is sufficient blood supply to the head through the ligamentum teres and periosteum, much of which remains attached to its circumference, to carry on its nutrition, still the impossibility of union taking place between the widely separated surfaces, and the possibility of great permanent deformity from eversion and shortening of the limb, render this advisable.

The same operation should be performed in older cases of displacement where a new acetabulum has not yet formed, and there is a hope of remedying deformity. The end of the bone will in all probability make a very efficient head, as exemplified by Professor Sayre's and Kocher's cases, quoted above. For this operation the anterior incision will be found preferable to the posterior.

Union of recent separations with displacement.—Fastening the fragments together by means of a steel pin has also been recommended. If attempted, the most rigid antiseptic and aseptic precautions should be carried out, otherwise suppuration may result as in the following case, recorded by C. A. Sturrock (*Edinburgh Hospital Reports*, vol. ii. 1894, p. 604). A boy of fourteen, when at play, fell and twisted his hip; his leg was examined shortly after the accident by several medical men, when the following points were made out—the presence of pain, unusual mobility, shortening, eversion of the leg, with absence of crepitus. The displacement was easily reduced, but at once recurred when the leg was let alone. The leg was subjected to prolonged and somewhat severe manipulations, and shortly afterwards the great trochanter was cut down upon and a rigid pin passed through it, the neck of the femur, and into the head. Unfortunately suppuration occurred in the wound, and the pin had to be withdrawn in two days. At the time of the report (1894)—i.e. some years after the accident—the leg was shortened and the thigh flexed, the patient walking with a marked limp.

Osteotomy for deformity.—When much deformity results from a separation which has been long overlooked and has united in a faulty position, osteotomy or some other operative measure is required to bring the limb into its normal position.

Professor Hoffa, of Würzburg, has performed osteotomy through the neck of the femur with success in these cases. In Dr. E. H. Bradford's case of osteotomy of the neck of the femur the deformity arising from the eversion of the foot was entirely corrected, but the shortening of one inch was not entirely overcome, although traction was continued for several weeks. The result, he states, was satisfactory, perfect movement at the hip-joint being re-established six months later.

CHAPTER III

SEPARATION OF THE EPIPHYSIS OF THE GREAT TROCHANTER

ANATOMY.—The cartilaginous mass of this epiphysis is separated from that of the lesser trochanter during the second year, although it is still blended with the head.

At the commencement of the fourth year, when it is almost isolated from the head of the bone by the growth of the neck, its centre of ossification appears. At an earlier date, however, during the first or second year, its site is often indicated by the appearance of a few bony granules. Two additional smaller centres are frequently met with close together, the anterior of which forms the anterior tubercle of the great trochanter; these soon unite, and about the fifth or sixth year join the main centre, which is placed more posteriorly. Up to the seventeenth year some cartilage is still to be found capping this epiphysis; beyond this date to the time of its final union with the diaphysis, from the eighteenth to nineteenth year, it is entirely osseous. Union usually takes place first towards the digital fossa.

This epiphysis is separated by its thin cartilaginous layer from the broad rough irregular surface on the upper end of the diaphysis; on the posterior aspect of the latter a distinct ledge is seen, which acts as a kind of buttress for the epiphysis and prevents its displacement in this direction.

Included in this epiphysis is the whole of the digital fossa with the insertion of the obturator externus, together with nearly the upper half of the posterior inter-trochanteric line. Above it slightly overlaps the upper border of the neck and corresponds to the limit of the capsule in this situation. Its lower border, joining the diaphysis externally, marks the insertion of the tendinous fibres of the vastus externus, and to its anterior, outer, and inner surfaces and upper border the powerful gluteal and other muscles are attached.

The line of junction of the epiphysis of the great trochanter with the shaft of the femur corresponds to the ' tubercle of the quadratus ' (Thane) situated on the posterior border of the great trochanter.

The lower edge of the epiphysial line where it joins the outer aspect of the diaphysis is 3 cm. 4 mm. below the upper margin of the trochanter at the thirteenth year; at the eighteenth year, 4 cm. 3 mm.

The antero-posterior width of the epiphysis at the thirteenth year is 3 cm. 5 mm.; at the eighteenth year, 4 cm. 2 mm.

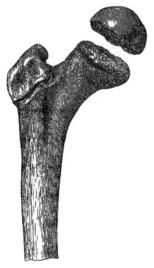

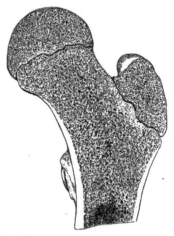

Fig. 203.—VERTICAL SECTION OF UPPER END OF FEMUR AT SIXTEEN AND A HALF YEARS. POSTERIOR HALF OF SECTION, SHOWING CANCELLOUS STRUCTURE OF THE EPIPHYSES ($\frac{2}{3}$-size)

Fig. 202.—ANTERIOR VIEW OF EPIPHYSES AT UPPER END OF FEMUR AT ABOUT THE FIFTEENTH YEAR. ($\frac{1}{2}$-size)

AGE.—From the anatomical condition of this epiphysis it would appear likely that separation should be most frequent between the thirteenth and eighteenth years. In seven out of ten recorded examples it occurred between thirteen and sixteen years of age. Out of twelve published cases the author has collected, ten were confirmed after death; of these the age is given in seven—viz. four at sixteen, two at thirteen years, and one at eight years. Of those in which the age is not stated with any accuracy, one occurred in a boy and two were old separations; in one of the latter the injury was supposed to have taken place between four and eighteen years of age. In two simple cases one occurred at thirteen years of age, and one in a young man.

From the anatomical condition it cannot occur beyond the eighteenth or nineteenth year.

ETIOLOGY.—It appears that this injury is almost always the result of **direct violence**, such as a fall on the hip or severe blow on the trochanter. In one or two the blow was not severe. Out of five cases observed during life, four were from this cause.

In Hutchinson's case it was also due to direct violence, a fall from a tree ; and in W. B. Savage's, of a little girl aged eight, it was caused by her little brother jumping upon her, as she lay upon her left side on a floor.

In Hilton's case the separation was produced by a kick from a man.

Packard draws especial attention to this (*International Encyclopædia of Surgery*, vol. iv. 1884, p. 199). '.The cause of fracture of the great trochanter would seem to be invariably direct violence ; and the majority of the subjects are distinctly stated to have been below the age at which this epiphysis becomes united to the shaft. In such cases it may reasonably be supposed that the separation takes place through the cartilaginous uniting substance, but that, as in separations of other epiphyses, it may in part run through true bone, detaching a layer of it of very irregular size, shape, and thickness.'

Muscular action.—From the number of powerful muscles attached to the epiphysis, it would appear at first sight that the action of these alone will be quite sufficient to cause it. Philipp Ingrassias alluded to a very doubtful case of separation of the great trochanter by muscular violence. A young man, whilst fencing with a halberd, is said to have torn off this process by a violent movement. This is the earliest record of this injury, but its exact nature was not proved by anatomical examination.

Dr. Roddick thought that the detachment in his case was due to muscular action, the boy being a very athletic subject.

PATHOLOGICAL ANATOMY. Pure separations.—A separation of this epiphysis is a rare one, and usually not complicated by any fracture of the neck of the bone. Some particles of the cancellous tissue of the diaphysis may, however, cling to the surface of the epiphysis.

The first authentic specimen on record is that of Mr. Aston Key's case, reported by Sir Astley Cooper (Sir Astley Cooper's *Fractures and Dislocations*, 6th edit. 1829, p. 166 ; *Cyclopædia of Practical Surgery*, vol. ii., art. on 'Special Fractures,' p. 375). There was no displacement of the epiphysis during life. A girl, about sixteen years of age, in crossing the street tripped, and in falling struck her trochanter violently against the curb-stone. She immediately rose, and without much pain or difficulty walked home ; on the fifth day, in consequence of the increase of pain on the inner side of the thigh, she was admitted into Guy's Hospital in 1822. Her constitutional symptoms being evidently more violent than those which usually arose from fractured femur, she was placed under the care of the physician, Dr. Bright, at whose request Mr. Key examined the limb. The right leg, which was the one injured, was considerably everted and appeared to be about half an inch longer than the sound limb.

It admitted of passive motion in all directions, but in abduction gave her considerable pain. She had perfect command over all the muscles except the rotators inwards. The fact that she had walked both before and since her admission into the hospital gave rise to some doubts as to the existence of a fracture, and the closest examination of the trochanter and body of the femur could not detect the slightest crepitus or displacement of bone. Mr. Key repeated the examination of the limb on the following day, but the result was equally unsatisfactory. She died nine days after the accident from irritative fever. At the post-mortem examination, wishing to ascertain the exact nature of the injury, Mr. Key previous to removing the soft parts moved the limb in every direction, fixing the trochanter and head of the bone, but could perceive no deviation from the normal condition, nor was the slightest crepitus under all the variety of movements distinguishable. There was no swelling of the thigh to be observed, and therefore the trochanter and head of the femur were as readily distinguished and examined as in a healthy limb.

A fracture was found which had detached the trochanter from the body and neck of the bone, but without tearing through the tendons attached to the outer side of the process. These so effectually prevented all movement of the fractured portion that, when they were dissected from the body, not the least motion could be produced except in one direction, upwards and downwards. It was the untorn condition of tendons which allowed this hinge-like motion, and it was evident that such motion could not have been produced by any direction given to the limb ; hence it is also manifest that the fracture could not have been detected during the life of the patient.

An abscess was also discovered in front near the pectineus, extending downwards towards the lesser trochanter and backwards behind the bone to the great trochanter. The specimen is in the Guy's Hospital Museum, Prep. 1195.

The precise condition of this lesion has also been established by several other post-mortem observations. The London Hospital Museum, Prep. No. 424, contains the very interesting specimen reported by Mr. McCarthy (*Trans. Path. Soc.* vol. xxv., 1874, p. 200 ; Hutchinson's *Clinical Illustrations*, Fasc. xix., Plate lxxi., fig. 1). The patient, a girl aged eight, was brought to the hospital with a large swelling over the back of the hip. She was considered by the house surgeon too ill for examination, and died a few hours afterwards.

The post-mortem examination revealed ' an abscess in the right sterno-clavicular articulation, pyæmic pericarditis, pleurisy and pneumonia, a large extra-peritoneal abscess in the pelvis, which was connected along the tendon of the pyriformis muscle with another abscess round the neck of the left femur. The trochanteric epiphysis was completely detached from the shaft, but held in position by tendinous attachments and the reflections of the capsule. The history of the case, as subsequently ascertained, was that the child, although not strong, had never had any illness, previous to a fall on her left side a week before while playing. Some days later a lump was observed on the left hip, and the child was kept in bed in consequence, but two or three days later she seemed to have such difficulty in breathing that she was brought to the hospital. Even then the child walked, holding by her mother's hand, for about half a mile, and did not complain of any pain.

Mr. Hutchinson (*Illustrations of Clinical Surgery*, Fasc. xix. vol. ii. 1888, p. 109) mentions a specimen from the Croydon Hospital exactly similar to Mr. McCarthy's. It was from a boy of thirteen, who was crushed between a railway carriage and the platform.

Dr. F. W. Warren (*Proceedings of the Pathological Society of Dublin*, N.S. 1876, vol. vii. p. 102; *Dublin Journal of Medical Science*, vol. lxii. 1876, p. 69) gives the description of a specimen obtained from the dissecting room of Steevens's Hospital, Dublin; consequently there was no history obtainable. It was removed from the extremely muscular body of a man aged about fifty. Before dissection nothing abnormal was observed. A distinct fracture of the base of the trochanter was then found extending precisely through the epiphysial line. The detached trochanter was firmly united by dense ligamentous tissue to the shaft, although drawn upwards and inwards so that its summit projected above the level of the head of the femur. When compared with a bone prior to the union of the trochanter to the shaft through its epiphysial line, the fracture was found to take a direction exactly corresponding to the epiphysial line. The tendinous expansion over this process was intact; the gluteus medius was inserted into its apex, and the gluteus minimus into its anterior margin. Dr. Warren thought that in this case the fracture had occurred through the epiphysial line between the ages of four and eighteen years. On section the neck of the bone was perfectly healthy, as was also the hip-joint itself, there being no appearance whatever of any fracture implicating the cervix femoris.

Professor Bennett informed Dr. Warren that there were three examples of this fracture in the Museum of Trinity College, Dublin.

Agnew (*Treatise on Surgery*, vol. i. p. 945) figures an example of this injury. The specimen was in his own collection, but he gives no details of the lesion beyond that ' there was present a considerable amount of granular callus around the circumference of the fracture, though there was none between the fragments.'

There was also in this case a fracture of the condyles of the femur.

Mr. John Hilton relates another case, which is also of interest to the medical jurist (*Guy's Hospital Reports*, 3rd series, vol. xi. 1865,

p. 342). A man, seeing, as he thought, one of his boys idle on his
estate in the country, 'kicked him, causing a separation of the
epiphysis of the great trochanter from the shaft of the femur. The
age of the patient is not stated. Suppuration ensued at the
injured part, and the boy died. The farmer was indicted for
murder, having produced the boy's death, according to the report of
the medical man who made the post-mortem examination, by
"fracturing the thigh bone." The counsel for the defence took
advantage of this verbal inaccuracy in the indictment, and used it
successfully in his client's favour, proving satisfactorily that it was
not a fracture, but a simple separation of portions of bone from
disease; and so the prisoner got off. The thigh bone, trochanter,
and adjacent parts were sent to Mr. Hilton in order to verify the
separation of the epiphysis; and as no doubt could be entertained
about the character of the accident, the indictment for murder
failed from the inaccuracy of the designation of the injury to the
bone.'

J. H. Ashton records (*Lancet*, February 13, 1875, p. 231) the
case of (A. R.) a well-developed boy, aged sixteen years, who had
been swung by the arms and legs and 'bumped' on the ground.
He was able to work for some days; pain and stiffness in the hip-
joint then came on. When seen the whole thigh and parts around
the hip were greatly swollen and tender; any movement of the
joint caused great pain. All movements were normal; no crepitus.
Tongue black, pulse rapid, weak, and irregular, and constant
delirium; after a fortnight the constitutional state improved, but
the limb had lengthened to the extent of an inch or more, and
fluctuation was apparent. An abscess was opened in the West
Norfolk and Lynn Hospital, and crepitus felt by grasping the
trochanter and moving the limb. A diagnosis of fracture of the epiphysis of the great trochanter was made by Dr. Lowe. A fortnight
later the boy died, and on post-mortem examination the trochanter
was found to be fractured and broken completely from the shaft.
The joint was destroyed, and the neck and upper part of the femur
were in a state of necrosis. The author has been unable to obtain
any further account of this specimen.

The author reproduces a photograph presented to him by Professor
J. G. Adami, of McGill University, Montreal. It shows a very pure
separation of the trochanteric epiphysis. In a note of this specimen,
kindly supplied by Professor Adami, he remarks: 'It shows the
trochanter major completely separated from the rest of the bone,
probably from fracture, for the head and the lesser trochanter are completely joined. The history of the case had been lost.' (See fig. 204.)

Separation with fracture.—Mr. Jonathan Hutchinson junior's
specimen in the Royal College of Surgeons Museum, No. 1021A,
shows separation of the epiphysis of the great trochanter in the
upper end of a femur, from a lad, aged thirteen, who fell between a

railway platform and the train.   The epiphysis, taking with it the attachments of the gluteus medius and minimus and the adjacent periosteum, is raised up; and the section shows that the line of separation followed the epiphysial disc exactly at the outer side, but passed above it on the inner (towards the neck of the bone) through the structure of the great trochanter upwards for a short distance.

The same surgeon exhibited, on December 3, 1895, before the Pathological Society, London (*Trans. Path. Soc.* vol. xlvii. p. 174), a specimen of traumatic separation of this epiphysis, given to him by Dr. Daniels, of British Guiana, and obtained from a native of the latter place aged sixteen. The lad had fallen from a tree to the ground, a distance of nearly twenty feet.   He survived for some eight weeks, dying from the effects of various internal

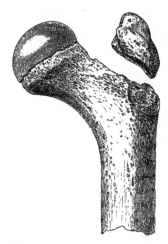

FIG. 204.—PURE SEPARATION OF GREAT TROCHANTER

(McGill University Museum, Montreal, Canada)

injuries, including rupture of the liver.   After the accident he had been able to stand and to raise the affected limb from the bed, so that a positive diagnosis was not made.   The post-mortem examination showed that the trochanter had been separated exactly at the epiphysial line, except at the lower and posterior corner, where a small portion of the diaphysis was also detached.   There was a decided interval between the epiphysis and the femur, but they were connected by the periosteum, which had been stripped off the shaft for some inches whilst still retaining its attachment below. No suppuration had occurred, and evidence of commencing repair was shown in the production of new bone in the neighbourhood of the injury.   The specimen is in the Royal College of Surgeons Museum, No. 1041H.

SYMPTOMS.—From the symptoms given in many instances by various authors the diagnosis is often a matter of considerable difficulty. As the usual signs pointing to fracture of the neck of the bone are absent, and as the shaft of the femur is uninjured, the patient might continue his occupation until pain and swelling come on—from irritation or inflammation of the surrounding structures. This was so in Ashton's case.

SEPARATION WITHOUT DISPLACEMENT.—On account of the dense tendinous and fibrous structures surrounding this epiphysis, *little or no displacement* may be present at first, the trochanter rotating freely with the shaft, through being held by the tendinous fibres of the muscles passing from it to the shaft, the very tough periosteum, and the outward prolongation of the fibres of the capsular ligament.

In fact, displacement may not be present at any time, so that the injury may be entirely overlooked.

The child may be able to stand, or even use his limb to raise it from the bed, or even walk, as illustrated by several of the recorded instances.

This fact may account in some measure for the peculiar mortality from suppuration and pyæmia in quite unsuspected cases, the irritation of movements of the epiphysial fragment upon the diaphysis producing severe inflammation and suppuration.

Pain at seat of injury, increased by movements of the limb tending to separate the fragments or by pressure on the great trochanter, and **some loss of the natural functions** of the limb, are present.

Inability to use the limb freely exists when the fragments are displaced. As this may be absent at first, only supervening in the course of a few days, the patient may even be able to walk for some time after the injury, as in Roddick's case.

Considerable swelling and extravasation are likely to be present over the trochanter, especially if the injury, as is the case most commonly, be caused by direct violence.

In relating his case, Professor Roddick (*loc. cit. supra*) says: 'The process being firmly held by the tendinous expansions covering it, the patient was able to walk with comparative ease for several days, until these suddenly gave way, either from ulceration or periosteal effusion. None of the ordinary symptoms of fracture were found at any time.'

For the same reason **muffled crepitus** is usually absent. It can only be elicited by fixing the thigh in the abducted position, and gently moving the trochanter to and fro, or by rotating the thigh very fully. Any severe manipulation would, however, only hasten a disastrous result; this sign, therefore, should not be sought for too persistently. In the same way the trochanter will move normally in rotating the limb.

Even supposing *some displacement* were present, its detection will be found very difficult on account of the distance-between the fragments and the surrounding extravasation of blood.

SEPARATION WITH DISPLACEMENT. **Deformity.**—The epiphysis will be drawn upwards and somewhat backwards and inwards by the powerful gluteal and rotator muscles attached to it, and a distinct cleft felt between the shaft and epiphysis.

There is no shortening or twisting of the limb, while loss of function of the limb, pain and swelling, may be even more marked than in separation without displacement.

If the displacement is great the trochanter will *not* follow the movements of the shaft; but it is improbable that the flattened upper end of the shaft can be felt, on account of the swelling present in these instances of severe injury.   The trochanter is fairly movable.

Crepitus.—The epiphysis will in this case have to be gently drawn downwards to obtain crepitus.

Eversion of the foot and limb, if present, will only be slightly marked.

Shortening of the limb, mentioned by Sir Astley Cooper, is impossible in an uncomplicated case of separation.

Packard says : 'There cannot be shortening of the limb, and in rotating the thigh the trochanter cannot describe a smaller arc than normal, but will either fail to follow the movements of the limb, or, if the fibrous coverings are untorn, will behave as under normal conditions.'

The late Mr. Alfred Poland (Bryant's *Practice of Surgery,* 4th edit. 1884, vol. ii. p. 446) had a case of deformity of the hip following separation of this epiphysis under his care in Guy's Hospital, December 1871, which was characterised by thickening and projection of the trochanter.

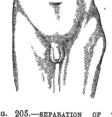

FIG. 205.—SEPARATION OF THE EPIPHYSIS OF THE GREAT TROCHANTER.   ALFRED POLAND'S CASE (T. BRYANT)

A. G., aged thirteen, ran up against a bar, striking his left hip.   Some swelling and pain were occasioned at the time, and were treated by blistering.   On examination four months after the accident, flexion and extension were found to be normal, but abduction, adduction, and rotation inwards and outwards were all limited. There was *projection,* with thickening of the great trochanter, the tip of which was the same distance from the anterior superior spine as that of the opposite side.   No shortening of the limb took place.   When out of bed the patient complained of much pain about the knee.

The following case, reported by Dr. W. B. Savage (*New York Medical Record,* 1895, xlvii. p. 690), differed from that of Sir A. Cooper and others, inasmuch as the epiphysial fragment was freely movable and drawn from its natural position by the gluteus medius and minimus muscles.

Ivy H., female, aged eight, on February 26, 1895, while playing with her little brother, was jumped on by him as she lay on her left side on the floor. The patient said that after the accident she had walked across the floor unaided, and her attention was called to her right hip 'by feeling something pricking her' at that point. Examination showed a portion of bone just protruding through the skin, over the site of the great trochantèr of the right side. This fragment was found to be freely movable beneath the skin, and apparently completely detached from the femur, and by moving it a little to one side a depression could be distinctly felt at the trochanteric site.

Upon pressing the fragment again in position, crepitus could be easily made out. Flexion and extension could be effected with the injured limb without discomfort, while abduction elicited pain. The wound in the skin made by the edge of the epiphysis was so small that it was deemed best to replace the piece of bone in position. To this end an extension by weight was hit on, both to overcome the eel-like tendencies of the child and to facilitate inspection of the surface wound; fixation of the epiphysis to the femur was made with bands of adhesive plaster and pads; the whole limb was then steadied between heavy sandbags. The surface wound was dressed antiseptically, and was completely healed six days later. On March 23, about four weeks after the receipt of the injury, the child was allowed to get up; at this time the epiphysis was completely united to the femur without any deformity.

DIFFERENTIAL DIAGNOSIS. Contusion of trochanteric region.— Where there is *no displacement*, as in Key's case, the diagnosis is one of great difficulty from the swelling and bruising being present in both. Mobility of the epiphysis is the only distinguishing sign, but even this must frequently be less marked than in the case of other epiphysial separations, on account of the closeness with which the tough periosteum and tendinous expansion bind it to the diaphysis. Muffled crepitus, if present, will be conclusive of separation.

Dislocation of the hip.— The epiphysis, if displaced, comes to occupy very much the same position as the femoral head in dorsal dislocation. The mobility of the epiphysis and the comparative rarity of dislocation in children are sufficient to distinguish it. Crepitus, if obtainable on drawing the epiphysis downwards, with the other signs is pathognomonic.

Packard says: 'When the trochanter is broken completely away from the shaft, it will probably be drawn upwards, inwards, and backwards by the action of the muscular fibres inserted into it; and in such a case it will be transferred from its normal place to that occupied by the head of the femur in backward and upward luxation.'

Stanley, speaking of the danger of confusion between these two lesions, urges 'the positive resemblance of the fractured portion of the trochanter to the head of the femur, the former occupying the same place which the latter would in dislocation; and if with these circumstances there should happen to be an eversion of the injuréd limb, the difficulty of the diagnosis must be considerably increased.'

Fracture of the neck of the femur (extracapsular).—Separation of the trochanteric epiphysis is readily distinguishable from this injury by the absence of shortening of the limb and neck of the bone, and by the absence of rotation of the epiphysis during the movements imparted to the shaft.

The latter symptom is only present when the trochanter is displaced, otherwise it may be held by the tendinous and periosteal structures to the shaft and rotate with it; but in this case it will describe the same arc on rotation of the thigh as on the uninjured side.

An anæsthetic should be administered in all cases to render the diagnosis certain.

PROGNOSIS AND RESULTS are favourable when there is but little displacement of the epiphysis, although from the twelve recorded cases it would appear to be a most fatal form of separation, two cases only in which it was diagnosed during life having recovered. Even more frequently than in other epiphysial separations displacement is absent, as we have seen in the above instances, and the injury probably remains undetected in many cases.

A considerable amount of callus formed in Agnew's and Hutchinson's specimens, indicating a great disposition to natural repair, but this apparently occurs less often than in other epiphysial separations.

In Mr. Alfred Poland's case deformity was present four months after the injury, with thickening and projection of the trochanter.

When there is great displacement, union will probably take place by fibrous tissue, or be delayed for a considerable time; this is likely due to the thinness of the periosteal covering, which will be more or less torn across in displacement of the epiphysis.

Complications.—Being more of an apophysis than a true epiphysis at the end of a long bone, *no arrest of growth* or important deformity of the limb or neighbouring joint need be feared.

Suppuration.—Separation of this process is perhaps of as much interest to the pathologist as to the surgeon. In three out of six cases suppuration with pyæmic symptoms rapidly ensued after the accident.

It is not clear why this epiphysis should be more prone than others to start infective disease after injury. It may be that (1) the bruising of the epiphysial junction is more considerable by reason of the greater amount of violence required to produce the injury; and that (2) the extensive stripping up of the periosteum from the very vascular upper end of the bone must of necessity occur.

It is remarkable that out of six cases seen during life, the injury in five (those of McCarthy, Ashton, Roddick, Hilton, Key) was rapidly followed by suppuration and death with pyæmic symptoms, as if the lesion to the epiphysial junction, whether from bruising or simply from the separation of the process, afforded a peculiarly favourable nidus for germs to develop and start this infective condition, which is not so often found in simple separations of the other epiphyses. Death from other injuries resulted in three out of the twelve cases.

Jonathan Hutchinson junior says (*British Medical Journal*, March 31, 1894, p. 671) : ' Out of eleven cases, no fewer than six were followed by suppuration (five of these ending fatally).'

Hamilton says : ' The cases reported would seem to show that in epiphysial separation of this process there is a peculiar tendency to the formation of pus and of general pyæmic infection, and which may perhaps find its explanation in the great vascularity of the bony structure at this point, and in the fact that the lesion of this spongy tissue especially exposes the patient to the absorption of the septic materials.'

This cancellous tissue forming the base of the great trochanter, which is in reality an apophysis, is certainly of a lighter and more spongy character than that in contact with the true epiphyses of the long bones. A considerable area of such structure is involved in this injury.

The great trochanter being entirely extracapsular, the hip-joint cannot readily be affected.

The most important case is reported by Professor T. J Roddick, of McGill University, Montreal, as having been caused by muscular action, the lad being very athletic (*Canada Medical and Surgical Journal*, November 1875-6, pp. 207–214 ; *London Medical Record*, January 15, 1876, vol. iv. p. 18). H. P., aged sixteen, thought he had sprained his leg the previous week while hurriedly leaping a fence in pursuit of a ball. This was followed on the fourth day by very considerable pain in the lower part of the left thigh and knee, with an aching sensation over the gluteal region, and inability to lie on the left side. There was pain on pressure and slight swelling over the outer side and front of thigh, so as to lead to a suspicion of periosteal inflammation. No lengthening or shortening of limb took place.

Severe constitutional disturbance set in with coated tongue, rapid pulse, rigors, swelling of both parotids, and pain in right ankle and great toe with slight redness (temp. 101·5°, pulse 116). Under chloroform a large abscess over the great trochanter was opened by a long incision, and a quantity of unhealthy-looking sanious pus excavated. The bone was found to be bare next day, and the exposed surface extended towards the neck of the femur. Pain and swelling of joints and parotid regions rapidly began to subside, and then disappeared (temp. 101°–103°). There was paralysis of the left arm on the tenth day, which Dr. Roddick thought might have been due to pyæmic abscess in the brain. Subsequently, five days later, on making a counter-opening above the original one, the great trochanter was felt to be loose, and drawn far away from the shaft of the femur, but still held firmly by the muscles inserted into it. The patient gradually sank, and died on the seventeenth day from pyæmic infection, thirteen days after admission to hospital. The epiphysis of the great trochanter was found entirely detached from the shaft, which lay in the centre of an immense abscess.

The periosteum was separated from the bone nearly to the junction of the lower with the middle third. The detached epiphysis was almost completely denuded of periosteum, so that it could be removed from its muscular attachments with little difficulty.

TREATMENT.—A carefully moulded splint of plaster of Paris or other material, well padded with cotton-wool, should be applied to the whole circumference of the pelvis and round the injured thigh, in all cases in which this lesion is believed to have taken place.

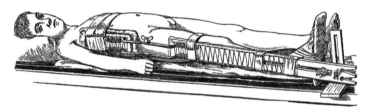

FIG. 206.—LONG EXTERNAL SPLINT WITH JOINTS IN CENTRE OF INTERRUPTION AT HIP PERMITTING ABDUCTION OF LOWER EXTREMITY. BY MEANS OF THE MOVABLE FOOT AND CROSS PIECE BELOW IT IS ADAPTABLE TO EITHER LIMB

If displacement is present, the fragment should be drawn down and secured in position by means of a semicircular collar or by compresses and strapping, and the limb fixed. The limb should be straight and slightly abducted, in order, if possible, to bring the lower fragment in contact with the upper if the epiphysis is much displaced. Malgaigne suggested abduction and eversion of the limb in similar fractures in the adult in order to bring the shaft towards the displaced fragment. Passive movement should not be commenced as early as in other epiphysial separations. Some surgeons might prefer a Thomas's hip splint, and its employment would certainly be of service in epiphysial separation without displacement, but in this case a surcingle as well should be applied round the hips (see fig. 198).

Should inflammatory signs present themselves, a free incision is to be made through the fibrous structures and periosteum, and the

x x

process thoroughly explored ; if it is found to be in any way bare, it should be *excised*.

Knowing the great tendency to suppurative inflammation in these cases, it is most essential that the limb should be kept at rest, even in the most simple case. In more than one case the movements of walking after injury to the trochanter rapidly produced an acute abscess and death.

A contrivance analogous to Malgaigne's patella hooks was suggested by Packard for keeping the fragments in position, and used by him for fractured olecranon. Seeing the great tendency to suppurative inflammation in these injuries in children, its employment might be attended with some danger. A safer method would be to fix the fragments together by carbolised silk, inserted in the tendinous structures under strict antiseptic precautions in an open operation.

SEPARATION OF THE EPIPHYSIS OF THE LESSER TROCHANTER

ANATOMY.—The cartilaginous process of the lesser trochanter is separated from the upper end by the second year. Ossification appears in its centre at the thirteenth year, but is sometimes delayed till the fourteenth. A small oval-shaped process is rapidly formed, convex on the outer side, and resting on a somewhat triangular prominence, which is flat on the surface.

This epiphysis joins on about the eighteenth year, somewhat earlier than the great trochanter.

Separation of this small osseous process can, therefore, only take place between the thirteenth and the eighteenth year.

In the only case of separation of this process which has been recorded the age was fourteen.

ETIOLOGY. — From its deeply buried position amongst the muscles on the inner and upper part of the femur, it is difficult to conceive that the lesser trochanter can be separated from the shaft of the femur except by violent muscular contraction, as in the case recorded below.

PATHOLOGICAL ANATOMY.—The only specimen of separation of this epiphysis is that in the McGill College Museum at Montreal, described by the late Dr. Fenwick, of Montreal, in his lectures on surgery.

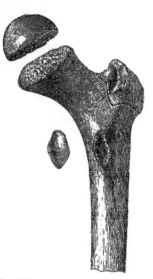

FIG. 207.—POSTERIOR VIEW OF EPIPHYSES AT UPPER END OF FEMUR AT ABOUT THE FIFTEENTH YEAR. (½-size)

Thirty years ago, his own son, aged fourteen, in climbing on to a fence, fell backwards on to his feet, twisting his leg. The violent strain of the psoas and iliacus tore away the lesser trochanter. This was verified by incision of an abscess which formed. The boy died, on the seventeenth day after the accident, of pyæmia, the direct result of the abscess occurring about the separated epiphysis. For the notes of this case the author is indebted to Dr. F. J. Shepherd, of Montreal, and for the photographs (from which the accompanying drawings were taken) to Professor J. G. Adami, of Montreal, who kindly placed them at his disposal, together with a number of photographs and notes of other cases of separation of the epiphyses from the McGill College Museum.

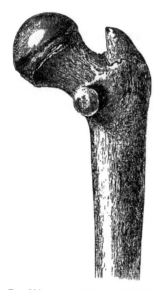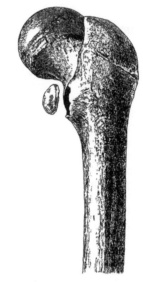

FIG. 208.—SEPARATION OF THE LESSER   FIG. 209.—SEPARATION OF THE LESSER
    TROCHANTER (POSTERIOR VIEW)   TROCHANTER (EXTERNAL VIEW)
            (From McGill College Museum, Montreal)

SYMPTOMS.—In a case of fracture of the lesser trochanter in an adult recorded by Julliard ('Fracture par arrachement du petit trochanter,' *Progrès Méd.* Paris, 1879, vii. p. 825), the symptoms were rotation outwards of the limb, as in fracture of the neck of the femur, the outer border of the foot lying on the bed; ecchymosis and swelling on the inner side of the thigh; inability to move the limb; deformity of hip and thigh. There was no shortening of the limb, swelling of the knee, or crepitus.

On account of the powerful action of the ilio-psoas muscle attached to the epiphysis, the retentive apparatus in the treatment of the injury must be kept on the limb for four weeks or longer before passive movement is commenced. If passive movement be commenced earlier, a fibrous union may be the result.

SEPARATION OF THE EPIPHYSIS OF THE THIRD TROCHANTER

Dr. A. F. Dixon (Roy. Acad. of Med., Ireland, *Lancet*, June 13, 1896, p. 1646) lately exhibited and described three specimens showing this special epiphysis.   In each example this epiphysis was small and scale-like, and was placed just above the groove present in the region of insertion of the gluteus maximus muscle.   The third trochanter is exactly like the lesser trochanter, consisting of a thin shell of compact tissue enclosing cancellous tissue within, while, according to Professor Birmingham, the contiguous gluteal ridge is composed altogether of layers of compact bone, showing that the ossification of the third trochanter was a special one.

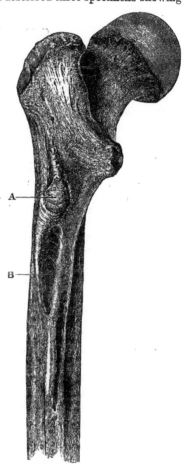

Mr. Luther Holden (*Human Osteology*, 4th edit. 1869, p. 183) was the first to point out that the ridge at the outer lip of the upper bifurcation of the linea aspera, to which the gluteus maximus is attached, is sometimes so prominent as to resemble the third trochanter of the lower animals.   It has now been conclusively proved by the investigations of Waldeyer, Fürst, Dollo, and others, that this epiphysis is really the survival of the third trochanter, and that it is found in about thirty-two to thirty-three per cent. of cases.

Fig. 210.—POSTERIOR ASPECT OF FEMUR OF ADULT MALE, SHOWING

A, third trochanter, and *B*, hypotrochanteric fossa. ½ natural size. (After Houzé)

For a complete account of this subject the reader must be referred to M. Houzé's paper: 'Sur la présence du troisième trochanter chez l'homme' (*Bull. de la Société d'Anthropologie de Bruxelles*, 1884, p. 21, Plate iii.).

CHAPTER IV

SEPARATION OF THE LOWER EPIPHYSIS OF THE FEMUR

ANATOMY.—This is the only epiphysis whose ossification begins before birth, with the exception of the occasional early appearance of the osseous nucleus in the upper epiphysis of the tibia. Ossification commences in the middle of the cartilaginous end above the intercondyloid notch from the second to the third week before birth.

By the eighteenth month this centre has increased to a considerable size, and is of an oval shape surrounded by osseous granules, especially at the sides, which assist in forming the condyles. The epiphysis at the fourth year is extensively occupied by osseous material, the projecting portions of the condyles on either side being still cartilaginous.

At the sixteenth year this enormous epiphysis is separated by its cartilaginous lamina from the diaphysis, the extremity of which presents a mammillated rounded surface divided by a slight furrow, running in an antero-posterior direction and corresponding to the intercondyloid notch.

The upper surface of the epiphysis is cup-shaped, with a central projection formed by the median centre of ossification and fitting into the furrow just mentioned on the diaphysis. Its anterior lip projects upwards, overlapping the front of the diaphysis, and, like the articular surface, which it includes, projects higher on the outer portion. The cartilaginous line of junction is at the outer portion of the anterior lip about one-eighth of an inch above the articular surface, and slopes downwards towards the lateral aspect of the condyles, and thus presents a sinuous outline ; behind it reaches the articular surface on each condyle and corresponds between these with the upper limit of the intercondyloid notch. The epiphysis is therefore seen to include the whole of the articular surface, both front and back.

Separation of this epiphysis with displacement means, therefore, injury to the synovial membrane of the joint. On a frontal section the conjugal cartilage presents a somewhat wavy outline, corresponding in direction very much with the articular surface of the epiphysis.

The adductor tubercle is attached to the extreme inner side of the diaphysial end close to its junction with the epiphysis.

The two heads of the powerful gastrocnemius are attached to the posterior limit of each condyle to some extent, but chiefly to the diaphysis of the femur. The plantaris is also attached to the diaphysis; these two muscles are stripped off the shaft with the periosteum and act solely upon the epiphysis when detached, and cause it to rotate upon its axis.

The popliteus muscle, together with the external lateral ligaments, is attached to the outer side of the outer condyle. To the inner side of the internal condyle is attached the powerful internal lateral ligament; while the anterior and posterior crucial ligaments are attached respectively to the inner and outer aspects of the external and internal condyles.

The medullary artery is directed upwards towards the proximal end of the bone.

De Paoli gives the following table of measurements of the lower epiphysis of the femur (in a median frontal section).

AGE	HEIGHT					
And principal periods	At the intercondyloid space	At the middle of the external condyle	At the middle of the internal condyle	At the outer edge	At the inner edge	Greatest BREADTH
Before birth (central osseous nodule)	10 mm.	16 mm.	19 mm.	16 mm.	19 mm.	30 mm.
1 year . . .	12 ,,	18 ,,	20 ,,	20 ,,	21 ,,	43 ,,
2 years . . .	12 ,,	20 ,,	22 ,,	25 ,,	21 ,,	48 ,,
4 ,, . . .	15 ,,	17 ,,	19 ,,	16 ,,	20 ,,	45 ,,
5 ,, . ?	16 ,,	23 ,,	25 ,,	19 ,,	23 ,,	50 ,,
	15 ,,	20 ,,	23 ,,	23 ,,	26 ,,	55 ,,
5½ ,, . . .	19 ,,	20 ,,	25 ,,	21 ,,	27 ,,	53 ,,
6 ,, . . .	15 ,,	21 ,,	23 ,,	23 ,,	26 ,,	58 ,,
7 ,, . . .	17 ,,	23 ,,	25 ,,	24 ,,	28 ,,	58 ,,
8 ,, . . .	17 ,,	22 ,,	28 ,,	27 ,,	32 ,,	62 ,,
9 ,, . . .	18 ,,	22 ,,	26 ,,	25 ,,	28 ,,	56 ,,
13 ,, . . .	17 ,,	24 ,,	30 ,,	28 ,,	36 ,,	68 ,,
14 ,, . . .	17 ,,	26 ,,	29 ,,	25 ,,	32 ,,	71 ,,
16 ,, (the ossification extends up to the lateral surfaces)	18 ,,	26 ,,	33 ,,	29 ,,	37 ,,	80 ,,
17 years . . .	16 ,,	26 ,,	25 ,,	19 ,,	28 ,,	62 ,,
20 ,, . . .	18 ,,	28 ,,	32 ,,	27 ,,	33 ,,	72 ,,

If the femur be sawn horizontally through at the level of the epiphysial line of junction of its lower epiphysis, the cut will pass below the upper edge of the cartilaginous surface of the articulation. In a well-developed boy of eighteen years of age its level will be found to be 1·2 centimetres below the highest point of the epiphysial line in front.

In a specimen taken from a subject of the same age, the author found the vertical thickness of the epiphysis at the middle of the intercondyloid notch to be 9·58 millimetres ; between the condyles, anteriorly, 1·3 centimetres ; at middle of internal condyle, 3·2 centimetres ; and at middle of external condyle, 2·7 centimetres.

König has also given similar measurements in his manual of surgery (*Lehrbuch der allg. Chirurg.* Berlin, 1883).

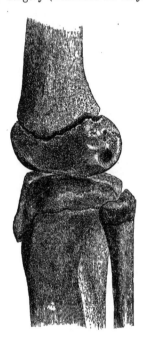

FIG. 211. — EPIPHYSES AT THE KNEE-JOINT AT THE NINETEENTH YEAR. OUTER SIDE (½ natural size)

Procknow also gives the height of the epiphysial line by placing a horizontal line along the lowest part of the articular surface of the epiphysis, and taking the vertical measurement from this along the edge of each condyle to the epiphysial line :

	In a girl 9 years of age	In a boy 7 years of age
Intercondyloid notch .	2·3 cm.	2·3 cm.
Internal condyle . .	2·7 ,,	2·7 ,,
External condyle . .	2·3 ,,	2·9 ,,

The author's own measurements confirm these precisely.

The height of the cartilage laterally at the fourteenth year is 3·4 centimetres from the lower edge of the internal condyle ; from the lower edge of the external condyle, 2·7. The height of the cartilage at the eighteenth year is 4·2 centimetres from the lower edge of the internal condyle ; from the lower edge of the external condyle, 3·5. All these measurements were found to be somewhat less in the female subject.

The thickness of the epiphysial or conjugal cartilage at about the ninth year is three to six millimetres.

This enormous epiphysis having been the first of all the epiphyses in the body to ossify, will be the last to join to the shaft, according to the usual law.

It unites with the diaphysis from the twentieth to the twenty-third or even twenty-fifth year.

The growth in length of the femur occurs to a great extent at this end of the bone. According to Ollier the growth from the lower end is about twice that from the upper.

It is only in front above the articular surface in the middle line and in front of each condyle, especially the external, that the epiphysial layer of cartilage is in close proximity to the synovial membrane of the joint.

Even here the membrane, which extends somewhat above the line of cartilage and overlaps the end of the diaphysis, would be protected from injury or laceration during the separation of this epiphysis by reason of the layer of loose fat which intervenes between it and the periosteum in this situation. The synovial membrane

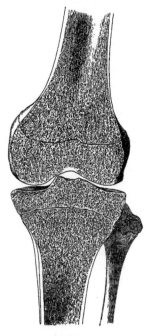

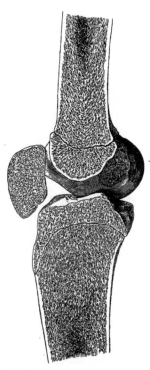

Fig. 212.—Frontal section of bones forming the knee-joint between the seventeenth and eighteenth years of life. Posterior half of section, showing cancellous structure of the epiphyses and ends of the diaphyses and the relation of the conjugal lines to the articulation ($\frac{2}{3}$-size)

Fig. 213.—Sagittal section of bones forming the knee-joint

approaches the diaphysis behind much nearer than it does at the sides. This relationship is well seen also in vertical sections through the middle of each condyle.

At the sides the attachments of the powerful lateral ligaments to the epiphysis widely separate the synovial cavity from the epiphysial line, so that on a transverse section of the knee-joint the synovial membrane is at a considerable distance from the diaphysis.

We may therefore say that the knee-joint is comparatively

secure against being opened in pure separations of this epiphysis without much displacement. The presence of the large bursa beneath the extensor tendon over the lower end of the diaphysis must not be forgotten, inasmuch as it communicates freely with the joint. It may escape injury, however, through the quantity of fat which separates it from the periosteum.

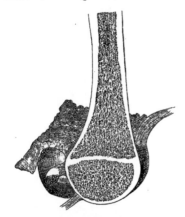

AGE.—Both age and sex appear to have a decided influence in separation of the lower epiphysis of the femur.

Out of *seventy-one specimens and cases verified by direct examination* (i.e. compound separations) sixty have the age clearly stated; of these no less than thirty-one were between the ages of 11 and 20 years: one at 20, two at 19, two at 18, two at 17, two at 16, five at 15, seven at 14, three at 13, four at 12, three at 11, one between 10 and 11, three at 10, two at $9\frac{1}{2}$, six at 9, five at 8, one at 7, two at 6, one at 5, four at 4, one at $3\frac{1}{2}$, and one at 2 years; one at 6 months, and one in a fœtus.

FIG. 214.—MEDIAN SAGITTAL SECTION OF THE LOWER END OF THE FEMUR, FROM A GIRL AGED FOURTEEN YEARS

The synovial membrane in front extends above the conjugal cartilage, a thick pad of fat intervening between it and the front of the diaphysis. Behind it passes off from the crucial ligaments (seen on section) at the level of the conjugal cartilage. The ligamentum mucosum is seen below.

Out of *nine other compound separations* not included in those just mentioned, and which terminated in recovery, the age is given in eight : in one at 15, one at $13\frac{1}{2}$, one at 12, one at 11, one at 10, one at $8\frac{1}{2}$, one at 7, and one at $6\frac{1}{2}$ years of age.

Taking *all which have been confirmed anatomically* of the total eighty, we find the age given in sixty-eight; of these, thirty-five instances were from 11 to 20 years of age.

The age is given in thirty-two out of thirty-four *simple cases*. The majority of these, twenty-three in number, took place also between 11 and 20 years of age: one at 20, four at 18, one at 17, four at 16, six at 15, one at 14, one at 13, three at 12, two at 11 ; one at 10, one at 9, one at 8, four at 7, one at 6, and one at 4 years of age.

Of the total 114 collected by the author, the age is given in 100, and of these the injury occurred in sixty-four between 10 and 20 years of age : two at 20, two at 19, six at 18, three at 17, six at 16, twelve at 15, eight at 14, one at $13\frac{1}{2}$, four at 13, eight at 12, six at 11, one between 10 and 11, five at 10, two at $9\frac{1}{2}$, seven at 9, one at 8½, six at 8, six at 7, one at 6½, three at 6, one at 5, five at 4, one at 3½, one at 2, one at 1½ years of age, and one in a fœtus.

Out of seventy-five cases the greatest number, twenty-eight, occurred between the ages of 15 and 20, precisely what would be expected in this epiphysis, which does not become completely united to the shaft until so late a period.

M. Delens, in his valuable paper on 'Traumatic Separations of the Lower Epiphysis of the Femur' (*Archives générales de*

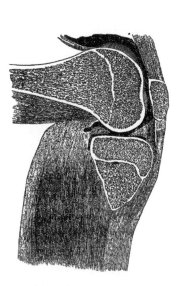
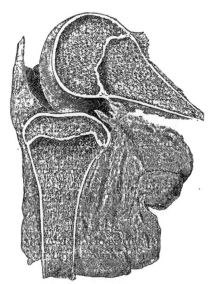

FIG. 215.—SAGITTAL SECTION OF THE LEFT KNEE-JOINT THROUGH THE OUTER CONDYLE OF THE FEMUR; THE KNEE IS IN THE FLEXED POSITION. OUTER SURFACE OF SECTION. FROM A GIRL AGED FOURTEEN YEARS

In front the synovial membrane passes off from above the conjugal line. Behind it forms a pouch in this position of the knee, and extends beyond the level of the conjugal cartilage, but in the extended position it reaches only as far as this point (½-size)

FIG. 216.—SAGITTAL SECTION THROUGH INTERNAL CONDYLE OF FEMUR AND INNER TUBEROSITY OF TIBIA IN A GIRL AGED FOURTEEN YEARS

Neither in front nor behind does the synovial membrane extend so far upwards as in the median line of the joint. In the extended position it passes off exactly at the conjugal line. (Above the outer condyle it extends somewhat above the epiphysial boundary.) Much more of the inner tuberosity of the tibia, anteriorly and posteriorly, is covered by the membrane than in the middle line (⅔-size)

Médecine, vol. cliii. March 1884, p. 272), has drawn attention to the same influence of age. Out of twenty-eight cases of this injury he found that nineteen were between 10 and 18 years of age.

The author has carefully excluded several examples mentioned by Professor Paul Bruns (*Archiv für klin. Chirurg.* Bd. xxvii. 1882) in his article on 'Traumatic Separation of the Epiphyses,' those related by Madame La Chapelle, and some other writers, mostly on account of the insufficient details rendering the diagnosis very doubtful, but some on account of separation being caused by putrefaction of the body or by disease.

In Madame La Chapelle's case traction of the foot during delivery caused a separation of this epiphysis, and a separation of the upper epiphysis of the tibia. The child was born dead.

The author has also omitted all cases of separation produced by the surgeon in the necessary manipulations for hip disease. Volkmann (*Virchow's Jahresbericht*, 1866, ii. S. 337) has three times separated this epiphysis in hip disease by traction in applying a plaster dressing, and by rotation in seeking for crepitus. It has also been separated in many instances by other surgeons in using very gentle force whilst applying a plaster-of-Paris bandage for the same disease.

Numerous cases of this accident have also been recorded by surgeons, produced by attempts to straighten limbs ankylosed in a rectangular or other bad position. Instances have been especially frequent during rectification of ankylosis of the knee (Callender, Chauvel; Spillmann, *Dict. Encyclopédique des Sciences médicales*, tome xxiv. art. 'Cuisse'). The author has carefully avoided these and such like cases of separation associated with a diseased condition, which Packard and others have included in their accounts of this injury. For example, Packard mentions the case of a girl, aged sixteen, communicated to him by Dr. W. B. Hopkins. She had bony ankylosis of one knee at a right angle, and had a fall, separating the lower epiphysis of the femur from the shaft. Under ether the limb was straightened and put up in plaster of Paris, and an excellent result was ultimately obtained.

Any constitutional tendency to rickets, syphilis, or tuberculous disease, or any liability to inflammatory change about the epiphysial line, may influence the normal time of union of the epiphysis, either accelerating or retarding it. We cannot therefore regard the age at which separation occurs in these cases as of any assistance in determining the limits in which it usually takes place in healthy subjects. Only a small amount of violence seems, under such conditions, to readily produce this separation. In this connection the following cases, which occurred at Guy's Hospital, are of interest.

Mr. Bryant had a case of this separation with marked rickets under his care at Guy's Hospital in 1882. The patient was a girl, aged two, who had fallen down stairs. There was no displacement, but considerable swelling above the knee, with dull crepitus and great pain on manipulation. A felt splint was applied, and the child slowly but completely recovered.

Mr. Birkett diagnosed a similar case in a girl, aged two and a quarter, under his care in 1874 at Guy's Hospital. Three days before admission she had fallen off a chair. Extension with lateral splints was applied, and the bones united in very good position.

Mr. Cock, at Guy's Hospital, May 1866, had a case of separation of this epiphysis in a boy (Fred. Wm. D.), aged nine, the subject of strumous diathesis. His leg had been caught between the spokes of a wheel; there was evidence of great contusion. The treatment adopted was a back splint with the limb bent at an angle.

The author has seen two other cases in rachitic children; in one of them, a girl aged three and a half, there was slight displacement inwards and backwards of this epiphysis, with dull crepitus and great pain above the joint. The knee-joint was normal: The child had been knocked over in the street, and fell on her hands and knees. Under chloroform a plaster-of-Paris bandage was applied; union slowly took place, accompanied by considerable thickening about the lower end of the femur.

Dr. Oscar H. Allis, of the Presbyterian Hospital, Philadelphia, has kindly sent the author the following notes of a case previously published by him (*Trans. Path. Society*, Philadelphia, 1878, p. 7).

The injury causing the separation of the upper and lower epiphyses of the right femur and partial separation of the lower epiphysis of the left femur 'was very slight,' and occurred in an unhealthy rachitic infant.

'J. K., eighteen months; about two weeks before its death the mother noticed that the child cried violently when she attempted to put on the right shoe. A week later Dr. Allis saw the child once and examined the ankle, knee, and hip, but did not detect any unusual symptoms. The child cried, but no more than when he examined the other limb or the abdomen. The child had a slight cold and was teething. The urine was dark and turbid. At death Dr. Allis was again sent for, and obtained permission to make an autopsy. The abdominal viscera were sound; the mesenteric glands swollen or enlarged. The ribs at their sternal ends were beaded and prominent. The head of the right femur was separated from the shaft with loss of substance. The condyloid epiphysis was separated from the shaft, and the periosteum free from the bone halfway up the shaft. The extremity of the shaft was injected with blood, and there was evidence that blood had been effused beneath the periosteum. There were no traces of inflammatory action, and it was therefore not easy to state at what time the traumatism occurred.

'On examining the left femur the neck was found intact, but a partial separation of the condyloid epiphysis was detected, without any evidence of effusion of blood. The mother attributed the injury to the fact that an elder sister (three years of age) was seen sitting on the infant two weeks before its death.'

In 1885, at Guy's Hospital, Mr. Howse had an instance of separation of the epiphysis nine years after excision of the knee for disease. The boy was now aged eleven, and the accident happened by his falling off a chair, catching his leg between the bars. The leg was found to be slightly bent backwards and inwards. There was no crepitus, but a quarter of an inch of separation of the epiphysis in front from the diaphysis. Consolidation rapidly ensued after the employment of straight splints.

The case of a girl, aged one and three-quarter years, is referred to in the *St. Thomas's Hospital Reports* for 1875 (N.S. vol. vi. 1875, p. 343) as having separated the lower epiphysis, recovery taking place in eighteen days.

In concluding this subject of age it will be seen that the opinions and statistics of the following writers are at great variance.

The author would regard the period from thirteen to eighteen years as that in which we find pure epiphysial separations of the lower end of the femur to be most common.

Packard's figures differ very considerably from those given above by the author. He says: 'As to the age of the patients, the average of forty-five in which it is stated was a little over seven years. The youngest was eighteen months, and the oldest eighteen years.'

Mr. Hutchinson says: ' The lower epiphysis of the femur may be detached at any age under twenty, but the accident usually occurs between eight and eighteen.'

Mr. Hutchinson junior has collected seventy-five cases, of which ten have not been previously published ; out of fifty cases, three of the patients had attained the twentieth year, the average being ten years.

A. H. Meisenbach, of St. Louis, U.S.A., in collecting the statistics previously published (*New York Medical Record*, December 15, 1894; *Annals of Surgery*, February 1895, p. 157), finds that traumatic separation of the lower end of the femur occurs in about one-fifth to one-third of all reported cases ; in the majority of instances previous to the sixteenth year, seldom later.

SEX.—With regard to sex Packard found in over sixty cases that there were nine in which the subjects are stated to have been girls ; and of these, strangely enough, three sustained their injuries by entanglement in the wheels of wagons, behind which they were clinging.

Delens observes that out of twenty-three cases where the sex of the patient was noted, twenty were males, and only three females.

In the author's figures, taking seventy-four examples there were only eight girls, but the statistics of the total separations of the lower femoral epiphysis are as follows :

Out of seventy-one specimens verified after death, the sex is stated in fifty-six. Of these, forty-eight occurred in males, and eight in females.

Of nine other compound separations, the sex is not given in one instance ; of the remaining eight, seven were in males, one in a female.

Of the total eighty verified by direct examination, nine occurred in females ; all of the latter were from fourteen years of age downwards—none above.

Of thirty-four simple cases, the sex is given in thirty-two. Of these, twenty-eight were in males and four in females; all the latter were below the age of thirteen years.

Of the total one hundred and fourteen, the sex is given in ninety-six, as eighty-three males and thirteen females.

It is not that this separation is more readily produced in males, but that they are more exposed than females to injuries of this kind. The natural muscular activity and the enterprising spirit of the boy lead him into greater danger. The modern tendency for the female sex to imitate the habits of the male may, however, in the future considerably modify the truth of this statement.

ETIOLOGY.—To separate so broad and thick an epiphysis as that of the lower end of the femur, it would appear that a very considerable amount of violence is required; but, as we shall see later on, in certain forms of this injury, and under peculiar circumstances, the violence may not be so very great, the tibia acting as a very powerful lever by means of the popliteus muscle and the crucial and other ligaments during hyper-extension.

Experimentally on the dead subject it is one of the epiphyses most easily separated.

Direct violence.—A broad line of distinction needs to be drawn in this as in other diastases between separations caused by extreme direct violence, such as violent contact with some heavy bodies, and those due to other causes. Of the former we may mention as examples the passage of a cart- or cab-wheel over the leg (five cases), a heavy weight, timber, or bale of rope falling on the knee, a kick by a horse. Eleven cases were produced in this way by direct violence.

The author finds several other examples in which direct causes are clearly stated, but the accounts cannot always be relied upon; it is often in these more indirect than direct, the exact mode or point of infliction of the violence being obscure.

Mr. A. W. Mayo Robson thinks that extreme direct violence is usually the cause; but Packard in one of his earlier papers gave an opposite opinion—viz. that in almost every case the cause of the injury was indirect violence.

Indirect violence.—In a record of sixty cases in which the cause of this diastasis is noted, the author finds that this occurred in fifty-three from indirect violence. It is probable that many others which at first sight seem to be due to direct violence—e.g. in Mr. Wheelhouse's case (*loc. cit. infra*), a fall of earth in a colliery accident—are in reality the result of indirect violence. The difficulty of exactly estimating all the factors of accidents of this nature is alone sufficient to raise a doubt as to direct violence being considered the cause. At any rate, we observe that the immense majority is certainly due to indirect violence.

Out of the fifty-three cases just mentioned, a large proportion (twenty-four) were produced by the entanglement of the leg in the spokes of a revolving carriage-wheel, the child, having climbed up or hanging on behind, letting the leg slip in between the spokes of the wheel. In three cases the child had fallen forwards with its leg fixed in a hole, or between the joists of a floor—e.g. M. Fontanelle's case (*loc. cit. infra*)—or else had got the limb entangled in some machinery. Separation occurred in one case from a fall from a height of eighty feet; in another from the patient—a boy—jumping from a steamboat and getting the limb entangled in a rope.

Packard found in twenty-seven out of sixty-eight cases which he had collected that it was produced by catching the leg in a carriage wheel.

In a few instances the violence, though indirect, has been less severe—e.g. a fall upon the curbstone of the pavement while running, the knee being violently struck. In two at least of these (Maunder's and Hilton's) the patient, after slipping, fell to the ground with the leg bent beneath him.

In one instance a push on the outer side of the leg when the patient was standing with his lower extremities wide apart was said to be sufficient to separate the lower femoral epiphysis. In another case a boy, whilst playing leapfrog, alighted on his feet, which were widely separated. A fall with the legs apart, a fall down stairs, and lastly a simple fall on the edge of a pavement, have all been mentioned as producing this injury.

This epiphysis is certainly placed at a great mechanical disadvantage. The knee-joint is the largest joint in the body, and the large articular ends which form it, being but little supported by bony cavities, are almost entirely dependent upon powerful and complex ligaments for their great strength and proper apposition. Any over-extension of the knee-joint is directly expended upon this huge epiphysis by the great leverage of the tibia, which is firmly connected to it by these powerful ligaments.

To this over-extension of the knee there is added some amount of twisting and traction upon the leg. Either the body or the leg at one end of the long lever may be the fixed point for the application of the extending force.

According to a case, which must be a rare one, recorded by Dr. E. E. Ware (*Lancet*, January 12, 1895, p. 92), it is possible, even under these circumstances, for the limb to give way and separate through the knee-joint without fracture.

A boy, aged seven years, was riding behind a four-wheeled cab when his thigh became impacted between the axle and the spring. In his struggles to extricate himself his leg became entangled in the spokes of the wheel. The cab was moving at a medium pace, and the boy's thigh being firmly fixed under the spring, and his leg forcibly wrenched by the moving wheel, his limb was torn off at the knee-joint. On examination at the East London Hospital for Children, it was found that the right leg had been completely severed from the thigh through the knee-joint. The skin of the lower third of the thigh was extensively bruised and lacerated, and the muscles exhibited torn and bruised ends, blood being extravasated into the sheaths. The femoral artery was occluded apparently by torsion, and was seen lying free in the remnant of Hunter's canal. The sciatic nerve was also ruptured. The patella was situated in the stump, and the ligamentum patellæ was not ruptured, but had been detached from the tibia by the separation of a small portion of the tubercle; the crucial ligaments also were entirely separated from their femoral attachments, and the lateral ligaments of the joint were completely torn away. The lower end of the femur was thus completely exposed, and the external and anterior surface of the bone had been denuded of periosteum. Under chloroform Dr. Ware performed immediate amputation of the thigh at about the junction of the upper two-fifths with the lower three-fifths. The wound healed by first intention, and recovery was uneventful.

On examining the leg it was found that the semilunar cartilages remained *in situ* and that the crucial ligaments maintained their attachment to the tibia. The long external lateral ligament was still attached to the fibula, and at the point of separation from the femur had denuded an adjacent extensive surface of bone of its periosteum. On dissection no fracture of the tibia or fibula could be detected, and there was no epiphysial displacement; the insertions of the hamstring muscles also remained uninjured.

M. Delens compares this separation with that of the lower end of the radius, and believes that the powerful posterior ligament of the knee in *forcible extension* of the limb plays the same part with reference to the femoral epiphysis as the anterior ligaments of the wrist do to the lower extremity of the radius in falls upon the palm of the hand.

The author would say that violent extension is the most important force in producing this lesion.

Many surgeons have separated this epiphysis as a means of straightening the limb in genu valgum, and the osteoclast of Collins has the same effect upon the lower end of the femur.

The exact mechanism in such cases has been ably described by Delore, and by V. Ménard (*La Revue de Chirurgie*, 1881, 'Recherches expérimentales sur le redressement brusque du genu valgum') and others. Ménard also gives the age at which such operations may be safely performed.

In straightening limbs for genu valgum by other methods, it is likewise the lower epiphysis of the femur which is usually detached.

M. Delore made an autopsy on a child, aged seven years, who had died of measles twenty-one days after an operation of this kind, and found separation of the lower epiphysis of the femur on either side, whilst there was on the left a separation of the upper epiphysis of the tibia; on the right there was a separation of the head of the fibula.

In these cases the force of torsion is replaced by a pushing force in an outward or inward direction—that is, by violent abduction or adduction of the leg on the thigh.

Violent torsion of the limb has produced epiphysial separation in ten cases, eight of them by the limb being caught by machinery in motion, two by the twisting of a cable round the limb on board ship.

Mr. Cock, at Guy's Hospital, in December 1866, diagnosed a case as separation of this epiphysis in a young man (Joseph H.) aged nineteen. While wrestling with another man he was thrown to the ground and his leg twisted, and he was unable to stand. The treatment adopted was a long outside splint and a short inner one. Great swelling of the knee occurred, and on his discharge two months later he was still unable to walk without crutches.

At the Medico-Chirurgical Society of Edinburgh, Mr. A. G. Miller showed, on December 19, 1888, a fracture of the lower epiphysis of the femur produced by torsion.

In fact, we may say that violent torsion, combined with forcible or hyper-extension, is the common agent in producing this lesion; this is probably the reason why we sometimes find a fragment of the diaphysis on the inner or outer side still attached to the epiphysis, while the remaining portion of the separation is clean.

Again, in compound separations there seems to be some proof of the existence of torsion combined with extension; for although the wound is frequently on the posterior aspect, it is sometimes found on the posterior, internal, or external aspects.

'Ce sont encore les torsions, les inclinaisons constatées sur le fragment épiphysaire' (Verneuil).

M. J. Colignon, in his doctoral thesis, 'De la disjonction traumatique des épiphyses' (Thèse de doctorat, Paris, 1868), brought forward a number of cases showing that separation of the lower epiphysis of the femur in newly born children could be produced by forcible extension or flexion. Twisting and lateral bending inwards at the knee produced the same results.

Bruns quotes a case in which he detached the lower epiphysis of the femur in correcting the deformity of chronic inflammation of the hip-joint. The girl was aged sixteen. Bruns agrees with the views the author has just stated. Although the epiphysial cartilage is at a distance from the disease for which the manipulation is required, and to all appearance is unaffected by disease, yet it cannot be said to be in a healthy condition—it must have undergone some pathological change. Its unhealthy condition predisposes to separation of the epiphysis. This is confirmed by the small amount of force required to separate so large an epiphysis as that of the lower end of the femur under such conditions.

It need scarcely be stated that **muscular action** alone cannot separate this epiphysis.

In an analysis of the seventy cases collected 'with a view to

determining the kind of violence most likely to produce this kind
of injury Dr. J. M. Elder, of Montreal (*Montreal Medical Journal*,
vol. xx. No. 9, March 1892, p. 645), gave the following results:
'Entanglement of the limb in a moving wheel (as of a carriage),
thirty-three cases; a fall while running, three cases; one case of a
fall from eighty feet; body thrown forwards while leg was in a hole
up to knee, two cases; one case while boy was playing leapfrog
and alighted with feet widely separated; direct blow to lower part of
limb (as in Dr. Elder's own case), four cases; run over by vehicles,
four cases; and finally, as result of surgical procedures for correction of ankylosis or deformities, five cases. In thirty-three of the
cases the compound character of the lesion is mentioned.'

PATHOLOGICAL ANATOMY.—G. C. Reichel and Bertrandi give
the earliest description of anatomical specimens of this injury. The
specimen figured by Reichel may, however, have been a united fracture in the adult or have been one due to disease.

The first (1824) authentic specimen of which we have an accurate
account and illustration is that by Sir Charles Bell, preserved in the
Edinburgh Royal College of Surgeons Museum.

From the number of specimens of separation of the condyloid
epiphysis of the femur now existing, it is evident that this accident
is by no means so rare as was a short time ago supposed. The
severity of the injury leading to a frequent fatal termination is
sufficient to account for this. Other separations—e.g. the lower
end of the radius—are less frequently noted or come under the
care of surgeons for operative treatment; more often they are
entirely overlooked.

From the specimens, twenty-two in number, which are preserved in the London Hospital Museum and elsewhere, it would, at
first sight, appear that separation of the lower epiphysis of the
femur was the most frequent of all epiphysial detachments. Bruns
(*loc. cit. supra*) has noted twenty-eight, the highest number, in his
table of 100 cases, but, as he remarks, this cannot represent the
exact relative frequency of the injury, by reason of the very serious
complications and secondary lesions which are so often met with
in this injury, and which necessitate immediate surgical interference.
These are the usual results of the great amount of violence which
alone can produce the displacement of so extensive an epiphysis.
It must also be remembered that Bruns has only taken into account
those cases in which the diagnosis was confirmed by direct anatomical examination or by an autopsy.

M. Delens collected twenty-eight cases, omitting several of those
recorded by Bruns on account of their doubtful diagnosis.

Manquat (*Sur les décollements épiphysaires traumatiques*, Thèse
de Paris, 1877) collected 130 cases of epiphysial separation, of which
twenty-three were of the lower end of the femur.

Many other writers have followed Bruns's statement that separation of this epiphysis is the most frequent of all separations. This view might be endorsed by the fact that the lower epiphysis of the femur is the largest in the body, and by the fact that it commences to ossify first, and remains one of the last unattached to the diaphysis. In the case of the lower femoral epiphysis a period of life is therefore reached when considerable muscular activity, agility, and restlessness, especially on the part of boys, are displayed. Such influential causations we do not find in the case of other epiphyses, which only remain separate from the shaft during the earlier periods of youth.

Dr. Joseph Prochnow, of Buda-Pest, writing in 1892 (*Traumás epiphysis-levdlds, Gyógydszat*, Buda-Pest, 1892, xxxiv.; abstract in *Pest. Med. Chir. Presse*, Buda-Pest, 1893, xxix. p. 389), makes the same observation.

The separation of the condyloid epiphysis of the femur which Maclise figures (*Fractures and Dislocations*, 1859, Plate xxxi. fig. 5), and which has been quoted as a case of traumatic separation, is probably the result of maceration. The figure represents a transverse fracture of the lower third of the shaft of the femur united in the angular position, while there is no evidence of the epiphysial separation—which is perfect and without the slightest evidence of fracture or displacement—having been due to the injury.

The length of the femur forming a very powerful arm of a lever, the early ossification, late union, and relative large size of this epiphysis, especially in young children, and the strength of the crucial and other ligaments binding it to the tibia, are all conditions most conducive to its separation. Although resembling the supracondyloid fracture of an adult in some points, it cannot, as we shall see later on, be considered as identical with it.

The whole limb has been known to have been torn off at this epiphysis. Mr. T. Bryant (*British Medical Journal*, May 31, 1884, p. 1044) reports the case of a girl, aged four, who was admitted into Guy's Hospital on August 14, 1882. Her leg had been caught in the driving-strap of a machine, and the limb torn off at the junction of the shaft with the lower epiphysis of the femur. There had not been much loss of blood. The knee-joint had been opened, and there was much contusion and damage at the seat of separation. Amputation was performed through the middle of the thigh. Temperature from 99·2° to 104°. Death took place on August 29. At the autopsy there was found suppurative meningitis and an acute abscess in the psoas muscle.

SEPARATION IN INFANCY may be of the **pure variety**; there is no specimen in the London museums.

Separation in infancy with fracture of the diaphysis is represented by a specimen in the Westminster Hospital Museum, No. 42 (*Catalogue of the Specimens in the Museum of Westminster Hospital*, 1892, p. 18). In the left femur of a full-term fœtus, the epiphysis has been completely separated by violence. The periosteum has been partly stripped off the middle of the shaft, which has been incompletely fractured transversely, the line of fracture being limited to the anterior and outer surfaces of the bone. There is no displacement of the diaphysis. In the account of the specimen, which was presented by Mr. Holthouse, it is not stated whether the lesion was the result of an experiment or occurred during life.

Pure separations.—In analysing the description of specimens in various museums, and after carefully examining all the specimens in the London hospitals and in other museums, the author found that they afforded some of the best examples of pure epiphysial separation.

In some few examples a few bony granules adhere to the circumference of the epiphysis, but are not in any way sufficient to justify the name of fracture. In the ordinary cases the separation has passed through the ossifying layer of the epiphysial cartilage situated between the epiphysis and the diaphysis.

In two instances the protruding diaphysial end is stated to have retained and been covered by the epiphysial cartilage. In Richet's case the appearance was that of a dislocation. In Coural's (Julia Fontenelle's) case the separation was through the middle of the cartilage, so that a layer of it remained attached to each osseous fragment. The specimen is described by Delpech, in whose possession it was.

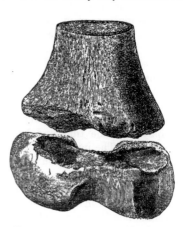

FIG. 217.—PURE SEPARATION OF LOWER
FEMORAL EPIPHYSIS

Mr. Cock's case. (Guy's Hospital Museum, ½-size)

In the museum of Guy's Hospital there are two preparations of pure separation; in one (*Guy's Hospital Museum Catalogue*, No. 1210⁶¹ and No. 1210⁶⁶) a few very small flakes remain adherent to the anterior edge of the separated epiphysis towards its outer side; in the other (*Guy's Hospital Museum Catalogue*, No. 1210⁴⁵) the epiphysis has a few granules of the diaphysis still attached to its inner part, but there is no fracture of the shaft.

The latter specimen (Mr. Cock's case, 1864) was taken from a boy (W. C.), aged seventeen, who was caught by the fly-wheel of some machinery and carried upwards to the wheel, where he was strangled. The specimen is figured in Mr. Bryant's 'Surgery.'

The London Hospital Museum (Mr. Ward's case) (*London Hospital Museum Catalogue*, No. G b, P. 54) contains a specimen of separation of the lower epiphysis of the femur (*Transactions Path.*

Soc. vol. xiii. 1862, p. 183). The detachment is clean, there being no fracture of the bone. The patient was a child two years old, who was run over in the streets. The lower epiphysis of the femur was completely detached and dragged forwards. With the epiphysis the periosteum has been extensively lacerated and detached in a sort of cup, thus leaving the lower end of the diaphysis quite denuded: The limb was injured beyond all chance of recovery, and the artery and vein were torn. Mr. Ward performed amputation at the hip-joint. The exposed surface of the epiphysis was covered with cartilage, but that of the extremity of the shaft showed no cartilage whatever. At the posterior border of the extremity of the shaft corresponding to the outer condyle some small spicules of bone had been broken off and dragged away with the epiphysis, but with this exception the exposed surface was whole and uninjured.

The museum of St. Bartholomew's Hospital (No. 982) contains another specimen, alluded to below, in which the end of the diaphysis is quite entire. It is an excellent example of a perfectly pure separation. In this case the epiphysis was displaced halfway off the shaft.

A specimen in St. George's Hospital Museum is also one of pure separation, and is figured by Holmes (*Diseases of Children,* 2nd edition, 1869, p. 259). The case is related fully later on. The lower epiphysis of the tibia and both epiphyses of the fibula were also separated. The injury to the lower end of the femur was compound, with extensive laceration of the skin of the groin. Death took place from pyæmia.

COMPOUND SEPARATION. - The same condition of pure separation has been found in many cases of compound separation where a direct examination has been made of the detached surfaces.

M. Richet (*L'Union Médicale,* Paris, 1876, 3rd series, vol. xxi. p. 426) describes a case of epiphysial separation of the femur, with protrusion of the end of the diaphysis through the skin.

A child, aged thirteen, under the care of M. Cusco, had his leg caught in the strap of a machine and violently twisted, so that it was bent upon the thigh to a right angle. The end of the bone, covered with epiphysial cartilage, protruded through a large wound on the outer aspect of the thigh at the lower part, and gave the appearance at first sight of a dislocation. The knee-joint was intact, and the femoral condyles and patella remained in normal relation with the tibia. There was no fracture of the diaphysis. Its narrower part was held by the soft parts like a button. Through the wound the condyles of the femur could be felt in position, as well as several small scales of bone still attached to the periosteum at the outer side of the separation, above the external condyle. Pulsation of the popliteal artery was also distinctly felt.

There was a shortening of seven to eight centimetres. Reduction was effected without chloroform after considerable difficulty. This was followed by delirium, elevation of temperature, convulsive attacks, and other signs of purulent infection.

Death took place on the sixteenth day from pyæmia. At the autopsy, metastatic abscesses were found in the right lung, and about seven ounces of recent sero-pus in the right pleura. The joints were normal. As a result of the convulsive movements, the end of the diaphysis was again displaced below and in front of the femoral epiphysis; it had perforated the synovial pouch, and penetrated the articulation, and was placed below the patella. There was no trace of fracture except what had been found before death. The condyles, imperfectly held by the lateral and crucial ligaments, were displaced backwards, so that their fractured surface looked towards the popliteal space; they were otherwise intact. The intra-articular fibro-cartilages and the tibia and fibula were uninjured.

Leisrinck (*Archiv für klin. Chir.* 1872, Bd. xiv. S. 436) reports the case of a boy, aged nine, who was caught and dragged along while stepping from a carriage. There was found complete separation of the lower epiphysis of the femur with very extensive laceration of the soft parts, and protrusion of the diaphysis for a distance of two inches from the wound. Amputation was performed through the upper part of the thigh.

Dr. John H. Owings records (*New York Medical Record*, 1891, xxxix. p. 11) a case of compound separation of the condyloid epiphysis in a girl aged ten years. The patient had had her left leg caught in a wagon-wheel. The wound being examined under an anæsthetic, it was found that the condyloid epiphysis had been separated from the diaphysis; the shaft had lacerated the soft parts, and was protruding through the skin fully five inches.

Attempts at reduction were made unsuccessfully, until three-quarters of an inch of the end of the shaft of the bone had been removed, when the bone was easily replaced.

The peculiar stellate radiations of the end of the shaft were found to be perfect, except the right upper or anterior portion, which had been ground off against the hub or spokes of the wheel. The wound was well washed with bichloride solution, and antiseptic dressings were applied. Professor N. R. Smith's anterior wire splint was the one employed. The wound sloughed a good deal, but healed completely after about three months. There was then good firm union, and considerable motion of the knee-joint, with only about one inch of shortening. The patient could walk without crutches, with very little limping, and with a firm elastic step and a good sound leg.

Dr. A. C. Post (*Medical News*, Philadelphia, 1883, xliii. p. 574) describes a similar case of a boy (W. D.) aged eight. He was riding in a wagon, when his left knee was caught between the spokes of the wheel and violently wrenched. The lower epiphysis of the femur was separated, and the end of the diaphysis protruded through an extensive wound on the outer side of the knee.   Amputation was recommended, but was refused by the parents.   Two months later, on September 16, 1883, the patient was examined under chloroform. The end of the diaphysis, detached from the epiphysis, still protruded from an extensive wound in a state of necrosis.   There were sinuses in different parts of the thigh, leg, and foot, and sloughs over the heel, exposing the os calcis.   The tibia was also exposed and superficially necrosed, and other suppuration existed about the foot. Amputation was performed through the middle of the thigh.   The femoral epiphysis was found to be *in situ*, but eroded and almost devoid of cartilage, and the head of the tibia was in the same condition. The knee-joint was completely disorganised.   Recovery took place.

Hamilton, in his *Practical Treatise on Fractures and Dislocations* (7th edit. 1884, p. 530), relates the case of a boy (W. S.), aged twelve; on August 11, 1877, he had his right leg caught in the spokes of a wagon-wheel, breaking his thigh at the junction of the lower epiphysis with the diaphysis, the lower end of the upper fragment protruding five inches through the flesh.   The end was nearly square.   His father, Dr. S. B. Smallwood, of Astoria, New York, the lad being under the influence of ether, reduced it within one hour by violent extension and flexion of the leg over his knee, one finger being in the wound and adjusting the fragments.   Lateral splints were employed.   The wound closed in about nine months, and in the meanwhile two small fragments of bone escaped.   The patient had also a sharp attack of synovitis. Professor Hamilton examined him on April 18, 1880, and found the leg straight, but shortened three-quarters of an inch.   There was complete ankylosis of the knee-joint, but the muscles of the leg were well developed, and he walked with very little limp.

Mr. Chas. Hawkins, in a discussion at the Royal Medical and Chirurgical Society on a case of dislocation of the knee on April 26, 1842 (*Lancet*, 1841–42, vol. ii. p. 202; *ibid.*, March 11, 1848, p. 286; Solly's *Surgical Experiences*, 1865, p. 334), related a case of this kind which occurred in St. George's Hospital many years before.   The patient was a boy, between ten and eleven years of age.   The accident happened by his getting his leg entangled between the spokes of the wheel when riding behind a carriage.   On admission, the end of the femur was situated in the popliteal space; there was a large wound through which the end of the bone had passed; there was great pain, but the vessels and nerves were uninjured. There was considered to be severe injury to the joint, and the leg was amputated.   On examining the limb, however, the joint was found to be perfect and intact; the end of the diaphysis had been torn from its epiphysis.   The boy did well.

At the same discussion Dr. Hocken mentioned a similar case he had seen at the Exeter Hospital, in which attempts at reduction were made, but failed.

Rutherford Alcock, in an article on 'Injuries of the Joints' (*Trans. of Med. Chirurgical Society*, vol. xxiii. 1840, p. 311, case ix.), describes the case of a boy, aged six and a half, whose leg was caught in the wheel of a cab behind which he was riding. A large lacerated wound extended across the ham from one condyle to the other, through which the shaft of the femur—separated from its epiphysis, and denuded of periosteum—protruded, projecting as far downwards as the middle of the belly of the gastrocnemius. The epiphysis was in position, and the patella uninjured. The capsule of the joint had probably been opened, on account of the synovial-like fluid which issued from the wound for some time. Reduction was found to be impossible; Mr. White therefore removed a portion of the protruding shaft with a saw, and reduced the remainder. The artery, vein, and nerve in front of the bone were intact. The bone was then easily replaced, and the limb was put in a semiflexed position on its side, with a splint. The next day the apparatus was disarranged, and the leg flexed upon the thigh. The progress of the case was slow. At the end of nine months the joint did not appear to have materially suffered. It was movable, but the leg was at an angle of 75° with the thigh. A large piece of the shaft was evidently undergoing exfoliation, a corner of dead bone projecting at the wound. The child could get about with crutches, and bear some weight on the leg.

A similar case is described by Mr. Gay (*Lancet*, 1867, vol. ii. p. 456)..

J. B., aged thirteen, was admitted into the Great Northern Hospital on May 29, 1867, having been caught and thrown with great violence by a carriage wheel. There was a simple fracture of the left femur about the middle, and a compound fracture of the right at the junction of its lower epiphysis. The end of the diaphysis, stripped of periosteum and cartilage, protruded to the extent of two inches through a very extensive transverse wound in the popliteal space. There was no evidence of any injury to the vessels or nerves. Under chloroform reduction could not be effected; Mr. Gay removed with a saw the protruding part of the shaft, and replaced the bone in its normal position. An interrupted iron splint was applied with very gentle extension. Some adduction of the upper fragment was overcome by applying splints and altering the position of the limb. On the fourth day there was effusion into the knee-joint, but this disappeared by the end of the third week. Complete recovery took place at the end of three months, so that the child was able to walk perfectly. There was firm consolidation of both bones, and no overlapping of the left femur. Measurement of the two limbs gave half an inch shortening on the right side. There was abundant callus.

Dr. R. H. Harte, of Philadelphia, cites (*Trans. Amer. Surgical Association*, 1895, vol. xiii. p. 396) the following instance of pure separation. It is also described by Dr. Packard.

William B., aged ten years, was admitted to the Episcopal Hospital, September 30, 1890. While clinging to the back of a vehicle his leg became entangled in the wheel. A compound separation of the lower epiphysis of the femur was produced, with a stripping off of a considerable portion of the periosteum. The lower epiphysis was completely separated, and carried with it the ossifying cartilage. The denuded shaft of the diaphysis projected through the large wound. So great was the violence of the injury that the leg was torn off below the knee. There was no rotation of the epiphysis, perhaps (Dr. Packard suggested) because the lower connection of the gastrocnemius was severed. The thigh was amputated in the middle third, and the patient made an uninterrupted recovery.

In Dr. Meisenbach's case of compound separation the detachment was perfectly smooth, no splinters being attached to the epiphysis.

A like pure separation of this epiphysis may occur at any age as the result of severe direct crushing violence, but such cases cannot be of so great value to the pathology of the lesions we are considering as those we have just considered.

Mr. Ward's case at the London Hospital, mentioned by Mr. Jonathan Hutchinson and described above, is an example of pure separation the result of complete smashing of the limb by direct violence.

M. A. Broca brought before the Société Anatomique in 1885 (*Bulletins de la Société Anatomique*, Paris, série iv., tome x. 1885, p. 228) a most interesting case of pure separation with rupture of the internal coats of the popliteal artery by direct violence. A child, aged five years, was brought to the Hôpital de la Pitié (under Professor Verneuil), having been run over and crushed by a carriage. The leg was almost completely separated from the thigh, for in front of the thigh there was a very large, irregular, and rugged wound, and an evident epiphysial separation of the femur. The lower end of the upper fragment was somewhat displaced outwards and completely separated from the patella. The femoral condyles could be seen in contact with the exposed articular surfaces of the tibia and presented their lower surface forwards, their posterior surface having been drawn downwards by the action of the gastrocnemii, and immovably fixed in this position by the postmortem rigidity of these muscles—for the leg was undoubtedly dead; it was quite cold, insensible, and without any trace of pulsation. There was no flow of blood from the wound of the soft parts—only a slight bloody oozing from the osseous surface, which continued till the following morning, when amputation of the thigh was performed. The child died the following day.

On dissection of the limb the following lesions were found: (1) There was a complete epiphysial separation of the lower end of the femur; this separation was remarkable in that, contrary to the rule, it was not accompanied by any fracture, but, on the other hand, some small cartilaginous processes remained adherent to the diaphysial surface. The periosteum was torn across two or three centimetres above the detached epiphysis, and formed a kind of irregular collar round the epiphysial excavation. The examination of the upper part of the femur, made after the death of the child, showed that the periosteum was detached from the shaft up to the great trochanter. The state of the popliteal vessels was particularly interesting. Their continuity was unbroken. Externally the vein seemed sound, but the artery presented a diminution in its calibre for about two centimetres in extent, and, on opening this vessel above, the two internal coats were seen to be lacerated and retracted. There was a clot in the upper end; the lower end was empty. Between the two ends the external cellular coat alone maintained the continuity of the vessel. The vein had resisted better than the artery, but that it had undergone some stretching was proved by a series of transverse markings or furrows on its internal surface.

The specimens from the case were placed in the Musée Dupuytren.

Mr. Symonds had a like case under his care at Guy's Hospital. Chas. A., aged nine, was admitted on April 9, 1886, his right leg having been run over by the wheel of a wagon. There was a very extensive lacerated wound eight inches long on the inner side, exposing the internal lateral ligament and opening the joint at the posterior part of its inner aspect. The tendons on the inner side of the knee were also much exposed, and the lower end of the diaphysis protruded into the wound. The epiphysial cartilage remained entirely with the diaphysis, and a sheath of periosteum was torn off the diaphysis for three and a half inches. The separation of the epiphysis was complete. Amputation of the thigh was considered necessary, and the patient recovered.

Although the report states that the whole of the epiphysial cartilage remained with the diaphysial fragment in this instance, it is open to considerable doubt whether this condition actually existed even as the result of the direct crushing violence. It must also be borne in mind that at the ninth year—the age of the patient—the cartilage which subsequently forms the conjugal disc is not yet a distinct structure from the cartilage forming the epiphysis.

Julia Fontenelle's and Rougon's cases (loc. cit. supra) may also be considered as examples of separation uncomplicated with fracture.

In Rougon's case the greater part of the cartilage remained adherent to the epiphysis, and Hutchinson says that the diaphysial end in his case bore no traces of it.

In Julia Fontenelle's case, at many points of the rugged extremity of the diaphysis, principally on the outer side, a white material was visible, of a glistening aspect, which appeared to be the ossifying cartilage; but the greater part of this had followed the condyles, which were surrounded by the capsule of the knee-joint and were continuous above with the periosteum.

Ménard, in his work, proves that the cartilage remains adherent to the epiphysis in these cases.

In Rathbun's case, quoted below, it was found that the line of separation followed the epiphysial cartilage throughout, and in no place did it traverse the osseous tissue.

Dr. H. R. Wharton mentions (*University Medical Magazine,* Philadelphia, January, 1889, vol. i. No. 4, p. 214) a case of pure epiphysial separation which he had seen. The lad had the shaft of his right femur cleanly separated from its lower epiphysis and driven through the skin by having his leg caught in a rapidly revolving wheel.

In a case of Fischer and Hirschfield the separation of this epiphysis, although a simple and pure one, was accompanied by other severe lesions (separation of the upper epiphysis of the tibia and both epiphyses of the fibula) of the opposite limb, which proved fatal from suppuration and necrosis. The separation of the lower epiphysis of the femur was found at the time of death, eleventh week, to be firmly consolidated, though with some rotation of the epiphysis. This was rotated so that its internal condyle ascended somewhat forwards, whilst the external condyle descended backwards. The knee-joint was not injured.

Another instance of pure separation is recorded by Jarjavay (*Traité d'anatomie chirurgicale,* 1852, tome i. p. 70) from the practice of M. Velpeau. A girl, aged nine years, had been knocked down in the street, and the wheel of an omnibus had passed over her thigh. The lower end of the diaphysis, entirely denuded of its periosteum, projected five centimetres on the outer side of the limb through a wound of the soft parts.

This end of the bone, which was resected, was preserved by M. Jarjavay, because in M. Guéretin's experiments the epiphysis always dragged away some portion of the diaphysis; in this instance the surface of the bone was slightly undulating, smooth, and without any trace of fracture.

Dr. J. M. Elder showed, before the Canadian Medical Association at Montreal, September 1891 (*Montreal Medical Journal,* 'Traumatic Separation of the Lower Epiphysis of the Femur,' March 1892, p. 643), the following case of compound separation in a youth.

· 'When seven years old he was standing on one foot, with the other resting on the hub of a wagon-wheel; a pile of lumber behind him fell forward and struck the standing limb just below the knee, driving the lower part of the leg violently forwards, and letting the lower part of the femur impinge on and perforate the popliteal space, through which the bone protruded for about three and a half inches, letting the boy down as it were. The two nearest medical men were at once summoned, and diagnosed compound dislocation backward of the femur, not noticing the absence of the condyloid cartilage on the protruding bone. Two different attempts under chloroform were made at reduction, but neither were successful, so amputation above the knee was advised. To this the boy's father strongly objected, and, failing this, they sawed off what they could not reduce (about an inch and a half), tucked in the remainder, and left the case in disgust at the obduracy of the father. It was hot weather, and before the days of modern antisepticism, so that the neglected wound soon became septic. The father (an intelligent French-Canadian blacksmith) then took the case in hand, and henceforward was the only one who acted as surgeon. He killed the maggots by pouring whisky into the wound, and improvised a sole-leather back-splint. In four weeks the lad was propelling himself around the garden, and in two months was walking, at first stiffly, but as time went on he got the perfectly good knee-joint which he then presented. The injured limb was shorter than the other by exactly the amount of bone removed thirteen years ago (one and a half inches), but in every other respect was as strong as its fellow, and he was able to do any kind of work. The specimen of bone was not quite perfect, owing to the father having singed it at his forge "to burn off the stink," but it could be plainly seen to be the lower end of the femur.'

From the above-mentioned evidence, museum specimens, and compound separations we see that the cartilaginous line of union generally remains adherent to the condyloid epiphysis, and that only a thin very fine layer occasionally adheres to the rounded mammillated end of the diaphysis. The end is somewhat of the shape of a wooden mallet, the separation occurring for the most part through the ossifying layer of Ranvier, but it may be observed that the separated cartilage more commonly drags off a few granules of the spongy tissue of the diaphysis in the form of small scales or flakes. Very frequently a somewhat larger chipping of the diaphysis takes place.

Pure separation without displacement.—The tough periosteum of the lower end of the diaphysis remains in this condition untorn, but stripped off the diaphysis to a greater or less extent.

Mr. Hutchinson junior's specimen at the Royal College of Surgeons from a lad aged fourteen is a good example; in this case there was also an intercondyloid fracture of the epiphysis, from which a small fragment was broken off.

The accompanying drawing is taken from a photograph kindly presented to the author by Professor J. G. Adami, of McGill University, Montreal. The specimen is in the McGill Medical College Museum. It shows a pure separation with little displacement. The epiphysis is only slightly rotated on its transverse axis, and a slight gap is left between the epiphysis and posterior edge of the diaphysis. Professor Adami notes that 'the condyles are completely separated from the diaphysis at the epiphysial line without any evidence of other injury to the bone. From the appearance of the parts separation had evidently occurred some time before death. Unfortunately there was no history.'

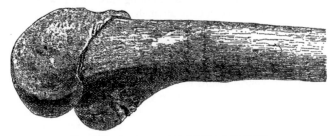

FIG. 218.—SEPARATION WITH SLIGHT DISPLACEMENT
(McGill University Museum, Montreal, Canada)

Separation with fracture of the diaphysis.—Although pure separation is not uncommon, on the other hand the separation is more often associated with a fracture of the diaphysis, which may be multiple or more or less extensive in character.

A careful and minute description has been given of the form and dimensions of the co-existing fracture in seventeen cases, in which a direct examination has been made. Six of these are museum specimens, eight were cases of compound fracture, and three were cases in which amputation was performed for subsequent gangrene or other complication.

The length of the portion of the diaphysis separated off from its end and remaining attached to the epiphysis varies very much, from one-third to two and a half inches. In others it is an insignificant spicule or two of bone. It may be from the *outer, inner, anterior,* or *antero-internal* part of the diaphysiary extremity, according to the direction of the displaced epiphysis and the violence causing it.

It is noticeable that in all six of the specimens in the London museums associated with fracture this has taken place on the *outer* side, and in the compound cases, mentioned above, four were combined with fracture on the inner side, one at the antero-internal part, and in one the situation is not stated. Of the three remaining cases one was fractured on the outer side, another at the anterior part, and in the third the position of the fracture is not stated. It is probable that the fragment of the diaphysis is always situated on the side of bone opposite to that upon which the violence first acts, consequently the epiphysis is first separated on the one side by the violence before the fracture takes place on the other.

The specimen in the Museum of St. Bartholomew's Hospital (*St. Bartholomew's Hospital Museum Catalogue,* vol. i. p. 110), No.

758, is the lower extremity of the femur of a boy, aged fourteen, showing a separation of the epiphysis from the diaphysis. In this specimen the epiphysis is not rotated. On its outer side there remains a small fragment of the diaphysis, about one-third of an inch long and nearly one inch in length, still adherent to it.

The specimen in the Charing Cross Hospital Museum, No. 391 (*Charing Cross Hospital Museum Catalogue*, 1888, p. 36), consists of portions of the bones of the knee-joint removed by excision.

Separation of the epiphysis has taken place quite cleanly through, about the inner three-quarters of epiphysial junction, but on the outer side a triangular piece of the diaphysis, one and three-quarters of an inch in width and one inch in thickness, retains its connection with the epiphysis. The patella and upper portion of the tibia are shown uninjured.

The case is described by Mr. E. Canton in the *Transactions of the Pathological Society* (vol. x. 1859, p. 232), and is figured in Treves's *System of Surgery* (vol. i. 1895, p. 847, fig. 291). A boy, aged eight years, when alighting from a cart, slipped, and, his foot becoming entangled between the spokes of one of the wheels, he fell to the ground. On examination at Charing Cross Hospital, Mr. Canton found the lower epiphysis of the femur torn from the shaft, with considerable contusion of the soft parts. The fragments were reduced and adjusted in the hope that union would take place. However, in the course of a few days, suppuration, sloughing, and severe constitutional disturbance necessitated the performance of excision of the whole articulation. Recovery rapidly ensued. The union of the soft parts was perfect, but the fibrous union between the bones permitted very considerable movement, so that the leg resembled a flail. At the end of five months, amputation, urged by the parents, was performed through the lower third of the thigh. Recovery. (*Dublin Quarterly Journal*, 1861, p. 74; *Lancet*, vol. ii. 1858, August 28, p. 231.)

The Museum of the Royal College of Surgeons of England (*Catalogue of the Royal College of Surgeons Museum*, Appendix I. p. 30) contains a specimen, No. 1041B, of the lower end of a femur and the knee-joint,

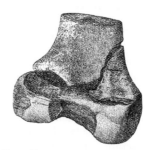

FIG. 219.—SEPARATION WITH FRACTURE OF THE DIAPHYSIS

(Royal College of Surgeons Museum, No. 1041B)

showing a separation of the lower epiphysis of the femur, associated with fracture of the diaphysis, presented to the museum by W. Spencer Watson, 1884. The separation is not a clean one, but a portion of bone (more than one inch in length) broken from the diaphysis is attached to the outer side. It was taken from a boy, aged twelve, who was severely injured one week before his death by being caught in some machinery. During life the lower end of the diaphysis of the femur projected on the inner side of the limb and nearly penetrated the soft parts; the periosteum covering the lower third of the shaft of the femur was separated from the bone by a collection of blood and pus. He died from exhaustion.

Another specimen, No. 1041A, in the Museum of the Royal College of Surgeons of England, presented by F. S. Eve, Esq., 1887,

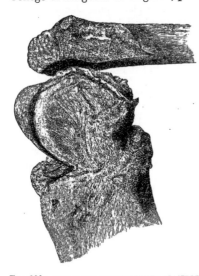

shows separation of the epiphysis with fracture of the diaphysis. The outer half of the epiphysis, corresponding to the external condyle, is cleanly separated; but at the level of the intercondyloid notch a dentate fracture extends upwards and inwards through the shaft, leaving a considerable fragment of it attached to the epiphysis. The part was removed by amputation from a boy, who sustained a severe injury to the limb by the wheel of a tramcar.

In Packard's case there was an extremely small portion of the diaphysis detached from the inner side.

FIG. 220.—SEPARATION WITH EXTENSIVE FRACTURE OF THE DIAPHYSIS
(Royal College of Surgeons Museum, 1041A, ½-size)

In some instances the fracture of the diaphysis may be so extensive and comminuted that the separation of the epiphysis can only be regarded as of secondary importance; but where the joint is involved as well, as in the following specimen from St. Bartholomew's Hospital, the lesion is increased so much more in its gravity.

The specimen in St. Bartholomew's Hospital Museum, No. 977, of the lower two-thirds of the shaft of a femur, shows a comminuted fracture of the lower end of the shaft and of the epiphysis, extending into the knee-joint. The fracture extends almost vertically along the centre of the shaft to the junction of the lower with the middle third; midway it is joined by a lateral fracture. The fractured surfaces are partially united. Above the upper limit of the fracture on the inner side is a projecting fragment of new bone, probably formed by a portion of uptorn periosteum. The condyles of the femur are separated, and the anterior portion of the articular surface is detached from them. On the outer portion of the fractured epiphysis none of the diaphysis adhered to the epiphysis. There is also new periosteal bone on both the lower fragments of the diaphysis, as if from the result of suppurative periostitis, and the cellular spaces of the whole of the shaft in the specimen are seen to be opening out and becoming rarefied.

In Mr. A. H. Tubby's specimen of separation of the lower epiphysis of the femur in the Royal College of Surgeons Museum, No. 1041G, there is extensive stripping off of the periosteum from the lower part of the shaft, probably the result of periostitis secondary to an injury. However, the epiphysial line of cartilage does not appear to have been destroyed by inflammation. The lower extremity of the shaft is displaced forwards, and is somewhat splintered. No history.

COMPOUND SEPARATION WITH FRACTURE OF THE DIAPHYSIS.— P. Bruns relates (*Archiv für klinische Chirurg.* 1882, Bd. xxvii. S. 240) the case of a girl, aged eleven years, who had been run over by a waggon loaded with hay. On the outer side of the knee there was a contused wound which exposed the outer condyle and opened the knee-joint. Death took place on the sixth day from exhaustion, primary amputation having been refused. The separation of the epiphysis on the outer side followed exactly the epiphysial junction as far as the middle line, and then passed upwards and inwards as a fracture through the spongy tissue of the diaphysis. The fragment of the diaphysis was still held in position by an unbroken portion, one centimetre in thickness, of the compact tissue on the inner side.

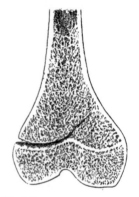

FIG. 221.—PARTIAL SEPARATION OF LOWER FEMORAL EPIPHYSIS, WITH INCOMPLETE FRACTURE OF DIAPHYSIS

(After Bruns, 'Deutsche Chirurgie,' 1886, S. 123)

Professor Jas. L. Little showed to the New York Pathological Society, May 24, 1865 (*New York Medical Journal*, vol. ii. 1865–6, p. 131; *The Illustrated Quarterly of Medicine and Surgery*, New York, vol. i. No. 1, January 1882, p. 23, plate iii.), a specimen obtained from his own practice. Willie B., aged eleven, while hanging on the back of a waggon, had his right leg caught between the spokes of the wheel, which was in rapid motion. A few hours after the accident, Dr. Little found a separation of the lower epiphysis, the upper fragment of the femur projecting three inches through an opening in the upper and outer part of the popliteal space—the upper fragment completely overlapping the lower—and considerable contusion and laceration of the soft parts. On examination, the wound did not appear to communicate with the knee-joint. The protruding part of the diaphysis was cleanly stripped of its periosteum. Under the

z z

influence of ether, the fragments were reduced by strong extension
of the limb and flexion of the leg upon the thigh, the reduction
occasioning a dull cartilaginous crepitus.   There was at the time no
pulsation in the posterior tibial artery, and the limb was cold.   The
hæmorrhage was free, but no ligatures were necessary.   The limb
was laid over a double-inclined plane.   The following day pulsation
and warmth returned, but the upper fragment had again become
displaced, and it was found that it could only be kept in place by
extreme flexion of the leg.   This position was maintained by the
application of plaster bandages, binding the leg to the thigh.

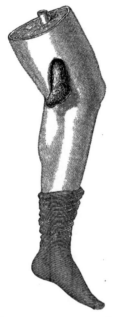

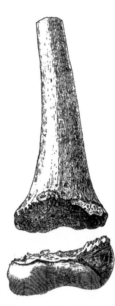

FIG. 222.—PROFESSOR J. L. LITTLE'S CASE OF
COMPOUND SEPARATION WITH DISPLACEMENT
INWARDS OF THE EPIPHYSIS

FIG. 223.—THE SAME AFTER AMPUTATION,
SHOWING SLIGHT FRACTURE OF THE
DIAPHYSIS

Considerable traumatic fever followed, with swelling, and on the
tenth day slight secondary hæmorrhage from the wound.   On the
thirteenth day serious secondary hæmorrhage occurred from the
anterior tibial artery near its origin, and it became necessary to
amputate.

The boy made a good recovery.   The specimen showed (a) the
synovial membrane involved and intensely reddened throughout and
an almost perfect separation of the lower epiphysis, which at one
point (b) however traversed the bony structure.

J. R. Reverdin has given (*Revue Méd. de la Suisse Romande,*
Genève, 1886, vi. p. 291, with figure) an accurate and detailed

account of an incomplete traumatic separation combined with fracture.

Marie B., aged four years and two months, while endeavouring to climb behind a carriage, had her right leg caught between the spokes of the wheel. There was a transverse lacerated wound right across the popliteal space, and the diaphysis, stripped of its periosteum, projected nearly four inches. Its end was convex, mammillated, and much soiled with dirt. The popliteal nerves were both exposed for a considerable distance, but appeared to be intact. On exploration, pulsation of the popliteal artery was felt on the inner side of the nerves, and a clean separation of the outer half of the epiphysis; at the inner part a largish pyramidal fragment of the diaphysis, three centimetres in height above the epiphysial line, was still attached to the epiphysis. Several loose scales of bone were also felt. Under chloroform, an attempt was made to preserve the limb. The soiled parts of the end of the diaphysis were soft enough to be removed with a knife, the wound was thoroughly cleansed with a five per cent. solution of carbolic acid, and iodoform dressings were applied. While a Volkmann's splint was being applied, the limb was noticed to be pale and cold. The next day the foot was still cold and insensitive. On the fourth day there was gangrene of the edges of the wound, ending at some distance on the inner side in the calf. On the sixth day the external popliteal nerve was found to be partially destroyed, the internal popliteal nerve reddened, and there was suppuration of the entire wound extending into the calf along the gangrenous part and into the thigh. There was also necrosis of the femur externally. Amputation was consequently performed. Recovery was rapid, and the wound healed in six weeks.

Examination of the amputated limb showed the popliteal artery full of pinkish grey clot, without any injury to its coats, and diffuse suppuration of the calf and thigh, also a small slough on the heel. It is probable that the vessel must have been compressed either by the epiphysis or the reduced diaphysis. Separation of the epiphysis, as previously seen, had occurred, and the pyramidal piece of the shaft was surmounted by a small fragment incompletely separated from the main piece. The epiphysial surface of the external condyle was formed of cartilage only at the margins; in the centre there remained adherent to the cartilage a thin granular layer of hard osseous tissue. A split with a slight interval between the epiphysis and the fragment of the shaft could be detected on slightly separating these portions of the bone. The periosteum was torn from the inner condyle behind at the level of the epiphysis, but in front one centimetre above this. The joint was opened by a small rent on the outer side, and behind, where the periosteum was torn off to the level of the cartilage, and contained a little sero-sanguineous fluid. The crucial ligaments were inflamed and of a pinkish colour.

Tapret and Chenet have reported a similar case (*Bull. de la Soc.*

Anatomique, Paris, January 8, 1875, 3ème série, vol. x. p. 25) in a boy aged nine and a half years. In climbing behind a carriage he had his right leg caught in the spokes of a wheel. The skin was transversely lacerated in the ham, and there was great articular effusion. Considerable hæmorrhage took place before his admission into the Hôpital des Enfants Malades. The limb was put up in an immovable plaster-of-Paris splint, leaving the popliteal region free; but after a few days sloughing ensued, and evacuation of a strip of muscle, which exposed the end of the shaft. Amputation was performed at the middle of the thigh by M. de Saint-Germain. On examination, the separation followed the line of union between the epiphysial cartilage and the shaft, but towards the inner side it deviated a little so as to include a small portion of the diaphysis at this part. The popliteal vessels were intact and the articular ligaments uninjured. Death ensued five days after the amputation. At the autopsy there were extreme muscular lacerations and collections of blood about the stump, some of which had suppurated.

M. A. Broca brought before the Société Anatomique, Paris, May 30, 1884 (*Le Progrès Médical*, Paris, 1885, 2ème série, vol. i. p. 170; *Bull. de la Soc. Anatomique*, 4ème série, tome v. 1884, p. 407) the case of a boy, aged three and a half, who had had his leg crushed by a tramcar, so that it was completely divided at the anterior tuberosity of the tibia. He was admitted into the Trousseau Hospital under the care of M. Lannelongue. The fibula was not fractured, but its upper end was detached at its articulation with the tibia, and protruded. The wound was greatly contused and pulped, and the lower epiphysis of the femur found to be movable. Amputation of the thigh was performed two and a half inches above the joint. Death ensued from shock the next morning. The epiphysial separation of the femur was combined with a fracture, which extended upwards and inwards from the inner third of the separated surface as far as the middle third of the diaphysis. This portion of the diaphysis remained connected with the epiphysis. The epiphysial cartilage was adherent to the epiphysis.

Mr. E. Canton reported a second case to the Pathological Society in 1860 (*Transactions of the Pathological Society, London*, vol. xi. 1860, p. 195, woodcut 10; *Dublin Quarterly Journal of Med. Science*, February 1861). W. J., aged fifteen years, was admitted into Charing Cross Hospital on October 21, 1859. He had received a violent kick from a horse on the left knee. On admission there was shortening of the limb, complete eversion of the foot, and slight flexion of the leg. The patella was directed outwards with considerable and general swelling around the knee, and with such distortion of the parts as to give the impression of the tibia being dislocated backwards and somewhat outwards. The inner femoral condyle appeared to project unduly, and the skin covering it was tense and abraded. On the outer side, and above the patella, a forward elevation of bone could be felt. Careful manipulation of the lower end of the femur elicited crepitus. By extension and counter-extension the parts were easily reduced and adjusted by means of splints, but towards the end of October they became displaced through the restlessness of the patient. There was also articular inflammation, and in two days' time a slough formed on the inner side of the knee, which allowed slight projection of the subjacent bone. Severe constitutional disturbance set in ; Mr. Canton, therefore, on November 3, excised the articulation. The boy recovered perfectly, and the bones were properly ankylosed when he was discharged.

The specimen showed a separation running through about three-fourths of the circumference of the epiphysial line, while the remaining fourth was still firmly held in its normal position. Thus an oblique fracture of the shaft commenced at its outer side and ran into the epiphysial separation below. There was also a comminuted portion of the shaft displaced into the popliteal space. The patient was able to walk a long distance. After being out of the hospital for about two months he had a fall, which was thought to have loosened the union between the bones. Amputation was performed at his own desire.

Mr. Holmes (*Surgical Diseases of Children*, 1869, 2nd edit. p. 260, fig. 45), in quoting the case, adds that the preparation at Charing Cross Hospital proves that there was really no reason for the amputation, and gives a figure showing the bones firmly ankylosed, in good position, and free from disease.

G. Marcano relates (*Bull. de la Soc. Anatomique*, 1875, 4ème série, x. p. 227 ; *Le Progrès Médical*, August 14, 1875, p. 460) the case of Chas. S., aged fifteen years, who was admitted into the Beaujon Hospital under the care of M. Dolbeau. His arm had been caught in the transmission strap of a machine and his body flung in all directions till his arm was completely torn off. Comminuted fractures of the left humerus and right femur were found, and at the inner side of the left knee, just above the joint (the movements of which were free), there was a large projection, presenting a sharp wrinkled edge.

There was soft crepitation, and reduction was easy by means of pressure on the upper fragment, but the displacement was reproduced as soon as the parts were left to themselves. Death occurred the next day. At the autopsy the epiphysial separation was seen to pass through the line of junction of diaphysis and epiphysis, except quite at the outer side, where there was a fracture of the diaphysis and a scale of bone detached, leaving an irregular surface for the extent of three centimetres on the anterior aspect of the femur. The periosteum was loosened at the inner side of the diaphysis for eleven centimetres in length by five centimetres in width, though it still adhered to the epiphysis.

Dr. Davis Halderman, Professor of Surgery in the Starling Medical College, reports (*New York Medical Record*, vol. xxi.–xxii. July 3, 1882, p. 600) a case in a mulatto boy, eighteen years old, caused by a violent blow over the front and lower part of the right thigh. Three hours after the accident the patient was brought to St. Francis Hospital, Starling Medical College. On examination there was great swelling about the knee; the leg and foot were cold, and the dorsalis pedis artery was pulseless. Numbness, too, was complained of below the joint, while in the latter excruciating pains were experienced. The limb was shortened two inches. Owing to the swelling the line of separation could be with difficulty made out, but it was finally located two inches above the articular plane in front, and the lower end of the shaft could be distinctly felt directly beneath the integument, in the popliteal space, on a level with the anterior tibial tuberosity. Efforts were now made with the aid of anæsthetics at adjustment, but without success; for although the limb, by means of extension and counter-extension, could be brought down to nearly its natural length and the projection in the popliteal space could be caused somewhat to recede, the moment the efforts were relaxed the displacement would recur. In view of this, and the crippled condition of the circulation, it was deemed advisable, for the time being at least, to place the patient in bed, with the limb slightly elevated and in as comfortable a position as possible, and await results.

At the end of twenty-four hours the swelling had increased; some slight discoloration over the foot and leg had set in, but the temperature was somewhat improved, and while the shock had been for the most part recovered from, the pains about the joint still seemed out of proportion for injuries of this kind, and the dorsalis pedis artery remained pulseless, as indeed it continued to the end. It was determined to place the limb in a flexed position upon a double inclined plane with moderate extension, and see if by this means suffering might not be lessened. In its adjustment the limb was brought down within half an inch of the length of its fellow, but no weight sufficient to keep it there could be borne. The patient from this time on felt easier, so far as the injured extremity alone was concerned. By next day, however—the second after the accident—considerable constitutional disturbance had supervened, pulse was 118, temperature 102°, and burning sensations in the foot and under side of the leg were experienced, while the toes and plantar aspects of the foot were dull on pinching and pricking. It was thus evident gangrene of these parts was threatening, but it was still thought the collateral circulation about the knee might arrest the morbid action below this point, a hope that was warranted by the natural warmth and sensibility over the upper part of the leg, and that was maintained to the last, which was three days later. Meantime the discoloration below this point spread and deepened;

phlyctenulæ finally formed over the lower, outer, and under part of
the leg and ham, and at the latter place also quite an eschar, from
the pressure of the end of the bone beneath the skin. The leg and
foot at last became cold and insensible to deep pricking, except near
the knee and along the inner aspect of the leg, corresponding to the
course of the great saphenous nerve, which, save at its termination,
remained intact. Accordingly, on the fifth day after the injury, the
limb was removed at the inferior part of the middle third of the
thigh, the damaged state of the tissues being such as to preclude
amputation lower down.

Dissection of the amputated limb revealed the fact that the tissues
about the injury had been severely damaged, the soft parts for some
distance around being extensively lacerated and pulped in the immediate vicinity of the fracture. Blood was widely extravasated up and
down the limb, and filled the joint cavity through a rent on its inner
side. The lower end of the femur was completely denuded of
periosteum, muscle, &c., and lay bare amid the *débris* of the injury,
as did also a mass of broken-off cancellous bone, about the size of
the end of a man's thumb. The detached epiphysis, still connected
with the popliteus and gastrocnemius muscles, was tilted backwards
by their action, and at the same time was overlapped at its posterior
and outer aspect by the shaft to the extent of several inches.
Between them, and on the anterior and inner aspect of the latter
bone, lay the internal popliteal nerve, and the popliteal vein and
artery were impinged upon by the fragments—that is, these parts, instead of being behind the bone, had been displaced to the front of it,
and were held there by the hook-shaped projection of the divided
internal condyloid ridge over which they had caught, so that any
effort at adjustment served only the more heavily to bear down
upon and closely embrace them, and thus to cut off the circulation and innervation beyond. The artery was contused and
inflamed. Its walls were thickened, its interior roughened and
filled with clotted blood. The vein was in the same condition, and
the nerve too, as concerned its pressure. The outer popliteal nerve,
although still sustaining its proper relation to the bone, was dragged
down and also pressed upon severely by the latter in its malposition.
Death occurred from pyæmia on the thirtieth day after amputation
and the thirty-fifth day after the injury.

M. Delens says (*loc. cit. supra*), in his analysis of cases, there
will be found twelve in which epiphysial separation is mentioned
without the question of fracture or splinters. In nine cases, on the
other hand, there existed a fracture in association with the separation, generally represented by one or more fragments from the
extremity of the diaphysis. 'But,' he continues, 'it is very likely
that these figures do not express the exact proportion of true
separations and separations with the existence of fracture. These
latter cases appear to me to be the most frequent, and no doubt the

observers of the cases above mentioned have more than once neglected to indicate the existence of small fragments when the separation had chiefly taken place in the line of the cartilaginous union.'

Separation with intercondyloid fracture.—Three specimens in the London museums show that this separation is sometimes accompanied by an intercondyloid fracture. It is somewhat surprising that this is not more frequently the case, seeing the comparatively thin condition of the epiphysis at the intercondyloid notch (see above).

Its existence has, however, been suspected in some cases of compound diastasis.

The specimen in the Guy's Hospital Museum, No. 1210[68], shows a vertical fracture of the separated epiphysis exactly in the

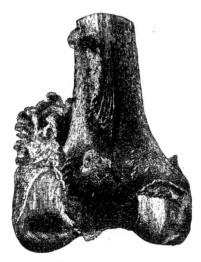

FIG. 224.—SEPARATION WITH INTERCONDYLOID FRACTURE
(St. Bartholomew's Hospital Museum)

centre. It was taken from a patient under the care of Mr. Durham, Cornelius McC., aged fourteen, who had been caught in the straps of some machinery and whirled round before it could be stopped. Three or four inches of the shaft of the left femur protruded through the skin. Death occurred the same day. There was found a fracture of the skull with meningeal ecchymosis, also fracture of the right tibia and fibula.

St. Bartholomew's Hospital Museum (*St. Bartholomew's Hospital Museum Catalogue*, vol. i. p. 140) contains a specimen, No. 981, exhibiting a separation of the epiphysis from the shaft of the femur, and a vertical fracture extending between the condyles into the knee-joint. The periosteum was stripped from the diaphysis to the extent of about six inches nearly all round, but remained partly attached to the condyles. The halves of the epiphysis are separated laterally for a distance of two inches in front, without any rotation of either fragment. The shaft protrudes through the muscles on the inner side of the thigh, and is intact. A line of new bone is formed on the anterior part of the shaft along the torn edge of that part of the periosteum which remained attached to the shaft. The injury was produced by a rope being entangled round the leg of a boy aged sixteen. Amputation was performed three weeks afterwards.

The specimen in St. George's Hospital Museum, No. 55A (*St. George's Hospital Museum Catalogue*, 1882, p. 12, No. 3443), shows a separation of part of the epiphysis combined with an oblique fracture of the diaphysis, and is figured in Holmes and Hulke's *System of Surgery* (3rd edit. 1883, vol. i. p. 1025).

The condyles are separated from each other by a longitudinal fracture through the intercondyloid notch.

The internal condyle is detached from the shaft by a fracture traversing the epiphysial line.

The external condyle is not separated at the cartilaginous junction ; this is still intact, but there is an oblique fracture of the lower end of the diaphysis, thus separating the external condyle with a portion of the diaphysis two inches in length. The specimen was taken from a boy, who was stated to be only fifteen, but who was fully developed and looked at least eighteen, judging from the size of the femur. He was a baker by trade, and caught his leg in the machine employed in bread-making. He was brought to the hospital, where there was found to be such laceration of the soft parts, conjoined with the fracture, that amputation was immediately performed. He died the same day.

Mr. Porter, in 1873 (*Proceedings of the Pathological Society of Dublin*, 1873–75, vol. vi. N.S. p. 117), exhibited at the Pathological Society of Dublin a similar specimen showing a separation of the lower epiphysis of the femur with a fracture between the condyles. There was also a fracture of the os calcis. The specimens were taken from a boy, aged thirteen years, who slipped in jumping on a tramcar and the wheel of the vehicle passed along his lower extremity, causing extensive laceration of the muscles with profuse hæmorrhage, for which the limb was amputated.

Mr. Mansell Moullin showed before the Pathological Society, on November 15, 1887 (*Pathological Society's Transactions,* vol. xxxix. 1888, p. 243), an interesting case of diastasis, associated with intercondyloid fracture and other lesions, which is quoted later on.

In the Royal College of Surgeons Museum, No. 1041D (Mr. Jonathan Hutchinson junior's specimen, 1888), there are transverse vertical sections of the left femur, from a lad aged fourteen, who sustained a severe crush of the leg between two carriages. Primary amputation was performed on account of the knee-joint being opened and the soft parts much torn. The patient recovered.

Owing to the periosteum retaining the epiphysis in its place, the detachment of the latter was not diagnosed before dissection. The line of separation has passed chiefly above the epiphysial disc, and in addition there is a vertical fracture of the epiphysis between the condyles, and a loose portion of the epiphysis, three-quarters of an inch long, at the intercondyloid notch. Some fragments of dirt are embedded in the epiphysis. As usual, the periosteum is here more extensively torn off the posterior than the anterior surface of the shaft, and there is little or no displacement of the epiphysis.

Displacement of the diaphysis is the usual accompaniment of this separation; it will be found to vary according to the causes producing the injury, which have been mentioned above. There have been various opinions up to the present as to the common direction of the displacement.

It usually takes place *backwards*—viz. into the popliteal space, as a result of violent overextension of the limb, from the leg being caught in the spokes of a wheel, or, as in Fontenelle's and Bell's cases, from the leg being fixed in a hole and the body thrown violently forwards; see also cases mentioned by Coural, Little, Voss, and Buck. Tillmans rightly states that in the majority of cases the epiphysis is pushed forwards, and the diaphysis backwards, into the popliteal space. König also distinguishes this same direction of the fragments, and the very exceptional opposite direction.

Among the museum specimens and cases of compound separation we find that thirteen were produced by the entanglement of the leg in the spokes of a revolving wheel; in eleven of these (Liston's, Bell's (second case), and those of Alcock, Gay, Hawkins, Little, Hamilton, Verneuil, Delens, Reverdin, Tapret) the displacement was backwards; in the other two it was outwards.

Among the same cases we find that the same displacement may occur from a fall from a height (eighty feet), from crushing of the leg, or by the leg being run over by a vehicle.

From these instances we also see that the diaphysis may be displaced *outwards* (Post's and Callender's cases, from the leg being caught in the spokes of a wheel)—slightly outwards in one of Broca's cases, being completely separated from the patella; or *inwards*, as in Watson's case (Royal College of Surgeons Museum), where the leg was caught in some machinery; or *forwards*, as in Adams's case (Royal College of Surgeons Museum); in a specimen (56A, Museum of St. George's Hospital), caused by twisting of rope round the leg; and in Richet's case, from twisting of the leg by the strap of a machine. In the last instance the end of the diaphysis had perforated the synovial membrane of the knee-joint, and entered the articular cavity, and was actually situated beneath the patella in front.

In this last mode of displacement, the diaphysis being thrust forwards on to the trochlear surface of the condyles, the popliteal vessels, as will be seen later on, are not so liable to be pressed upon, being protected by their normal relations and retained in their position in the intercondyloid notch of the condylar fragment.

The author has cursorily sketched out the directions of displacement of the diaphysial end, since separation of the lower femoral epiphysis has been described in this manner by a few writers. It is, however, better to follow the plan adopted in the case of most of the other epiphysial separations, and classify according to the displacement of the epiphysis rather than of the diaphysis.

Displacement of the epiphysis forwards.—The most common position for the epiphysis to be displaced is upon the front of the femur. The forcible extension of the limb causes rotation of the epiphysis upon its transverse axis, so that its separated surface looks backwards. The obliquity of the epiphysial surfaces will facilitate its progress in this direction.

The powerful muscles of the leg keep up the displacement or render it more marked when once the epiphysis has been displaced by the violence of the injury. Although the gastrocnemius muscle is not entirely attached to the epiphysis, but is partly above the epiphysial line, yet the action of the muscle in displacing the epiphysis forwards is very complete; for the whole of the muscle becomes torn off with the periosteum attached to the epiphysis, which is very dense at this point—the epiphysial junction. In cases of less severe violence, without great stripping of periosteum, the fact of the partial attachment of the muscle alone might tend to counteract the ill effects which overextension might otherwise have..

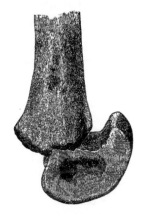

FIG. 225.—INCOMPLETE DISPLACEMENT OF EPIPHYSIS FORWARDS OFF THE DIAPHYSIS

(St. Bartholomew's Hospital Museum, No. 982. ½-size)

The epiphysis may be displaced forwards and upwards, only halfway off the diaphysis, as in a specimen in the Museum of St. Bartholomew's Hospital, No. 982 (*Catalogue of St. Bartholomew's Hospital Museum*, vol. i. p. 140). The lower epiphysis of the femur is rotated on its transverse axis and displaced forwards and upwards, halfway off the diaphysis, so that the inferior surface looks forwards and downwards. The popliteal vein was pressed upon by the projecting lower extremity of the shaft, which is entire, and gangrene was thus produced. The separation is a perfectly pure one.

The Museum of St. George's Hospital (*Catalogue of the Museum of St. George's Hospital*, 1866, p. 45; *Trans. Path. Soc.* vol. xiii. p. 187) contains a preparation [No. 56B (138)] showing complete separation of the lower epiphysis from the shaft, with a few osseous fragments of the diaphysis still adhering to its anterior lip in front of each condyle, and slight rotation upwards and forwards on its transverse axis; this was said to be more marked when the parts were fresh. There is also an opening into the knee-joint, exposing the posterior part of the outer condyle, and communicating with a large wound in the ham. The injury was caused by a fall of about eighty feet. The patient, Thomas R., aged sixteen, recovered after primary amputation.

In many other instances the epiphysis is displaced forwards completely off the diaphysis, so that its upper fractured surface is in contact with the front of the diaphysis, as in McDiarmid's case and Fontenelle's case.

A specimen in the Museum of the Leeds Infirmary, No. 1099 (*Brit. Med. Journal*, vol. ii. 1869, p. 610, woodcuts; *Liverpool Medico-Chirurgical Journal*, vol. iii. 1883, p. 262; Hutchinson's *Illustrations of Clinical Surgery*, 1878, fasc. xi. plate xl.), shows a complete and clean separation of the lower epiphysis of the femur with rotation. The lower end of the diaphysis has been displaced backwards and downwards into the popliteal space, and the nerves and vessels are visible tightly stretched over its edge, whereas the detached epiphysis is seen lying in a flexed position, with its fractured surface on the front of the femur, its articular surface looking forwards, and its anterior margin upwards, its posterior downwards. The periosteum has been completely stripped from the end of the shaft and left as a sleeve in connection with the epiphysis. The gastrocnemius is attached to the diaphysis.

A boy, A. B., aged fifteen, under the care of Mr. Wheelhouse, had his leg crushed in a colliery accident. The circulation in the leg was impeded from the first, and on the forty-third day amputation of the thigh was performed for gangrene. The boy died of pyæmia nine days later.

Mr. Wheelhouse mentions (*British Medical Journal*, March 7, 1885) a preparation showing a separation of the lower epiphysis of the femur taken from a patient in the Leeds General Infirmary. The patient was a youth, aged about seventeen, who had been caught in some machinery, and had been violently twisted round. A fracture very low down in the shaft of the femur was diagnosed, and it proved impossible to rectify the displacement which had taken place. When Mr. Wheelhouse took charge of the case, a few days later, gangrene was found setting in both in foot and leg, and the limb was amputated above the fracture. The lower epiphysis of the femur had been torn from its connection with the shaft, and had remained, with but little displacement, almost *in situ*. The shaft had been driven down into the popliteal space, and had so stretched the vessels, both artery and vein, and the popliteal nerve, that gangrene was inevitable; and it was clear that no power would have sufficed to replace the fragments in position. Recovery ensued.

Since then Mr. Wheelhouse had seen an almost identical case in the hands of Mr. Atkinson, and a knowledge of what had taken place in his case enabled a correct diagnosis to be formed from the first concerning it. Mr. Atkinson, to begin with, endeavoured to excise the displaced epiphysis, but without success, and was compelled, as Mr. Wheelhouse had been, to resort to amputation, which, as in Mr. Wheelhouse's case, proved successful so far as the life of the patient was concerned.

The same museum contains a second similar specimen, No. 1067 (Mr. Mayo Robson's paper on 'Separation of the Lower Epiphysis of the Femur,' *Liverpool Med.-Chirurgical Journal*, July 1883; *London Medical Record*, 1883, vol. xi. p. 422), of complete separation of the lower epiphysis.

F. C., aged six, was run over by a cab and brought to the infirmary under the care of Mr. T. Hey. It was found that compound diastasis of the lower femoral epiphysis had occurred, with severe laceration of the soft parts. The lower end of the diaphysis projected for three inches through a wound in the popliteal space, whilst the epiphysis was displaced forwards. Primary amputation of the thigh was performed with a good result.

These specimens just described are now in the museum attached to the Medical Department of the Yorkshire Collége.

Mr. E. Atkinson gives (*Brit. Med. Journal*, July 14, 1883, p. 70, woodcut; *Liverpool Medico-Chirurgical Journal*, vol. iii. 1883, p. 262) an account of a case in which he resected the knee-joint and this epiphysis, which had been displaced and united on to the front of the femur.

Chas. F., aged fifteen, whilst adjusting a belt, was caught up and whirled round the shaft several times. On being brought to the Leeds General Infirmary the next day, February 3, 1883, he was found to have such extensive swelling of both legs and thighs that no diagnosis could be made for a time. Obscure crepitus was felt about the head of the left tibia, and absence of pulsation below the knees. Back splints were applied to both legs. Swelling of the left knee subsiding at the end of a week, a fracture of the left tibia was clearly demonstrated. On February 13 the right knee was aspirated, and two and a half ounces of dark fluid blood removed. On March 1 the right leg was thought to be dislocated forwards, the condyles of the femur apparently projecting backwards. On March 14 pulsation in the tibials was fairly perceptible. On March 21 epiphysial separation was diagnosed from the shortening of the thigh (one and a half inch) and the projection of the lower end of the shaft into the popliteal space, which was felt as a sharp margin, with a prominent pointed angle at each extremity. The epiphysis was displaced anteriorly on to the front of the shaft of the femur, and could be felt as a large irregular mass of bone beneath the patella; there was also considerable œdema of the leg.

On April 26, with full antiseptic precautions, Mr. Atkinson made the usual incision for excision of the knee, removed the patella, which was lying upon the upturned condyles, and by means of a chisel and mallet detached the condyles from the front of the femur, where they had become firmly fixed by callus. He then sawed off the rounded end of the diaphysis and the articular surface of the tibia, wiring the cut surfaces together.   Complete recovery took place.

A specimen in the Royal College of Surgeons Museum, No. 1041c, from Guy's Hospital, 1889, shows the lower extremity of a femur with separation of the lower epiphysis, displaced slightly forwards and to the inner side.   The periosteum is detached from the whole circumference of the diaphysis to a height of two and a half inches.

The patient, a boy aged nine, was injured by the passage of two wheels of a van over his leg.   There was a large wound on the inner side of the knee, through which the lower end of the diaphysis of the femur protruded.   The knee-joint was open.

The epiphysis in this specimen appears to be only displaced directly forwards about half an inch, and there is but little appearance of its rotation.

Examples of the same displacement are seen in the specimens in the Museums of St. Bartholomew's, St. George's, and the London Hospitals, and in the Museums of the Royal College of Surgeons of England and Edinburgh (*loc. cit.*), and in Fontenelle's case.

Wright and Ashby (*Diseases of Children*, 1889, p. 644) also allude to a case of compound separation of the lower epiphysis with similar displacement.

Dr. A. H. Méisenbach reports (*New York Medical Record*, October 5, 1895, p. 475) a case of compound separation of the lower epiphysis of the femur in a boy (W. P.), aged eleven, who had his left leg caught in the revolving wheel of a vehicle.   The femur protruded about four inches through a wound on the outer side of the popliteal space.   The arteries were intact.   With great difficulty, under chloroform, the dislocated epiphysis was reduced.   The wound was treated antiseptically, a drainage tube introduced, and the limb placed on a posterior splint.   Dr. Meisenbach saw the case the next morning, but did not advise amputation, taking into consideration the fact that the separated epiphysis had been perfectly reduced, and that there was no evidence of injury to the vessels.   The patient's general condition was good.   A plaster dressing was applied the same evening, but 'delayed shock' having appeared (fourteen hours after the injury), the patient did not rally, and death ensued within forty-eight hours after the receipt of the injury.   At the autopsy the separated epiphysis was completely reduced, and there was considerable difficulty in evulsing the femur so as to separate it.   The femur was stripped of its periosteum for about four inches, and the soft parts of the popliteal space were much lacerated.   The knee-joint was not involved, the capsule was intact, this being shown by an absence of effusion of blood in the joint.   The separation from the shaft was perfectly smooth, no splinters being attached to the epiphysis.

In some instances the epiphysis has undergone vertical rotation in its displaced position on the front of the diaphysis. In one, that of Atkinson's, one condyle was placed directly above the other.

Displacement of epiphysis backwards.—The epiphysis has rarely been found displaced backwards.

In Richet's case of compound diastasis, the condyloid epiphysis, imperfectly held by the lateral and crucial ligaments, was found displaced backwards, so that its fractured surface looked directly backwards towards the ham. The diaphysis appeared through the skin at the inner and lower part of the thigh, penetrating the joint as described above.

In Coural's specimen, described by Delpech (*Chirurgie Clinique*, t. i. 1823, p. 252), the lower fragment or epiphysis was displaced backwards, so that the two surfaces were not in contact.

Mr. Hutchinson thinks that the usual displacement of the epiphysis is backwards. He says: 'If the epiphysis has been completely disengaged from the shaft, the tendency will be for it to be displaced by the gastrocnemius into the position of full flexion at the knee; this is the position shown in the woodcut. Much must, however,' he adds, 'be allowed for the direction in which the violence has been applied.'

The same author figures (*Archives of Surgery*, January 1893, p. 287) a clean and complete separation of the lower epiphysis of the femur. The muscles of the leg have been dissected in order to show the relation of those of the calf to the epiphysis itself. The lower half of the femur has been cleaned, in order better to exhibit the form of its epiphysial end. The specimen was obtained by a primary amputation in the case of a boy, aged fourteen, under Mr. Hutchinson's care some years ago in the London Hospital.

The displacement of the epiphysis here appears to be the backward displacement so frequently seen in fracture of the femur above the epiphysial junction. In adults the lower end of the upper fragment penetrates the broad tendinous expansion of the quadriceps extensor just above the patella, and effectually prevents reduction and union. It usually necessitates operative measures and suture of the fragments under strictest aseptic procedures, since the joint is generally involved.

Dr. White at the Westminster Hospital had a similar case, in which, however, the bone protruded in front. The extremity of the protruded bone was sawn off, and the parts put in apposition. The joint was uninjured. The limb was thereby saved, and resulted in a useful one.

Hermann Lossen believes (*Deutsche Chirurgie*, 'Die Verletzungen der unteren Extremitäten,' 1880, S. 110) that this displacement of the diaphysis forwards is the more common form of injury, and that the converse rarely takes place—namely, the displacement of the diaphysis backwards.

Displacement of the epiphysis laterally.—This displacement in an unmixed condition has rarely been found after death. During life the epiphysis is often found to be rotated when displaced laterally, so that one condyle is above the other.

The epiphysis may therefore be described as *displaced outwards*, and *rotated* upon its vertical axis, as well as slightly through its transverse axis, so that the outer end of the shaft impinges against the hollow of the condyle, the internal condyle presenting in the popliteal space, the external condyle on the outer side. In this position the cup-shaped epiphysis will be found to move with a see-saw motion, 'mouvement de bascule.' This to-and-fro movement of the distal on the proximal fragment serves to explain the frequent absence of the characteristic 'muffled crepitus,' for no gliding movement of the diaphysis is then allowed upon the epiphysis. It undoubtedly shows the difficulty of reducing such a displacement without operative measures; in fact, it would be impossible to effect this reduction without unlocking, as it were, the two fragments.

M. Dolbeau reported a case to the Société de Chirurg., Paris, on March 28, 1866 (*Gazette des Hôpitaux*, 1866, p. 162; *Bulletin de la Société de Chirurg. de Paris*, 1867, 2ème série, vii. 120), in which this condition was present.

Jules A., aged twelve, was knocked down by a bale of ropes, which fell from a second story and struck him on the lower part of the left thigh. He was unable to rise, and was taken to the Hôpital Saint-Pierre de la Martinique, under the care of Dr. Rougon. The next day the whole limb was swollen; on its outer side there was a bony projection elevating the skin and threatening to perforate it. In the popliteal space there was a bony projection pressing upon the popliteal vessels. The condyles of the femur and the tuberosities of the tibia were felt to be in their normal relationship. It was found to be impossible to reduce the deformity. Six days after the accident a slough, which had formed at the upper part of the popliteal space, separated, and some foul bloody serum discharged. There was some constitutional disturbance. Amputation at the middle of the thigh was performed the following day. Examination of the amputated limb showed severe pulping and laceration of the soft tissues. The knee-joint was intact, but contained about five ounces of bloody serum. The epiphysis was completely separated with the epiphysial cartilage, without any osseous connections, and moved readily over the tibial tuberosities. This mobility, together with the see-saw movement (*mouvement de bascule*), made it not only difficult, but almost impossible, to reduce the epiphysis over the projecting edge of the upper fragment and place the latter in its epiphysial cavity. It was the external condyle which projected on the outer side, and the internal condyle which was felt in the popliteal space.

St. George's Hospital Museum contains (*St. George's Hospital Museum Catalogue*, 1866, p. 43, No. 56A) a third specimen of separation of the lower femoral epiphysis. It was displaced outwards and backwards, and the diaphysis was on the inner side.

Anthony W., aged eighteen, was admitted into the hospital on July 29, 1849, with considerable deformity of the knee, presenting very much the appearance of a partial dislocation inwards of the condyloid portion of the femur, with extensive laceration of the lateral and crucial ligaments. There was also a compound fracture of the leg at its lower third, as well as extensive laceration of the skin of the inguinal region. The limb was quite cold below the knee, and there was a good deal of swelling, especially about the knee, foot, and ankle. The accident happened a short time before admission; it appeared that the foot had been caught in the ropes of a ship; the rope, in twisting round the lad's leg, threw him into the water, where he remained some time. Amputation of the thigh was immediately performed, and a complete separation of the condyloid epiphysis was found. The outer portion of the end of the diaphysis was in contact with the internal condyle, and projected forwards and inwards; the periosteum was separated off the lower third, but remained adherent to the epiphysis, forming a fold behind, which hindered reduction. The epiphysial cartilage adhered to the condyles, to which here and there some minute fragments of the diaphysis were still attached.

The posterior ligament was slightly torn at the internal part; the other ligaments were intact. A quantity of blood was present in the articulation. There was laceration of the middle and internal coats of the popliteal artery, the lumen of which was obliterated by blood clot; the nerves were intact.

Death occurred on August 12 from pyæmia; pus was present in the femoral vein. In this case both epiphyses of the fibula and the lower epiphysis of the tibia were said to have been separated.

Reichel figures (loc. cit. p. 34, and tab. ii. figs. 1 and 3) a specimen representing a separation of the lower epiphysis completely displaced towards the outer side, and there united by osseous material. As Reichel supposes, the separation was probably the result of disease, as distinct traces of caries were to be seen on the articular surfaces, and numerous osteophytic formations, produced by periosteal inflammation extending a considerable distance upwards on the diaphysis.

An instance of marked lateral displacement outwards of the epiphysis is quoted by Dr. R. H. Harte. On admission it was reported to be a lateral dislocation of the knee. Extensive suppuration ensued, and the thigh was amputated (vide infra). The separation was a pure one.

Displacement of the epiphysis inwards.—Halderman's case is the only one in which, after death, the epiphysis has been found on the inner side. It appears to have been lodged above the inner side of the shaft in such a way that it would have been impossible to displace it by traction during life ;ᵣhowever, the description given is somewhat vague : ' The epiphysis was tilted backwards, and also overlapped at its posterior and outer aspect by the shaft to the extent of several inches.'

An instance of lateral displacement, confirmed by dissection after removal, ·is quoted by Dr. R. H. Harte, of Philadelphia (*Trans. Amer. Surg. Association*, Philad. 1895, vol. xiii. p. 396).

Edward H., aged fourteen years, was admitted to the Episcopal Hospital,· March 23, 1894. While employed as a polisher in a glass factory he became entangled in belting. On admission it was found that he had sustained a fracture of the left femur, with a compound comminuted fracture of the bones of the right leg, and an epiphysial separation of the lower end of the femur in the same limb. The deformity was very great, so that the knee and condyles could be slipped to either side of the diaphysis, simulating lateral displacement of the knee. As an amputation of the leg at a high point was demanded, it was deemed expedient to amputate through the thigh. On exposing the separation above the lower condyle, the diaphysis was observed to be clearly separated from the epiphysis and denuded of a large portion of its periosteum, particularly over the popliteal surface. The patient made an uneventful recovery.

Displacement of the epiphysis forwards and inwards.—M. Chassaniol resected in 1863 (*Gazette des Hôpitaux*, 1864, p. 39) the end of the diaphysis in a case of complete separation with displacement forwards and inwards of the epiphysis. The child (B.), a boy aged nine and a half years, who was a perfectly healthy child, fell off a door to the ground, striking, it is said, the inner and lower part of the thigh. The lower end of the femur, deprived of its epiphysis and periosteum, projected on the outer and posterior aspect of the joint through a·large laceration in the integuments on the outer side, which also extended into the popliteal space. The leg· was slightly flexed, and the protruding femur made a very obtuse angle with the direction of the wound. Notwithstanding the length of the wound (four centimetres), its oblique direction made all efforts at reduction quite unsuccessful, even after the administration of chloroform. Amputation of the limb was proposed, but refused by the parents. Three and a half centimetres of the protruding diaphysis were therefore removed by means of an ordinary saw. The femur was immediately reduced, and the marked deformity of the knee which was present vanished on making extension of the limb. The epiphysis remaining in its place, it was thought that the knee-joint had not been opened or the lateral ligaments ruptured. The limb was put up in the extended position with two long splints, which were replaced by a starch bandage on the fifteenth day. On the twenty-second day the end of the femur appeared again in the wound, and a second resection was attempted under chloroform, but abandoned when it was found that consolidation had taken place throughout the greater part of the diameter of the bone.

Although the end of the femur was not in the centre of the epiphysis, good union ultimately took place, and the child was able to walk with a raised heel.

The resected specimen was placed by M. Ange Duval in the anatomical museum of the school at Brest.

Dr. F. J. Shepherd, of Montreal, says (*Montreal Medical Journal*, vol. xviii. 1890, p. 199) that he had seen two cases of this accident.

In both the accident had occurred several years before, and the patient had good use of the limb.

In one case, under the care of one of his colleagues at the McGill University, the diaphysis had been displaced outwards, and caused a remarkable obliquity and deformity of the lower end of the femur which interfered with the lad's progression. The limb was straightened by Macewen's osteotomy.

The other case was that of a boy, aged seven, who fell and injured his leg. The lower end of the femur was found to be projecting through the skin on the outer side of the popliteal space. Amputation was advised by the doctors, but this was refused, and on failing to reduce the protruded bone they sawed off two inches. The boy ultimately did well, and was able to go about in three weeks. At the time of this report, ten years after the accident, he had perfect use of his leg, and the knee had as wide a range of motion as the other. He walked with only a slight limp, and measurement gave some two inches of shortening.

Partial separation with fracture of one or other condyle.—It is quite possible for a partial separation of the epiphysis to be associated with a vertical or oblique fracture into the joint between the condyles, in this way separating one or other condyle off without displacing it.

Verneuil met with such an accident in the adult (specimen in Dupuytren's Museum), but no specimen exists showing its actual occurrence during youth.

In the account of the following case reported by Quain (*Lancet*, March 11, 1848, p. 286) there is no positive evidence of a true separation of the epiphysis.

It was under the care of Mr. W. P. Brookes, of Cheltenham, and there was said to have been a compound fracture of the external condyle of the femur, laying open the knee-joint, and complicated with a simple transverse fracture of the lower third of the same bone.

The boy was aged eleven and a half years, and, in getting up behind a coach, fell with his left leg entangled between the spokes of the hind wheel in motion. There was a compound fracture of the femur, extending obliquely downwards through the external condyle, which was movable with the lower portion, projecting through a wound in the popliteal space, and the leg was twisted inwards.

The capsular ligament was lacerated and synovia escaped. Amputation was refused, and the limb was therefore adjusted and treated with straight splints. The lad recovered the entire use of the limb, and could bend the knee to a right angle. There was also no shortening.

COMPLICATIONS.—Complications are very numerous and frequent, on account of the great violence usually required to effect separation of the lower epiphysis of the femur, and from the close proximity of important structures (e.g. Halderman's case). They are *primary* or *secondary*, i.e. occurring at a *later* period.

Packard, in Ashhurst's *Encyclopædia of Surgery*, 1884, vol. iv. p. 216, mentions two specimens in the Museum of the Pennsylvania Hospital (*Pennsylvania Hospital Museum Catalogue*, p. 31, No. 1132). In one there was separation of the lower epiphysis of the femur, with transverse fracture of the middle third of the femur, caused by the patient being run over by a railroad-car. In the other specimen there was epiphysial separation only, without history.

Wounds.—Separation of the lower epiphysis of the femur is very frequently complicated with a contused or lacerated wound, occasionally very extensive in character.

The author has collected fifty compound separations. In a large proportion the laceration of the skin was in the popliteal space, and the result of the over-extension of the limb, or was caused in a large measure by indirect violence—i.e. by the diaphysial end penetrating the soft parts from within outwards. In some it was placed towards the upper and outer part of the ham, and more seldom towards the inner side of the knee; in all the violence appears to have been very severe. In Post's case it existed on the outer side of the knee. In others we find a contused wound with lacerated muscles caused by direct violence.

The plate given by Professor J. L. Little shows the situation of the wound in his case at the upper and outer part of the popliteal space.

In Rathbun's case the rent in the skin was oblique, and extended right across the popliteal space, commencing two inches above the internal condyle and terminating below at the head of the fibula.

In Owing's case the end of the diaphysis, with its peculiar stellate radiations, protruded through the rent in the skin for fully five inches, and in Hamilton's case it projected for the same distance.

Hæmorrhage may occur and recur from the wound without laceration of the principal vessels of the limb. It may proceed from the diaphysial end if this has been fractured, as it often is. It may prove to be so serious as to be an important factor in determining the question of preservation of the limb.

Oozing of blood from the osseous surface was seen in one case in which the separation was a pure one, and the plugging of the popliteal artery prevented any loss of blood from the soft parts. It continued for some hours until amputation was performed. It is possible that the blood may delay or even cause serious interference with union, by producing separation of the detached surfaces.

Dr. John A. Macdougall records (*Edinburgh Medical Journal*, vol. xxxvi. Part ii. March 1891, p. 826) the following case, in which hæmorrhage recurred from the wound and the limb was amputated.

E. D., aged nineteen, while driving the horses attached to a threshing mill, unfortunately slipped the heel of his right boot into the cogs of the driving wheel. At once realising his danger, he threw himself violently to one side in order to escape it. On examination immediately afterwards there was found a markedly oblique fracture of the lower part of the thigh, and with this a deep and ragged tear of the soft parts, passing from one condyle to another across the popliteal space. This wound, from which there had been free hæmorrhage, after being thoroughly cleansed, was brought together, and the limb was placed in a retentive apparatus. Late on the day following the accident severe arterial bleeding occurred from the wound, the source of which could not be found, and which it was difficult to check.

Early next day Dr. Macdougall saw the patient, and his condition was then as follows : a pale and very exsanguine lad, with a small, quick, and feeble pulse, with a temperature of nearly 103°, and with a very exhausted look. The injured limb was much swollen, and in the general fulness the calf of the leg was notably prominent. Pulsation in the tibial was quite perceptible. On removal of the sutures from the popliteal wound much sanious matter escaped. Examination with the finger passed deeply into the popliteal space detected bare bone, and, following this up, there was no difficulty in entering the fracture gap. This examination led to a renewal of the arterial bleeding, demonstrating pretty conclusively what was its source.

In the knee-joint itself there was considerable effusion. This, coupled with the facts that the fracture was low down and very oblique, that the lad was under twenty, and that the limb had been violently twisted, led to the belief that the epiphysis had shared in the injury, and that the joint itself was probably involved.

In all the circumstances of the case it seemed to Dr. Macdougall the wisest course to remove the limb. Although externally there seemed little deformity or displacement, the space between the fractured ends was nearly two inches wide, and it was filled with a dense blood-clot. This clot extended downwards into the muscles of the calf, and gave rise to the prominence in that region already referred to. The periosteum, fairly closely adherent to the upper fragment, was completely stripped from the lower portion, and widely separated along the line at which the epiphysis had given way.

Dr. Macdougall adds the following note : ' The specimen thus obtained is fraught with interest, for although at the time of its removal it was believed by all who saw it that the line of fracture passed obliquely through the epiphysis, it was ultimately found that this was not so, that only on the outer third did the line of separation trench upon, but did not pass through, that of the epiphysis, and that this structure, although gravely implicated, was still attached to the femoral condyles.' Recovery took place.

Detachment of the periosteum.—In all compound separations the end of the diaphysis projects from the rent in the skin—always stripped of its periosteal covering, sometimes to the extent of four to five inches—and is often much soiled by dirt.

In one of the specimens in St. George's Hospital (56A) the periosteum was stripped from the lower third of the shaft, and was found to have formed a fold behind, which hindered reduction. In other instances the detachment has been noted as high as the middle third, while in two cases the periosteum is said to have been torn off as high as the trochanter.

Mr. Hutchinson mentions (*London Hospital Reports*, vol. i. 1864, p. 88) a specimen removed by amputation from a boy of twelve, in which the lower end of the femur had been detached from the epiphysis. The latter remained in position with the tibia, and the knee-joint was uninjured. The lower three inches of the shaft of the femur were quite bare of periosteum.

The extent of the stripping of the periosteum with the protrusion of the diaphysis will vary with the degree and direction of the violence. It has also been found detached to a greater or less extent from the diaphysis in the simple cases in which operative interference has been considered necessary—e.g. in one simple case of Dr. R. H. Harte's in which suppuration occurred.

That detachment of the periosteum occurs in all cases of displacement of the epiphysis, even though they may be only simple and not compound, and generally from the posterior aspect, is proved by Professor Little's case. In this case it was found that the vitality of the bone was not interfered with by this detachment.

The periosteum is never torn off the peripheral surface of the cartilaginous disc or of the epiphysis, on account of the thick and dense attachment it has to both lying beneath it.

The periosteum, as usual in epiphysial separations, remains adherent to the epiphysis, and the diaphysis directed downwards by the violence penetrates the periosteum in a buttonhole manner, which is stripped off, and the end of the bone is then thrust through the skin. In some few examples it has been found torn more or less away from the epiphysis, as in Reverdin's case, where it was detached from the epiphysial margin behind, corresponding to the portion of the detached shaft, and also to a slight extent in front of this.

The periosteum will not only be detached but lacerated in the direction of the displacement of the diaphysis, and the extent of this laceration usually corresponds to the amount and nature of the displacement of the diaphysis. The laceration of the periosteum was well marked in one of Broca's cases.

From the results of compound separations we find that, as a rule, the periosteum becomes adherent again in the diaphysis, and no ill results from its separation.

In some few cases, however, suppuration may ensue, and even pyæmia, for which the periosteal detachment is largely responsible.

Injury to popliteal vessels.—These vessels are sometimes pressed upon by the posterior margin of the femoral diaphysis in backward displacement, without laceration of their coats.

Little, Tapret, Atkinson, and Wheelhouse note the absence of pulsation in the posterior tibials below, without any lesion of the popliteal vessels. In some instances these vessels are but slightly stretched. In Reverdin's case, pressure upon the artery gave rise to thickening and clotting in its interior, plainly demonstrating that it is not necessary for the coats to be ruptured for occlusion to take place. Halderman states that the artery in his case was contused, inflamed, thickened, and filled with clot, and that the vein was in the same condition, from pressure by the anterior edge of the displaced diaphysis. Between the epiphysis and the diaphysis, on the anterior and inner aspect of the latter, lay the internal popliteal nerve and popliteal vein and artery, which were pressed upon by the fragments, and held there by the hook-shaped projection of the divided internal condyloid ridge, over which they had caught.

The artery, vein, and nerve anterior to the bone were uninjured in Rutherford Alcock's case.

On the other hand the artery and vein have been found completely lacerated in some instances by the diaphysial end impinging on them ; in some they have been only partially lacerated. In others only the inner and middle coats have been divided, these being rolled up to a greater or less extent ; clotting soon takes place in the interior, and leads to complete occlusion.

M. A. Verneuil relates (*Mémoires de Chirurgie*, vol. iii. p. 400) the case of Ferdinand S., aged eight, who was admitted into the Lariboisière Hospital on July 9, 1868. He had climbed behind a carriage, and caught his left leg in the wheel. There was an extensive wound of the leg, with contusion of the soft parts and bones. In the thigh there was a wound and separation of the soft parts, with rupture of the popliteal artery. M. Verneuil performed amputation of the thigh the next day, and discovered complete separation of the lower epiphysis of the femur, to which the epiphysial cartilage adhered. The lower end of the diaphysis had completely divided the popliteal artery and vein, and, displacing the internal popliteal nerve outwards, protruded through the transverse rent in the skin. The periosteum was separated from the end of the bone, but remained adherent to the soft parts and to the epiphysis.   The knee-joint was uninjured.   Recovery took place.

The artery and vein were lacerated in both of Mr. Hutchinson's cases.   The second is described by him in the *Transactions of the Pathological Society*, vol. xv. 1864, p. 206.

A lad, aged twelve, was brought to the London Hospital, having been run over in the street.   At first sight it was supposed that there was a compound dislocation of the left knee-joint, and the soft parts were severely injured.   The projecting bone was found to be the end of the shaft abruptly and completely detached from its epiphysial extremity ; the latter was still connected with the tibia, and the joint uninjured.   Primary amputation was performed by Mr. John Adams.   The popliteal artery and vein were found to be torn across, and the periosteum very extensively stripped from the lower part of the shaft.   The epiphysis, by the action of the gastrocnemius, had been displaced so that its separated surface looked directly backwards into the popliteal space.

The popliteal vessels were ruptured in Dr. W. T. Davison's case, mentioned by Gross (*System of Surgery*, 1882, vol. i. p. 1019), while in Clutton's case the artery was ruptured and the vein pressed upon.

In one of the specimens in St. George's Hospital Museum, described above, rupture of the internal and middle coats of the artery took place with the formation of coagulum obliterating its lumen.

And in another case (Broca), which was caused by direct violence, the popliteal artery was obliterated, and the two inner coats torn across and retracted, the external coat holding the ends in continuity. In this instance the popliteal vein had undergone stretching, and its inner coat was furrowed by transverse markings.

Dr. A. McDiarmid records a similar case of a simple clean separation with displacement forwards of the epiphysis, and complete laceration of the popliteal artery (*Northern Lancet*, Winnipeg, 1891-2, vol. v. p. i).

A boy (Allen W.), about eight years of age, had his right leg caught in the front wheel of a wagon, and on examination seven hours later it was found that ' the condyles were still in contact with the head of the tibia, but only by an edge, the whole epiphysis being rotated so that the articular face looked forwards and the detached surface backwards.'   The skin being unbroken, and the precise condition of the soft parts uncertain, an attempt was made to save the limb.   Chloroform was therefore given, the tendo Achillis divided to allow coaptation of the fragments, and the limb put up moderately flexed.   Nearly twenty-four hours later, as the limb was found to be cold, amputation of the thigh was performed.   The patient made an excellent recovery.   The popliteal artery was found to be completely divided by the rough margin of the femur, and there was great contusion of the soft parts.

In the following additional examples verified by dissection, the popliteal vessels were seriously injured.

At the Birmingham and Midland Counties Branch of the British Medical Association, December 14, 1893 (*British Medical Journal*, January 6, 1894, p. 21), Mr. Haslam showed a specimen of a separation of the lower epiphysis of the femur, which had been complicated with rupture of the inner and middle coats of the popliteal artery and bruising of the vein, causing gangrene of the limb, in a lad aged nineteen, apparently the result of injury.

M. Ardouin (*Bulletins de la Société anatomique de Paris*, tome xi. 5me série, 1897, p. 539) exhibited before the Société Anatomique the lower epiphysis of the femur taken from a young man, aged sixteen, who had met with a serious injury on March 16, 1896. The patient, a printer, had his leg seized in a transmission band and was taken to the Hôpital Broussais. Although there was extensive laceration of the integuments, and a large opening through which the diaphysis of the femur, completely separated from the epiphysis, protruded, an attempt was made to preserve the limb. For fifteen days the condition was satisfactory, but at last amputation of the thigh had to be performed. On dissection, there was found a perforation of the popliteal vein, which had given rise to extensive extravasation of blood, and an abscess in the coats of the popliteal artery. On the femoral epiphysis all the depressions and eminences could be seen which corresponded to similar eminences and depressions on the diaphysis. The patient recovered.

It is remarkable that the popliteal vessels have escaped laceration or bruising in so many of the recorded cases, even of compound separation. No doubt this immunity from injury may be explained in some instances by the peculiar character of the lesion, the epiphysis with the limb below being twisted at the time of the accident off the diaphysis, which is more or less fixed. The popliteal vessels and nerve in this twisting of the limb will follow its movements, and tend to glide over the posterior margin of the diaphysial end instead of being pressed upon by it, as would be the case were the epiphysis thrown directly forwards off the diaphysis.

At the Philadelphia Academy of Surgery, on February 2, 1891 (*Medical News*, March 21, 1891, p. 339; *Annals of Gynæcology and Pædiatry*, November 1890; *Archives of Pediatrics*, 1891, p. 318), Dr. J. H. Packard showed specimens of separation of the lower epiphysis of the femur, taken from a boy nine years of age, who was admitted to St. Joseph's Hospital on April 16, 1889, having had his right leg caught in the wheel of a wagon behind which he was clinging. From the appearance of the anterior aspect of the limb, a forward luxation of the knee might have been suspected; but upon examination the true nature of the lesion was at once apparent. At the lower and back part of the thigh there was a large oblique wound, through which protruded the end of the diaphysis of the femur, bare of periosteum; the condyles were still partly in contact with the tibia, but the whole epiphysis was rotated so that its articular face looked forwards, and the upper cup-shaped surface backwards. This was due to traction by the two heads of the gastrocnemius muscle. The patella was not materially displaced, being still in relation with the joint, but was tilted up by the action of the quadriceps muscle. Ether was given, and a careful examination showed that although there was great bruising and laceration of the soft parts, the vessels had not been torn, but, along with the nerve, had slipped aside around the end of the diaphysis; they were, however, sharply stretched, and the blood in the artery was coagulated, so that there was a probability of the limb becoming gangrenous. Reduction of the protruding bone was found to be impossible, and an attempt to save the limb by resection seemed to be attended with so much risk, in view of the damage to the soft parts, that amputation was performed, about an inch and a half of the shaft being removed. The boy made a perfect recovery. Upon dissection it was found that the epiphysis had been almost cleanly separated; entirely so, but for a very small splinter detached from the end of the diaphysis on the inner side. The specimen is in the Museum of the Pennsylvania Hospital.

In the following case described by Dr. John A. Macdougall (*Edinburgh Medical Journal*, vol. xxxvi. Part ii. March 1891, p. 826), the vessels escaped injury, although there was very great displacement backwards of the epiphysis.

C. G., an active young fellow of twenty, was, while superintending some work, caught in the coils of an endless rope, and his right leg was very violently twisted round. The surgeon, who did not see him for some little time after the accident, found all the marked signs of fracture close above the knee. The lower fragment was small, and was very acutely drawn back, so much so as to stretch the integuments over it, but there was no great displacement of the upper portion of the bone. An attempt to reduce the displaced fragment was not very successful, and the surgeon in attendance ultimately succeeded in placing the limb in a MacIntyre splint fixed at a not very acute angle. About a month after the accident, Dr. Macdougall saw him. There was then still such pronounced displacement of the lower fragment existing that the skin had ulcerated over it, and the whole condition, owing in a measure to the shrunken state of the limb, left no doubt as to what the true nature of the injury was. The absence of all attempt at union—for union in the circumstances was wellnigh impossible—tended to confirm the diagnosis of diastasis. Amputation was advised and performed, and what it demonstrated was a transverse separation running almost entirely through the epiphysial line, and the rather striking fact that, in spite of the long stretching to which the popliteal vessels had been subjected, they were quite uninjured.

In Dr. Donovan's case, although there was very extensive laceration of the skin and soft structures, the popliteal artery escaped laceration; it was displaced by the backward escape of the lower end of the femur. Recovery took place in this case after resection of two and a half inches of the diaphysis.

In Meisenbach's case, although the diaphysis protruded for four inches on the outer side of the popliteal space, the vessels were uninjured.

In Clutton's compound case the popliteal vessels appeared to have been ruptured by the backward displacement of the diaphysis.

The special danger in these cases of injury to the popliteal vessels is that the large veins may become, most frequently in compound separations, the seat of infective thrombosis, leading to pyæmia and the death of the patient.

In one instance the anterior tibial artery was torn open.

Injury to nerves.—The popliteal nerves may be contused, lacerated, or exposed for a considerable distance.

In Dr. Donovan's case the nerve trunks were injured, and resulted in paralysis of the extensor muscles of the leg, although good union had taken place. Tuberculous disease occurred in the limb and necessitated amputation.

Pressure upon popliteal nerve.—Where the displacement has not been reduced in simple cases, the upper fragment, being thrust downwards and backwards, may stretch the internal popliteal nerve, as well as the popliteal vessels over its edge.

In a case related by Professor J. L. Little (*Illustrated Quarterly of Medicine and Surgery*, vol. i. No. 1, January 1882, p. 24), under Dr. McBurney's care at St. Luke's Hospital, N.Y., the internal popliteal nerve was so stretched, the pain so intense, and the deformity so great, that amputation was resorted to. The case was of two or three months' standing, and strong bony union had taken place. The patient died of tetanus. The periosteum was completely stripped from the end of the shaft, although the case was not compound and union had taken place before amputation. The vitality of the bone was not interfered with by this loss.

In other instances the internal popliteal nerve may, like the vessels, escape the pressure of the lower end of the diaphysis by slipping to one side of it.

Dr. J. B. Roberts (Philadelphia) had seen a case (*Annals of Surgery*, February 1896, p. 201) in which nerve injury was accompanied by epiphysial separation, and he wanted to operate, but delayed, finally finding it unnecessary. The child had been injured about six weeks before. There had apparently been an epiphysial separation of the lower end of the femur, with displacement backwards into the popliteal space. The lower fragment could be easily located, and there was 'foot drop,' showing injury of the external popliteal nerve. He advised operation to release the nerve from pressure, but the other physicians preferred to wait. The child obtained perfect use of its foot from regeneration of the injured nerve, and could then (October 1895) walk well and had no paralysis.

Gangrene of the limb, more or less extensive, is a frequent consequence of pressure upon the vessels; it occurred in the cases described by Little, Reverdin, Tapret, Halderman, Wheelhouse (on the forty-third day), Canton, and others.

Reverdin thought that the application of a 2½ per cent. solution of carbólic acid to the exposed popliteal nerves contributed to the subsequent gangrene in his case.

Gangrene was present in one of the specimens in St. Bartholomew's Hospital from pressure on the popliteal vein by the displaced diaphysis.

A case is mentioned by S. Laugier in the *Nouveau Dictionnaire de Médecine et de Chirurgie Pratiques*, Paris, 1869, tome dixième, art. ' Cuisse,' which was produced by the leg falling into a hole nearly to the knee while the body was carried forwards. The inferior fragment turned backwards, so that its broken surface rested on the anterior aspect of the femur; the lower end of the shaft of the bone descended behind, and pressed out the popliteal space with its vessels and nerves to an extreme degree. Gangrene ensued, and amputation did not save the patient.

The following is the earliest case of injury of the lower epiphysis of the femur reported in a detailed manner: gangrene ensued on the eighth day.

M. Julia Fontenelle relates (*Archives Générales de Médecine*, 1ème série, tome ix. 1825, p. 267 ; Roux (Brignolle), *La Presse Médicale*, No. 55, 12 Juillet 1837, p. 436; also quoted by Guéretin, *La Presse Médicale*, 1837) the case of a boy (J. M.), aged eleven, who had plunged his right leg into a hole up to his knee and fell forwards, separating the lower epiphysis from the shaft, and at the same time driving the shaft into the popliteal space. The child remained two days without receiving any attention. He was taken to the hospital on the third day, and there was found shortening of the limb with projection forwards of the condyles. The lower end of the shaft pressed upon the vessels and nerves, and the epiphysis became tilted in such a manner that its lower extremity was directed forwards. There was considerable swelling of the limb. The limb was put up in an ordinary apparatus, as reduction could not be effected and the parents refused amputation. On the fourth day there was numbness of the limb, pain in the joint, swelling, and coldness of the foot. On the seventh day the foot was livid, and small incisions were made. On the eighth day gangrene was evident, and diarrhœa set in ; the parents still refused amputation. On the eighteenth day the gangrene was limited at the knee, and there was general emaciation. On the twenty-third day the foot separated from the leg; the bones of the leg were bare at certain points. On the twenty-fourth day (September 26) Dr. Coural, of Narbonne, amputated four inches above the condyles. The patient left the hospital cured on December 10.

Delpech describes (*Chirurgie Clinique*, tom. i. 1823, p. 252) as follows the specimen of separation of the lower femoral epiphysis in Coural's case, which was in his possession, whilst Roux made several coloured drawings of it: 'The epiphysis has been separated from the shaft in the middle of the cartilaginous layer, so that a layer of it remained attached to each osseous fragment. The two surfaces are thus invested with soft material, and the lower fragment had been displaced backwards, so that the two new surfaces were not in contact.'

The popliteal vessels in Clutton's case were ruptured, leading to gangrene of the foot, amputation, and death from pyæmia.

In Dolbeau's case pressure of the internal condyle of the epiphysis upon the popliteal vessels and skin produced ulceration and sloughing in the upper part of the popliteal space, thereby converting a simple into a compound diastasis.

Ulceration of the skin and protrusion of the diaphysis are also mentioned in Bell's, Voss's, and Halderman's cases.

Secondary hæmorrhage.—Severe hæmorrhage from the anterior tibial artery, due to an injury close to its origin, occurred on the thirteenth day in Little's case, and compelled him to amputate.

Mr. C. F. Maunder mentions (*London Hospital Reports*, vol. iv. 1867–8, p. 239) the case of a male child (F. J.), aged six years, who was run over, and sustained a simple fracture of the left thigh bone, and also a compound separation of the lower epiphysis of the femur. The wound was transverse in the popliteal space, and the finger introduced found the lower end of the shaft of the femur stripped of periosteum to the extent of at least an inch; a small fragment only of the femur was adherent to its epiphysis. The limb was put up with the knee in the flexed position. The case progressed fairly well, but with profuse discharge, until suddenly copious hæmorrhage arose from the depth of the wound.

As the little patient could not afford to lose blood, being already much exhausted, amputation was at once performed. Symptoms of pyæmia, including swelling of the opposite thigh, with deep fluctuation, supervened, and death took place on the eighteenth day after amputation.

Articular lesions.—Contrary to what we should expect to find from the close proximity of the articulation and the actual contact of the synovial membrane in front with the epiphysial line, the joint is but seldom seriously involved. The crucial and other ligaments uniting the epiphysis to the bones of the leg are far more powerful than the cartilaginous bond of union between the epiphysis and the diaphysis, and are but rarely injured. The crucial ligaments were, however, in R. Adams's case, torn from the femur, carrying with them small portions of the bone.

In several examples—e.g. Rathbun's case—it was especially stated that the articular cavity was not opened, although in this particular case the posterior ligament of the joint was slightly torn at its upper part.

In Meisenbach's case of compound separation with displacement backwards and outwards of the diaphysis for four inches, the knee-joint was not involved, and the capsule was intact, as shown by the absence of blood in the joint.

Injury to the articulation has, however, been occasionally observed in pure and uncomplicated separations— e.g. Bruns mentions that the contused wound in his case opened the knee-joint, whilst Rutherford Alcock thought that the capsule of the joint had probably been opened in his case, on account of the synovial-like fluid which for some time issued from the wound.

In two of the specimens in St. George's Hospital the joint has been injured: in one, of displacement of the epiphysis backwards and outwards, the posterior ligament was slightly torn at the internal part, but the other ligaments were intact; in the other, of displacement forwards of the epiphysis, there was an opening, exposing the posterior part of the outer condyle.

In Halderman's case of displacement of the epiphysis inwards and backwards there was laceration on the inner side of the cavity of the knee-joint, which contained some blood.

In an article on 'Abnormal Conditions of the Knee-joint' (*Cyclopædia of Anatomy and Physiology*, R. B. Todd, M.D., 1839–47, vol. iii. pp. 68, 69), Robert Adams describes a case of simple separation in a boy, aged thirteen. The femoral condyles were detached at their normal line of junction with the shaft, and where they are covered with synovial membrane; the anterior and posterior crucial ligaments were separated from the femur, and had carried with them small portions of this bone. The result of the secondary amputation is not recorded, but the specimen preserved in the Museum of the Richmond School of Medicine shows, besides the injuries of the bones, traces of the very acute inflammation which followed, particularly on the surface of the synovial membrane; the latter was covered with lymph. The periosteum of the femur in the vicinity of the fracture was much thickened, and detached all round from the femur.

At the Philadelphia Academy of Surgery in 1889 (*Med. News*, Philadelphia, May 1889, p. 552) Dr. John H. Brinton exhibited a specimen presented seven years previously to the Jefferson Medical College by Dr. Willis T. Davison, of Pennsylvania.

The patient was a boy, twelve years of age, who, while riding on the back of a buggy, had his left foot caught between the spokes of the wheel and carried forwards, producing a separation of the epiphysis, with a slight nipping off of one portion of the edge of the diaphysis. There was an oblique wound, four or five inches long, extending across the upper portion of the popliteal space. The skin, superficial fascia, and muscles were severely lacerated, and there existed copious venous hæmorrhage and extensive extravasation around the joint and upper part of the leg; no pulse could be felt in the posterior tibial artery. The boy was able to turn over and imperfectly raise the knee from the bed. An unsuccessful attempt was made to save the limb, but amputation was necessary on the fourth day, and the patient made a good recovery.

Careful dissection of the amputated limb showed that the epiphysis had been torn from the diaphysis, and the artery injured in such a manner that a probe could with difficulty be passed through it. It was also found that there was a rupture at the posterior part of the synovial membrane, opening the knee-joint.

Packard says: 'The epiphysial line is just above the boundary of the knee-joint, and when a separation takes place exactly through it, that cavity will not be involved, although it may become so secondarily.'

Blood in the joint has been found in two cases of simple diastasis —viz. Dolbeau's and Atkinson's cases; and in Reverdin's case of compound injury the articulation contained a little sero-sanguineous fluid, and the crucial ligaments were inflamed and of a pinkish colour, without any lesion of the joint being discovered.

It is probable that in some instances besides the one just alluded to the crucial or other ligaments have been partially lacerated.

Great articular distension from effusion may ensue without any discoverable lesion to account for it, beyond the close relationship of the epiphysial line to the joint.

It has been especially noted by Hamilton, Tapret, Harte, and others.

Fracture of the upper end of the tibia.—A transverse fracture of the upper end of the tibia complicated separation of the lower epiphysis of the femur in Dr. F. D. Rathbun's case (*St. Louis Courier of Medicine*, vol. xi. No. 3, March 1884, p. 211).

On November 20, 1883 (C. S.), a boy, aged ten years, while attempting to climb into the rear end of a wagon in motion, caught his right leg in the spokes of the wheel in such a manner as to over-extend the leg upon the thigh, thereby separating the lower epiphysis of the femur, and driving the lower end of the shaft backwards through the popliteal space. The lower end of the shaft was found to present a broad slightly roughened extremity, which clearly showed its separation from the epiphysis, and protruded from a wound which communicated with the point of separation. The rent in the skin extended obliquely across the popliteal space, beginning two inches above the internal condyle and terminating over the head of the fibula, and the tissues were very much lacerated.

By flexing the leg upon the thigh, the separated surfaces could be brought into accurate apposition. There was considerable venous hæmorrhage, which was, however, easily controlled. On the following morning the patient's general condition was good, and no shortening of the limb existed while in the position of flexion. Some swelling supervened, and the temperature of the limb was about normal. No pulsation could be felt in the posterior tibial artery. After ether had been administered and the limb straightened, the fragments became displaced, with marked shortening; the lower extremity of the shaft projected backwards and outwards, but did not protrude from the wound until the leg was carried forwards considerably beyond a straight line with the thigh. By pressing the finger into the wound the separated surfaces could be clearly felt, the shaft of the bone being denuded of its periosteum to the extent of nearly three inches. The tissues in the popliteal space were greatly lacerated. Amputation of the thigh was performed, the femur being divided four inches above the line of separation. The patient made a good recovery.

After removing the soft parts it was found that the line of separation followed the cartilage throughout. In no place did it traverse the bone tissue. In addition, a fracture of the upper extremity of the shaft of the tibia was discovered that had not been previously suspected; it was situated just below the epiphysial line, and was nearly transverse in direction, being directed from without inwards, slightly downwards and forwards. There was no displacement of the fragments whatever. The posterior ligament of the joint was slightly torn at its upper part. With this exception, no laceration of ligaments occurred. The joint cavity was not opened.

Other severe lesions.—Dr. J. A. Donovan, of Lewiston, U.S.A., has kindly furnished the author with the notes of a severe case of compound separation of the lower femoral epiphysis accompanied by other extensive injuries to the body (*Transactions of the Maine Medical Association*, 1884, vol. viii. part ii. p. 345).

On November 13, 1882, Dr. Donovan was called to T. B., a lad, aged ten, who had met with a severe accident twenty to thirty minutes before, and was lying in an apparently lifeless condition. After some hypodermic injections of brandy had been administered, a careful examination under an anæsthetic showed a fracture of the left parietal bone, with extensive infiltration of blood. The left femur was fractured just below the trochanter major. The condyloid epiphysis was separated and the intervening shaft much comminuted. Notwithstanding such complete breaking of the whole femur, the skin was not torn, but was rendered very tense from bloody effusion. A large and extensive wound across the popliteal space of the right limb was found, through which the lower end of the femur projected about four inches. The epiphysis was separated and retained its proper relation with the knee-joint. The popliteal wound was so extensive that only about three inches of skin on the front of the limb remained intact. The laceration of connective and muscular tissues was very extensive. The inner hamstring tendons were stripped of their investments. The saphenous vein was exposed, and the popliteal artery, though it escaped laceration, was displaced by the backward escape of the lower end of the femur.

The accident resulted from the boy becoming entangled in a belt, which carried him round its pulley about forty times, the limbs and head striking adjacent timbers at each revolution. Although but little hope was entertained that the patient could survive the profound shock of the injury, amputation of the right femur was advised as the best course, but determinedly refused by the friends. Two and a half inches in length of the shaft of the femur were removed. So much was taken for two reasons : that the periosteum was entirely separated as high as the point of section, and that the sharp edges left by cutting the expanding shaft would probably have injured the adjacent popliteal vessels. The limb was put up in an anterior splint to afford an opportunity of dressing the wound. The boy rallied fairly from the ether and the shock of the injury, and, although in a very critical condition for several days, made an uninterrupted recovery. No cerebral symptoms followed the cranial injury. The left femur, that was so thoroughly comminuted, united well, no apparent deformity resulting. Five months after the injury the wound of the right limb was completely healed, and firm bony union had occurred between the cut shaft of the femur and the separated epiphysis, which had been allowed to remain in relation with the knee-joint. Two years later (1884) the boy had grown and developed well. There was good motion at the knee, and the growth was in keeping with its fellow. But for the unfortunate circumstance that the nerve trunks affording supply to the extensor muscles of the leg were injured, leaving these muscles paralysed in motion, the boy would scarcely have suffered serious loss by his injury.

Dr. Donovan, in a letter to the author dated October 31, 1893, says : 'The very flattering condition in which the above report left him did not very long continue. The boy grew rapidly, and the right limb failed to keep pace with the left, which recovered fully. He became "knocked" in the right knee. I confined him to his bed with a correcting splint. The deformity was in part relieved, but the limb became tuberculous and I amputated at the mid portion of the femur. The young man subsequently did well.'

Fracture of shaft of femur.—Packard, in Ashhurst's *Encyclopædia of Surgery*, 1884, vol. iv. p. 216, mentions a specimen in the Museum of the Pennsylvania Hospital (*Pennsylvanian Hospital Museum Catalogue*, p. 31, No. 1132) in which there was separation of the lower epiphysis of the femur, with transverse fracture of the middle third of the femur, caused by the patient being run over by a railroad-car. Fracture of the shaft of the femur as a concomitant lesion has been noted in one other case.

Severe general symptoms, such as pallor, collapse, coldness, with compressible pulse and other signs of general prostration, usually accompany this injury in its more serious forms, of which the instance quoted above is a good example.

LATER COMPLICATIONS. **Suppuration.** — Diffuse suppuration appears to be a frequent result, especially in compound separations. Dr. Voss, at the same meeting of the New York Pathological Society at which Dr. Little communicated his case (*New York Medical Journal,* vol. ii. 1865-6, p. 133), remarked that he had met with a similar one. The fracture was simple at the time of the accident, but subsequently an abscess formed and the upper fragment protruded. In this condition Dr. Voss saw the case, and was compelled to amputate. Dr. Buck mentioned a similar case of separation of this epiphysis in a boy, aged fourteen, whose legs had been caught by the spokes of a revolving wheel and twisted. Dr. Buck could not recollect whether the fracture was compound or not.

Mr. Jonathan Hutchinson junior's specimen (1888) in the Royal College of Surgeons Museum, No. 1041E, shows the lower end of the right femur divided vertically from side to side. It displays detachment and partial crushing of the epiphysis, the epiphysial disc having been *destroyed by suppuration.* The periosteum is stripped off the back of the diaphysis, but adheres in front ; the popliteal vessels are uninjured, and the two heads of the gastrocnemius are attached to the displaced epiphysis and periosteum. No trace of the epiphysial disc remains. Several pieces of the epiphysis were broken off at the time of the injury.

The patient was a child, aged four years, whose thigh had been run over by a van-wheel five weeks before death. The injury was compound, but so little was the displacement that the separation was not at first diagnosed. Amputation became necessary at the end of ten days ; the cause of death was thrombosis of the vena cava.

Acute periostitis and necrosis.—Acute periostitis is clearly exhibited in not a few specimens. Necrosis of the diaphysis more commonly ensues in compound than in simple separations.

The Museum of the Royal College of Surgeons of England contains a specimen, No. 1041A (*Catalogue of the Museum of the Royal College of Surgeons,* Appendix I.), presented by Mr. W. Adams, showing epiphysial separation followed by acute periostitis. In this specimen the separation is through the greater part of the epiphysiary junction, except for about the outer third, where a vertical fracture passes upwards for one and a quarter inch, separating off this part of the diaphysis, which remains firmly connected to the epiphysis below. The end of the diaphysis projects forwards and inwards, and the epiphysis is slightly rotated; otherwise its connections with the tibia are normal. The joint also appears to be normal.

Suppuration beneath the periosteum had taken place in another specimen in the Royal College of Surgeons of England, No. 1041B (see page 703).

A specimen in the Museum of the Royal College of Surgeons of Edinburgh, No. 139, xx. c., and figured by Charles Bell in his *Observations on Injuries of the Spine and Thigh Bone* (1824, Pl. IV. fig. 2), shows evidence of suppurative and septic periostitis or osteomyelitis, for on the anterior aspect of the shaft, two inches above the end, a considerable amount of new periosteal bone is to be seen; below this the bone is bare, and appears about to exfoliate (see fig. 12, p. 120). A small wedge-shaped piece, one inch by half an inch, of the diaphysis has been split off from its front and outer aspect. The case was that of a boy, aged thirteen, who fell through an open floor, between the joists, in such a manner as to twist his leg, causing thereby what was supposed to be a fracture near the knee-joint. The joint suppurated, and the restlessness of the patient brought about ulceration of the skin and a protrusion of bone which was readily recognised as the extremity of the diaphysis. There were deep sloughing spots upon the inner side of the knee.

The patient died some weeks after the accident, before amputation could be performed.

The dissection exhibited great suppuration within the knee-joint, and an immense abscess or cavity communicating with the articulation and extending up the bone nearly to the hip. The periosteum could be torn with the fingers from half the length of the bone.

C. W. Cathcart adds (*Descriptive Catalogue of Museum Royal College of Surgeons of Edinburgh*, 1893, p. 134, specimen No. 3, 248) a similar note on the condition of the bone.

'The surface of the shaft at the lower end has at some places a considerable crust of new periosteal bone, while at others the vascular pores are opened out. A similar opening out is seen all the way up the shaft. At the front of the neck a patch of the surface is eroded. These changes have evidently been due to septic osteomyelitis, an accidental consequent of the injury.'

Suppurative periostitis was probably the cause of the deposit of new bone and the rarefaction of the old shaft in one of the specimens in St. Bartholomew's Hospital, No. 977. There was extensive comminution of the shaft and fracture of the epiphysis into four pieces (see page 704).

Mr. E. Willett had under his care at St. Bartholomew's Hospital (Walsham, 'Surgical Consultations,' *St. Bartholomew's Hospital Reports*, 1888, vol. xxiv. p. 288) a lad, aged nine, who had received a fracture of the lower end of the femur about six months previously. A piece of the femur, which had necrosed and separated, showed clearly that the fracture had occurred through the epiphysial line.

The knee-joint was healthy. On the outer side of the thigh, just above the knee, was a mass of prominent granulations, an inch and a half in diameter, covering a protruding portion of bone. The parts around were excessively tender. It was considered that he had sustained a separation of the lower epiphysis of the femur, with much unreduced displacement; that, owing to the outward protrusion of the diaphysis, the integument had ulcerated, exposing the bone ; and that, subsequent to the necrosis of a portion of the lower end of the femur, the bone had united in a faulty position, leaving the lower end of the upper fragment projecting on the outer side. An incision was made over the prominence, and an inch or so of the protruding portion of bone cut away. The patient made an excellent recovery.

Dr. Post's case of compound separation likewise terminated in necrosis of the diaphysis.

Dr. R. H. Harte, of Philadelphia, narrates (*Trans. Amer. Surg. Assoc.*, Philad. 1895, vol. xiii. p. 397, and the *American Journal of the Medical Sciences*, June 1896, p. 689) a simple case of epiphysial separation with marked lateral displacement, terminating in extensive suppuration, for which amputation was performed. Harry H., aged sixteen years, was admitted to the Episcopal Hospital May 4, 1894. While running round a pile of heavy sheet iron, used in shipbuilding, which was standing upon its edge, a plate fell, striking the side of his leg a little above the knee, and producing a marked lateral displacement, which on admission was reported to be a lateral dislocation of the knee. On examination (under ether) there was found to be much effusion in and about the knee-joint, with distinct softening and a hæmatoma over the lower end of the vastus internus muscle. All deformity could be readily corrected by extension and lateral support, but under lateral pressure, in which the thigh was fixed and the lower or condyloid portion pressed, the deformity would recur, simulating lateral displacement of the knee. On careful examination the sharp outline of the diaphysis of the femur could be distinctly outlined through the softened or ruptured vastus internus muscle. Crepitus of a soft or moist character could be readily detected. Extension was applied, and long lateral splints with bran bags on either side of the limb. With these the ends of the bones were kept in perfect apposition, although with much effusion about the knee. In the course of a few days there was evidence of suppuration in the region of injury, which was opened and drained. Through the incision, made on the inner side of the thigh, the line of separation could be distinctly outlined in perfect apposition. A large portion of the lower end of the femur was divested of its periosteum. Extensive suppuration followed, and in order to prevent a fatal termination the thigh was amputated in the middle third. From that time the patient made an uneventful recovery. The drawing from a photograph which accompanies Dr. Harte's report, taken from the dried specimen in his possession, displays a pure separation of the epiphysis and manifest traces of suppurative periostitis. Dr. Harte thought that the subsequent discharge of several pieces of bone might be connected with the periosteum; that these pieces might have been developed from the osteogenic layer of the denuded periosteum, as there was found a number of such fragments attached to the separated periosteum.

Dr. J. Prochnow, of Buda Pest, relates ('Traumás epiphysis-leválás,' *Gyógyászat*, Budapest Nov. 1892, 546 ; abstract *Pester medizinisch-chirurgische Presse*, Budapest 1893, April 389) a case of displacement backwards of the epiphysis, followed by necrosis of the skin and the end of the diaphysis, in a boy ten years old. The separation was at first a simple one.

The patient, whilst running (June 12, 1891), fell upon the curb-stone of a pavement and violently struck his left knee. He was unable to stand, and had to be carried home. The doctor called in detected a fracture, and sent him to the hospital. There was at once seen a notable displacement of the knee outwards and backwards from the thigh, causing an angular appearance of the limb. At the lower part of the inner side of the thigh, in the normal situation of the internal condyle, the skin was bluish, and stretched over the sharp edge of the femur. This became more tense with every movement. The lower fragment or epiphysis was displaced backwards, the upper fragment inwards and forwards. The knee was somewhat swollen, but the patella could be easily made out, being placed towards the outer side. Both condyles were easily identified, but the lower fragment could not readily be fixed. With every movement crepitus was perceptible. Flexion of the knee failed to adapt the fragments accurately. The upper end of the fracture projected completely forwards ; this became very marked on extension, but less so on moderate flexion. The limb was therefore put up in this position on an inclined plane. However, the skin necrosed from the pressure of the bone, which, bare of its periosteum, became exposed, and protruded for one to two centimetres. The protruding end of bone gradually necrosed, and a moderate amount of suppuration delayed the progress of the case. The inclined plane was continued for many weeks, when the limb was placed upon a cushion, as there was no movement at the seat of fracture. On September 27 the necrosed bone came away, and two smaller pieces on November 2 and 21. On February 6, 1892, the patient left the hospital perfectly recovered, and, as Dr. Prochnow afterwards learned, walked well, and up to the time of the report no alteration in the length of the extremity had occurred.

The following account of a case of compound separation of the lower epiphysis of the femur by Dr. E. H. Nichols (*Medical and Surgical Reports*, Boston City Hospital, U.S.A., 1896, 7. S. p. 118),

examined by him at the Sears Pathological Laboratory of the
Harvard Medical School, gives an interesting description of the
appearances subsequently found in the traumatic osteomyelitis
which existed.

P. McD., a schoolboy, aged thirteen years, was admitted on
June 19, 1895. One hour previously he had tried to jump upon the
tailboard of a moving wagon, and his left leg was caught in the
revolving wheel. The boy's general condition was good, and he
showed little evidence of shock. There was a compound separation
of the lower epiphysis of the left femur from the diaphysis, the end
of which projected through the wound about eight centimetres, and
was denuded of periosteum for about five centimetres. The joint was
not opened, and the dorsalis pedis artery pulsated. Under ether it was
necessary to enlarge the superficial wound before the bone could be
reduced. The wound was cleaned, and a drain inserted at the
lower angle, the opening being closed by interrupted sutures. The
leg was put up in a plaster dressing, which extended from the toes
to the groin. The wound was dressed again on the second day on
account of staining of the dressing. In about a week the boy began
to lose ground, and two weeks after the first dressing pus was seen
in the wound. The patient steadily growing worse, amputation
was advised and refused. The discharge increased, and various
sinuses, leading down to dead bone, were formed. Seven weeks
from the day of admission there was sudden profuse hæmorrhage
from the sinuses, which was controlled by packing. Hæmorrhages
recurred almost daily for nearly two weeks. Finally the parents gave
reluctant consent to amputation; this was performed fifteen centimetres below the hip. Even then the flaps had to be trimmed and
curetted to free them of the infiltrated tissue. Improvement immediately took place, and the patient was discharged four weeks later. On
examination the surface of the end of the shaft was roughened and
eroded, while its lateral surfaces for a distance of three to five centimetres were entirely denuded of periosteum, which had been stripped
back like a glove finger. Beginning at the level of the periosteal
detachment, the shaft was enlarged and irregular from new bony
formation. The fractured surface of the epiphysis was rough, shreddy,
and slightly eroded, and a small osseous fragment was torn from the
internal condyle. The articular surface was normal. Section of
the shaft showed the lower three centimetres to be spongy, with large
irregular areolar spaces. Above this area there was an irregular
transverse dense white band, and above the band the shaft was
apparently normal, except for a considerable layer of newly formed
periosteal bone outside the original dense walls.

On microscopical examination the articular cartilage appeared
normal. The marrow of the epiphysis, in which the cell elements
predominated (' red marrow '), was normal to within five millimetres
of the epiphysial line. At that level the areolar spaces began to be

filled partly with young connective tissue containing numerous large vessels ('granulation tissue'). Then came a transverse band of dense fibrous tissue, completely filling the areolar spaces. Between this fibrous band and the line of fracture was a layer of lymphoid cells and of polynuclear leucocytes.

The shaft of the femur for the distance of over three centimetres above the epiphysial line was entirely necrotic, the cells were fused into a faintly staining granular mass, and the trabeculæ showed neither laminæ nor bone cells. This necrosis was less marked the greater the distance from the epiphysial line. Above the area of necrosis was an irregular obliquely transverse band of dense fibrous tissue, the fibres of which completely filled the areolar spaces, while the trabeculæ were mostly necrotic. In places the fibrous tissue was œdematous, and enclosed large numbers of lymphoid cells and polynuclear leucocytes.

Outside the original shaft of the femur, beginning a little below the level of the band of fibrous tissue just described, was a wide layer of newly formed periosteal bone, having numerous trabeculæ, whose surface was covered by many bone-forming cells (osteoblasts), while the areolar spaces were filled with young connective tissue cells and osteoblasts. Above the transverse band of fibrous tissue the marrow was normal. With Weigert's stain many colonies, large and small, of cocci, apparently staphylococci, could be seen scattered throughout the necrotic lower end of the shaft. In the transverse band of fibrous tissue no such colonies could be seen, nor did·they appear in the normal marrow above the band. In the epiphysis only a very few colonies could be found, and in all cases the colonies were outside the band of fibrous tissue.

From a consideration of this case it seemed certain to Dr. Nichols that it would have been impossible to avoid infection. The lower end of the shaft, stripped of periosteum, its blood supply cut off, and its vitality lowered by injury, inevitably must have become necrotic, he says, and been separated as a sequestrum. This necrotic bone yielded easily to a slight infection. It is probable that, if the periosteum had not been stripped, the bone would have been able to resist infection, for the epiphysis did resist infection, except directly along the edge of the line of fracture, while the shaft at the level where the periosteum was intact completely walled off the bacteria. The walling-off of so extensive and active a process indicated that the infection came late, after the process of repair was well advanced.

The case suggested to Dr. Nichols that it may be desirable, in such a case of extensive stripping of the periosteum, to attempt to replace the lacerated periosteum, or, if that is impossible, to excise the denuded bone, since the resulting shortening would be of less consequence than the practically certain infection with its attending dangers.

Inflammation and suppuration of the knee-joint.—Suppuration of the joint and popliteal space occurred in one instance three years after the accident, when the epiphysis had united in its malposition on the front of the femur. The specimen from the museum of Robert Liston is now in the Museum of the Royal College of Surgeons of England, No. 1041, and is figured by this surgeon in his *Elements of Surgery* (second edition, London, 1840, p. 721), and by many other surgical authors. The patient, a girl, was fourteen years old when her leg was caught between the spokes of a wheel and the epiphysis separated. After the accident the knee remained painful and swollen, and she halted a little in walking; but nothing particular ensued for three years after her apparent recovery from the accident, when a large abscess formed in the ham and lower part of the thigh, and communicated with the knee-joint. For this the limb was amputated, and the patient recovered. The epiphysis has been displaced forwards and upwards about halfway on to the front of the femur, and the diaphysis forced downwards and backwards. In this position firm and smooth reunion has taken place, with very little shortening or distortion of the limb.

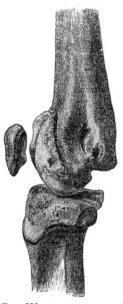

Fig. 226.—SEPARATION AND DISPLACEMENT FORWARDS OF THE LOWER EPIPHYSIS OF THE FEMUR. UNION IN THIS POSITION WAS FOLLOWED BY SUPPURATION OF JOINT AND POPLITEAL SPACE

(Royal College of Surgeons Museum.)

Suppuration of the joint may occur as the result of direct injury or laceration of the articular structures, or from suppuration extending to it from the vicinity of the epiphysial lesion. Dr. Harte says that this articulation was implicated in one of his cases (Edward H.), possibly the result of secondary infection.

Septic suppuration of the joint is particularly prone to ensue in compound separations.

Mr. Charles Hawkins, at the Royal Medical and Chirurgical Society in April 1842 (*loc. cit. supra*), mentioned a case of compound separation in Westminster Hospital where the end of the bone was sawn off. Suppuration formed in the joint, which became ankylosed.

Septic phlebitis and pyæmia are mostly represented in compound separations.

An interesting example of compound separation with rupture of the popliteal artery, followed by amputation, pyæmia, and death, is published by H. H. Clutton (*St. Thomas's Hospital Reports*, N.S. vol. xxii. 1894, p. 13).

Jane B., aged eight years, was admitted into St. Thomas's Hospital on October 28, 1893. She had been running behind an undertaker's cart, and had her left leg caught between the spokes of one of the wheels.

On admission the left leg was held in a flexed position by the child, who seemed in great pain. There was a hollow just above the patella at the lower third of the thigh in front. An inch and a half above the upper edge of the patella, on the outer side of the thigh, was a wound which looked almost like an incised wound, about one inch in length, extending through the deep fascia and into the muscle, which was exposed. There was an extensive hæmatoma on the outer side of the thigh. Under an anæsthetic there was found a separation at the epiphysial line, with displacement of the epiphysis forwards, so that the lower end of the diaphysis was pressing against the popliteal vessels. The deformity could only be reduced with difficulty, and reappeared on omitting extension. The arteries could not be felt at the foot either before or after reduction, and with a finger in the wound it was thought probable that the popliteal artery was ruptured. As there was no hæmorrhage, an attempt was made to save the limb. The blood-clot was cleared out of the popliteal space, and by constant irrigation the wound rendered as aseptic as possible. A dressing of cyanide gauze was applied, and the whole limb and abdomen enveloped in plaster of Paris, with a window opposite the wound. The foot, which had been previously cold and blanched, became warmer and redder. Extension was kept up till the plaster had set, when it was found that the deformity did not recur. Unfortunately a clove-hitch was then applied to the ankle, and from this a weight suspended over the end of the bed. The discharge from the wound became offensive and the foot gangrenous; a back splint in place of the plaster of Paris was applied. Amputation of the thigh was performed on November 10 at the line of the wound on the outer side of the thigh. It was found necessary to remove a small portion of the femur. Septic absorption still went on, and the temperature varied from 99° to 103°. The flaps retracted and exposed the end of the femur, which was apparently dead. Mr. Clutton thought a septic osteomyelitis was taking place, and therefore on November 18 removed the end of the femur. There was no pus in the medullary canal, and the section of femur exposed was healthy. Suppurative arthritis of the left shoulder-joint and many other signs of pyæmia occurred, and the patient died on November 30. At the autopsy there was suppurative thrombosis of the left femoral and external iliac veins as high up in the vena cava as the entrance of the renal veins. There was a similar clot softening here and there in the right iliac and femoral veins, with a small collection of pus at the apex of

Scarpa's triangle. The lungs were a little œdematous, and with the exception of a drachm of thick pus in the left shoulder-joint, there were no other changes indicative of pyæmia, and Mr. Clutton considered that success would probably have followed a ligature of the left femoral vein at the groin at any time before the thrombosis had extended beyond Poupart's ligament. Before death, on November 24, thrombosis of the right femoral vein became apparent, followed by great swelling of the whole of the right thigh and leg, but, as Mr. Clutton says, it was recognised too late to consider the advisability of arresting the progress of pyæmia from suppurative thrombosis by ligature of the vein on the cardiac side of the furthest limit of the clot.

Aneurism.—The presence of the end of the diaphysis in the popliteal space by pressure on the popliteal artery may cause an aneurism to develop, in after years, from ulceration or rupture.

This is well shown in a specimen in the Museum of the Royal College of Surgeons, Edinburgh, No. 138, xx. c., of separation of this epiphysis, united in its displaced position ; a beautiful illustration of the same specimen is given by Sir Charles Bell (*Observations on Injuries of the Spine and Thigh Bone*, 1824, p. 86 ; *Medico-Chirurgical Review*, N.S. vol. viii. 1825, p. 49). (See p. 122, fig. 13.)

A boy, age not stated, in getting on to the back of a carriage, caught his leg in the spokes of the wheel, twisting off the epiphysis from the extremity of the diaphysis. Union took place after this accident, but the broken portions united irregularly, and a point projected. About twenty years after this accident the patient, now grown into manhood, in jumping down from a chair, felt something snap, and very soon after a pulsating tumour formed, which was found to be an aneurism brought about by rupture of the popliteal artery, occasioned by the projecting extremity of the shaft. The epiphysis is seen to be firmly, though somewhat irregularly, united to the anterior aspect of the shaft, with its articular surface looking forwards and slightly downwards, and its back part projecting downwards. The end of the diaphysis presents backwards into the popliteal space behind the epiphysis, and is rough and irregular. Although the epiphysis and the shaft are in bad position, the union between them has been exceedingly solid. (*Catalogue of Pathological Specimens in the Royal College of Surgeons of Edinburgh*, 1893, p. 134, specimen No. 3, 249).

Mr. C. Mansell Moullin showed before the Pathological Society (*Transactions of the Pathological Society*, vol. xxxix. 1888, p. 243) in 1887 a somewhat similar case, though the artery had ulcerated through at a much earlier date.

The patient from whom the specimen was obtained was admitted into the London Hospital at Christmas 1886. About a year before, when he was fifteen years old, he sustained a compound fracture of the lower end of the femur. From this he recovered completely, and was able to get about again fairly well, with a slight amount of deformity and a certain degree of stiffness about his knee-joint. A few days before admission this stiffness began to increase, and he found not only that he was unable to bend the joint, but that the attempt was exceedingly painful.

On examination the popliteal space was found to be occupied by a tense swelling, in which a slight degree of pulsation could be detected, especially on the inner side. There was a scar on the front of the limb; the joint could not be bent to a right angle, and even that was exceedingly painful. A faint bruit could be heard at times where the pulsation was most distinct; the limb itself was fairly well nourished, but colder than the other, though the tibial arteries could scarcely be felt. Pulsation was checked at once by pressure on the femoral, but no change of any kind could be produced by direct pressure. An incision was made into the popliteal space, rather to the inner side of the middle line, and a very large quantity of recent coagulum turned out; the end of the upper fragment was found projecting backwards and pressing upon the popliteal artery, in which there was a small opening with rounded edges, evidently formed by gradual ulceration. The vessel was isolated as well as it could be, and tied above and below, the projecting fragment being removed by means of a chain saw. About the fourth week the knee-joint began to enlarge, and finally suppurated, and the limb was amputated.

After maceration the epiphysis was detached, and the line of fracture could be followed on the posterior surface of the shaft, along the intercondyloid notch, and upon the anterior surface of the epiphysis. Evidently the condyles had been separated and were united again; but while the cartilage still persisted between the epiphysis and the shaft over the whole of the rest of the surface, along the line of fracture it was replaced by bone, and this had to be broken through before the epiphysis could be detached.

PROGNOSIS AND RESULTS.—The prognosis would seem at first sight to be extremely serious, if we consider the number of reported cases in which amputation had to be performed.

Out of 125 separations of the lower epiphysis of the femur collected by the author, although many compound separations were complicated by extensive bruising and laceration of the soft parts, or serious lesion of the vessels, and demanded immediate amputation, yet it is impossible to deny the fact that many of these limbs would now be saved by the antiseptic precautions of modern surgery.

Secondly, amputation would also be less frequent in simple as well as in compound separations at the present day, when free resection or reduction of the displaced epiphysis or diaphysis can be safely and successfully carried out in those cases which would formerly have been followed by gangrene, secondary hæmorrhage, or other complication.

Again, a very large number of simple cases are unpublished, or not even diagnosed. This is particularly true when displacement of the fragments is not present.

The mortality following separation of this epiphysis with displacement will necessarily remain high, by reason of the numerous complications with which it is so commonly combined, but will certainly in the future be greatly diminished from the present high rate.

Delens observes with regard to this, that it is possible to obtain relatively favourable results even in the most complicated cases, and quotes his own case in proof of this. With the exception of unavoidable shortening, the result in great measure of the resection of the end of the diaphysis, the movements of the articulation were rapidly and completely re-established.

In Alcock's and Gay's cases also, primary resection of the diaphysial end was followed by an excellent result.

Union.—It is certain that in *simple separations* in which displacement has not taken place or has been reduced, rapid consolidation ensues, without impairment of the joint.

In Liston's case, and probably also in Bell's case, the separation was not detected at the time of the accident, and the epiphysis became displaced; consolidation then took place with the shaft in its malposition, and this impaired not only the usefulness of the limb, but also was the cause of further disease in and around the articulation. But even in these cases it is surprising how much rounding off and moulding of the parts takes place; in Liston's case there was stated to be but little distortion of the limb.

In many others that have been properly observed and treated accordingly, good union has occurred in a few weeks, with a straight limb and free movement of the knee-joint, without atrophy.

In Callender's patient union took place in six weeks, and six months later there was no sign of shortening.

Even in cases of severe displacement where reduction has been fully carried out and maintained, there may, as in Mayo Robson's case, be no deformity. This surgeon alludes to another, diagnosed early, in which reduction was easily effected, and the ultimate result was very good.

In Puzey's case, eight months after the accident there was a good straight limb and perfect movement of the knee-joint. At the time of the injury the condyloid epiphysis was displaced incompletely off the diaphysis, so that the leg was in the position of genu valgum.

In Sturrock's patient, thirteen months after the accident the circumference of the knee was only a quarter of an inch greater than that of the sound knee. No definite thickening could be felt, but the knee seemed bulkier; as regards length, both limbs were absolutely the same. The range of movements was perfect, the boy walking without a limp. In this instance the epiphysis had been displaced backwards.

Out of twenty-eight simple cases collected by J. Hutchinson junior, sixteen were got into good position and recovered with very useful or perfect limbs, while of the remaining twelve, in which perfect replacement was not obtained, six were followed by sloughing or suppuration. In four of these amputation had to be performed, one recovered after excision of the knee, and one after resection of the diaphysial end. In one case a popliteal aneurism formed twenty years after, and led to amputation. The remaining cases recovered with more or less useful limbs, the displacement persisting.

Ankylosis of joint.—Some stiffness of the joint may be expected, even though the displacement has been corrected, and an otherwise satisfactory recovery takes place from the injury.

In one of Hamilton's compound cases, complete ankylosis of the knee-joint resulted, with shortening of the limb three-quarters of an inch. He had had a 'sharp' attack of synovitis after the injury.

Bryant says that these epiphysial separations 'are serious on account of the joint complication, as some stiffness of the joint generally, but not always, follows; this result depending upon the amount of inflammatory action that takes place after the injury.'

Spillmann quotes (*Dict. Encyclopédique des Sci. Méd.* tome xxiv. art. 'Cuisse,' 1880, p. 252) a case seen by Chauvel in 1872, in which the separation had been produced by direct violence. The patient was a youth, aged eighteen, whose leg was ankylosed to the thigh at a right angle. The limb was straightened without any great violence, but was followed by suppuration, septicæmia, and death. A separation of the lower epiphysis of the femur, which was still connected with the tibia, was found after death.

The knee-joint being so seldom damaged in separations without or with little displacement, no loss of function follows as a consequence.

Deformity.—The character of the deformity of the knee varies (1) according to the nature of the separation, whether simple, or combined with a fracture of the epiphysis or diaphysis, and (2) according to the displacement of the fragments, especially if they are allowed to remain unreduced, or continue in their locked condition.

M. U. Trélat describes (*Progrès Médical*, August 1875, p. 470) a deformity of the knee arising from forward displacement of the epiphysis; but it was only seen by him four years after the accident.

A girl, aged eighteen, was admitted into the Hôpital de la Charité with pain in the left knee and difficulty in walking. At the age of fourteen she slipped on the edge of the pavement and fell on her knee, and was unable to rise. This was followed by acute pains and swelling of the knee, and she remained in the Hôpital Sainte-Eugénie under the care of M. Marjolin for one year, the limb being kept fixed for four months in different forms of splints. She had been lame ever since and the knee was somewhat deformed, but movements of flexion, adduction, and abduction were free and without pain. There was also a little fluid in the joint, and the patella was displaced a little inwards, but it was not dislocated, since it preserved its natural relation with intercondyloid space. At the level of the upper border of the patella, a series of projections belonging to the intercondyloid notch of the displaced femoral condyles was felt, so that the external aspect of the condyles had become more anterior, their internal aspect posterior. The epiphysis was firmly united. Just below the middle of the popliteal space, the projection of the lower end of the femur was felt as a hard mass, and had evidently undergone a 'kind of rotation' from within outwards and backwards. There was shortening of the limb to the extent of four and a half centimetres.

In other cases which have not been treated or recognised, the deformity may become more and more marked as the child walks about, the epiphysis being gradually displaced off the diaphysis—e.g Liston's case.

The knee may assume the *varus position*, from displacement inwards of the epiphysis.

Dr. R. Winslow, Professor of Surgery, Baltimore, U.S.A., relates (*Maryland Medical Journal*, Baltimore, June 21, 1884, p. 142) the following case of diastasis of the inferior epiphysis of the femur, causing genu varum.

On February 25, Mrs. F. brought her son to the hospital in order to obtain treatment for a deformity of the left leg. The history of the case was as follows : About four weeks previously, S. F., aged eleven years, was struck by a large 'double-decker' sled. According to his own account the sled did not pass over the limb, but in some way mashed or jammed it. He suffered pain, and, being unable to walk, was taken home and put to bed, but received no medical attention. He remained in bed two weeks, and at the end of that time got up and began to use the limb. At first progression was painful and difficult, but the soreness gradually subsided, and at the expiration of four weeks from the time of the accident he walked nearly a mile to the clinic. An examination made at that time revealed the following conditions. The right leg was perfectly straight and normal, but there was a marked bowing of the left leg, so that the knees were separated two or three inches, and could not be made to touch each other. At the same time there was slight shortening of the left limb and some outward rotation of the foot.

The patient walked easily, scarcely limping, and only experienced pain after long walking. There was no bruising of the integument of the knee, little or no tenderness upon pressure, and no effusion within the capsule of the joint. The knee appeared somewhat broader than normal and unduly prominent. The condyles of the femur preserved a normal relation to the tibia, and flexion and extension were unimpaired. The patient could not stand alone upon the hurt leg. The patella was in its proper position, and was freely movable. The leg presented a marked varum, the knees being two inches apart. Upon the outer condyle, about one inch above the tibia, was a slight angular projection, and upon the inner side a corresponding depression existed, the rotundity of the vastus internus muscle being entirely destroyed. Immediately below this depression the projection of the inner condyle could be felt. The mother positively declared that no deformity existed previous to the accident.

Taking into consideration the youth of the patient, the direct injury to the knee, the peculiar deformity, and the fact that the motions of the joint were unimpeded, the diagnosis of separation of the epiphysis was arrived at, with a sliding of the epiphysis inwards, or a displacement of the shaft outwards, in which position union had taken place. The nature of the lesion was explained to the mother, and her sanction to infraction or subcutaneous osteotomy was obtained.

On March 3 the boy was anæsthetised, and with the assistance of Professor Jay it was found possible by the exhibition of considerable force to completely break up the adhesions between the fragments, and to restore the bones to their proper position. When this was done the knees could be easily brought together, and all deformity disappeared. The limb was now well padded and encased from the foot nearly to the pelvis in a nicely fitting plaster-of-Paris splint. The boy was placed in bed, and a sufficient amount of morphine administered to relieve pain. The next morning he was sitting up and clamouring to be taken home. Within a week he was seen standing upon the splint, though against orders, and without any discomfort. The apparatus was removed March 31. The limb was found to be slightly shorter than normal, but the two knees could be easily placed together.

Arrest of growth.—Many instances of separation of the lower epiphysis of the femur have been recorded which have not been followed by arrest of growth when examined some time after the accident, so it must be reckoned that this is an unusual occurrence.

Callender, in the *St. Bartholomew's Hospital Reports* (1873, vol. ix. p. 34), mentions the case of a boy, F. W. P., aged eleven. Whilst hanging on behind a cart he got his leg entangled in the wheel. There was a lacerated wound on the inner side of the knee leading down to the separated epiphysis. Firm union took place in six weeks without shortening. Sixteen months later there was no arrest of growth in the length of the femur.

J. Hutchinson junior alludes to a case under his own care in which there was no arrest of growth. A lad, aged twelve, with very

marked forward and lateral displacement of the epiphysis, the diaphysis pressing on the popliteal artery so as to almost stop the pulse.
Reduction under anæsthetic, MacIntyre's splint, and perfect recovery
is the brief history of the treatment and its results. When the patient
was seen last, one year after the accident, there was no shortening
whatever.

Although bony union may have taken place, it is always to
be feared that the growth of the length of the femur may be subsequently interfered with by the premature ossification or permanent
interference with the function of the epiphysial junction cartilage
consequent upon the injury. The proper proliferation of this
cartilage is mostly responsible for the growth in length of the bone.

Uffelmann was the first to direct attention to arrest of growth
(*Anat.-chir. Beiträge z. d. Lehre v. d. Knochen jugendl. Individ.*
1865) following separation of this epiphysis.

The cases alluded to by Professor Humphry, König, Paschen,
and others show that very grave disturbances in the growth of the
femur and tibia follow resection of the knee-joint when the
epiphysial cartilage of either bone has been removed.

Turgis (*Bull. de la Soc. de Chir.* t. iv. 1878, No. 10, p. 787)
mentions the case of a boy ten years old who had been injured by
machinery ; amongst other lesions he received there was a separation of the lower epiphysis of the femur. When seen after the
lapse of twelve years the thigh was shortened three centimetres.

Delens gives a most accurate and detailed account (*Archives
Générales de Médecine*, vol. cliii. 1884, p. 272) of a case which he
had observed and taken measurements of during ten years—a case
of compound separation of the lower epiphysis of the right femur
with protrusion of the diaphysis, in which the lower end was
resected on account of the impossibility of reduction.

R. L., aged eight and a half, on January 15, 1873, when
climbing behind a carriage in motion, had his right leg caught
between the spokes of the wheel. He was seen by M. Delens
within an hour. The lower end of the femoral diaphysis, characteristic in shape and covered with a thin yellowish layer, protruded through a wound at the outer angle of the popliteal space.
There was no great hæmorrhage, and pulsation of the posterior
tibial artery was felt. Exploration of the popliteal space by the
finger in the wound could not detect any pulsation of the popliteal,
but the condyles of the femur were felt in contact with the tibia.
Slight crepitus suggested intercondyloid fracture, but this was not
proved to exist. The periosteum was stripped off the lower end of
the diaphysis. Even after the patient had been placed under chloroform it was found impossible to reduce and replace the fractured
surfaces. This was again repeated the following day, with a similar
result. The protruding portion of the diaphysis was therefore
removed by means of a saw and bone forceps, and the bone easily

reduced. On the antero-internal aspect of the diaphysial end a triangular fragment two centimetres in height had been detached. The limb was then put up in a trough splint. On February 3 an enormous abscess was found occupying the whole of the outer part of the thigh, extending almost to the great trochanter. This was incised, and a drainage tube passed through to the popliteal wound. From this time the wounds rapidly healed and the bones quickly united, so that at the end of two months, on March 16, the wounds had almost quite healed and the bones firmly united. An immovable splint was applied, and the child allowed to walk on crutches. In about another five weeks' time, on April 24, the splint was finally removed, and it was found that the shape of the limb was perfect with only a moderate amount of callus above the condyles. The wound was now healed, and the child could move its knee and walk easily with the aid of a stick. There was from four to four and a half centimetres shortening. After June the movements of flexion of the knee were perfect; the heel could be placed in contact with the buttock.

The patient could walk about without limping, using a boot raised two centimetres, but there was a marked tendency to rotation of the foot inwards. After this time he was seen only at long intervals for the purpose of measurement. On March 15, 1874, it was noted that the limb had almost regained its normal size, and the position of the foot was good. Measurement of the two limbs from the anterior superior iliac spine to the tip of the external malleolus: left side, 65·5 centimetres; right side, 62·5 centimetres. On April 8, 1875, the measurement was: left side, 67·5 centimetres; right side, 64·5 centimetres. On April 24, 1876: left side, 70 centimetres; right side, 66 centimetres. On April 27, 1877: left side, 77 centimetres; right side, 72·5 centimetres. On January 3, 1878: left side, 80 centimetres; right side, 74 centimetres. So that in the five years following the accident the shortening, which was at first about 4 centimetres, had increased to 6 centimetres. The patient was seen again ten years after the accident, on July 30, 1883; he was then a robust young man, and came to ask if he could enlist as a soldier. From his gait it was impossible to perceive that he had undergone such a severe operation; there was only a slight dragging of the leg. On measurement the left side was 89·5 centimetres, and the right 80 centimetres, giving nine and a half centimetres shortening. During the ten years the sound limb had increased 24 centimetres and the resected limb 17½ centimetres. The difference was entirely in the femur, for the tibiæ had exactly the same length—38 centimetres. The growth of the right femur had taken place mostly through the upper epiphysial cartilage; the lesion of the lower epiphysial cartilage had only produced a decrease of about six centimetres in the total length of the bone.

In Dr. Donovan's case of severe compound separation the

3 c

epiphysis united to the diaphysis after resection of two and a half inches of the latter. The femur appeared to keep pace in its growth in length with its fellow for about two years. The limb, however, subsequently became knock-kneed, and failed to increase in length. Tuberculous disease set in, for which amputation was performed.

The following case of shortening came under the observation of J. Hutchinson junior. A medical student, when aged fifteen, had his knee severely injured at football. On examination at the age of twenty-three there was fibrous ankylosis of the knee with one and a half inch shortening.

Table of cases in which shortening followed separation of the lower epiphysis of the femur

Surgeon	Age of patient	Sex	Amount of shortening	Date of measurement after injury	Remarks
Gay . . .	18	Male	½ inch	9 months	Compound. Resection of end of diaphysis. Simple fracture of opposite femur
Trélat . .	18	Female	1¾ inch	4 years	Displacement of epiphysis forwards and slightly inwards
Callender . .	12½	Male	None	16 months	Compound
Delens . .	18½	Male	9½ cm.	10 years	Compound. End of diaphysis resected
Turgis . .	22	Male	8 cm.	12 years	Simple ?
Puzey . .	19	Male	1 inch	8 years	Simple ? Displacement outwards of epiphysis
Hutchinson jr..	23	Male	1½ inch	8 years	Fibrous ankylosis of knee
Poland, John .	11	Female	8 inches	9 years	Genu varum. Adduction of leg

Professor Nicoladoni, of Innsbruck, relates a very remarkable case of deformity of the knee and lower extremity following gradual obliteration of the epiphysial cartilage from behind forwards, the result of injury.

A young man (L. A.), aged sixteen years, strong and well developed both as to his muscles and bones, came under this surgeon's observation in 1882 with marked flexion of the left lower extremity, so that he had to get about with an addition of about twenty-five centimetres to the sole of the left boot. The left lower extremity was remarkably short as compared with the right, and kept in a flexed position as regards the knee-joint. Flexion of the knee could be effected to an unusual extent, so that the muscles of the calf came in contact with the very muscular upper part of the thigh. Extension was possible only up to an angle of 95° to 98°. However, within this range of movement the patient could easily and very powerfully move his leg. There was no other diseased condition about the knee-joint, and the muscles of the left thigh, leg, and foot were apparently as strong as on the right side.

The left leg and thigh were considerably shortened, the tibia bent concavely inwards at its upper part, and the head of the fibula more than two centimetres above the level of that of the tibia. The left hip-joint and buttock were perfectly normal, and the trochanters of the two limbs on the same level. The left os innominatum appeared to be much more developed than the right. The knees being placed in similar positions, the measurement from the anterior superior spine to the patella was forty-two centimetres on the left side and fifty-two centimetres on the right, and from the head of the tibia to the inner malleolus thirty-six centimetres on the left and forty-five centimetres on the right.

After his memory had been assisted the patient stated that, according to his mother, he fell at the age of seven—that is, nine years previously—from his bed on to his left knee, but that nothing abnormal was ever noticed about the joint as the result of this fall; that from this time (seventh year) it was certain the knee became more and more flexed. Professor Nicoladoni believed that premature ossification of the epiphysial cartilage of the lower end of the femur and of the upper end of the tibia had given rise in the course of nine years to a shortening of the thigh for ten centimetres, and of the leg for nine centimetres.

At the same time that this shortening of the femur took place there was a peculiar contraction of the knee-joint, consisting principally of its range of movement being continually forced towards the side of flexion, whilst the free mobility of the joint was unaltered. In the figure the condyles of the femur are seen to be bent backwards, and the patella (disregarding the flexed portion of the knee) rises in a very striking manner above the level of the articular projections of the femur. This condition he thought had been brought about by the gradual obliteration of the epiphysial cartilage, commencing at the posterior part, i.e. that from behind forwards premature ossification of this structure had taken place; so that the femoral condyles had come in this way to be attached to the posterior aspect of the shaft, and to be directed backwards, while the range of movement of the joint was completely preserved on the side of flexion; the range of movement of extension was limited to the same degree. Both these movements were affected in proportion as the condyles became displaced backwards, and it was to be hardly considered a contraction of the knee-joint, but rather a bending of the femur close to the condyles with the convexity to the front. At the same time the upper epiphysial cartilage of the tibia became

3 c 2

obliterated, that of the fibula remained unaltered, and the inequality of its growth with relation to the tibia resulted in a bending over of the latter bone towards the inner side.

Professor Nicoladoni also draws attention to the fact that similar contractions of the knee-joint have been alluded to by König as the result of premature ossification from before backwards of the epiphysial cartilage after excisions of the knee-joint in young persons, although the whole of the epiphysial cartilage was preserved in these cases.

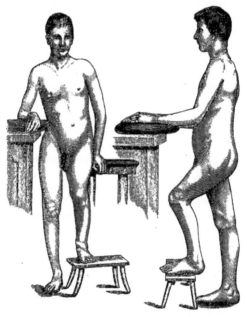

Fig. 227.—ARREST OF GROWTH OF THE FEMUR AND TIBIA WITH CONTRACTION OF KNEE FOLLOWING INJURY TO THE LOWER EPIPHYSIS OF THE FEMUR AND UPPER EPIPHYSIS OF THE TIBIA NINE YEARS PREVIOUSLY. (AFTER NICOLADONI)

The following unique instance of arrest of growth of the femur with a varus position of the knee came under the author's care at the City Orthopædic Hospital in October 1897. The girl (C. S.), aged eleven, was sent to the Hospital by his Grace the Duke of Fife. The history of injury was somewhat indefinite—that the mother had placed the child when about two years old in the country under the charge of some friends, and that on its return home it was noticed to limp. This lameness had increased gradually up to the present time. She had been to more than one hospital in London for treatment, but nothing certain appears to have been detected; at any rate, no advice was offered as to the remarkable condition, and she had not worn any boot or other appliance to correct the deformity, which now existed in the right lower extremity. The whole limb was shortened for four inches, and much smaller than the left. When she stood upright the right knee was thrown outwards into the varus position, the pelvis tilted downwards on this side, and the spine much curved (see fig. 228). On placing the spine and pelvis in their normal position by raising the foot four inches, it was discovered that the femur was rather more than three inches, and the tibia rather less than one inch, shorter than the left (see fig. 229). The knee-joint could be freely flexed and extended, but considerable movement was permitted in a lateral direction by adducting and abducting the leg. During ab-

duction a very considerable gap could be seen and felt on the inner side of the knee between the internal condyle of the femur and the inner tuberosity of the tibia. This was due to the slightly oblique direction of the lower epiphysis of the femur, and its ill-developed condition. The external condyle was the most prominent of the two condyles, and projected downwards lower. This had probably been brought about by the upward pressure of the tibia upon the internal condyle during progression. This upward displacement of the internal condyle was a very notable feature, especially when the leg was adducted, the inner tuberosity placed in contact with the inner condyle, and the shortening of the limb corrected. The limb placed in this position was across the front of the left, so that the right

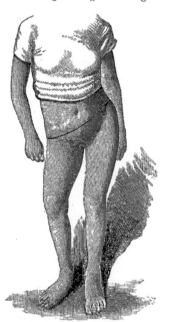

FIG. 228.—ATTITUDE OF PATIENT FROM ARREST OF GROWTH OF LOWER EXTREMITY FOLLOWING INJURY TO LOWER EPIPHYSIS OF FEMUR

knee was just above the left (see fig. 230). The wasting and smallness of the tibia on the affected side was probably the result of the small amount of use that had been made of this limb. The hip-joints were normal. The shaft of the femur, especially at its lower end as well as its lower epiphysis, was felt to be small and atrophied as compared with the opposite side, and between the internal condyle and the diaphysis a concavity could be felt. The skiagraphs revealed the fact that the lower end of the diaphysis of the femur was almost one inch less than the left in width just above the epiphysial line, and that the chief atrophy of the diaphysial end as seen in a lateral view was in the antero-posterior direction.

The skiagraphic view of the leg placed almost in a line with the thigh displayed the moderate gap in this portion between the internal condyle and the inner tuberosity of the tibia. The femoral diaphysis is also seen to be curved forwards and outwards at its lower third.

Supracondyloid osteotomy was successfully performed just before the time of this report.

SYMPTOMS.—From the severity of the injury and the numerous complications often present, separation of the lower epiphysis of the femur engages the attention of the hospital surgeon perhaps

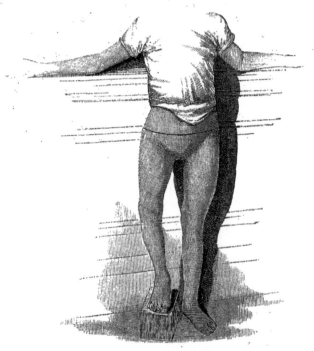

Fig. 229.--THE SAME PATIENT WITH LIMB ELEVATED FOUR INCHES

more than any other epiphysial separation. These injuries differ in their symptoms very considerably, both from the variety of the displacement and the numerous complications attending them.

We may at once dismiss the consideration of those examples of compound injury where the square-shaped, rammerlike protruding end of the femur, somewhat flattened from before backwards, with its mammillated surface devoid of epiphysial cartilage, stripped of periosteum, allows us to make a sure diagnosis, or where it is possible to explore the fragments through the wound.

Some separations present much the same symptoms as those of

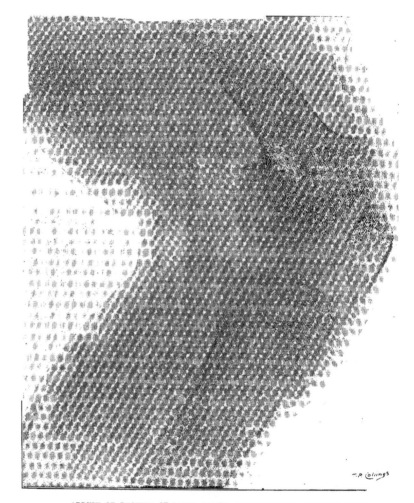

ARREST OF GROWTH OF RIGHT FEMUR AFTER INJURY. LATERAL VIEW.

Author's case.

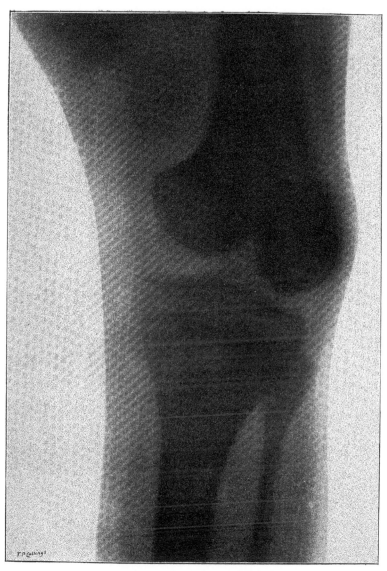

ANTERO-POSTERIOR VIEW OF SAME CASE.

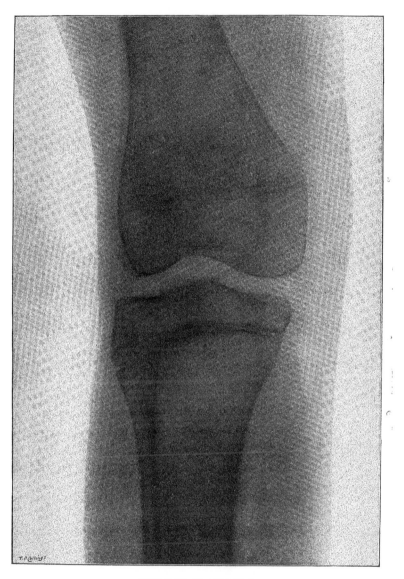

LEFT KNEE OF SAME CASE.

transverse portions of the lower end of the femur ; the author therefore cannot but agree with Dr. Packard when he says that many of
the published cases have been so carelessly reported as to leave room
for doubt · whether they were not simple supracondyloid fractures
instead of simple separations.

In some forms the group of symptoms is perfectly pathognomonic of separation ; while in others the greatest difficulty is
present, there being little to
direct the surgeon in making
an exact diagnosis.

PURE SEPARATION WITHOUT
DISPLACEMENT.—Here the diagnosis must always be a matter
of considerable difficulty. In
this condition the surgeon can
be guided solely by the age of
the patient, by the manner in
which the injury has been received, by the presence of abnormal mobility of the epiphysis
at the conjugal line, and by the
existence of more or less acute
pain, especially at the same
point. Crepitus may· be absent,
and the patient be even able
to use the limb ; yet in some
cases the limb may be rendered
powerless.

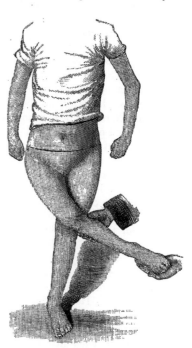

The author believes these
to be far from uncommon, but
curiously they had, as far as he
is aware, never been alluded to
by writers previous to his paper
on ' The Diagnosis of Traumatic
Separation of the Epiphyses,'
read before the West Kent

FIG. 230.—THE SAME PATIENT SHOWING POSI-
TION OF LIMB WHEN THE INNER TUBEROSITY
OF TIBIA WAS PLACED IN CONTACT WITH THE
INTERNAL CONDYLE OF FEMUR

Medico-Chirurgical Society in 1886, in which special attention was
directed to the probable frequent occurrence of separation of the
lower femoral epiphysis without displacement.

Mr. Howard Marsh (since the above paper was written) agrees
with this opinion (art. 'Fract.' of Femur,' Heath's *Dict. of Pract.
Surgery,* 1887, vol. i. p. 534), when he says that ' sometimes the
displacement is so slight that the injury may easily escape notice,
or be mistaken for a mere traumatic synovitis.'

Packard thought that separation of the lower epiphysis of the
femur was a rare accident, but adds ' although perhaps it sometimes
occurs without being recognised.'

The violence producing separation without displacement appears to be less than that which causes displacement of the epiphysis ; still, there will be found some stripping up of the periosteum from the diaphysis, as in the more serious displacements.

SEPARATION WITH SLIGHT DISPLACEMENT.—Instances in which the displacement exists to a slight extent are yet more common than separations without displacement.

At Long Island College Hospital, New York, in 1860 (*American Medical Times*, August 18, 1860, p. 116), Professor F. H. Hamilton had under his care a girl, aged four, who had fallen down a flight of steps. On examination of the left leg one hour after the accident, swelling was found about the ankle-joint, and distinct crepitus, more like that occasioned by the friction of cartilage than of bone. The lower epiphysis could be moved slightly upon the diaphysis. There was, however, no displacement, and the treatment adopted was simple rest in bed without splints. A week later the limb was still in good position and all crepitus ceased, but the ankle remained swollen, as if from effusion into the joint. The same treatment was continued.

A similar case was under the care of Mr. Howse at Guy's Hospital in 1866. Walter K., aged eight, was running behind a cab, when he caught his left leg between the spokes of the wheel.

There was great pain in the line of junction of the lower epiphysis of the femur, but no shortening or displacement. There was considerable swelling about the knee, and some fluid in the joint. The patella was in its normal relations. A double interrupted splint was applied, and the patient left the hospital seven weeks later without any deformity or noticeable callus around the seat of injury.

Dr. R. H. Harte, of Philadelphia, records (*Trans. Amer. Surg. Association*, 1895, vol. xiii. p. 399 ; *American Journal of the Medical Sciences*, June 1896, p. 683) an instance of only slight displacement.

Louis S., aged fifteen years, was admitted to the Episcopal Hospital, June 14, 1895. While he was hanging on the back of a wagon, a leg became entangled in a revolving wheel. On admission there was effusion into the knee-joint, and marked softening over the internal condyle. Crepitus of a moist character could be detected, although with slight displacement. Extension by means of a weight and firm lateral support, with bran bags and long lateral splints, were employed. The patient made a good recovery, and left the hospital, cured, in fifty-seven days. The mobility of the joint was unimpaired.

That separation of the lower epiphysis of the femur can occur without giving rise to many definite symptoms is also corroborated by the following case of F. W. Elsner's (*Australasian Med. Gazette*, July 20, 1895, p. 266).

A boy (C. W.), aged twelve years, was kicked on the left thigh, a hand's breadth above the knee, on Christmas Day, 1894. On examination of the limb the next morning there was nothing but increased mobility and a peculiar moist crepitus—no pain, no shortening whatever, and not a trace of hæmorrhage or swelling. With the exception of the foot rolling outwards whenever it was let go, there appeared to be very little the matter. A few rotatory movements were sufficient to replace the parts in position. A long Liston with a short inside splint was applied. On removing these a fortnight later there was found half an inch of shortening; the limb was therefore placed on an inclined plane. Four weeks after the injury the boy was able to lift his leg without pain off the bed, and could a fortnight later get about well on crutches. On account of immediate union having taken place, there was no distinct callus along the femur, and the shortening was now (July 1895) less than half an inch.

Displacement may occur subsequently.—Although deformity will be absent in separations without displacement, it is not impossible that some displacement of the epiphysis may take place at a later period than the accident. In Liston's case the true nature of the injury was evidently overlooked at the time, there being no displacement, and the patient merely halting a little in walking. It is probable that in this case (*loc. cit. supra*) the displacement forwards of the epiphysis occurred for the most part subsequent to the accident.

In Elsner's case just mentioned, in which there was no displacement or shortening at the time of the injury, a fortnight after it had been placed on a Liston's splint half an inch of shortening appeared; the limb was then placed on an inclined plane.

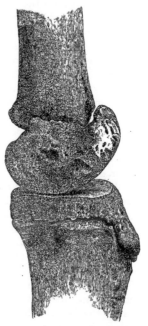

FIG. 231.—NORMAL EPIPHYSES OF THE KNEE-JOINT AT THE NINETEENTH YEAR, VIEWED FROM THE INNER SIDE. (HALF NATURAL SIZE.) DIAGRAM TO SHOW COMMENCING ROTATION AND DISPLACEMENT FORWARDS OF THE LOWER FEMORAL EPIPHYSIS

In others there may be felt, if the patient be seen soon after the injury and no swelling be present, a slight projection of the epiphysis commencing to be displaced into the popliteal space.

However, after the lapse of some hours, swelling takes place with rapidity around the fragments, and is accompanied with effusion around and beneath the separated periosteum, entirely obscuring any projection of the diaphysis or epiphysis that might have been detected previously.

Although in the adult and uninjured youthful bone only a small part of the two heads of the gastrocnemius muscle is attached directly to the epiphysis, yet the whole of this muscle will act upon the epiphysis or lower fragment, by reason of the great detachment of the periosteum, to which the gastrocnemius is intimately connected. The epiphysis thereby tends to be thrown backwards by the action of this muscle, which no longer has any hold upon the diaphysis.

Mr. Durham had under his care in Guy's Hospital in 1884 (when the author was Surgical Registrar and had the opportunity of carefully examining the case) a boy (Alfred B.), aged twelve, who was struck on the left knee by some wood and knocked down. There was a good deal of swelling about the knee, and some mobility, but no crepitus. The movements of the joint were normal; an ordinary back splint was applied. About three weeks later a projection was felt in the popliteal space of the lower epiphysis of the femur, commencing to rotate and be displaced backwards by the action of the popliteus and gastrocnemius muscles. The limb was placed on a double-inclined plane, and consolidation rapidly took place in a few weeks without any displacement or shortening.

Dr. Clement Dukes, medical officer to Rugby School, relates (*Brit. Med. Journal*, vol. ii. 1874, p. 402) the case of a youth, aged eighteen, which he diagnosed as condyloid separation of the femur.

While playing in the close at school, he was pushed on the outer side of his right leg, his legs being extended laterally from the median line, when he suddenly felt acute pain above the knee and fell down, the limb becoming powerless. On examination the knee-joint was not swollen, and no distortion was perceptible to the eye. The leg lay powerless on the bed, but the foot was neither twisted nor everted. The limb was slightly shortened, and on taking hold of it no crepitus could be elicited, nor any abnormal movement, though pain was felt whichever way it was moved. On slightly flexing the leg, a rub as of two gliding smooth surfaces was felt, with a slight depression about two inches above the knee. The lower fragment formed a slight prominence posteriorly at the upper part of the popliteal space, being rotated a little backwards by the gastrocnemius.

A long outside and a short straight-back splint, with pad over the situation of the epiphysis, were employed, with extension by weight. At the end of six weeks there was firm union without shortening, and there was not the slightest thickening at the seat of injury, so that it was impossible to tell there had been any separation.

SEPARATION WITH DISPLACEMENT.—Mr. Hutchinson (*Archives of Surgery*, vol. iv. January 1893, p. 288) says : 'Fortunately the complete displacement of the shaft from the epiphysis is rare, even in cases where the separation is quite complete. The surfaces separated are large, and that of the shaft does not usually leave the whole of that of the epiphysis.'

Strong dissent must be expressed from the opinion given in a recent text-book on surgery that 'the wide surfaces are seldom completely separated.'

Should this opinion be accepted and the treatment recommended carried out, a very disastrous result may ensue. 'The treatment consists simply in supporting the limb for a few days on a back splint till the swelling has subsided, when a starched bandage or plaster-of-Paris splint may be applied.'

Displacement in a very marked degree, with its accompanying deformity, is met with in a very large proportion of cases, and its precise location is due chiefly to the character and direction of the force applied; a careful study, therefore, of the different osseous projections should furnish us with signs not only for an exact diagnosis but also for the necessary treatment.

Mayo Robson thinks that 'the direction of the displacement probably partly depends on the direction in which the violence has been applied, but also on the attachment or otherwise of the gastro-cnemius tendon to the lower end of the upper fragment.'

As a broad rule it may be said that the lower fragment or epiphysis usually retains its normal connections with the head of the tibia; at the same time, it is often rotated on its transverse or vertical axis.

Displacement forwards.—The most common displacement of the epiphysis is forwards, more or less completely off the diaphysis, on to the anterior aspect of the lower end of the latter, so that the lower aspect of its articular surface is in contact with the patella. This is largely due to the action of the heads of the gastrocnemius tilting the epiphysis forwards, the nature of the violence being that of forcible extension, which may be combined with rotation or twisting, while one or other end of the limb is fixed.

The quadriceps extensor in front, and the hamstring muscles behind, by their action will displace the diaphysial end backwards and downwards into the popliteal space.

Mr. A. F. McGill described a typical case before the Leeds and West Riding Medico-Chirurgical Society, May 1884 (*Med. Times and Gazette*, London 1884, vol. i. p. 695) in a strong, well-developed boy, aged fifteen, who was admitted into the Leeds General Infirmary. While sitting at work with his feet on the ground, a heavy iron plate struck the lower part of the femur just above the knee. He was unable to walk, and his left leg was slightly flexed and everted. There was general swelling of the knee-joint, with well-marked deformity. The anterior aspect of the patella was one inch and a half in front of that of the femur, and behind the patella a mass of bone the shape of the lower epiphysis of the femur was felt in front of the lower end of the diaphysis. The popliteal vessels were displaced backwards, and were felt beating directly under the skin.   The circumference of the left limb at the upper border of the patella was fourteen inches and seven-eighths, while that of the right was thirteen inches.   The ilio-patellar line was shortened five-eighths of an inch. Pulsation in the tibial arteries below was unimpaired.   Under ether the deformity was easily reduced by forcible flexion of the limb till the heel touched the buttock.   A back splint was applied, and the case did well.

Mr. Mayo Robson alludes (*Annals of Surgery,* July 1893, p. 2) to six or seven cases which he had seen, in all of which the displacement of the epiphysis was forwards.

The readiness with which the diaphysis is placed backwards into the

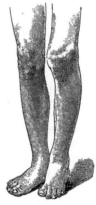

FIG. 233.—DISPLACEMENT OF
EPIPHYSIS FORWARDS
(Ashby and Wright)

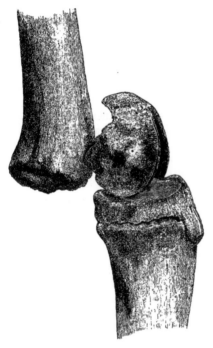

FIG. 232.—DIAGRAM OF COMPLETE DISPLACEMENT OF THE EPIPHYSIS FORWARDS AND ROTATION ON ITS TRANSVERSE AXIS

popliteal space may also be explained by this being in the direction of the least resistance towards the loose tissues of the space, while on the front aspect there are the quadriceps extensor, the patella, and the ligamentum patellæ.

Combined with forward displacement there is often observed some *rotation of the leg and foot outwards,* as in one of Mayo Robson's cases.

In some the leg and knee roll completely outwards, and rest on their outer side.

The leg is usually semiflexed.—Mr. G. A. Wright, of Manchester, figures (Ashby and Wright, *Diseases of Children,* 3rd edit. 1896,

p. 755) an example of separation of the lower epiphysis of the left femur, in which the epiphysis is displaced forwards and the knee flexed.

Swelling about the joint may be very considerable. It has led to error in diagnosis in several instances.

In one instance mentioned by Mayo Robson (Atkinson's) the swelling was so great at the time of the injury that it prevented a diagnosis being made until a fortnight afterwards, when reduction could not be effected, so that excision of the joint had to be performed, as it was necessary that pressure should be removed from the popliteal vessels. In this case, at the time of the injury, Atkinson says the extensive effusion into and about the joint completely obliterated the natural outline, so that none of the bony landmarks—not even the superficial outline of the patella—could be defined.

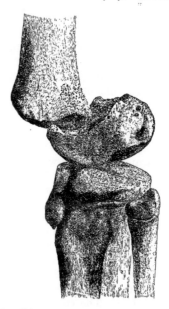

Mr. Canton makes special mention of very great swelling of the lower part of the thigh and knee in one of his cases.

Displacement backwards. — When the epiphysis is beginning to rotate forwards on its transverse axis, its posterior border will be the projection felt in the popliteal space ; this was so in Mr. Durham's case. This rotation is largely due to the attachment of the heads of the gastrocnemius to the posterior part of the epiphysis.

When the displacement is not very great, the popliteal vessels retaining their normal

FIG. 234.— DIAGRAM TO SHOW INCOMPLETE DISPLACEMENT OF EPIPHYSIS BACKWARDS (½-size)

relation to the intercondyloid notch will not be so liable to be pressed upon as when the diaphysis is displaced backwards. When the displacement is greater, the posterior margin of the condyloid notch or either condylar margin may press upon and injure the vessels ; this is the more likely to occur if any vertical rotation of the epiphysis has taken place.

A few cases are recorded where the epiphysis is entirely displaced backwards and the diaphysis forwards.

Mr. J. Hilton describes a case (*Medical Times and Gazette,* February 12, 1859, p. 163) in which this form of displacement was diagnosed.

John H., aged eighteen, was admitted into Guy's Hospital on May 20. In carrying a hod of bricks down the slope of an embankment, he slipped and fell with his legs doubled under him and the whole weight of his hod on his shoulder. After the fall he felt severe pain in the left knee, and on attempting to rise was unable to straighten the limb. The left thigh and knee were greatly swollen, the knee semiflexed, and the foot slightly everted. One and a half inches above the upper border of the patella the well-defined anterior edge of the diaphysis could be distinguished projecting forwards. In the popliteal space a considerable projection was easily felt; the outline of the parts was not ascertained, but it was clear, however, that the condyles of the femur projected considerably beyond the lower end of the diaphysis. No crepitus was felt. Mr. Alfred Poland attempted reduction, but found it impossible either to flex or alter the abnormal position of the fragments. Chloroform was given, and the limb was straightened by means of extension, but some projection in front still remained. The following day, the deformity having recurred, chloroform was again administered, and Mr. Hilton reduced it by extension and by forcibly pushing the shaft of the bone backwards. A back splint was then applied. On the 27th the apparatus was disarranged, and the same displacement again took place. Reduction was again effected with some difficulty by means of the same measures. Back and side splints were applied, the limb elevated, and the thigh flexed on the pelvis. In another three weeks, at the end of the seventh week after the accident, the apparatus was removed. There was firm union without any thickening about the bone, and the movements of the knee-joint were perfect.

Dr. C. E. Sheppard gives a note (*St. Thomas's Hospital Reports*, vol. viii. N.S. 1877, p. 436) of the case of a boy, aged fifteen, the subject of hæmorrhagic diathesis, who was in St. Thomas's Hospital under Mr. Simon in 1875. The separation was caused by the boy stumbling while running uphill and falling with his leg doubled up under him. The end of the shaft projected forwards, and a back splint was applied with the limb in a flexed position.

In one of Macdougall's cases (*loc. cit. supra*) the displacement of the epiphysis backwards was so great and the skin so tightly stretched over it that it ulcerated. Secondary amputation was performed a month afterwards for deformity, which was still present from the displaced epiphysis. Union was impossible from the position of the fragments.

In Prochnow's case the displacement backwards and outwards of the epiphysis was very marked, the diaphysial end being very plainly felt on the inner side. Here also the skin was so tightly stretched that sloughing of it ensued, with necrosis of the end of the diaphysis.

In Fischer and Hirschfeld's case (see under UPPER EPIPHYSIS OF THE TIBIA) the diaphysis was somewhat forwards, the epiphysis being rotated so that the internal condyle ascended a little in front, whilst the external condyle descended a little backwards.

C. A. Sturrock gives (*Edinburgh Hospital Reports*, vol. ii. 1894, p. 605) a marked case of displacement backwards of the epiphysis.

H. C., æt. eleven, was admitted to the Royal Infirmary, Edinburgh, under the care of Mr. Hodsdon, on August 25, 1892, and gave the history that a cab had run over his left knee. On inspection the knee, which was very painful, was flexed, and showed an abnormal gap above the patella, with a marked prominence immediately above. The leg felt cold, and appeared slightly œdematous. When the patient was anæsthetised, an unusual prominence could be felt in the popliteal space, which was apparently the epiphysis, while the lower extremity of the shaft of the femur could be distinctly felt lying in front of it ; the separation appeared to be perfectly horizontal ; the condyles could be moved while the femur was fixed, producing smooth crepitus. When the leg was flexed, and traction made upon it, the deformity was reduced, but on extending the limb it again recurred. The limb was accordingly put up in splints, with the thigh at right angles both to the abdomen and to the leg, and by partially swinging the leg it was hoped to exercise a slight amount of extension on the fragments. The limb was thus retained for four weeks, and in the extended position for four more weeks, when a plaster-of-Paris case was applied for a short time. Within a month after the removal of the plaster case—during which time passive movements, friction, and douching were regularly employed —the patient could walk without a limp. On examining the leg thirteen months after the accident it was found that the circumference of the injured knee was a quarter of an inch greater than that of the sound knee ; that no definite thickening could be felt, but the knee seemed bulkier ; that as regards length both limbs were absolutely the same ; that the range of movements was perfect, and that the boy walked without a limp.

Displacement backwards and outwards.—An example of displacement backwards and somewhat outwards is described by C. E. Sheppard (*loc. cit. supra*, p. 433, Plate VIII.) in his Solly Medal prize essay, 1878.

Charles S., aged fifteen, was admitted into St. Thomas's Hospital under Mr. Sydney Jones, April 9, 1877. He was riding behind a cab in a sitting position, with his back towards the cab, when his left leg became entangled in the spokes of the rapidly revolving hind wheel. He was thrown violently into the road, and found he was unable to stand. The left leg was slightly flexed, with considerable displacement of the knee inwards (abduction of leg on thigh). On the front and inner side of the 'knee' there was a rounded smoothish prominence, evidently the lower cartilaginous end of the diaphysis. Below and to the outer side of this prominence could be felt the patella and its ligament in normal relation to the tubercle of the tibia. The articular ends of the femur and tibia were felt in normal relation to one another. The knee-joint was uninjured. The epiphysis of the femur apparently projected into the popliteal space, but could not be felt. The whole knee-joint, including the femoral epiphysis, was displaced outwards and backwards, the shaft projecting forwards and inwards. This position of the fragments was to be accounted for by the nature of the accident. The boy was sitting with his back towards the vehicle, and the leg as a lever, being caught between the spokes, was forced upwards against the spring or rail of the cab as a fulcrum. The epiphysis would in this way be dragged backwards. The leg could be abducted on the thigh to a right angle, and on extreme flexion could be brought nearly parallel to it. Some distinct crepitus was felt during manipulation. Genu valgum was present on the other side. Reduction of the displacement was effected after considerable difficulty by means of traction with the limb in the flexed position and the hand behind the head of the tibia, combined with gentle manipulation of the end of the diaphysis. Liston's back splint was applied in the slightly flexed position. On April 10 there was slight projection of the diaphysis, with some effusion into the knee-joint. On April 11 a long outside splint was applied, with 4 lb. extension. A month later the splint was removed, and there was no trace of the deformity, this limb being straighter than the other. On May 25 (seven weeks after the accident) the patient left the hospital; the movements of the limb were nearly perfect, and he could flex the knee almost to a right angle.

Displacement outwards.—Many instances of this lateral displacement have been recorded; the deformity gives rise to an appearance of the limb similar to *genu valgum*. Mr. Chauncey Puzey, in relating two cases of this injury (*loc. cit. infra*), questions the cause of the fixation of the limb in this position; at first he was disposed to think it was due to impaction of the shaft into the epiphysis, but afterwards considered it was due to the separation of the epiphysis not having been complete at its outer portion, and that here a vertical tear of the lower and external expanded shaft took place, resembling a greenstick fracture. He alluded to the two specimens in St. George's Hospital Museum, related above, in which the separation was complicated by a limited fracture of the diaphysis, and thought, from the manner in which the accident occurred in his two cases, that this limited fracture would be accompanied by a certain amount of impaction of the fragments; and that, this being the case, the fixation of the limb would be readily accounted for.

As stated above, there cannot be impaction in the true sense of the phrase, but rather an impingement of the outer part of the diaphysis in the hollow of the epiphysis, rendering reduction almost impossible by reason of the see-saw movement which has been referred to above.

It is quite possible, however, that the fracture of the diaphysis at the outer part may be incomplete and a greenstick one, but this is not borne out by pathological facts.

With reference to the signs present, the knee is kept a little flexed, and the foot slightly everted while the patella looks a little outwards.

The anterior and inner edge of the end of the diaphysis is to be felt towards the inner side of the patella.

The adductor magnus and the other powerful adductor muscles act strongly on the shaft, and are powerful agents in producing this form of displacement.

In many cases, as mentioned above, the outer and anterior part of the diaphysis is lodged in the cup-shaped hollow of the epiphysis—this shape of the epiphysis especially pertaining to young children before twelve years of age—and consequently the epiphysis undergoes the see-saw movement during manipulation.

In this form of displacement, as in the last described, the lower angular margin of the diaphysis will be placed against or penetrate the front or inner portion of the vastus internus, and may possibly be felt in this position if the effusion is not too extensive.

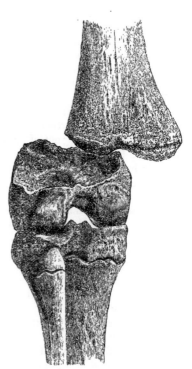

Fig. 235.—DIAGRAM OF DISPLACEMENT OF EPIPHYSIS AND LEG DIRECTLY OUTWARDS BEFORE ABDUCTION TAKES PLACE. THE LIMB MUST BE BROUGHT INTO THIS POSITION BEFORE REDUCTION CAN BE EFFECTED. (⅓-size)

As early as 1837 Mr. John Grantham, of Crayford, Kent (*London Medical Gazette*, N.S. vol. i. 1838, p. 799; *Facts and Observations in Medicine and Surgery*, 1844), diagnosed a case of detachment of this epiphysis by the unusual extent of the deformity, the knee lying on its fibular side. S., aged twelve years, had his right thigh run over by the wheel of an unloaded timber cart. On making gentle extension, the limb appeared straight and the fracture adjusted; but on placing it over a pillow the knee fell again to the

3 D

outer side, as if it moved on a pivot. A transverse separation about an inch above the patella was detected, and attended with a soft inaudible crepitus. The femur was also fractured obliquely through its middle, and the great trochanter separated, which conveyed the same sensation as the separation above the condyles. The limb was placed on a double-inclined plane, and anterior and lateral splints adapted to the thigh. On the fourteenth day the union of the epiphyses was found to be firm, and at the end of the fifth week the boy was permitted to use the limb gradually.

In Marcano's case the displacement was very pronounced, for on the inner side of and above the articulation a projection could be felt about the nature of which there could be no possible mistake.

Mr. Puzey's first case is described (*Liverpool Med. Chirurg. Journal*, 1885, vol. v. p. 42; *Brit. Med. Journal*, 1882, vol. ii. p. 788) as follows :

Arthur L., aged sixteen, was playing at leapfrog, and, on alighting with his legs rather further apart than usual, fell, and on attempting to rise found his knee ' out of joint,' and was at once brought to the Liverpool Northern Hospital (November 30, 1881). When seen lying in bed on his back, he looked as if he was the subject of well-marked genu valgum of the right knee, the limb lying flat on the bed, but the leg being fixed at an angle of 130° with the thigh. There was considerable fulness about the joint, more especially at the inner side, and any attempt at movement appeared to cause great pain. The patient was etherised, and it was then found that the ordinary movements of the joint could be freely carried out, showing that no true dislocation existed ; and in spite of the swelling it was ascertained that the inner condyle bore its normal relation to the head of the tibia, but the leg remained fixed laterally in its extraordinary position.

The lower end of the thigh was now steadied, and by pushing the leg firmly towards the middle line the limb was straightened ; in so doing there was felt the soft crunch or crepitus which is generally noticed in straightening out a ' greenstick' fracture ; and further examination made it evident that what had occurred was a separation of the condyloid epiphysis, not quite complete at its outer aspect. The limb was put on a MacIntyre's splint. Considerable swelling occurred around the lower part of the thigh, and there was also some effusion within the joint, which passed away in the course of a week or two. After seven weeks the boy was allowed to move the knee, and he returned home on January 30, having fair movement of the joint. Six months later he was seen again, and had a good straight limb, with perfect movement of the knee-joint. On December 10, 1884, three years after the accident, he had an absolutely sound limb ; but careful measurement showed that the femur of the injured limb was nearly one inch shorter than the other.

Mr. Puzey's second case. is given in the same volume of the *Liverpool Med. Chirurgical Journal* (*loc. cit. supra*, p. 439).

John M:, aged fifteen, was admitted into the Northern Hospital on June 2, 1884. The description of this case exactly coincided with that just given, but in this instance the skin over the inner condyle was much bruised, and the lower part of the inner aspect of the thigh much swollen from extravasated blood. Any attempt at lateral movement of the limb caused pain, but the knee could be gently flexed to a considerable extent.

The patient was anæsthetised, and the joint found perfectly movable. With some difficulty, owing to the swelling, the inner condyle.was made out holding its normal relation to the head of the tibia, and above this a gap evidently existed. Reduction was effected by pushing with some force the leg towards, and even a little beyond, the middle line, and was accompanied by a sensation of rustling or slight tearing under the hand. An ordinary long external splint was applied. There was articular effusion for a considerable time and swelling above the joint, evidently due to extensive deep extravasation of blood, probably caused by laceration of the vastus internus. This was to be accounted for by the manner in which the injury was caused—i.e. by direct violence. The lad was walking along a wall, and fell on to the low wall of an ash-pit, with which the inner side of his knee came in contact, thus sustaining laterally the whole stress of the fall. On July 16 the limb was put up in plaster of Paris, and the patient.was discharged from the hospital on July 23 with very slight stiffness of the knee-joint; on December 10, 1884, there was no difference between the two limbs, except that the inner condyle was more prominent than that of the other limb. At the time of the report there was no shortening, and the movements of the joint were quite restored.

Mr. Maunder relates (*Lancet*, 1870, vol. i. p. 192) the case of a lad, aged twenty, in the London Hospital, who slipped and found himself on his back, with the leg bent upon the thigh and unable to be straightened. As he lay upon the bed the limb had a position of genu valgum; he could flex the thigh slightly on the pelvis, and in doing so the knee-joint appeared to be higher up the thigh than usual. However, the condyles of the femur, the head of the tibia, and the patella held their normal relations, and the loss of continuity corresponded to the junction of the condyles with the shaft of the femur. A soft crepitus was easily elicited.

Mr. Davies-Colley had a similar case under his care in Guy's Hospital.

Henry T., aged seven, was admitted on February 14, 1884, having been run over by a cab, and was at first thought to have fractured his right femur. The knee was swollen, and there was mobility apparently three or four inches above the joint, but no crepitus. Ether was given to determine the diagnosis. The condyles could be displaced one inch and a half outwards, and at the inner side of the patella the inner and anterior edge of the lower extremity of the diaphysis could be felt, but no crepitus or even 'rubbing.' The lower epiphysis seemed to rotate round an antero-posterior axis, three to four inches up the femur. Mr. Davies-Colley explained this by the curved surfaces upon which it moved. A 'Croft' combined with a Hodgen's splint was applied. On May 8 the patient was wearing a trough splint to the outer and posterior aspects of the limb. On June 30 he could walk well. There was no lateral movement and no deformity. The injured leg was slightly the longer of the two.

Dr. Henry Wallace (*The Railway Surgeon*, Chicago, 1897, November 2, p. 283, and *Brooklyn Medical Journal*, 1897, vol. xi. p. 686) also reports the following case of separation with displacement outwards of the epiphysis.

The patient (S. O'D.), aged seven years, was brought to St. John's Hospital, Brooklyn, on March 31, 1897. He said that he had caught his left leg between the spokes of a revolving wheel while jumping from the backboard of a wagon. On examination the next morning, the leg was seen to be much swollen and discoloured in the vicinity of the knee-joint, which was partially flexed and in the position of genu valgum. There was decided interference with the circulation, as shown by the colour and temperature of the toes. Ether was administered, and a diagnosis of epiphysial separation easily made. Reduction by traction in the position of complete extension of the leg proved ineffectual. Traction on the semiflexed leg, combined with manipulation, succeeded in completely reducing the displacement. There was no tendency for the fragments to become displaced after they were once completely reduced. The entire limb was then put up in a plaster splint in the position of slight flexion. As soon as the plaster had set, the splint thus formed was divided into anterior and posterior sections. The anterior being removed, the limb was now resting on a perfectly fitting posterior splint. For several days the injured limb was decidedly cold, with marked ecchymosis at the seat of injury. The interference with the circulation was probably due to the hæmatoma which gradually formed in the popliteal space. On the fortieth day the limb was put up in a complete plaster splint. On the fifty-second day all dressings were removed, passive movements were commenced, and the patient allowed full use of the limb. He made an uninterrupted recovery, with the prospect of perfect function of the knee-joint. Measurement showed the injured limb to be three-eighths of an inch longer than the other, the probabilities being, Dr. Wallace thought, that it was originally the longer and that no shortening resulted from the accident. The hæmatoma had been absorbed. A fluoroscopic examination showed good apposition of the fragments and some callus in the popliteal space.

Displacement outwards and forwards.—A case of separation of the lower femoral epiphysis, with displacement laterally and forwards, is described by Mr. Mayo Robson in the *Annals of Surgery,* vol. xvii. part 7, July 1893, p. 4.

J. C., aged fourteen, recovering from a severe compound fracture of the right leg, for which a splint was still being worn, fell, September 6, 1888, while getting about on crutches, with the left leg under the splint of the right. Something in the neighbourhood of the left knee was felt by the patient to have given way. When seen he was sitting on the ground, pale, and complaining of intense pain in the left knee. The left thigh was flexed on the abdomen and the leg flexed on the thigh, the whole limb being rotated outwards. On measuring from the anterior superior spine of the left ilium to the lower border of the patella, there was found to be slight lengthening on the left side. There was considerable swelling of the joint, and immediately above the upper border of the patella there was a depression. No fracture of the shaft of the femur was made out. The relation of the femoral condyles to the head of the tibia was found to be normal, but the whole joint could much more than normally be moved laterally, and especially outwards. This movement was accompanied by a soft cracking sound. The limb was straightened and placed on a back splint, lead lotion being applied to the knee, which was much swollen. September 7 : no pain ; knee still swollen. September 8 : on examination under ether, half an inch of lengthening ; knee

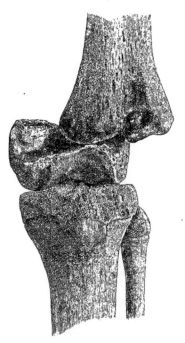

Fig. 236.—DIAGRAM SHOWING DISPLACEMENT DIRECTLY INWARDS AT THE AGE OF SEVENTEEN AND A HALF YEARS. ($\frac{1}{2}$-size)

swollen, distinct soft crepitus felt, and extensive lateral displacement just above the knee-joint. Separation of lower epiphysis of femur, with lateral displacement, diagnosed. Reduction effected, and limb placed on back splint. September 15 : on admission to the Leeds Infirmary Mr. Robson found that there was still a good deal of effusion into the knee-joint, and reapplied the back splint. September 25 : very little swelling ; back splint removed, and limb put up in plaster from ankle to groin. October 20 : plaster removed. On December 15 patient could walk well, and there was no deformity. On May 25, 1893, no sign of the injury could be discovered.

Displacement inwards.—The violence producing this form of displacement is usually of a twisting, or rather lateral, character, or at right angles to the axis of the limb.

The lower end of the shaft is felt and seen on the outer side of the knee.

Mr. T. Bryant records (*Brit. Med. Journal*, May 31, 1884, p. 1044; *Practice of Surgery*, 4th edit. 1884, vol. ii. p. 384, fig. 464A) a case in which the epiphysis had been displaced inwards, and also rotated in the same direction (see figure 237).

William B., aged six, was admitted into Guy's Hospital on August 15, 1882. The patient was riding behind a brougham when he slipped on one side, and his right leg became entangled in the spokes of the wheel. The right leg was considerably deformed, the lower epiphysis was wrenched off, and the diaphysis abducted, with its lower end nearly projecting through the skin on the outer side.

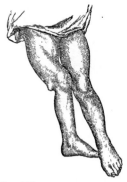

The epiphysis with the tibia was driven upwards and inwards, and the head projected on the inner side. The limb was shortened about two inches, and the foot inverted. There was also considerable effusion into the knee-joint, with much pain. A Macintyre's splint was applied after the parts had been restored to their normal position by manipulation and extension. On September 12 the bones had united and the limb was in good position. On September 20 there was felt to be a little thickening on the outer side of the lower end of the femur, firm union, and a quarter of an inch shortening.

FIG. 237.—DISPLACEMENT INWARDS AND ROTATION OF LOWER EPIPHYSIS OF FEMUR. (T. BRYANT)

On October 19 the patient could walk with the aid of a crutch.

The late Mr. Alfred Poland had under his care at Guy's Hospital in 1868 a girl, Margaret S., aged thirteen years. She had fallen down three or four steps, and afterwards was unable to stand. On admission, June 4, separation of the lower femoral epiphysis was diagnosed, with displacement inwards and a little backwards. The lower end of the diaphysis could be felt beneath the skin just above the anterior, upper, and outer part of the joint. A long outside splint with extension was used, and on July 30 a gum and starch bandage applied. A good recovery resulted.

Dr. F. J. Shepherd, of Montreal, alludes to an instance of this form of displacement in which Macewen's operation had subsequently to be performed for the obliquity and deformity of the lower end of the femur.

In one of Canton's cases the projecting end of the diaphysis could be felt on the outer side of the knee above the patella.

Dr. J. C. Reeve describes and figures (*Cincinnati Lancet and Clinic*, 1878, N.S. vol. i. No. 21, November 23, p. 385) a case under his care.

The patient, a German boy, aged sixteen, became entangled in a belt, and was carried over a shaft between it and the floor above. He received the following injuries—viz. compound fractures of the right forearm and arm, with extensive laceration of the soft parts, and separation of the lower epiphysis of the left femur. Under A.C.E. mixture the arm was amputated at the upper third, and on examining the lower extremity there was found to be extreme deformity; from the knee downwards the limb was rotated inwards, so that the foot and patella looked directly towards the opposite side, the line of fracture was immediately above the knee-joint, the condyloid portion of the femur projected inwards nearly its whole breadth, looking as if the knee might be dislocated, and on the outer side, just below and behind the normal position of the joint, a point of bone protruded through the skin, making a wound about the size of a finger-nail. The limb was restored, as much as possible, to its normal position and shape by applying very considerable force. A long outside splint was applied to the leg and trunk, and extension (of sixteen pounds) to the foot for about ten days, when an immovable bandage of plaster of Paris and thick pasteboard was applied, the knee being kept in a slightly flexed position, as that was considered the best position if ankylosis should occur. This was removed in about two weeks' time, when it was found that the patient had considerable power of flexion of the knee-joint, and ultimately had nearly as good a limb as the other. He could walk well without the use of a stick, and had full use of the joint except for extreme flexion.

Displacement forwards and inwards.—An instance of this displacement inwards and slightly forwards came under the care of Mr. Durham at Guy's Hospital in September 1886. A child, Harry N., aged seven years, was run over by a butcher's cart, and received a simple fracture of the left femur at the upper third, with separation of the lower epiphysis, which was displaced forwards and inwards. There was half an inch shortening. A double interrupted outside splint was applied with extension, and after seven weeks a plaster-of-Paris dressing; there remained a quarter of an inch shortening.

Mr. John Birkett had a like case at Guy's Hospital in April 1867. A girl, Fanny S. W., aged seven, was thrown backwards with her leg doubled up beneath her. The limb was shortened one inch, and there was a prominence in the popliteal space. Under chloroform the end of the femur could be felt at the under and outer side of the space, and a depression of the thigh caused by the backward displacement of the femur could be seen and felt just above the patella. There was some effusion into the joint; a long outside splint was applied, and a month later a starch bandage. At the end of May the patient could walk without the assistance of a crutch, but turned the foot inwards a little in walking.

Projecting diaphysis.—The end of the diaphysis in many of these forms of displacement, especially when it projects forwards, may be felt beneath the skin as a somewhat expanded flattened mass.

The patella is freely movable as a rule, but may be fixed if the displacement of the fragments is very extreme.

Shortening can usually be recognised whenever there is any overlapping of the epiphysis on the diaphysial end, and its amount depends upon the extent and form of the displacement.

It may not be present at the time of the accident, not until the epiphysis has undergone rotation by the action of the gastrocnemius and popliteus muscles. Although the greater part of the former is attached to the diaphysis, yet this muscle is stripped off from the bone with the periosteum.

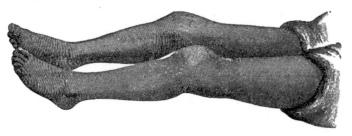

Fig. 238.—DISPLACEMENT FORWARDS AND INWARDS OF LOWER EPIPHYSIS OF FEMUR
(Guy's Hospital Museum.   Mr. Birkett's case)

At Guy's Hospital Mr. Cooper Forster treated a case of this separation in a boy (Chas. R.), aged sixteen, by means of a Hodgen's splint. The injury occurred on November 4, 1878, by the patient's leg being run over by the wheel of a light cart. The separation was accompanied by three-quarters of an inch shortening, and but little bruising. Effusion into the joint subsequently ensued, and the boy left the hospital on December 29 with the movements of the knee fairly free, but with much thickening of the lower end of the femur.

Crepitus is a most variable and inconstant sign.

It may be present in its typical form of a 'muffled character' when the surface of one fragment glides over that of the other, and is often felt in compound separations, the finger being in the wound, during reduction of the displacement.

In the majority of cases the crepitus has not the characteristic smoothness, but partakes more of the nature of crepitus in fracture, from the frequent presence of a more or less extensive fracture of the diaphysis or an intercondyloid fracture.

As in other forms of fracture, the presence of shreds of the periosteum or muscle between the fragments is sufficient to account for the total absence of this sign ; though in this case locking of the fragments may also be partly responsible.

Again, we may find crepitus absent from the loss of contact between the separated surfaces, due to the complete displacement of the epiphysis.

Pain is frequently very severe in some cases, but in a few simple separations it may be almost entirely absent.

In other instances the intense pain may be attributable to the stretching of the popliteal nerves, especially the internal.

Dr. R. H. Harte states, though the author does not know upon what grounds, that ' the pain that is elicited in the production of crepitus is not so severe as would be found in fractures of the femur higher up.'

Mobility.—Abnormal mobility of the epiphysis exists in all cases of this separation, with or without displacement, and consequently is the most trustworthy of all the symptoms.   In fact, the presence of this symptom alone is quite sufficient in youth to suggest an epiphysial separation.

It is felt to be situated above the knee-joint.   It may be slight in the antero-posterior or lateral direction, or may be marked, so that the limb can be carried into any position.   This is the case when the two separated surfaces glide one over the other when they are not completely displaced apart.   If complete displacement of the epiphysis has taken place, if the fragments are. locked in one another, or if the epiphysis is much rotated, mobility is but little marked.   Free lateral movement occurring at the epiphysial line, without marked crepitus, should at once suggest the nature of the injury.   At a superficial examination it might from the mobility appear that the knee-joint was higher than normal.   In this connection it should be borne in mind that the line of epiphysis slopes slightly downwards and backwards.

If a separation of one condyle with intercondyloid fracture has occurred, the looseness will be confined to that condyle.

The size of the lower fragment and the exact distance of the seat of mobility from the lower edge of each condyle will materially assist in forming a correct diagnosis.   They both differ according to the age of the patient (see under ANATOMY).

Dr. R. H. Harte gives (*Trans. Amer. Surg. Association*, Philadelphia 1895, vol. xiii. p. 398) the following instance in which lateral mobility was a notable feature.

Thomas M., aged eighteen years, was admitted to the Episcopal Hospital, June 8, 1894. While he was riding in a freight car, and lying on his back, with his leg extended out of the car door, the leg came in contact with a telegraph pole, bending it round the edge of the door laterally.   On admission there was effusion about the knee, and marked softening of the vastus internus muscle. Crepitus and deformity could be elicited by moving the knee with the condyles and diaphysis of the femur in opposite directions. When the deformity was reduced there was little or no shortening. Extension with bran-bags and long lateral splints, and an ice-cap over the knee, were used. The effusion gradually subsided, but the softening over the internal condyle was persistent for nearly a month. The patient was discharged cured August 14, 1894, with fair motion in the knee-joint.

A more severe injury was recently diagnosed by Dr. F. W. Schmidt (*The Railway Surgeon*, Chicago, U.S.A., vol. iv. June 29, 1897, p. 54) as an example of separation of the lower epiphysis of the femur, with intercondyloid fracture from the free mobility and separation of one condyle from the other. It is interesting to note in this case that skiagraphs were taken one year after the accident, and that by observing them closely the lines of fracture could be noted. The patient, male, aged fifteen years, slim and anæmic, a machinist, while crossing a slippery floor, fell, striking his knee and doubling up his limb, so that the weight of the entire body bore down upon it. The limb had been placed on a double-inclined splint, and when Dr. Schmidt saw him four hours afterwards the knee was so œdematous that he decided not to remove the splint until the following day. The limb was then gently extended, and a long sandbag placed on each side of it, with cooling applications to the joint. In this position it was left until the third day, when it was found that the swelling had sufficiently subsided to permit a thorough examination under an anæsthetic. The condyles could be freely moved and separated from each other, the diagnosis being made of intercondyloid fracture with separation of the lower epiphysis. A plaster-of-Paris dressing from the heel to the hip was then applied. Counter-extension had to be discontinued after several hours, owing to the intense pain which it caused. As on the following day the patient became very feverish and delirious, and complained of great pain about the joint, a fenestrum was made into the dressing and several bluish black spots were discovered. The fenestrum afforded immediate relief. Five weeks after the accident the dressing was removed, and passive motion attempted under an anæsthetic. It was found that very extensive adhesions had formed, and considerable force had to be used in flexing the limb. The dressing was reapplied loosely, and daily massage employed. A few days later the dressing was finally removed, and the patient commenced to employ passive motion himself. He was placed on crutches, and in the course of four months could walk with a support; and he was subsequently able to walk long distances after his day's work. There was ultimately one inch shortening and only partial ankylosis, but the lower fragment seemed to be rotated posteriorly.

Dr. Schmidt thought that, considering the fact that amputation had been proposed before he saw the case, the patient had every reason to be grateful for this apparently poor result.

Detachment of the periosteum.—Allusion has already been made to the fact that detachment of the periosteum probably occurs in all cases of separation of the epiphysis, however simple they may be. Although the stripping up of this membrane may be at first only to a slight extent, subsequent hæmorrhage beneath it, either from the primary injury or from undue manipulation, may greatly increase its limits.

The periosteum was completely stripped from the diaphysial end in McBurney's case, although the injury was a simple one..

This stripping of the periosteum is, even in simple cases, followed by much thickening of the lower end of the femur during the process of union.

The stripped-up periosteum remains mostly continuous with the epiphysis ; this is an important fact, especially as regards treatment of the displacement. The presence of a thick band between the fragments adds very greatly to the difficulties of reduction.

It is undoubtedly true that extensive periosteal detachment will in great measure be responsible for suppurative periostitis and suppuration, which sometimes occur even in simple cases. Sub-periosteal suppuration may extend the denudation of bone, and lead to necrosis of the bone, small though it often is, through failure of nutrition.

COMPLICATIONS.   **Pressure on vessels.**—When the lower end of the diaphysis projects into the popliteal space, it generally presses upon the popliteal vessels, interferes with the circulation of the limb, and later produces great œdema or gangrene of the leg.

If to this important sign of compression of the vessels we add shortening, and the deformity arising either from the displacement of the epiphysis on to the front of the diaphysis or from its partial overlapping and the presence of the diaphysis in the popliteal space, we find a group of symptoms perfectly *characteristic* of this form of separation.

The displacement of the epiphysis backwards, although it does not occur usually to a very great extent, may possibly cause, in some cases, pressure upon the vessels. The popliteal vessels commonly escape by reason of the retention of their normal relation with the condyloid notch, and their consequent protection from pressure This will not, however, be the case if the epiphysis has rotated.

In McGill's case the vessels, although much displaced and pressed upon by the diaphysis, were not occluded ; for the popliteal vessels were displaced backwards, and could be felt beating under the skin, but pulsation in the posterior tibial and dorsalis pedis arteries was unimpaired.

In J. Hutchinson, jun.'s, case of a boy, aged twelve, the pressure of the diaphysis upon the popliteal artery almost stopped the pulse. Reduction was effected under an anæsthetic, and perfect recovery ensued.

Mr. Bryant had under his care at Guy's Hospital (November 1876) the case of a boy, Thomas C., aged seventeen, in which œdema of the leg indicated a certain amount of pressure on the popliteal vessels. The accident happened by the boy's leg being caught in the wheels of some machinery and violently twisted. There was also effusion into the knee-joint. He was treated by means of a Hodgen's splint, and he left the hospital at the end of six weeks with limited movement in the knee-joint.

In June 1884 Mr. Waren Tay mentioned to the author a case (at that time in the London Hospital) of separation of the lower epiphysis of the femur, with pressure on the popliteal artery.

The following case came under the care of Mr. Mayo Robson at the Leeds Infirmary in December 1885 (*Annals of Surgery*, St. Louis, vol. xi. 1889, p. 107).

A labourer (F. V.), aged sixteen, was admitted on account of injuries produced by an unshod horse, which had kicked him above the outer side of the left knee-joint two days previously. He fell down, and was unable to rise. He was seen by a surgeon, who applied evaporating lotions and sandbags. On admission there was considerable swelling, with fluctuation round the knee. The leg and foot were enormously swollen, due to œdema and venous congestion ; the foot was everted, and the leg rotated outwards. No pulsation could be felt in either the anterior or posterior tibial arteries, the circulation being arrested by the sharp edge of the lower end of the diaphysis, which was pressing on the popliteal vessels and making the skin bulge in the popliteal space. The leg and foot were quite numb, but the patient suffered intense pain when movement was attempted. The injured joint was in a state of semiflexion, and extension could only be effected at the expense of great pain. A marked depression existed above the patella, beneath which could be felt a movable mass with rounded edges. The heads of the tibia and fibula appeared to be normal. The limb was shortened to the extent of about one inch and a quarter. A diagnosis of epiphysial separation being made, the patient was placed under ether ; when the limb was fully flexed on the thigh by an assistant, another assistant placed his locked hands round the femur, drawing it forwards. The epiphysis was then forced into position and the leg extended. After two attempts the length of the leg was fully restored, and the parts bore a proper relation to one another. A MacIntyre's splint was adjusted, and evaporating lotions applied. Pulsation at once returned in the tibial vessels, the engorged veins emptied themselves, and normal sensation was restored to the limb within a few hours. The swelling of the leg gradually subsided. Nine days later a double-inclined plane was substituted for the MacIntyre's splint, and twenty days after this a Liston's long splint, there being no tendency to displacement, and the effusion into the knee-joint having almost disappeared. A fortnight later the splint was removed, there being firm union. At the end of February the patient could raise the limb without pain, and a Thomas's knee splint was applied. This he left off a month later, and was allowed to use the limb. When seen two months afterwards the joint was capable of being fully flexed, there was no deformity, and the left leg was as useful as the right.

Another case of separation of the lower femoral epiphysis, with displacement upon the front of the femur and pressure upon the popliteal vessels, is recorded by Mr. Mayo Robson (*Annals of Surgery*, Philadelphia and London, vol. xvii. Part 7, July 1893, p. 2).

J. W. M., aged fifteen, was admitted to the Leeds General Infirmary, December 11, 1891. The same morning the patient had been struck over the lower part of the left thigh by a metal roller, six feet long and five inches in diameter, weighing several stone; he at once lost all use of the limb. On admission a few hours later there was very great swelling of the left knee, with evident displacement forwards of the lower extremity of the femur, and projection backwards into the popliteal space of the lower end of the upper fragment. The lower segment could be felt riding altogether in front of the upper portion, with its flat surface applied to the front of the lower end of the femur. The lower end of the upper fragment evidently compressed the vessels and arrested the circulation in the leg, which was livid, cold, and swollen. There was an inch and a half of shortening. The head of the tibia and the patella were carried forward with the condyles of the femur. No crepitus was obtainable.

Ether having been administered and the limb fully flexed, an assistant locked his hands behind the femur and exerted traction upwards, and another, grasping the foot, drew the leg downwards. Mr. Robson was then able to manipulate the epiphysis, which slipped into position with a distinct sound. The length of the limb was then found to be normal, and the circulation was immediately resumed in the leg and foot. The limb was put up in a suspended MacIntyre's splint. On January 18, 1892, the limb was taken off the splint, and the bone found to be in very good position and firmly united. Plaster of Paris was applied to fix the joint and removed at the end of three weeks, when gentle massage was employed. January 29, 1892, the patient walked to the infirmary, and there was neither deformity, shortening, nor impairment of use in the limb. On May 5, 1893, no sign of the injury could be made out.

Mr. Mayo Robson alludes (*Annals of Surgery*, Philadelphia, vol. xvii. Part 7, July 1893, p. 5) to a similar case, in which reduction was successful and a useful limb resulted. The displacement of the epiphysis forwards was incomplete.

Dr. R. H. Harte regarded the following case under his care as an epiphysial fracture, its termination being similar to that of cases quoted by Wheelhouse and others.

A lad, with ankylosis of the knee-joint and marked flexion, fell, producing a fracture above the condyles. The limb was treated in the extended position, rotating the detached lower fragment. A fatal termination ensued in the second week, from hæmorrhage due to pressure on the popliteal vessels. The diagnosis was not verified by an autopsy.

Provided reduction can be effected, and other circumstances are favourable, even laceration of the popliteal artery does not necessarily demand amputation.

Pressure on nerves.—In backward displacement of the diaphysis the internal popliteal nerve is the one most likely to be pressed upon, as in Mayo Robson's case.

DIFFERENTIAL DIAGNOSIS. Dislocation of the knee-joint.—Dr. R. H. Harte says: 'In two of my own cases the idea of dislocation would naturally be suggested by the distortion of the limb. In fact, the displacement was so like what would be expected in lateral luxation that it took some minutes to convince my house surgeon to the contrary.'

Mr. C. Holthouse mentions (Holmes, *System of Surgery*, 2nd edit. vol. ii. 1870, p. 915) the following case in discussing the diagnosis of dislocations of the knee.

'A little boy, four years of age, was riding behind a cart, when his left leg got between the spokes of the wheel, and he was brought into Westminster Hospital with an apparent dislocation of the tibia inwards. With very slight extension of the limb, the deformity was removed and distinct crepitus elicited; the existence of this sign, then, is conclusive as to the nature of the injury, viz. separation of the lower epiphysis of the femur.'

The only difficulty in distinguishing between dislocation of the knee and separation can arise when displacement has occurred. The deformity has been described in many such cases as resembling a dislocation of the knee backwards and outwards, or directly inwards. In the absence of any very great swelling about the knee, a careful examination of the deformity, the different bony prominences of the tibia, femur, and patella, the more or less normal motion in the joint, and abnormal mobility corresponding to the epiphysis, should be sufficient to distinguish it from dislocation. Dislocation, besides being of so rare occurrence in young subjects, is accompanied by fixation of the limb at the knee-joint, so that the movements of flexion and extension on the thigh are very restricted. Crepitus is so often absent that it cannot be relied upon.

The swelling about the knee occurs sometimes so rapidly and to such an extent that some weeks have elapsed before an exact diagnosis has been made, the osseous projections being entirely obscured.

In compound epiphysial separations such a mistake could scarcely occur, on account of the character and shape of the protruding bone ; yet in one case (Richet's) the diaphysial end, covered with epiphysial cartilage, protruded through a large wound on the outer aspect of the thigh and gave the appearance at first sight of a dislocation.

In the more simple cases of displacement forwards of the epiphysis there can be but little difficulty of diagnosis from (1) the shortening of the limb, (2) the projection of the end of the diaphysis in the popliteal space, and (3) the presence of the epiphysis in front of the femur—to which may be added the signs of pressure upon the popliteal vessels.

Supra-condyloid fracture.—Besides being exceedingly rare in children, the end of the upper fragment is more pointed and oblique than in separation, and is more distant from the articulation. The character of the crepitus cannot be relied upon on account of the frequency with which the separation of this epiphysis is accompanied by a certain amount of fracture of the shaft. In this case the separation will very closely simulate a fracture.

The characteristic soft crepitus, if present, is pathognomonic of separation.

Separations, except the more simple cases, are much more difficult to reduce and maintain in position than similar fractures about the same situation.

In transverse fracture of the lower end of the femur it is often the lower fragment drawn backwards by the gastrocnemius which presses upon the vessels, and not the lower end of the diaphysis, as in epiphysial separation. This is, however, only true in instances of great displacement ; in the more simple cases, where the lower fragment or epiphysis is commencing to rotate, its posterior edge is the first to project into the popliteal space.

Packard writes : ' The age of the patient and the characters of the fracture, its want of obliquity, its nearness to the joint, and the smoothness of the fragments, will be the chief points to be relied upon in distinguishing this lesion from ordinary supra-condyloid fracture.'

In cases of *old separations* in which a considerable time has elapsed after the occurrence of the injury, difficulty may at first sight be experienced, as in the case of old separations of the epiphysial head of the femur, in distinguishing it from distortions of the joint from chronic disease, especially those of a tuberculous nature.

TREATMENT.—There is no question of the gravity of the injury, says Dr. R. H. Harte, as nearly half of sixty cases terminated in amputation.

Cases of simple separation without displacement or complication are best treated by immediately placing the knee in the position of slight flexion. A MacIntyre's splint or a Croft's lateral plaster-of-Paris splint should be applied to keep the fragments at rest, and prevent any subsequent displacement of the epiphysis by the action of the gastrocnemius and other muscles. The plaster splint has this advantage, that it allows inspection from time to time without disturbing the fragments.

Where displacement has occurred from rotation of the epiphysis on its transverse axis, and reduction has · been effected under an anæsthetic (which procedure might be facilitated by division of the tendo Achillis), the same treatment in the flexed position on an inclined plane or otherwise is essential.

In some cases reduction has apparently been effected after considerable difficulty by pushing the diaphysis forwards, or by traction of the leg. in the flexed position when the epiphysis is in front of the femur.

In all cases, under an anæsthetic, the leg and epiphysis should be gently pressed in the opposite direction to which it has been

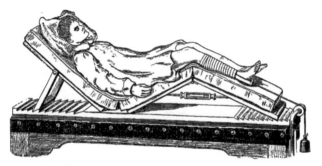

Fig. 239.—DOUBLE-INCLINED PLANE WITH EXTENSION ON LEG

displaced, combined with gentle manipulation of the end of the diaphysis.

Under ether Mr. McGill easily reduced the deformity in his patient by forcibly flexing the leg until the heel touched the buttock.

In Dr. R. H. Harte's two simple cases the deformity was corrected by extension, with the leg in the extended position.

The deformity does not readily recur in the more simple cases, when the reduction has been easily and completely effected and a suitable splint applied.

In simple displacement outwards or inwards, reduction and the application of a plaster dressing, with or without an outside or inside splint, are quite effectual, especially if they are a little bent, so that the knee may be maintained in the slightly flexed position.

Mr. Hutchinson (*London Hospital Reports*, vol. ii. p. 347, 1865), in a note on the best position of the limb in cases of this separation, advocates this plan of treatment by flexion.

Some prefer the extended position, or the use of a weight combined with Liston's long splint.

Agnew (*Surgery*, vol. i. 1878, p. 969) recommends that the limb should be placed in the extended position, and the ham well supported by a compress of oakum, covered with an immovable dressing, but admits that this position may be changed for the semiflexed one should there be any difficulty in properly adjusting the fragments. .

Among the Guy's Hospital cases the author finds the case of a boy (C. M.), aged four years, who had his right femur fractured in its upper third, with separation of its lower epiphysis. The patient was under the care of Mr. Cooper Forster in 1874, and was treated with a long outside splint and extension by weights to the foot. Forty-one days after the accident there was said to be only a quarter of an inch shortening, and on his discharge nine days later the patient was commencing to walk.

In Elsner's case, there being no displacement, the treatment adopted was a long Liston's splint. This was followed at the end of a fortnight by half an inch shortening. A MacIntyre's splint was then applied. A straight splint may, therefore, be even prejudicial.

Some writers recommend the same mode of treatment as in supra-condyloid fracture—viz. by suspension in Hodgen's splint, Smith's anterior splint, or plaster-of-Paris dressing. If plaster of Paris is applied, lateral pieces should be used in the slightly flexed position as just mentioned. Dr. R. H. Harte knew of a case in which a fixed plaster-of-Paris dressing had been employed after reduction, but had to be removed owing to pressure, as it caused gangrene of two of the toes.

Mr. Davies-Colley had under his care at Guy's Hospital a boy (Geo. B.), aged nine, who was admitted on March 11, 1885. His right knee had been struck by timber falling from a passing cart.

The knee was slightly flexed and slightly displaced backwards. There was also some crepitus of a blunted wooden character, and free lateral passive movement, but no shortening. Under ether, when the knee was extended and the tibia displaced outwards through 50°, a depression could be felt above the internal condyle, bounded below by a distinct ridge, which disappeared entirely on adducting the tibia to its proper position. A 'Croft' and straight trough splint were applied, the latter composed of straight outside and back pieces joined together at a right angle. On March 23 there was still some abduction; the trough splint was therefore alone applied. On June 11 the legs were both straight and equal in length, and without deformity.

Packard advocates the straight position as the one in which the limb should be placed if an effort is to be made to save it; he says: 'Something must probably depend upon the chances for a movable knee; if this is out of the question, there can be no doubt that the straight position is the best. And where the epiphysial fragment is rotated so that the condyles look upwards—the patient lying on his back (and this rotation in my case was very obstinate), flexion of

the knee would, of course, carry the head of the tibia further away
from the articular surface of the condyles, unless the rotation is
overcome, and the condyles well brought down into place. But if
the natural relations of the parts can be restored, it seems to me
that, after a few days, flexion may be gently and cautiously tried,
and gradually increased, with passive movements, so as to prevent
the necessity for the breaking up of adhesions at a later date. For
the retention of the parts in shape, a "back splint" has been
generally employed, but I should prefer the application of sheet zinc
or of binder's board moulded along the whole length of the outer
and inner sides of the limb, well lined, and held in place by a very
accurately laid bandage. When flexion is to be made, fresh splints
with suitable angles should, of course, be prepared. Suspension
might very well be employed, and may add to the comfort of the
patient.'

The action of the gastrocnemius upon the epiphysis is so constant
that it is difficult to see how proper coaptation of the separated
surfaces can be effected and maintained without flexion of the limb.

Mr. Hutchinson says (*Archives of Surgery*, January 1893):
'It may be quite impossible to alter the position of the epiphysis;
the best chance of doing so will be by first effecting reduction, with
the knee bent at right angles, and then partially straightening the
limb. The treatment of such cases is, however, extremely difficult
and unsatisfactory.'

Reduction of the displaced epiphysis must be *immediately and
completely* effected, and the limb put up in the flexed position.
Any great eversion or inversion of the leg or foot should be carefully
guarded against by means of a foot piece.

Mr. Robson thinks that reduction under ether would be the best
plan to try at first; and this, he believes, will be certainly facilitated
by division of the tendo Achillis. After reduction he recommends
either the long splint, with weight and pulley, or the double-inclined
plane.

Whatever form of splint be employed, it should be kept on for
three or four weeks. The foot and toes should be carefully watched,
especially during the first few days, for any discoloration indicating
obstruction of the circulation or commencing gangrene.

Effusion into the knee and other inflammatory action should be
dealt with by evaporating lotions, ice-bag, &c.

Passive movement may be commenced at the end of four weeks
in simple cases. It should at first be of the most gentle character.
The ultimate mobility of the knee-joint in the more simple cases
should be unimpaired.

In displacements of the epiphysis, after firm consolidation has
taken place, and there is little or no deformity remaining, it will
likewise be found necessary to gently manipulate the joint should
any stiffness remain.

These attempts should be made with or without an anæsthetic, and accomplished with the greatest caution. Even as early as the fifth or sixth week gentle daily movements of the knee may be carried out in these instances. The following statistics of simple separations of the lower epiphysis of the femur can be considered as anything but a credit to surgery in the past. They prove conclusively that operative measures should be undertaken much more frequently than has been the case hitherto.

'Out of twenty-eight cases (uncomplicated by wound) recorded by Hutchinson junior, sixteen were got into good position, and recovered with very useful and perfect limbs; whilst of the remaining twelve in which perfect replacement was not obtained, six were followed by sloughing or suppuration. In four of these amputation had to be performed, one recovered after excision of the knee, and one after resection of the diaphysial end. In one case a popliteal aneurism formed twenty years after, and led to amputation. The remaining cases recovered with more or less useful limbs, the displacement persisting.'

Among the author's collection of sixty-two cases of separation which were not complicated by a wound the three cases treated by open incision mentioned below may be excluded from the following analysis. Of the fifty-nine cases, in twenty-six the fragments were able to be replaced in good position, and the patients regained most serviceable limbs without deformity. In one instance, after satisfactory replacement, the patient died from shock, the result of other injuries. Of the remaining thirty-two cases, recovery took place in fourteen with a somewhat distorted though useful joint from more or less persistent displacement of one or other fragment; and one recovered after excision of the epiphysis. In two cases primary amputation was performed, one terminating in recovery, the other in death from pyæmia due to other severe injuries. In one case death resulted from pyæmia, but it was not stated whether amputation was performed, and in another death ensued from exhaustion after sloughing and suppuration. In thirteen cases secondary amputation was performed for sloughing, ulceration, suppuration, gangrene, injury to nerves, aneurism, &c.; of these, four ended in death, three from pyæmia and one from tetanus. In eight cases recovery took place after amputation, one of them being a case in which excision of the knee had been previously performed, and in one case the result was not stated.

Replacement by open incision.—In cases uncomplicated with a wound operative interference may be necessary, and the form the operation should take will depend on the relative position of the separated surfaces and on the condition of the joint and surrounding soft parts.

In all displacements, on account of the danger to the popliteal vessels, the precise condition of the latter must be ascertained;

reduction may be effected, even where pressure exists upon these vessels, and recovery may ensue.

In other cases of simple separation, where, from the locking of the fragments or the interposition between them of a piece of periosteum or muscle, reduction appears to be impossible even after the administration of an anæsthetic, or where retention of the fragments in their normal position is unattainable, an open operation should be undertaken and the displaced fragments completely and at once reduced. An incision being made four inches in length, down to the bone, along the outer border of the tendon of the biceps, under strict antiseptic precautions, the epiphysial fragment or fragments should be reduced, and fixed in position on the diaphysis by means of pegs or sutures. Removal of a portion of the diaphysial end may be required in addition, and the epiphysis and diaphysis secured in position in the same way by wire or other sutures. The limb should be afterwards put up on a double-inclined plane after careful irrigation of the wound with perchloride of mercury or some other antiseptic solution and closure of the wound.

If the epiphysis be allowed to remain in its displaced position, sloughing of the skin—rendering the injury a compound one—suppuration, gangrene, or subsequent great deformity may result. The truth of this statement and the dangers of imperfect reduction are amply verified by the statistics just quoted of cases of separation uncomplicated by a wound.

As late as the twenty-first day after the accident an open operation has been successfully carried out for simple separation. It must be stated, however, that in the following case related by F. W. Elsner (*Australasian Med. Gazette*, July 20, 1895, p. 265) the diagnosis was not exactly made out before incision, and repeated attempts at reduction had been ineffectual.

A little boy (B. M.), aged thirteen, was admitted to the Tamworth Hospital on October 1, 1893, having been kicked by a horse just above the knee on the outer side. On admission the right leg was drawn up on the inner side of the shaft of the femur, the end of which protruded externally as if about to perforate the skin ; the tibia, fibula, and patella were all intact, but pulled together upwards and inwards by the powerful muscles of the thigh. The leg, with the femoral parts attached, was freely movable in all directions, but there was no crepitus. There was enormous swelling, effusion, and great ecchymosis from hæmorrhage around the femoral protuberance. A lengthy and unsuccessful attempt was made under chloroform to reduce the displacement, the shortening recurring to the amount of several inches. The leg was then put up in a long Liston's splint, with weight at the foot and counter-extension. A week or so later another attempt was made at reduction under chloroform, the tendo Achillis being divided, and the limb placed on a MacIntyre's splint. Very little improvement having been obtained—the femoral projection still threatening to perforate the skin, while the diagnosis was not exact—an incision was made over the protruding bone. It was found that the condylar epiphysis of the femur had become detached, but was securely attached to the head of the tibia, whilst the protruding part was the end of the femur, rough and bare, but unlike an ordinary fractured surface. Even with the fracture exposed it was impossible to bring the surfaces into apposition ; this was only effected after two inches of the femur in successive discs had been removed with a Butcher's saw. The limb after dressing was placed on a back splint with foot-piece. Union took place rapidly, and the boy was soon able to get about without inconvenience in a plaster-of-Paris splint, putting his foot to the ground. On his discharge, February 2, 1894, there was a perfect limb and a fractional shortening. The report on January 24, 1895, was ' that he walked without a limp, but a little lameness could be noticed when he ran.' The limb developed well.

Walther has recently (*Rev. de Chir.* May 1895) carried out most successfully this treatment by suture in the case of an adult. It was a severe injury to the knee, in which the lower end of the femur was broken into three fragments, and the tibia with the internal condyle was displaced backwards. Functionally the result was perfect.

Dr. Charles McBurney, of New York, reports (*Annals of Surgery*, vol. xxiii. No. 5, May 1896, p. 506) two cases which possessed some precisely similar characters. The deformity was exactly the same, and in both all attempts at reduction by simple manipulation were impossible. After the operations no deformity was left, and in one there was only very slight limitation to flexion.

CASE I.—David M., nine years of age, came under his care at the Roosevelt Hospital on November 16, 1895. The boy had fallen from a height, alighting upon the feet, and had injured the left limb near the knee. The case was brought to his notice on the twentieth day after the injury. A considerable anterior displacement of the leg forward at or about the knee-joint was noted. Externally at the extreme lower end of the shaft of the left femur a sharp angular projection of bone could be felt. This was clearly continuous with the shaft. Anterior to this there was a considerably firm tumour elevating the soft parts over the point of the femur and practically continuous with the leg. Holding the tumour with one hand and the femur with the other, false motion could be made between the two without crepitus. Motion of the tibia—that is, flexion and extension —was normal in quality and took place between the tumour and tibia. The diagnosis of separation of the lower epiphysis of the femur was deemed probable, and with the aid of anæsthesia attempts at reduction were made. Extension in the straight and flexed positions, over-extension with pressure from above upon the epiphysis, and lateral angular motions were all made without success. Partial reduction without crepitus was accomplished, but redisplacement immediately took place. An incision was then made about five inches long, beginning on the outer side of the limb just below the projecting angle of the lower end of the shaft. The incision passed vertically upwards. The soft parts were divided down to the bone, and the lower end of the shaft was exposed. It was quite bare, the periosteum having been stripped up from its face for several inches. When the soft parts were still more freely lifted the whole lower end of the diaphysis could be seen, and the characteristic appearance when separation through a conjugal cartilage has taken place was plainly recognised. The epiphysis could now be lifted on the fingers. A superior, somewhat excavated, quite smooth surface could be felt across its whole width. The epiphysis lay quite anterior to the lower end of the diaphysis, markedly to the inner side, thus accounting for the angular projection of bone externally already mentioned. Even now there was difficulty in making reduction, which was only successful with powerful extension, and at the same time, with the aid of a periosteal elevator, the posterior lip of the epiphysis was pushed over the anterior edge of the shaft.

After the reduction no difficulty existed in maintaining the epiphysis in place when the leg was partially flexed. Full extension reproduced the deformity. Partial flexion was therefore maintained, the wound closed, and the limb put up in plaster of Paris. No fever or other interruption to wound-healing occurred, and the position remained good.

CASE II.—Thomas B., five years of age, received an injury to the region of the right knee, having been run over by a vehicle on December 16, 1895. He was brought to the Roosevelt Hospital on the same day. The knee was swollen, very tender to touch, and the leg partly flexed. No voluntary movement of extension could be made. The general appearance of the limb was such as would be produced by an anterior dislocation of the leg. Externally, and just above the position of the external condyle, was a prominent angular point of bone which was continuous with the shaft. In front of this, and somewhat to the inner side, was a movable tumour, evidently consisting of the articular end of the femur. This could be moved laterally without crepitus. On this tumour the leg could be partly flexed and extended. The ligamentum patellæ was markedly tense. Efforts at reduction of the displacement, similar to those made use of in the preceding case, were carefully made. That is to say, extension in the straight and flexed positions, over-extension with pressure from above upon the epiphysis and lateral angular movements with extension and pressure, were all carefully practised and all failed. An operation, precisely similar to that done in the first case, was then at once performed, and reduction was readily accomplished. After reduction only soft cartilaginous crepitus could be produced by motion of the lower upon the upper fragment. The wound was then closed with catgut stitches and drainage, and the limb immobilised in a slightly flexed position by means of plaster of Paris. Wound-healing was entirely perfect, and took place under the primary dressing. The position and the general condition of the limb were most satisfactory.

The report on April 1, 1896, states that in the younger of the two patients the result was perfect in every particular; while in the other case, which first came under observation twenty days after the injury, a minute necrosis of skin and bone at the extreme outer

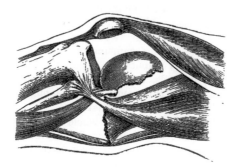

Fig. 240.—Diagram of complete displacement forwards of epiphysis and pressure upon popliteal vessels

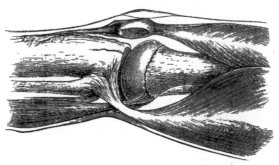

Fig. 241.—Diagram; the same after reduction

angle of the diaphysis took place. In other respects the result was perfect, excepting that voluntary flexion was limited just after the right angle is passed.

Such operative interference as above described is therefore imperative whenever there is evidence, by absence of pulsation of the vessels below, of pressure by one or other fragment on the vessels and nerves; for, if the fragments are not reduced, gangrene of the foot and leg may result, even when at first the vessels are not severely pressed upon, or traumatic aneurism may develop later on, while many examples afford abundant proof that, under favourable circumstances, the limb can be saved, and that with but little detriment to the powers of locomotion. The removal of a part or even the whole of the diaphysial end does not produce so much decrease in length of the femur as might be supposed, provided that of course the epiphysial cartilage remains adherent to the epiphysis.

Packard, Mayo Robson, and others suggest division of the two heads of the gastrocnemius muscle when difficulty is experienced in reducing the epiphysis, due to the contraction of the heads of this muscle, causing its rotation, either through the wound if this be very large, or, if not, by a subcutaneous incision on either side.

Excision of epiphysis.—Mr. Canton (*loc. cit. supra*) successfully excised the whole epiphysis in two cases of simple separation— in one after a few days for suppuration and sloughing; in the other it was followed by amputation.

Mr. Atkinson, of Leeds, attempted in one case (*loc. cit. supra*) to excise the epiphysis for threatened gangrene, but without success, and was compelled to resort to amputation.

Resection of the epiphysis or the whole knee-joint is not to be recommended. It is only in exceptionally unfavourable cases as an alternative to amputation that it may have to be considered. Amputation will be the safer course to pursue.

Massage is a useful adjunct to after-treatment. A light millboard or other moulded light splint may be applied during the intervals, especially when the patient first gets about on crutches.

COMPOUND SEPARATION.—If the epiphysial separation is complicated with a wound of the soft parts, but without laceration of the vessels or other serious complication, *reduction* must always be effected, and an attempt made to save the limb. The wound, or even the periosteal rent, should be enlarged, and the diaphysial end freed from dirt, all soiled portions removed with a stout knife, and the recesses of the wound thoroughly cleansed with antiseptic solution. By the use of antiseptic dressings and a carefully moulded apparatus, or MacIntyre's splint, the limb should be maintained in the best possible position.

Resection of the diaphysial end is further necessary in cases where the protruded diaphysis is irreducible, or where it is locked in the epiphysis. Perfect drainage of the wound should also be carefully attended to.

Delens thinks that the limits of the periosteal detachment should generally indicate the point where the diaphysis should be divided, and that even when the denudation of the bone is high up, resection may be effected up to this point, and not limited to the terminal part of the shaft. This seems to be an unnecessary procedure, for the periosteum will rapidly again become adherent to the shaft, and the nutrition of the bone will not be interfered with to any extent. It would also entail much shortening of the bone subsequently.

No more of the diaphysis should be removed than is necessary for reduction, unless it be soiled by dirt, &c. If the joint has been opened, this as well as the wound should be rendered thoroughly aseptic.

Three-quarters of an inch of the diaphysis was removed in Owing's case, and the bone replaced; good firm union resulted at the end of three months.

Whatever the precise lesions may be, they are sure to be pretty extensive. Diffuse suppuration and septic infection must be carefully guarded against by the complete and thorough disinfection of the wound and removal of all soiled portions of the bones by means of a chisel or strong knife. The author is confident that inability or neglect to render the wound absolutely aseptic satisfactorily explains the unfavourable termination of a great number of cases which have occurred in the past; and not a few of those at the present day. Amputation has been, and is still, far too frequently recorded.

It must be remembered however that owing to the age of these patients the employment of powerful antiseptics is not always without danger, and constitutes in compound separations, as in Reverdin's case, a great difficulty. In this instance the subsequent gangrene was thought to be due, in part at least, to the action of the carbolic acid upon the exposed popliteal nerves.

The increase in length of the femur, although affected by resection of the diaphysial end, is not arrested. Delens's and other cases are examples of this.

In the cases collected by Reverdin, in only two instances was the attempt to save the limb successful after compound separation.

In the author's own collection of fifty cases of compound separation, in seven the diaphysis was resected and reduction effected, the patient regaining a very serviceable joint and limb. In nine others, reduction was effected without resection; of these five recovered with an equally satisfactory result, while death resulted in four, one from pyæmia and three from shock. In one of the last-mentioned amputation had been refused by the parents. In one instance the whole epiphysis and joint were excised without loss of life. Of the remaining thirty-three compound separations, in twenty-one cases primary, and in twelve secondary, amputation was performed.

Packard found that 'reduction was successfully accomplished in fourteen cases except in one instance (Richet's), in which the patient died of purulent infection on the fifteenth day. One boy recovered with a stiff knee; two had good motion; of seven it is merely said that they did well, or had useful limbs, while in two it is only stated that consolidation occurred.'

Mr. W. Philpot Brookes, of Cheltenham, recorded (*London Medical Gazette*, N.S. vol. iv. 1847, p. 56) a case of compound fracture of the external condyle, with rupture of the capsular ligament, followed by recovery without amputation. It was probably an instance of compound separation of the femoral epiphysis combined with an intercondyloid fracture, and has been already alluded to on page 723.

Henry T., aged eleven and a half years, while getting up behind a carriage, had his left leg caught in the spokes of the hind wheel. He was admitted into hospital June 28, 1845. On examination there was found a compound fracture of the thigh extending into the popliteal space, and the lower end of the femur protruded. The capsular ligament of the knee-joint was ruptured, and there was an oblique fracture through the external condyle of the femur. There was also a transverse fracture above the articulation, but the vessels were intact. Two days later the finger could be passed between the external condyle of the femur and the head of the tibia, through the wound. Preservation of the limb was attempted, with the result that at the end of a month the wound was almost healed. Two months later a small piece (one inch long) of necrosed bone came away. When seen, December 1846, he had very good motion of the joint, so that he could flex the leg completely on the thigh, and could walk well with the aid of a stick, bearing the whole weight of the body on the injured limb.

A similar case with almost as extensive lesions is described in Sir Astley Cooper's work on Fractures. A child, Michael D——, was admitted into St. Thomas's Hospital, under the care of Mr. Travers, on September 17, 1816, his leg having been entangled in the wheel of a carriage in motion. There was a transverse fracture of the lower end of the femur above the joint, complicated with a fracture extending in the direction of the axis of the bone. There was considerable displacement of the fragments, and a small wound opposite the external condyle. The external condyle was movable, and displaced as if by twisting of the limb inwards. The limb was placed in a fracture-box in a semiflexed position.

The skin over the external condyle ulcerated, exposing its articular surface. Two months later the protruded fractured surface of the femur— viz. the external condyle with its articular surface—became necrosed and exfoliated. The patient left the hospital three weeks after this. On December 1 the use of the limb was almost entirely recovered, extension and flexion were painless, and the wound healed. In the following February he could walk without any support, and all movements of the knee were recovered.

Many compound separations will therefore recover without amputation—e.g. Owing's, Gay's, Delens's, Elder's, Chassaniol's, Shepherd's, and Donovan's cases.

'Out of thirty cases of compound separation collected (*British Medical Journal*, March 31, 1894, p. 672) by Hutchinson junior, four died from shock, &c.; in eight reduction was more or less effected, with four subsequent amputations and three deaths from pyæmia. The remaining case recovered after suppuration and some necrosis. In thirteen cases amputation was performed soon after the injury, with at least three deaths (in one the limb was removed at the hip-joint).'

Ligature of femoral vein.—The timely ligature of the femoral vein in compound separations for infective thrombosis may arrest a pyæmic process, and possibly avert death.

Resection of the whole epiphysis and joint will be rarely required; it will be necessary only in exceptional cases where extensive suppuration of the joint and soft parts may be expected, after severe lesions to them; otherwise the joint will almost always completely recover its normal movements.

Arthritic inflammation from contiguity with the separated epiphysis will often be seen, or even some local suppuration, but these need not necessarily destroy the function of the joint in these young subjects.

Primary amputation is a very grave question, and its advisability can only be determined by consideration of the particulars of each case; it is necessary only when there exists laceration or irreparable injury of the popliteal vessels in either simple or compound separations, or in severe and extensive injury to the soft parts of the limb.

The condition of the foot and leg should in all cases be carefully watched for any interference with the circulation and consequent danger of gangrene.

Dr. McDiarmid found that primary amputation was performed in eleven out of nearly fifty cases, with four recoveries and three deaths, and in four the result was not stated.

Primary amputation was performed in two of Dr. R. H. Harte's cases; in one the separation was compound and the leg torn off below the knee, in the other the separation was simple, but accompanied with a compound comminuted fracture of the bones of the right leg and a simple fracture of the opposite femur.

In the total of sixty-eight cases, Packard found that amputation had been performed in twenty-eight. In twelve it was primary, in nine secondary, in five it was effected at a very late period, and in two the time is not stated. In a number of the cases there were other injuries, causing death in a short time, and in many others the diagnosis was not satisfactorily established.

In the author's collection of fifty cases of compound séparation, twenty-one necessitated amputation at or soon after the time of the accident. Of these no results are stated in six, while of the remaining cases twelve recovered and three died, one from pyæmia and two from shock.

Secondary amputation.—Should the judicious treatment above indicated be carried out, secondary amputation for gangrene, extensive suppuration of the limb, suppurative periostitis, pressure upon the internal popliteal nerve, aneurism, or deformity from impossibility of keeping the fragments in position, will be less frequent than they have been hitherto in simple separations.

Secondary amputation has also been sometimes resorted to in compound separations for profuse suppuration, pressure upon vessels and nerves, secondary hæmorrhage, and suppuration of the knee-joint.

Secondary amputation was performed (in Canton's, Atkinson's, and other cases) for accidental fracture after resection, and at the request of the patients' friends.

In these instances recovery not infrequently ensues. Dr. McDiarmid however found secondary amputation performed in five out of nearly fifty cases, with only one recovery, one death, and three results not stated.

In Dr. McBurney's case, quoted by Little, secondary amputation was undertaken, two or three months after compound separation, in order to relieve the intense pain and deformity. Death ensued from tetanus. In this instance strong bony union had taken place, and the internal popliteal nerve was discovered to be stretched over the edge of the diaphysial end of the femur.

In one of Dr. R. H. Harte's cases secondary amputation was performed for suppuration after simple separation.

In Dr. Halderman's case amputation for impending gangrene had to be performed, although the circulation through the main artery and vein was greatly crippled, if not abolished, from the commencement; in this example also both popliteal nerves were paralysed from pressure, the joint cavity opened, and the surrounding tissue badly damaged and the bone comminuted. All this condition of affairs existed without a breach of integument.

By reason of the peculiar incarceration of the vessels between the fragments, it is improbable that any manipulation or operative interference in this case would have succeeded in freeing the popliteal artery and vein, even though the adjustment of the fragments had been accomplished.

Mr. Morven Smith, of Baltimore (*American Journal of Med. Sci.* 1838, 4th Fasc.), describes a somewhat similar example of secondary gangrene following the injury, which was not diagnosed at the time as a separation of the lower epiphysis of the femur.

A youth, aged nineteen, had a sack full of goods, which was being let down from a vessel, fall on his knee. A ' fracture ' of the femur near the condyles was detected, and at the end of five days the limb was attacked with gangrene and amputation was performed. The popliteal artery and vein had been flattened by the edge of the upper fragment, which was displaced backwards.

Among the author's collection of fifty cases of compound separation, twelve underwent secondary amputation for one or other of the conditions just mentioned. Of these the result is not stated in one, and of the remaining cases six recovered and five died, two of pyæmia, one of tetanus, one of thrombosis of the vena cava, and one from shock.

Treatment of deformity some time after the accident.

Lateral displacement of the epiphysis, producing genu valgum and genu varum, may be corrected by osteotomy of the femur above the condyles.

In a case described by F. J. Shepherd the displacement of the diaphysis outwards caused a remarkable obliquity and deformity of the lower end of the femur, which interfered with the lad's progression. The accident had occurred several years before. The limb was straightened by MacEwen's operation, and the patient had good use of the limb.

In the author's case of severe genu varum and arrest of growth of the femur, following epiphysial injury in infancy, osteotomy was performed upon it just before the time of the report for correction of the deformity with success.

In displacement of the *epiphysis forwards*, osteotomy also may be desirable in severe deformity.

If seen at an earlier period—a few weeks after the accident—forcible replacement of the fragments may be attempted, and the soft uniting osseous material broken through.

It required considerable force in Winslow's case to break up the adhesions between the fragments four weeks after the injury. The marked varus position—the knees being two inches apart—was completely corrected, and at the end of four weeks the limb was found to be slightly shorter than its fellow, but the knees could be easily placed together.

CHAPTER V

SEPARATION OF THE UPPER EPIPHYSIS OF THE TIBIA

ANATOMY.—Both ends of the tibia are usually cartilaginous at birth. The ossific centre is distinguishable in the upper cartilaginous end about two weeks after birth, but its appearance may be delayed till the sixth or even as late as the twelfth month. On the other hand, it may sometimes appear just before birth.

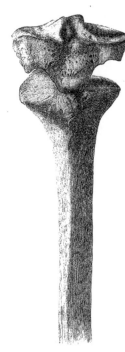

It is situated exactly in the centre of the cartilaginous end, rather towards its lower limit, and surrounded by scattered osseous granules, which are most developed immediately beneath the articular depressions above. These rapidly coalesce with the main centre during the first year, and form this wide expanded epiphysis composed of the two tuberosities.

The tubercle of the tibia is usually developed in front in an extension downwards of the cartilaginous epiphysis, ossification proceeding from the main centre forwards and downwards. It is often, according to Béclard, Sappey, and others, ossified by a separate centre, as in many of the lower animals, forming from about the eighth to the twelfth year (thirteenth year, Sappey), and rapidly extends upwards, joining the epiphysis above later—that is, about the sixth or eighth month after (Sappey)—and a short time afterwards blends with the diaphysis. By the fourteenth or fifteenth year the upper epiphysis with the tubercle is almost completely ossified, concave below, and merely separated from the diaphysis by a thin layer of cartilage above and in front.

Fig. 242.—UPPER EPIPHYSIS OF THE TIBIA AT THE SIXTEENTH YEAR (½-size)

It is half an inch in thickness, and its outer tuberosity presents at the posterior and outer aspect the whole of the articular facet

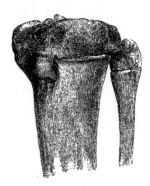

FIG. 243.—ANTERO-LATERAL VIEW OF THE FULLY FORMED EPIPHYSES OF THE TIBIA AND FIBULA AT THE NINETEENTH YEAR (Half natural size)

for the head of the fibula, and affords attachment to the capsular ligament of the superior tibio-fibular articulation. The upper end of the diaphysis is generally slightly convex, but a little depressed towards the centre. The junction of the epiphysis with the diaphysis occurs from the twentieth to the twenty-second year, at times as late as the twenty-third year. Eighteen to twenty years, and even as late as the twenty-fourth, are given by Sappey.

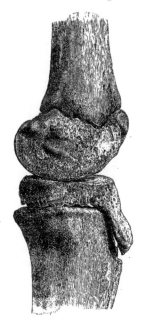

The conjugal line of cartilage at the fourteenth year is half an inch below the level of the upper articular surface of the tibia on the inner side, and five-eighths of an inch on the outer. At the eighteenth year it is five-eighths of an inch below it on the inner side, and three-quarters of an inch on the outer. The epiphysis overlaps the diaphysis much more on the outer than the inner side; consequently the line pursues a longer course downwards on this side.

FIG. 244.—EPIPHYSES OF THE KNEE-JOINT AT THE NINETEENTH YEAR. INNER SIDE (Half natural size)

The *synovial membrane* of the knee-joint at no part of its circumference extends down to the epiphysial cartilage of the upper end of the tibia, so that it is at a considerable distance from the diaphysis.

The epiphysial line, however, on the outer side approaches the superior tibio-fibular articulation—a layer of periosteum and some fibrous tissue, belonging mostly to the capsule of this joint, separating the two.

The epiphysial line being directly below the tibio-fibular joint, this joint is likely to be opened in separation of the upper epiphysis of the tibia. As the synovial membrane of the former joint not infrequently communicates with the large bursa beneath the tendon of the popliteus, which is an extension of the synovial membrane of the knee-joint, an indirect opening of the knee-joint may take place on the outer side in separation of the upper tibial epiphysis.

The following table of measurements of the upper epiphysis of the tibia and fibula in individuals of various ages is given by De Paoli from frontal sections :

	TIBIA					FIBULA	
AGE	HEIGHT				BREADTH	Height (at the external margin)	Breadth
	At the outer margin	At the inner margin	At the middle of the external tuberosity	At the middle of the internal tuberosity			
Before birth	9 mm.	9	9	8	26	7	8
1 year .	11 ,,	10	10	9	36	—	—
2 years .	12 ,,	10	9	8	38	9	11
4 ,, .	10 ,,	10	12	11	39	8	12
5 ,, {	12 ,,	10	18	11	45	6	13
	15 ,,	12	14	12	48	9	15
6 ,, .	14 ,,	11	12	11	48	10	15
7 ,, .	12 ,,	11	10	11	48	10	14
8 ,, {	18 ,,	16	15	18	60	12	15
	14 ,,	12	18	11	55	9	15
9 ,, .	15 ,,	18	14	18	58	9	15
18 ,, .	20 ,,	18	16	14	61	—	—
14 ,, .	20 ,,	19	15	13	66	—	—
16 ,, .	20 ,,	15	18	15	68	10	20
17 ,, .	16 ,,	14	12	11	62	—	—
20 ,, .	16 ,,	14	15	18	59	—	—

ETIOLOGY.—The disjunction of this epiphysis can only be effected by great violence, and that for several reasons : its great breadth, the fact that its somewhat cupped inferior surface with tonguelike process in front fits on to the diaphysis ; the presence of powerful internal lateral and other ligaments, the semimembranosus and other tendons, and the way in which it is attached to the diaphysis by the tough periosteum.

In the recorded examples the violence has usually been *direct*, from some severe crushing force, such as the passage of a wagon-wheel over the leg. In Ashhurst's case the boy was crushed between the buffers of a railway carriage. The author found this mode of violence to be the common cause in experiments on the dead body, but separation could be more readily produced between the ages of eight and fifteen years than later.

According to Poncet, the epiphysis of the tibia projects so little at the knee that it does not allow direct violence to have much play upon it.

In others the injury appears to have been *indirect*.

In Peulevé's case the leg was completely torn off at the level of this epiphysis, having been caught in the spokes of the revolving wheel of a carriage.

Verneuil (Lariboisière) saw a leg, which had been completely torn off at the level of the epiphysial cartilage of the tibia, of a child

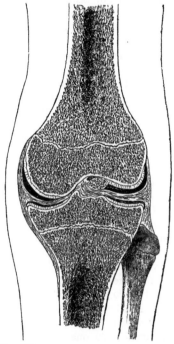

FIG. 245.—DIAGRAM OF FRONTAL SECTION OF KNEE-JOINT, SHOWING RELATION OF SYNOVIAL MEMBRANE TO THE EPIPHYSIAL LINES AT THE EIGHTEENTH YEAR. POSTERIOR HALF OF SECTION (Half natural size)

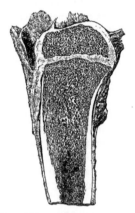

FIG. 246.—MEDIAN SAGITTAL SEC-
. TION OF TIBIA IN A BOY AGED
THIRTEEN AND A HALF YEARS

The synovial membrane does not extend so far anteriorly or posteriorly over the upper surface of the tibia as it does over the tuberosities. The bursa under the ligamentum patellæ is seen in section in front of the epiphysis and tubercle of the tibia, separated from the knee-joint by a cushion of fat (⅔-size)

six years old. The limb had been caught in the spokes of a wheel. This is probably the same case as Peulevé's, the age being given the same in both instances.

In Blasius's case the complete separation of the epiphysis and displacement backwards of the diaphysis were effected by the boy's right foot being caught in a threshing machine.

In Mr. Marsh's case the youth had been caught in the belt of a machine and received other very extensive injuries. Mr. Marsh thought that the blows on the os calcis, with the weight of the

3 F

body moving in the opposite direction, were the cause of the separation.

When the same force acts upon the epiphyses at the knee-joint, as in straightening knock-knees, it almost always happens that the lower end of the femur gives way rather than the upper epiphysis of the tibia.

Monteggia and Bertrandi are both said by M. Rognetta to have seen separation of this epiphysis in children, following a fall upon the knee. Rognetta questions the mechanism of the separation which these two authors describe. He does not think that separation of the tibia can occur in this way, but that the force in falling upon the knee is received entirely upon the femur, and not upon the tibia.

Guéretin separated this epiphysis on the bodies of newly born infants by hyper-extension of the knee.

AGE.—Mr. Hutchinson junior collected the records of ten cases (including three unpublished ones) mostly happening from wrenches of the leg. The youngest patient was twelve months, the oldest sixteen years.

In a total of twenty-four cases the author has brought together the age ranged from three up to twenty years: one at 20, two at 17, one at 16½, one at 11, one at 9, four at 8, two at 6, two at 4, one at 3½, and two at 3 years of age. Of the remaining seven, in four the age was not given, in one it occurred in a boy, another in a youth, and a third in a porter. Of the seventeen in which the age is stated, no less than twelve occurred between 3 and 9 years of age, and out of these five were between 8 and 9 years of age.

Of *thirteen cases* verified by *direct examination*, one only was *compound*, and terminated in recovery (girl, age not stated). Of the other twelve, in which death occurred or the limb was amputated, two occurred at 17, one at 16½, one at 11, two at 8, one at 6, and one at 3 years of age (female); one occurred in a boy, one in a porter, one in a youth, and in one the age was not stated.

Of the *eleven simple cases*, one occurred at 20, one at 9, three at 8, two at 4 (one in a girl), one at 3½ (girl), one at 3 years of age, and in two the age was not stated.

SEX.—The sex is given in twenty out of the twenty-four cases; sixteen occurred in males, and only four in girls.

Among the thirteen cases verified by direct examination, two were in female, the rest in male subjects.

PATHOLOGICAL ANATOMY.—The upper epiphysis of the tibia is remarkably easy to separate experimentally in the dead subject, especially in infants.

Separation of the epiphysis *in infancy* was first carefully considered during the second part of the present century.

However, the often-quoted case of the newly born infant recorded by Madame Lachapelle (*Prat. des Accouch.* tom. ii. p. 225, and tom. iii. p. 180) cannot be relied on, inasmuch as the child was born dead. The upper epiphysis of the tibia and the lower epiphysis of the femur were separated by traction of·the foot during parturition. In all probability there was some morbid condition of bone present.

Delore separated the upper epiphysis of the tibia and lower epiphysis of the femur on the one side, and the upper epiphysis of the fibula and the lower of the femur on the other, in straightening the knees of a boy affected with genu valgum. Death occurred from measles twenty-one days after the operation.

Separation of the upper epiphysis of the tibia is a rare form of injury according to the number of specimens in existence, yet there have been thirteen examples verified by direct examination out of a total of twenty-four.

. The leg is sometimes completely torn off at this epiphysis, like the lower femoral epiphysis.

M. Peulevé, before the Société Anatomique, Paris (*Bull. de la Soc. anat.* 1865, tom. x. 2 Sér. p. 305), described a case where this had taken place, and showed the relative specimens. There was complete separation of the epiphysis from the shaft, and destruction of the superior tibio-fibular articulation. The knee-joint, however, was quite intact.

The patient, a boy aged six years, had climbed behind a carriage and caught his left leg in the revolving wheel. Amputation was performed on account of the severity of the injury, and was followed by recovery.

PURE SEPARATIONS.—The tongue-like process of the tubercle goes with the epiphysis. Mr. Durham's specimen mentioned below, in which the tubercle was broken off and remained attached to the diaphysis, is therefore exceptional. There are several specimens of this pure form of injury in the London museums. In those instances the injury was caused by the limb being run over by the wheel of a heavy vehicle, and was accompanied by severe lesions of the soft structures and laceration of the skin.

The specimen (No. 541) in the London Hospital Museum (*Catalogue of the London Hospital Museum*, 1890, p. 119) was taken from a girl, aged three years, a patient of Mr. Jonathan Hutchinson's. The upper epiphysis of the tibia has been completely and evenly detached, taking with it also the tubercle. The epiphysial cartilage goes with the epiphysis, as also a thick sleeve of periosteum detached from the upper end of the shaft; .on the inner side a flap of the periosteum was found doubled in so as to cover the under surface of the epiphysis and prevent its coming in contact with the shaft. The external lateral ligament is entire, and, the fibula being uninjured and still connected with the epiphysis, no great displacement could be effected at this part. On abducting the foot, the line of separation gaped widely at the inner side, where all periosteal fibres, &c., had been torn through. No doubt the direction of the original violence

was such as to force the leg outwards. The injury was compound,
and was attended with great damage to the soft parts, requiring
primary amputation. A wagon had run over the limb in the street.
The left forearm was also so injured as to require amputation.

The specimen in Guy's Hospital Museum (No. 1210[46]) shows a
complete separation of the lower femoral epiphysis as well as of the
upper epiphysis of the tibia. In both the periosteum has been torn
off the adjacent portions of the diaphyses, while retaining its connection with the epiphysial ends. The popliteal artery was occluded by
laceration of its internal coats, and there was a greenstick fracture
of the upper end of the fibula on the same side. The patient,
George S., aged eight years, was under the care of Mr. Davies-Colley
in July 1886. He had fallen off a hearse, and a wheel passed over
his right knee. Amputation was performed on account of the
severity of the injury, and recovery took place.

There is another specimen in the same museum (No. 1260)
where the epiphysis was thought to have been loosened, from the
appearance of the preparation after it had been dried. . Examination
of the specimen does not seem to supply much evidence of separation of the epiphysis, but its anterior lip, forming the tubercle of the
tibia, has been broken off. The tibia was grazed by the wheel of a
railway carriage.·. The patient, a porter, had his limb amputated for
the great injury to the soft parts (July 1863).

In one of the specimens in St. George's Hospital, referred to under
SEPARATION OF THE LOWER EPIPHYSIS OF THE FEMUR, there is
besides this lesion a separation of the upper epiphysis of the tibia.

Messrs. Ashhurst's and F. Marsh's. specimens may also be considered as pure separations ; the small scale of the peripheral border
of the diaphysial end in the latter's case was not sufficiently large
to constitute it a fracture of the diaphysis.

The tibia may sometimes give way, not through, but at a short
distance below, the epiphysial line, as in Rathbun's case of separation
of the lower epiphysis of the femur. In addition to the femoral
separation, there was in this instance discovered after death a
fracture of the upper extremity of the shaft of the tibia that had
not previously been suspected. It was situated just below the epiphysial line, and was nearly transverse in direction, being directed
from without inwards, slightly downwards, and forwards ; there was
no displacement of the fragments whatever.

Separation with displacement forwards of the epiphysis.—In Hirschfeld and Fischer's case, related below, the displacement of the
diaphysis was backwards.

In St. Bartholomew's Hospital Museum, No. 990B, to show a
splendid instance of pure separation, there is the upper part of a
tibia which has been divided by a sagittal section of its upper epiphysis. The specimen shows marked displacement forwards for
three-eighths of an inch of the epiphysis from the diaphysis. Union,

however, fibrous in nature, was extremely firm. There is no fracture of the epiphysis. The separation is perfectly pure, there being no fracture of the diaphysis or of its anterior process which forms the tubercle. The periosteum, ligaments, and tendons surrounding the upper epiphysis present great displacement.

The leg was removed by operation (1895) from a boy, aged sixteen, who was admitted on account of his being caught by a machine; gangrene of the leg followed, and the leg was amputated thirty-six days after the injury.

Mr. F. Marsh showed a specimen of complete separation of the shaft of the tibia from the upper epiphysis (*British Medical Journal*, January 27, 1894, p. 216) before the Birmingham and Midland Counties Branch of the British Medical Association, taken (*post mortem*) from a youth, aged seventeen, who had been caught in the belt of a machine, and received very extensive injuries. Separation at the line of the epiphysis was complete, the left knee-joint was uninjured, and the left fibula was intact. Mr. Marsh pointed out the extreme rarity of the specimen, and the difficulty in this instance, the fibula being intact, of satisfactorily explaining the mechanism of the separation.

Subsequently this surgeon very kindly furnished the author with the following detailed account of the case.

The specimen was taken from a youth, æt. seventeen, who had been caught in the belt of a machine, and had received the following injuries. The left arm was almost torn off above the elbow-joint, and there was also a compound fracture of the humerus in its upper third; both bones of the right forearm were badly comminuted; the right femur was fractured; the tissues over the heel and sole of the left foot were stripped off, and the os calcis was split into three or four pieces; the shaft of the left tibia was separated from the upper epiphysis and displaced backwards; the head, trunk, and extremities were also much bruised. The condition was diagnosed when the youth was anæsthetised, and Mr. Marsh was about to amputate the foot. On raising the leg he noticed some unusual mobility in the region of the knee-joint, and on examining found what was evidently a separation of the epiphysis. The displacement of the diaphysis was directly backwards, and was complete and very marked. The reduction was easy, but the condition was as readily reproduced. Supra-malleolar amputation of the left foot, and amputation through the surgical neck of the left humerus, were performed, and the patient rallied fairly well for a time, but died thirty-six hours later, apparently from shock. The *post-mortem* examination showed that no other injuries except those enumerated had been received. Examination of the left leg showed that the separation of the epiphysis was complete, that the knee-joint was uninjured, and that the fibula was intact.

The youth was well developed and very muscular. Mr. Marsh

was inclined to think that the blows on the os calcis, with the weight of the body moving in an opposite direction, caused the separation.

The specimen which Mr. Marsh also kindly sent the author showed a very small flake of the diaphysis broken from the front of the diaphysis; the separation was otherwise quite pure. The specimen is in the Mason College Museum.

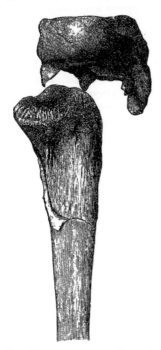

Displacement forwards and out-wards of the epiphysis. — Blasius records (Poncet, *Nouv. Dict. Méd. et de Chir.* t. 19, p. 513; also E. Gurlt, *Handbuch der Lehre von den Knochenbrüchen*, 1 Theil, 1862, S. 87) the case of a boy, aged sixteen and a half years, who was injured by his right foot being caught in a threshing machine. The upper epiphysis was com-pletely separated from the shaft exactly at the epiphysial line, even to the tongue-like process in front : the diaphysis being displaced back-wards and inwards an inch beyond the epiphysis, and large lacerated wounds produced in the flexure of the knee. The fibula was also fractured below the head, and the capsule of the joint was perforated towards the posterior aspect by a small splinter of compact tissue detached from the inner side of the diaphysis of the tibia. After death, on the sixth day, fœtid pus was found in the knee-joint, and the skin of the lower part of the

Fig. 247.—Mr. Frank Marsh's specimen (½-size, Mason College Museum, Birmingham)

thigh and part of the leg was gangrenous.

Displacement backwards of the epiphysis.—No instance has been recorded of this form of displacement.

Lateral displacement of the epiphysis.—A specimen of separation from a crush of the leg, in which the extensive laceration of the soft parts required amputation, is figured by Ashhurst (*Principles and Practice of Surgery*, 3rd edit. p. 269, figs. 132, 133, Philadelphia, 1882).

The specimen is in the Museum of the Episcopal Hospital, and was taken from a boy, eleven years old, who was caught between the buffers of railway cars.

Dr. Ashhurst very kindly furnished the author with the following drawings of the case (figs. 248, 249).

SEPARATION WITH FRACTURE OF DIAPHYSIS.—A fracture of the diaphysis often accompanies separation of the upper epiphysis of the tibia in experiments on the dead subject.

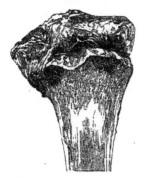 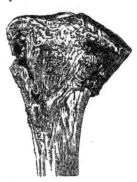

FIG. 248.—LATERAL DISPLACEMENT OF UPPER
EPIPHYSIS OF TIBIA. POSTERIOR VIEW
(After Ashhurst)

FIG. 249.—THE SAME SPECIMEN.
ANTERIOR VIEW

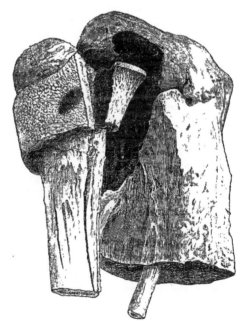

FIG. 250. —SEPARATION OF THE UPPER EPIPHYSIS OF THE TIBIA, WITH
FRACTURES OF THE DIAPHYSIS
(Royal College of Surgeons Museum)

The Royal College of Surgeons Museum contains a specimen, No. 1110A, showing upper extremity of a tibia with separation of the epiphysis. The diaphysial end is broken up into several large fragments, and a longitudinal fracture extends downwards into the shaft. The epiphysis of the tibia remains firmly attached to the head·of the fibula. The fractures are mostly of the posterior·part of the diaphysis, which are displaced backwards, while the anterior part has been displaced forwards. Mr. A. H. Tubby says: ' Unfortunately no history was obtainable in this case, as it was found among a number of discarded specimens given to me from a private collection' (*Annals of Surgery*, March 1894, p. 316)..

Mr. Durham had the case of a boy, aged eight, under his care at Guy's Hospital in April 1885, who was injured by the wheel of a tramcar passing over his leg. Primary amputation was rendered necessary on account of the extensive laceration of the skin on the outer and front part of the leg, laying bare the gastrocnemius muscle and upper part of tibia. The upper epiphysis was completely separated from the shaft, but not displaced; the portion forming the tubercle was broken from the epiphysis, which was otherwise intact, and remained attached to the shaft. The upper end of the diaphysis had been fractured vertically in three pieces, the innermost piece being quite loose. The joint, fibula, and large vessels and nerves were uninjured. The patient rapidly recovered. .

Lefort gives the description (*Bull. de la Soc. de Chir.* 1865, p. 529) of the case of a girl in whom there was a compound separation of the upper epiphysis of the tibia, accompanied by a fracture of the diaphysis. Through a wound of the upper part of the leg a movable fragment could be distinctly felt, so that the fragments were completely separated. M. Guérin removed the fragment of the diaphysis, one surface of which presented a mammillated appearance, corresponding to the epiphysial cartilage ; the other aspect was rough, like fractured bone.

The patient completely recovered.

COMPLICATIONS.—Laceration of the capsular ligaments and opening of the knee-joint is not a necessary accompaniment, even in compound cases, although some effusion into the knee-joint must be expected in all. In Blasius's case of compound separation the capsule of the joint was perforated towards the posterior aspect by a small splinter from the inner side·of the diaphysis, and led to suppuration of the knee-joint, discovered at death on the sixth day.

In Peulevé's specimen and in F. Marsh's the joint was intact, yet in the former the leg had been completely torn off at the epiphysial junction.

Dr. H. Fischer and Dr. E. Hirschfeld record (*Berliner klinische Wochenschrift*, 6 März 1865, ii. S. 93) a case in which there occurred separation of the lower epiphysis of the right femur, upper epiphysis of the left tibia, and both epiphyses of the left fibula, exactly at the epiphysial line. As regards the separation of the lower epiphysis of the right femur, the injury was a simple one. The epiphysis was rotated so that the internal condyle ascended somewhat forwards and the external condyle descended backwards, the upper fragment being also a little forwards. Soft crepitus was distinct, and abnormal mobility slight. The right knee-joint appeared normal. On the left side the lower fragment of the tibia was displaced backwards and upwards, forming an angular projection behind, and being overlapped in front by the upper fragment. This projection was plainly visible on hyperextension of the knee-joint, and disappeared on flexion. These movements were accompanied by distinct crepitus. The upper fragment formed a small prominence in front, which ended a little below the tubercle of the tibia; its shape could be accurately made out. At the upper and lower epiphyses of the fibula, soft, yet distinct, crepitus was felt, with some abnormal mobility of the epiphyses; there was, however, no displacement. The knee- and ankle-joints appeared to be free.

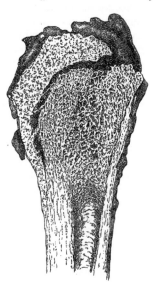

Fig. 251.—DISPLACEMENT FORWARDS OF UPPER EPIPHYSIS OF TIBIA. UNITED AT THE ELEVENTH WEEK

(After Fischer and Hirschfeld)

Under . chloroform the displacement of the tibia of the left leg was reduced, and the limb put up in a plaster splint. But in spite of careful treatment, in the eleventh week amputation through the upper part of the thigh was obliged to be performed for necrosis of the whole separated lower epiphysis of the fibula, partial necrosis of the upper epiphysis of the fibula, and suppuration of the knee- and ankle-joints. The latter was quite destroyed, having been opened from the outer side. The epiphysis of the tibia was found to be again displaced forwards, and was firmly united in this position, covering over the upper part of the tibia like a cap.

The patient was a lad, aged seventeen years, who was injured by being caught in the driving shaft of a threshing machine, and violently twisted round by it. Recovery took place, and the fracture of the right femur consolidated, though with some displacement and rotation of the epiphysis.

Suppuration and necrosis result most frequently in compound cases.

Suppuration of the knee-joint.—This occurred in Blasius's case of compound separation, in which the capsule was opened at the posterior aspect. Gangrene of part of the leg and thigh ensued, terminating in death on the sixth day.

PROGNOSIS.—Union has resulted in two instances—in Fischer and Hirschfeld's, and in the St. Bartholomew's Hospital Museum specimen—a firm union, although only a fibrous one, notwithstanding the fact that gangrene of the leg supervened in both, and necessitated amputation in the first case at the eleventh week, in the second on the twenty-sixth day.

C. A. Sturrock records (*Edinburgh Hospital Reports*, vol. ii. 1894, p. 605) a case in which no trace of the injury could be seen eleven months after the accident.

A. L., aged eight, was admitted to the Royal Infirmary, Edinburgh, on January 27, 1893, under Professor Annandale's care. When swinging, he got his foot caught and fell to the ground. On admission, some time after the accident, the swelling round the knee was so considerable that the precise nature of the injury could not be ascertained; when in three days the swelling had in great measure disappeared by means of evaporating lotions, it was found, on grasping the tibia, that the tuberosities could be moved from side to side, and slightly from before backwards, cartilaginous crepitus at the same time being elicited. There appeared to be no other injury to the neighbouring bones, though there was some synovitis. The most comfortable position was a flexed one, and it was with considerable difficulty that the leg could be straightened and placed in a box splint. It was retained thus for seventeen days, and encased in plaster of Paris for three weeks. When heard of eleven months after the accident the boy had no limp, and no trace of the injury was to be seen.

Good union likewise resulted in Heuston's case without much displacement.

Ankylosis of the knee-joint and fixation of the tibial epiphysis to the femur may ensue as the result of the synovitis due to direct injury of the joint, or as the result of extra-articular inflammation following the severe injury.

Deformity.—There will be no trace of deformity in separation without displacement provided the injury be judiciously treated, as in Bryant's, Annandale's, and Birkett's cases. In other separations the deformity after reduction will be inappreciable—e.g. Heuston's case. It has been stated that if the separation remain undetected, the epiphysis may unite with displacement inwards and inversion of the knee-joint, but that this *valgus* condition may result from rotation of the leg and foot without any lateral displacement. M. Rognetta alludes to a case observed in 1625 by the celebrated Severino at the Hospital for Incurables at Naples. In this case twisting inwards of the knee took place in consequence of separation of the upper epiphysis of the tibia.

Arrest of growth.—Some arrest of growth may take place after separation of the upper epiphysis of the tibia, but since the lower epiphysis also has a share in the growth of the tibia, the extent of the shortening following injury to its upper end is uncertain ; the amount contributed by each epiphysis has not yet been determined, although it appears from the experiments of Vogt that the increase in length of the tibia takes place mostly through the upper epiphysial cartilage, and this is borne out by the frequency with which arrest of growth of the limb is met with after disease about this epiphysis.

The truth of this is also often seen in the comparatively rapid increase of the tibia in amputation of the leg in childhood, producing a conical stump, and necessitating the removal of the end of the quickly growing shaft.

Mr. Bryant (*Practice of Surgery*, 4th edit. 1884, vol. ii. p. 458) figures a well-marked case of arrest of growth in the shaft of the right tibia for one inch, with bowing of fibula, following injury to the upper epiphysis two years before. At the time of observation the child was aged eight years.

The growth of the fibula continuing unchecked, it becomes bowed outward, as in this instance, and hypertrophied, or else displaced upwards ; see fig. 252.

Volkmann records another case of three centimetres shortening after injury to the upper end of a tibia.

A boy, aged three, had been severely knocked about by his drunken father. At the age of four he began to limp, and subsequently the tibia ceased to grow at its upper end, so that the shortening finally amounted to three centimetres. A ridge could be felt, as

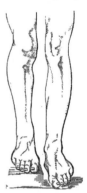

FIG. 252.—ARREST OF GROWTH OF TIBIA TWO YEARS AFTER INJURY TO UPPER EPIPHYSIS (Bryant)

though the diaphysis had been displaced somewhat inwards and forwards. It must be stated, moreover, that the femur and foot of the same side, in fact the whole lower extremity, were less developed than those of the opposite side (Hutchinson junior).

Mr. J. Jones reported (*London Medical Record*, 1883, vol. xi. p. 228; *Lancet*, March 1883, p. 403) a case of separation of this epiphysis during traction by extension in hip disease, followed by arrest of growth for one and a half inches in the bone two years after the injury. However, this case must be considered as somewhat inconclusive, inasmuch as the separation, as well as the subsequent rapid arrest of growth, was possibly much favoured by the diseased condition of the patient.

SYMPTOMS. Separation without displacement.—Probably many instances of separation of this epiphysis without displacement are overlooked.

Helferich is of the same opinion. He thinks that wherever there has been a severe direct injury to the upper end of the tibia in a child, our attention should be directed to the possibility of this injury.

An accurate diagnosis can only be made under an anæsthetic, when abnormal mobility and characteristic cartilaginous crepitus may be detected. The presence of the fibula on the outer side attached to the epiphysis and articulating with it, and the tongue-like process in front forming the tubercle, tend to prevent displacement.

Among thirty-seven instances of traumatic separation of the epiphyses, Guéretin found only two of the upper epiphysis of the tibia.

Separation with displacement of the epiphysis.—In milder cases the displacement may be insignificant, especially if the fibula, which is connected wholly with this epiphysis, be not fractured, and the internal lateral ligament intact. A gap between the epiphysis and diaphysis may be felt on the inner or outer side on carefully abducting or adducting the leg.

In Hutchinson's there was no displacement, but the periosteum was tucked in between the fragments, being detached from the diaphysis. This detachment is seen in the Guy's Museum specimen, and is a constant complication in this injury, even in the less severe cases, and may be followed by acute periostitis.

The displacement of the epiphysis in the more severe cases may be completely *forwards*, and the diaphysis behind press upon or lacerate the popliteal vessels.

Incomplete displacement forwards was found in Fischer's case. The deformity is very prone to be reproduced.

In some instances, as in the cases of Lefort, &c., fracture of the diaphysis complicates the injury.

Displacement of the epiphysis forwards and outwards occurred in the case of Blasius; *directly outwards* in the case of a youth, aged twenty, under the care of Mr. Howse at Guy's Hospital in March 1888. The patient, Arthur R., was thrown off a bicycle in Cheapside, and in falling the crank axle of the bicycle struck the inner side of his left knee. On examination there was to be felt below the knee, on the inner side, a distinct rounded edge, apparently the upper edge of the diaphysis of the tibia, and a good deal of effusion into the knee. Under chloroform, on applying pressure inwards to the outer side of the knee, the upper fragment moved over the shaft, and the projection on the inner side disappeared. This manipulation was accompanied by slight cartilaginous crepitus. A 'Croft's' plaster-of-Paris splint was applied to the limb, and firm union took place at the end of a month. The case is also mentioned by Dr. E. P. Manby (*British Medical Journal*, September 22, 1888).

Mr. Durham had a similar case at Guy's Hospital in November 1877.

The patient (John H.), aged nine, got his right leg entangled in the wheel of a cab, and was dragged along the ground for some distance. The leg was found to be much twisted inwards, and a projection felt just below the knee, the result of the displacement of the epiphysis of the shaft. He was treated by a back splint, and left the hospital at the end of six weeks able to walk with some support.

Displacement of epiphysis inwards.—For displacement directly inwards to occur, the upper epiphysial junction of the fibula must be broken or the ligaments uniting the fibular head with the outer tuberosity of the tibial epiphysis lacerated.

Swelling.—The amount of swelling is usually very considerable.

It was so great in Annandale's case that the precise nature of the injury could not be ascertained for three weeks, when the swelling had in great measure disappeared.

Mobility of the epiphysis, most noticeable in the lateral direction, is the most trustworthy sign in this as in other epiphysial separations with incomplete displacement.

In Annandale's case there was slight mobility of the tuberosities from before backwards, as well as from side to side.

Dr. F. T. Heuston, surgeon to the Adelaide Hospital, Dublin, relates (*British Medical Journal*, vol. ii. July 21, 1888) the case of R. L., aged eight years, under his care. The boy, while running in school, was caught between two desks, and injured his leg in attempting to wrench it free. At the time there was little pain, and he was able to walk home. Considerable swelling supervened in a few hours. On examination six days later there was acute synovitis of the knee-joint, while free movement was obtainable between the superior epiphysis of the tibia and the shaft, there being, however, no crepitus.

Crepitus of the usual muffled character can be detected in many of the simpler cases in which mobility of the epiphysis is present.

Mr. Bryant, at Guy's Hospital in 1885, diagnosed separation of the upper epiphysis of the tibia from the dull crepitus and mobility of this epiphysis in a girl (D. W.), aged three and a half, who had slipped and fallen backwards. The injury was treated by a posterior and two lateral splints, the patient being discharged three weeks later with a ' Croft's ' plaster-of-Paris splint.

Under an anæsthetic the joint will be found to be perfectly movable and free.

COMPLICATIONS. **Articular lesions.**—Some effusion into the knee must be expected in all forms of severity of separation of the upper tibial epiphysis.

It was marked in Annandale's case. In other instances the knee-joint has been directly or indirectly opened at the time of the accident.

DIAGNOSIS.—**Dislocation of the knee** in childhood is scarcely known ; besides, the free movement of the joint in cases of separation is quite sufficient to distinguish it from this injury, while the mobility below the articular interline at the epiphysial level is conclusive.

When little swelling is present and displacement marked, but little difficulty will be experienced in the diagnosis.

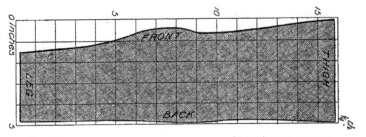

FIG. 253.—PATTERN OF LATERAL SPLINTS FOR KNEE (CROFT'S). FOR A BOY OF FIFTEEN YEARS

Reduced to one-quarter size on scale of inches

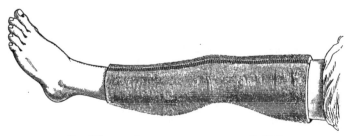

FIG. 254.—CROFT'S LATERAL SPLINTS APPLIED TO KNEE

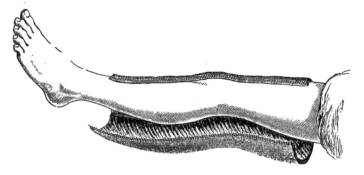

FIG. 255.—THE SAME WITH OUTER PIECE LAID ASIDE AFTER CUTTING THROUGH GAP IN FRONT

When, however, there is little or no displacement or mobility, the injury may be mistaken for a sprain of the knee-joint.

TREATMENT.—Separation without displacement should be treated according to general rules with a simple retentive apparatus.

In simple separation with displacement reduction can be easily effected with the use of anæsthetics, the limb afterwards being placed in a trough splint composed of posterior and lateral pieces, or by ' Croft's ' lateral plaster-of-Paris splints.

In severe displacements of the diaphysis backwards or laterally the leg should be flexed upon the thigh, and gentle pressure made upon the diaphysial end in the opposite direction to which it has been displaced. After the diaphysis has been restored to its normal position, the limb should be placed in the flexed position in a trough splint, or one composed of foot, thigh, and leg pieces with lateral pieces and hinge at knee.

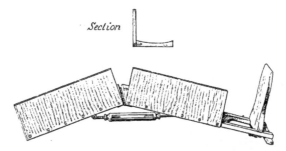

Fig. 256.—POSTERIOR SPLINT FOR THIGH AND LEG WITH FOOT-PIECE AND HINGE AT KNEE. FOR SEPARATION OF EITHER OF THE EPIPHYSES FORMING THE KNEE-JOINT. VERTICAL EXTERNAL OR INTERNAL LATERAL PIECES ARE EMPLOYED ACCORDING TO DISPLACEMENT OF THE EPIPHYSIS INWARDS OR OUTWARDS

Mr. Bryant and Mr. Birkett had each a case of this separation, at Guy's Hospital, in 1872 (H. L.) and 1868 (T. M.) respectively, and both were treated successfully by posterior and lateral splints. In both the child was four years of age and did well.

Primary amputation is necessary only in exceptional examples of compound separations, owing to the severity of the laceration to the neighbouring parts.

If there be but little destruction, more especially if it is caused by indirect violence, an attempt should always be made to preserve the limb, and there is little doubt that this may be usually done.

Secondary amputation.—Amputation was resorted to in Fischer's case in consequence of necrosis and suppuration in the knee- and ankle-joints. In the St. Bartholomew's Hospital specimen amputation was performed on the thirty-sixth day, and in Fischer and Hirschfeld's in the eleventh week, in both cases for gangrene of the leg.

CHAPTER VI

SEPARATION OF THE EPIPHYSIS OF THE TUBERCLE OF THE TIBIA

ANATOMY.—Although the cartilaginous tongue-like prolongation of the upper epiphysis in front usually ossifies by a downward extension of ossification of the upper epiphysis, yet the tubercle of the tibia has sometimes an entirely separate centre of ossification, and forms a distinct epiphysis, which may be detached by direct violence, or by the violent action of the quadriceps extensor.

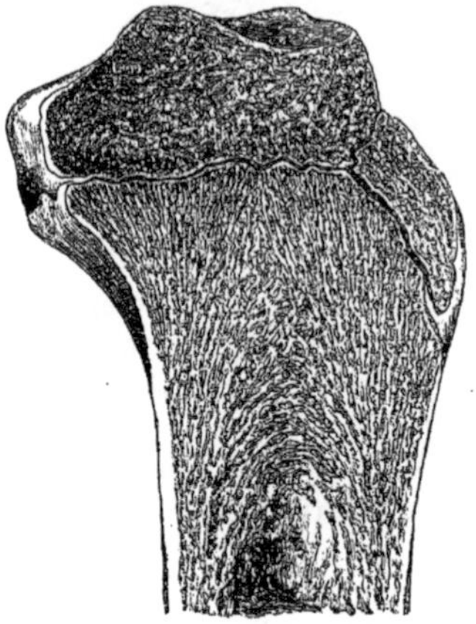

FIG. 257.—VERTICAL SECTION OF THE UPPER END OF THE TIBIA BETWEEN THE FOURTEENTH AND FIFTEENTH YEARS

The upper epiphysis is completely ossified, and there is a separate epiphysis for the tubercle. The latter still presents some cartilage at the lower part. Both epiphyses are separated from the tibia and from one another by a thin layer of cartilage (After Rambaud and Renault)

This centre appears, according to Béclard, about the eighth or tenth year, but is no doubt often of later date—about the twelfth or fourteenth year (thirteenth year, Sappey). This osseous nucleus rapidly invades the whole of the cartilaginous tubercle, spreading upwards towards the thick epiphysial plate above, and finally joins with it (six to eight months later, Sappey) and shortly afterwards with the diaphysis. The tubercle serves for the insertion of the powerful quadriceps tendon at the lower part, while at the upper end there is a smooth surface for the bursa—between the tendon and the bone.

Mr. Quain saw one instance only of a separate epiphysis for the tubercle.

It is quite possible, therefore, for the epiphysis when formed by a separate centre to be torn off without any fracture—a true separation of the epiphysis—but more commonly it is detached at its upper end or neck, where it joins the front portion of the upper epiphysis of the tibia, and therefore the epiphysial separation is accompanied by a fracture.

The relation of the synovial membrane of the knee-joint to the upper end of the tubercle of the tibia is a very close one. Its anterior aspect, as just stated, is covered by the bursa beneath the ligamentum patellæ. This bursa is separated from the cavity of the knee-joint by a pad of fat. Professor Macalister states that the bursa and knee-joint communicate in eight per cent. of limbs.

ETIOLOGY.—Of the ten cases recorded, we find that nine occurred by violent muscular action of the quadriceps, powerfully contracting and detaching the tubercle, and in male subjects. Three of. these patients were gymnasts, and the injury took place when they were vaulting the horse or jumping from the spring-board. In five out of the ten cases the injuries were caused by jumping and in one by an attempt to save the body from falling, and in one the injury was simply stated as due to a fall. With the exception of De Morgan's patient, who was said to have been very scrofulous, all were powerful and muscular young men.

All the three instances in which the injured side is stated were on the right.

De Morgan notes that this injury is allied to fracture of the patella, being, in fact, a tearing away of the attachment of the rectus, taking with it a portion of the bone into which it is inserted.

Although in Lauenstein's case the knee was directly struck against the vaulting horse, it does not appear that this could have been the sole cause of the detachment, and, as Müller states, Lauenstein did not consider it as caused by direct violence.

In Weinlechner's case the detachment does not appear to have been due to the action of the quadriceps, but to an overstretching of this muscle during excessive flexion of the knee. The patient in this case fell with his buttock resting on the calf of the leg.

The first recorded instance of detachment of the tubercle of the tibia is De Morgan's (*Medical Times and Gazette*, N.S. vol. vi. 1853, p. 268). It was produced by the muscular action of the rectus femoris. The patient (J. C.), aged seventeen years, was a very scrofulous lad, with scars on his head and extremities, evidently connected with diseased bones. Whilst walking in the street he slipped, and saved himself from falling by catching hold of the railings. He felt something give way in the knee, and immediately found he was unable to walk. On admission into the Middlesex Hospital, April 7, 1852, the left knee was much swollen, the swelling taking the shape of the joint, but extending downwards some inches over the inner surface of the tibia. The patella on the injured side was drawn up a quarter of an inch higher than on the other side. The tubercle of the tibia, with a piece of bone about an inch long, could be felt as if chipped off from the head of the tibia, the fragment remaining attached to the ligamentum patellæ, and being drawn up with it.

On holding the fragment between the fingers and moving it upon the bone beneath, distinct crepitus could be felt. The limb was placed in the extended position and raised, the thigh being flexed on the body. After several attacks of inflammation of the knee-joint, the effusion had quite disappeared at the end of three weeks. After seven weeks the patient was able to get about with a posterior splint, and a week or two after this he could walk and bend his knee. Two months later he was discharged from the hospital; some necrosis of the fourth metatarsal bone followed, and was removed. In December he had completely recovered the use of his leg. The fragment was perfectly firm; the union being osseous, with some thickening of the bone around it.

Dr. E. Müller relates (*Beiträge zur klin. Chirur. zu Tübingen*, 1888, S. 257) a case from Bruns's clinic.

A. H., a gymnast, sixteen years of age, fell down whilst exercising, as he was about to jump from the spring-board. He immediately experienced acute pain in the right knee, and was unable to move. On admission to the hospital, the right leg remained powerless in the extended position, the knee-joint was swollen all round, and the patella floated slightly. Over the upper end of the tibia in front of the knee the skin was rendered prominent by a triangular fragment of bone, with the base upwards measuring five centimetres, parallel with the articular interline. Its apex was downwards, the inner side measuring three centimetres, the outer side five centimetres. The fragment moved freely both laterally and from above downwards, but with pain to the patient; and the motion was accompanied by crepitus. The patella was about two centimetres higher than on the left side. The fragment, which was clearly the detached tubercle of the tibia, was drawn slightly downwards, and fixed in this position by means of a bandage and plaster of Paris reaching from the toes to the upper third of the thigh. On removing the plaster bandage eight days later, the tubercle was still movable, but fourteen days afterwards it had firmly united and the effusion into the joint had disappeared. The plaster-of-Paris bandage was finally removed six weeks after the injury; the tubercle of the tibia and the patella were one centimetre higher than the left. Three weeks later the functions of the limb were perfectly normal, and no difference whatever could be observed between the two knees.

Müller records a second case observed by Lauenstein, of Hamburg.

A gymnast, eighteen years of age, during his exercises, whilst springing upon the vaulting horse, knocked his right knee against it, and was unable to use his leg from that time.

Fracture of the patella was at first diagnosed, but on the second day Lauenstein found the knee swollen, though without effusion into the joint; and three fingers' breadth below the apex of the patella he found a fragment of bone over the head of the tibia, which could be moved laterally with crepitus. The patella was drawn downwards by strapping, and the tubercle pressed towards the tibia by the same means. A plaster-of-Paris bandage was also applied, and allowed to remain on five weeks. Perfect restoration of the functions of the leg resulted.

AGE.—In eight of the ten recorded instances of detachment of the tubercle the age is clearly stated. Two were verified by operation, and all were between sixteen and eighteen years of age—viz., one at 18 years, four at 17 years, and three at 16 years of age. Of the two remaining cases, in one the injury occurred to a young man, and in the other the age is not stated.

The whole ten were in male subjects.

PATHOLOGICAL ANATOMY.—A few examples have been verified by operative measures. J. Landsberg reports (*Medicinsk Revue*, 1889, Juli (Norwegian) ; *Centralblatt für Chirurgie*, September 28, 1889, S. 704) a case of avulsion of the tuberosity of the tibia in a lad, sixteen years old, by muscular effort in jumping.

The patella was displaced upwards for ten centimetres, and at about the same distance below there could be felt a small movable piece of bone ; an erroneous diagnosis of fracture of the patella was made, and, because of the supposed wide separation of the fragments, it was determined to wire them. A transverse incision was made, and then the actual condition was recognised. A longitudinal incision was carried downwards from the transverse one, and the tuberosity was fastened in place by a nail ; this was removed at the end of a fortnight. Complete recovery followed.

A case of fracture of the tubercle of the tibia is recorded by J. C. Ogilvie Will (*British Medical Journal*, January 22, 1887, p. 152), in which the signs of fracture of the patella were so exactly simulated that it was mistaken for this before the operation, which consisted in fastening the detached tubercle to its shaft by means of a steel pin. The result proved eminently satisfactory, so that the patient could at the end of three months execute all the ordinary movements of the joint as readily as on the uninjured leg. The functions of the limb were completely restored.

G. W., aged seventeen, a fairly muscular lad, a stonecutter, was admitted to the Aberdeen Royal Infirmary on August 28, 1885. He stated that a short time previously, when jumping with a pole, he felt something give way in the region of the knee-joint when he had risen about two feet from the ground. A diagnosis of fracture of the patella was made, for the joint was largely distended with blood and painful. There were two bony tumours with a considerable interval between them, one at the upper, and the other, the smaller, at the lower aspect of the joint, whose outlines could only be indistinctly made out on account of the swelling. The power of extension was entirely lost. The slightest movement caused the greatest pain. On exposing the patella by a vertical incision, this was ascertained to be intact, whilst the ligamentum patellæ was found to have torn away the bony prominence into which it was inserted. The portion of bone was about the size and shape of a small oyster shell, and its fractured surface was turned upwards from muscular contraction. It was readily replaced and fixed in position with the steel pin of an Archimedean drill. The joint was then thoroughly cleared of clots, and a stiff bandage applied with antiseptic dressings. On September 17 the pin was loose, and therefore taken away. On November 2 the union was quite firm, and the splint was removed. The patient completely regained the use of his knee, and could walk without any limping.

From the rough diagram and the description given by Will, it would appear that some of the surrounding diaphysis was torn away with the epiphysis, especially from the upper part of the tibia intervening between the tubercle and the articular surfaces of the tibia.

Pitha says that it is exceptional for the ligamentum patellæ to rupture; that it usually does so at, or even in, its insertion, and that a portion of the spine of the tibia remains hanging to the ligament itself.

Injury to knee-joint.—The bursa lying between the upper part of the tubercle, the front of the tibia and the lower portion of the ligamentum patellæ must always be lacerated in detachment of tubercle. From the proximity of the tubercle to the front of the synovial membrane of the knee-joint a laceration of the latter is very likely to occur. In Will's case the joint was full of blood clots.

Although in less severe lesions the knee-joint may escape direct injury, yet it must always be remembered that only a small amount of tissue intervenes between the articular cavity and the injured bursa, and that inflammation of the knee-joint is likely to follow; while the possibility of a communication existing between the bursa and knee-joint, though rare, deserves consideration as well.

SYMPTOMS.—The symptoms very closely resemble those of fracture of the patella, more especially those transverse or oblique fractures which so commonly occur in the lower third of the bone.

At the time of the injury the patient experiences a tearing sensation or crackling at the knee-joint.

Inability of the patient to extend the leg at the knee-joint from the time of the accident is a prominent sign.

The patella is drawn upwards to a greater or less extent. In Vogt's case this occurred to the extent of between two and two and a half centimetres.

If the swelling be not too great, the natural outline of the patella may be made out above the fragment, indicating that this bone is not fractured.

The detached epiphysis or **fragment of bone** can be felt beneath the skin, movable more or less freely in all directions. The size of this fragment varies very much in the recorded clinical cases.

In Vogt's case a piece of a triangular shape with a base measuring two centimetres, and a piece in one of Müller's five centimetres, was detected. The height of the fragment in Müller's was three centimetres.

A fragment or flake of the outer layer of the shaft below, or of the front of the upper epiphysis of the tibia above, may remain attached to this process. The outline of the detachment will therefore not exactly resemble the shape of the epiphysis.

Just below (quarter to half an inch) the apex of the patella the fragment may be felt still attached to the ligamentum patellæ, and movable both laterally and vertically. In Vogt's instance the mobility in the vertical direction was slight or entirely absent.

Crepitus has been present in the majority of the published cases, due probably to the small amount of displacement of the epiphysial fragment.

Effusion into the joint almost always takes place.

In Vogt's case there was thought to be considerable effusion of blood into the joint, and in Will's case at the time of operation the joint was full of blood-clots.

Possibly in more than one instance the tubercle was not a distinct epiphysis, but the upper end of this process was connected to the upper epiphysis, and its separation was therefore only effected by fracture caused by more severe violence.

It cannot be supposed, however, that the articular cavity must necessarily be involved in all instances, notwithstanding the close proximity just mentioned of the upper end of the tubercle to the knee-joint.

DIAGNOSIS. Transverse or oblique fracture of the lower part of the patella.—This accident closely resembles separation of the tubercle of the tibia. Fracture of the patella never occurs in childhood, and is as rare as separation of the tubercle during adolescence. There are, however, some distinguishing features at the latter period of life which should render the diagnosis an accurate one. In separation the patella above may be felt to be intact. Below the apex of the patella and over the upper end of the tibia a fragment of bone can be detected. Crepitus is detected in separated tubercle by drawing this fragment downwards, in fractured patella by drawing it upwards.

In both of the cases operated upon by Landsberg and Will the lesion was mistaken for fracture of the patella, and suturing of the fragments was undertaken. This in each case led to the recognition of the actual lesion.

TREATMENT.—In exceptional simple instances of *little or no displacement* the treatment is similar to that for fractured patella : the leg should be extended on the thigh and elevated, the body at the same time being supported. The fragment should be held firmly in position by strapping or by a bandage of plaster of Paris carefully applied.

The retentive apparatus must be kept on for four weeks, on account of the action of the quadriceps extensor attached to the epiphysis. *Passive motion* may then be commenced.

In the majority of instances, however, the treatment will differ very considerably from that of fracture of the patella in its common form at about the age of seventeen; for in the former *operative measures* are imperative, otherwise the utility of the limb will be greatly impaired.

Under careful aseptic and antiseptic methods the upper end of the tibia should be exposed by means of a flap incision, and all blood-clot and shreddy tissue removed from the osseous surfaces. The tubercle should be firmly attached to the tibia by means of needles or pins, as in Landsberg's and Will's cases. In Will's case the result was most satisfactory, and it was thought that in no other way, apart from operation, could it have been obtained.

PROGNOSIS.—The result differs from that of fractured patella inasmuch as osseous union may always be expected if the fragments are brought well into apposition.

Mr. A. Shaw has recorded (*Path. Soc. Trans.* vol. v. 1853, p. 253) the case of a boy, aged seventeen, who fell and tore the tubercle, along with the ligamentum patellæ, from the tibia; the tubercle, being an epiphysis, had not been firmly united to the shaft. He thought it was owing to this and the immobility of the patella from spurious ankylosis that the violence directed on the front of the joint produced diastasis of this tubercle. Union occurred as in ordinary fracture.

In P. Vogt's case ('Ein Fall von Abreissung der Tuberositas tibiæ durch willkürliche Muskelcontraction,' *Berl. klin. Wochenschr.* 1869, vi. 225; (abstr.) *Deutsche Klinik*, Berl. 1869, xxi. 217) the patient was a gymnast sixteen years old. When about to jump over the vaulting horse he slipped, with his right foot on the spring-board, and endeavoured with a violent effort to save himself from falling backwards. This he succeeded in doing, but felt at the same time a sudden intense strain at the knee, and then observed that he was not able to put his foot forwards or to move from the place. Half an hour after the accident, there was found considerable effusion of blood into the right knee-joint, and there could be felt, six centimetres below the lower end of the patella, the apex of a triangular osseous fragment, the bone of which was two centimetres in extent, its inner margin perpendicular, and with an oblique edge; the apex was nearly two centimetres distant from the tibial crest. The fragment was movable laterally with crepitus. The patella was displaced upwards a distance of 2·5 centimetres. The limb was placed on an inclined plane, and a plaster-of-Paris bandage applied for five weeks. This was replaced during the next three weeks by a simple posterior splint. Towards the end of this time the tubercle of the tibia was still somewhat movable. A year afterwards there was firm osseous union of the tubercle and complete return of function in the limb, the only trace of injury being a small osseous projection one centimetre in height from the tibial crest.

Müller quotes a case (Bruns, *Beiträge*, iii. 1888, S. 261 ; *Wiener medicin. Blätter*, 1881, Nr. 51), observed by Weinlechner, of a student, aged seventeen years, who in jumping over a vaulting horse fell in such a manner as to rest upon the calf of his left leg. There was swelling of the knee-joint, and below the patella a movable piece of bone as large as a walnut. The treatment consisted in drawing the patella towards the tibia by means of a bandage and in the application of extension. Four weeks after the accident a silicate bandage was applied, which was removed after six weeks. Good use of the limb was re-established in this case.

Pitha saw a case ('Verletzungen und Krankheiten der Extremitäten,' *Handbuch der allg. u. speziell. Chirurgie*, von Pitha-Billroth, 1868, iv. Bd. 2 Abthlg. S. 268) many months after the accident ; the use of the leg was greatly impaired, a loose band only connecting the displaced tubercle with the tibia. He gives the following account. A guide (age not stated), while jumping a puddle, tried to save himself from falling backwards on the other side. The ligamentum patellæ was completely detached, and the tubercle of the tibia and the patella drawn upwards four fingers' breadth. A loose connection only united the quadriceps muscle with the tibia, and the whole extremity, particularly the quadriceps, was wasted. Walking was possible only with the aid of a stick and a strong knee-cap to the joint. An osteophytic outgrowth on the tibia indicated the locality of the detached bone.

F. Stabell ('Fractura Tuberositatis (spinæ) Tibiæ,' *Tidskr. f. prakt. Med.*, Kristiania, 1887, vii. 111–115, and *La Semaine Médicale*, 1887, No. 18) mentions the case of a 'young man' who, in making a 'dangerous leap,' suddenly felt a rupture at the level of the knee, and then found himself unable to hold himself upright. Beneath the skin below the knee a hard rounded body could be seen projecting. The patella was drawn upwards, and a detachment of the tibial tuberosity diagnosed. The fragment of bone was drawn downwards and held firmly in position by means of a silicate bandage. The ultimate result was that consolidation took place, and the patient obtained the perfect use of the limb.

In five examples out of nine which were treated in the recent condition, a perfect restoration of the use of the limb with firm union resulted in a longer or shorter period. In Müller's case the period was two months ; in Will's three months ; in Vogt's a year. In three cases the mode of union was said to have been an osseous one. In Pitha's case, seen for the first time several months after the accident, the tubercle was drawn up for four fingers' breadth and ununited.

CHAPTER VII

SEPARATION OF THE LOWER EPIPHYSIS OF THE TIBIA

ANATOMY.—The lower epiphysis of the tibia is developed from a single osseous nucleus, which appears in the centre of the horizontal portion of the cartilaginous extremity about the eighteenth month.

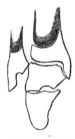

Fig. 258.—FRONTAL SECTION THROUGH THE LOWER END OF TIBIA AND FIBULA BEFORE BIRTH

(After Küstner)

During the second year nearly the whole of this portion of the epiphysis is ossified, and osseous granules appear in the malleolar portion and rapidly coalesce with the main nucleus.

By the fourteenth or fifteenth year the whole lower end of the tibia, comprising the internal malleolus and articular surfaces, is com-

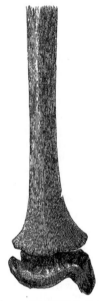

Fig. 259.—LOWER EPIPHYSIS OF THE TIBIA AT THE SIXTEENTH YEAR

Epiphysis removed to show the stellate appearance of its diaphysial surface (½-size)

pletely osseous. Its upper surface is more or less flat, and presents elevations and depressions of a somewhat peculiar arrangement, corresponding to similar irregularities on the lower end of the diaphysis. There are four prominent ridges, with depressions between, radiating in a stellate manner from a central point to each angle of this quadrilateral-shaped epiphysis. They are well marked at the sixteenth year. At this age the plate of bone is about three-eighths of an inch thick in the centre.

This epiphysis unites with the diaphysis in the eighteenth or nineteenth year. (Sixteenth to eighteenth year according to Sappey.).

Béclard has once seen and described a special centre for the internal malleolus immediately joining the principal portion, but the author has never seen a distinct epiphysis, and its occurrence must be extremely rare.

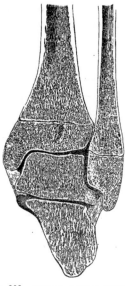

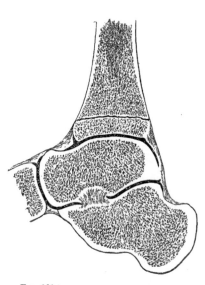

FIG. 260.—FRONTAL SECTION THROUGH THE BONES OF THE ANKLE-JOINT AT SEVENTEEN AND A HALF YEARS. POSTERIOR HALF OF SECTION. RELATION OF EPIPHYSIAL LINES TO THE SYNOVIAL MEMBRANES (⅔-size)

FIG. 261.—SAGITTAL SECTION THROUGH BONES OF THE ANKLE-JOINT AT SIXTEEN YEARS

On the outer side the epiphysial cartilage passes immediately above the inferior tibio-fibular joint, eight millimetres above the articulation of the ankle-joint, and comes in relation with the pouch-like extension upwards of the synovial membrane between the tibia and fibula, but is separated from it by the periosteum, continuous here with the epiphysis. In infants this synovial pouch of the inferior tibio-fibular joint is often but little marked.

Neither in front nor behind does the synovial membrane of the ankle-joint come in contact with the epiphysial line, although it overlaps the lower edge of the epiphysis a little in front. This holds good for children of younger or older age.

In front the epiphysial line is half an inch above the level of the ankle-joint, and posteriorly ⅝ inch. In the centre of the epiphysis it is only $\frac{3}{8}$ inch above the articular surface. On the outer side it is from $\frac{1}{4}$ to $\frac{5}{16}$ inch above this level from the fifteenth to eighteenth year.

On the inner side, from the apex of the internal malleolus, it is distant at the twelfth year about $\frac{5}{8}$ inch, at the fifteenth year about 1 inch, at the eighteenth year about $1\frac{1}{4}$ inch; while on the outer side it is above the apex of the external malleolus rather more than $\frac{7}{8}$ inch at the eighth year, $1\frac{1}{8}$ inch at the twelfth year, and at the eighteenth year $1\frac{3}{5}$ inch.

De Paoli gives the following table of measurements of the lower epiphysis of the tibia and the fibula in a frontal section (i.e. dividing them in halves, anterior and posterior).

AGE	TIBIA				FIBULA		
	Height			Maximum breadth	Height		Breadth
	At the internal malleolus	At the outer edge	At the middle		At the external malleolus	At the internal edge	
Before birth	11 mm.	2·5 mm.	3 mm.	16 mm.	13 mm.	3 mm.	9 mm.
1 year { Appearance of the osseous points in both bones }	13	3	5	21	12	7	10 ......
2	14	3·5	6	23	15	7	10 ......
4	14	5	7	25	13	6	10 ......
5	18	6	8	27	18	7	13 ......
5½	16	5	7	27	16	11	13 ......
6	18	5	9	29	15	12	13 ......
7	18	8	8	33	20	11	15 ......
8 { The ossification penetrates the base of the internal malleolus }	20	6	8	34	16	11	12 ......
	20	8	9	32	21	11	16 ......
9	20	6	7	31	16	11	11 .. ...
13	22	8	9	38	21	9	16 ......
14	24	8	11	38	19	16	17 ......
16 { The ossification reaches the lateral aspect of the tibia and the fibula }	....	....	....	....	20	15	16 ......
17	21	6	8	38	20	12	15 ......
20	22	9	9	40	25	13	15 ......

AGE.—The period between eleven and eighteen years appears to be the time in which this separation is most likely to occur.

Of twenty-two cases in which the separation was compound, or in which the limb had been amputated for extensive lesions of the soft parts, and thus the separation verified by direct examination, the age is known in eighteen and ranged from the ninth to the nineteenth year; sixteen were between the tenth and nineteenth years.

Of eleven specimens and cases *verified by direct examination*, the age is given in seven—viz. one at 19, one at 18, one at 17, one at 15, one at 13, one at 9, and one at 5 years of age.

The eleven *compound separations* were as follows: one case at 15, two at 14, four at 13, one at 11, and three at 10 years of age.

Of sixteen *simple separations*, ranging from three to seventeen years of age, we find that eleven were between the ages of eleven and seventeen years; one was at 17, two at 16, one at 14 and 9 months, two at 14, one at 13, one at 12, three at 11, three at 10, one at 6½, one at 6, and two at 5 years of age.

In *eight cases* of arrest of growth, the date of the injury producing it is stated in four—two at 10, and one each at 9 and 8 years of age.

Of the total *forty-six* cases the age is given in thirty-eight; of these, thirty took place between the ages of 9 and 17 years.

Fracture of the lower end of the fibula or separation of the epiphysis of the fibula is noted in twenty-three of the total (forty-six) recorded examples. In two of these combined lesions the age is not recorded, but of the remaining twenty-one the greatest number, fifteen, occurred between 10 and 15 years of age: viz. one at 19, one at 18, one at 17, two at 15, three at 14, four at 13, three at 11, three at 10 (two in females), one each at 9, 6, and 5 years. Distinguishing now between fracture of the fibula and separation of its epiphysis, we find twelve of the former and nine of the latter lesion; out of the former, eleven were between 9 and 17 years of age; while six of the latter were between 10 and 15 years of age.

The author has rejected the often-quoted cases described by Champion (*Journal complément. du Dict. des Sc. Méd.*, 1818, p. 325) and Carus (*Gem. Deutsche Zeitschr. f. Geburtskunde*, 1828, Bd. ii. 31), the former being one of separation of this epiphysis of the tibia in an infant, due to violent traction on the foot during parturition. In the other the injury was caused in a fœtus of four months by a fall of the mother upon the abdomen from a height. The diaphysis protruded through a wound at the inner ankle. Death took place on the thirteenth day after birth.

Other cases recorded of separation of this epiphysis by midwives during delivery are best omitted as untrustworthy.

SEX.—The injury mostly occurs in boys; all the seven pathological specimens in which the age is given occurred in males, and the same sex was noted in the whole of the eleven compound separations. The female sex has only been recorded in two instances of simple separation among the total forty-six cases mentioned above; both occurred at ten years of age, and were associated with solution of continuity of the fibula—one being a fracture, the other a separation of the lower end of this bone.

ETIOLOGY.—Indirect violence is the most common cause of separation of the lower epiphysis of the tibia.

It is commonly produced by the foot being fixed and the leg violently flexed or extended. The history often given is that the child, while in the act of jumping or climbing over a fence, has caught his toes and fallen forwards; or the foot has been fixed between a cart and the spokes of the wheel, and the leg violently twisted between the spokes. At other times the injury may result from a fall from a height on to the feet, the foot being doubled beneath; or the foot has been injured in the same manner by machinery, by being twisted by a ship's cable, or by a simple fall with the foot doubled beneath and forcibly extended or twisted on the leg. Again, a heavy blow on the side of the leg above the ankle may produce the same effect if the foot be firmly placed on the ground.

In two cases at Guy's Hospital the injury was caused by a fall, in one of them the patient falling down stairs and 'wrenching' his foot. This case of separation of the lower epiphysis of the tibia was under the care of Mr. Cooper Forster in January 1872, and the boy (W. D.) was aged twelve. The other was under the care of the same surgeon in April 1876, and was aged six years. Both were treated with wooden posterior splints, and left the hospital in between two and three weeks' time; there was good union, and the patients were able to walk without assistance.

The author cannot agree with the opinion that separation of the lower epiphysis of the tibia combined with fracture of the fibula, or with separation of the lower epiphysis of the fibula, may practically be said to take the place of Pott's fracture in young subjects, and may occur either from extreme inversion or eversion. The mechanism is not entirely of the same description, for in separation of the lower epiphysis of the tibia the foot and epiphysis are fixed, whilst the body is violently thrown to one side. Moreover, the amount of violence requisite to separate the lower epiphysis of the tibia is considerably greater than that causing Pott's fracture.

Severe twisting of the foot, however, may cause fracture of the fibula or separation of its lower epiphysis, combined with separation of a part of the tibial epiphysis; but in these instances the violence is never so great as that which produces separation of the whole of the tibial epiphysis with displacement.

Experimentally this epiphysis has been separated by forcible flexion.

M. Curtillet produced separation by letting a weight of fifty-seven kilogrammes fall on the sole of the foot of an amputated limb which rested by the tuberosities of the tibia firmly on the ground, thereby combining powerful flexion with vertical shock, analogous to that which is met with in a fall from a height on to the heels.

In Guéretin's experiments upon the ankle in infants and children, the fibular epiphysis was separated as well as that of the tibia.

The lower epiphyses of the tibia and fibula have a few times been separated during forcible straightening of very severe club foot (Helferich).

In his article, 'L'Entorse juxta-épiphysaire,' in the *Revue de Chirurgie*, t. i. 1881, pp. 795 and 797, Ollier gives two figures to represent the lesions of juxta-epiphysial sprain he has produced on the lower end of the tibia in infancy by forcible adduction and abduction of the foot. (See figs. 262 and 263.)

Direct violence has in a few examples separated the lower epiphysis of the tibia alone. Messrs. Durham, Howse, and Cooper Forster at Guy's Hospital had cases of separation of the lower epiphysis of the tibia, caused in the first two cases by the passage of a cart-wheel over the ankle, and in the third by the fall of some blocks of wood on to the leg, the foot being turned outwards.

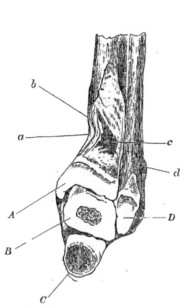 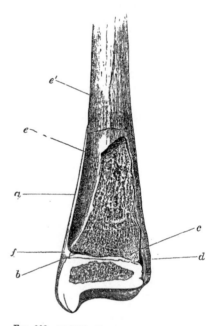

FIG. 262.—JUXTA-EPIPHYSIAL LESIONS PRO-DUCED BY FORCIBLE ADDUCTION OF THE FOOT. FROM A SLIGHTLY RACHITIC SUBJECT EIGHT MONTHS OLD

A, lower epiphysis of the tibia; B, astragalus; C, os calcis; D, lower epiphysis of the fibula; a, deep juxta-epiphysial notch at about one centimetre above the conjugal cartilage, the result of bending inwards of the compact tissue of diaphysis; the latter is covered in by the periosteum, b, which conceals it from sight, but does not prevent its being felt on pressure; c, site of trabecular fractures; d, bending of the fibula inwards. (After Ollier)

FIG. 263.—LESIONS OF THE TIBIA PRODUCED BY FORCIBLE ABDUCTION OF THE FOOT. OBLIQUE SECTION. FROM AN INFANT TWO YEARS OLD

a, periosteum on the inner aspect of the tibia, not lacerated, but detached from the bone; b, diaphysis separated from the epiphysis for one-third of its width; c, crushing and compression of the spongy tissue towards the outer aspect of the bone; d, periosteum on outer aspect of diaphysis; e, subperiosteal extravasation of blood extending up to e'; f, continuity of the periosteum with the conjugal cartilage. (After Ollier)

Their ages were respectively four (E. T., 1875), seven (C. P., 1885), and three years (T. H., 1879).

In another recorded example separation was the result of a fall of a wall on the ankle.

Direct violence is always the cause of the more severe forms of separation of the lower epiphysis of the tibia accompanied with displacement, and fracture of the lower end of the fibula, or separation of the lower fibular epiphysis.

PATHOLOGICAL ANATOMY.—Separation of the lower epiphysis of the tibia alone is a much more rare form of injury in the living subject than separation of the lower epiphysis of the tibia with separation of the lower end of the fibula or with fracture of the lower part of the shaft. Yet in experiments on the dead subject separation of the lower epiphysis of the tibia is effected with the greatest ease, although the solution of continuity is often transversely through the diaphysis immediately above the conjugal line.

In the London Hospital Museum (*London Hospital Museum Catalogue*, 1890, p. 115, No. 506) a preparation has been made showing that in young persons fractures near to the extremities of the bones do not always follow the line of the epiphysis, being at the same time an instance of intra-periosteal fracture and of fracture with

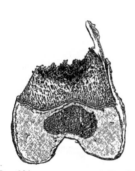

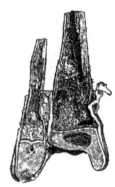

FIG. 264.—EXPERIMENTAL SPECIMEN (Royal College of Surgeons Museum, No. 1110B)

FIG. 265.—EXPERIMENTAL SPECIMEN (Royal College of Surgeons Museum, 1110B)

impaction. The tibia is fractured transversely half an inch above the junction of the epiphysis. The portion of bone between the epiphysial line and the fracture shows a vertical split about half an inch from the anterior surface, which extends, though less distinctly, through the epiphysis itself to the articular cartilage. The periosteum is everywhere entire, but the fibula is fractured four inches above the outer malleolus. The foot and lower fragment have been displaced forwards to a slight extent.

An experimental specimen in the Royal College of Surgeons Museum (No. 1110B) by Mr. Jonathan Hutchinson junior consists of the lower ends of the femur and of the bones of the leg from the same subject. The diaphysis of the femur has been broken across about three-quarters of an inch above the epiphysial disc. That of the tibia has been partially detached at the inner side from its disc, the fibula being broken within the periosteum somewhat higher up.

There is no displacement of the tibia, and the lesion is of the severe type of juxta-epiphysial sprain, while that of the femur is a fracture of the lower end of the diaphysis well above the epiphysial line, both of which forms of injury are commonly met with in experiments on bones of infants.

The lower epiphysis with the foot is often torn off at the epiphysial line in severe crushing accidents to the foot, &c.

There are three specimens in the London museums of separation of the lower tibial epiphysis. Two of them are accompanied by fracture of the diaphysis. The specimen in St. George's Hospital Museum, No. 56A, is described by Mr. Holmes (*Trans. Path. Soc.* xiii. p. 187), and has been already quoted (under LOWER EPIPHYSIS OF THE FEMUR). There was a compound separation of the lower epiphysis of the tibia, with fracture of a small part of the posterior aspect of the lower end of the diaphysis, one inch long and a quarter of an inch broad, and separation of both epiphyses of the fibula ; also detachment of the lower epiphysis of the femur, with laceration of the popliteal artery and fracture of the shaft of the tibia. Death occurred from pyæmia after amputation in this case of a boy, aged eighteen years. (See also Holmes, *Dis. of Children*, 2nd edit. 1869, p. 263, fig. 44.)

The preparation in the Museum of the Royal College of Surgeons of England (*Catalogue of the Museum of the Royal College of Surgeons of England*, vol. ii. p. 176, No. 1103) consists of portions of a tibia from a patient of Sir Astley Cooper. The lowest portion, which appears to be the separated lower end of the shaft, protruded and was sawn off. The other portions, it is probable, were afterwards exfoliated.

The London Hospital Museum contains a specimen of the lower epiphysis of the tibia and fibula, together with the upper two-thirds of the astragalus, which are said to have exfoliated after what was probably a compound separation of the epiphysis ; but no history was obtainable. Firm ankylosis of both malleoli to the articular surface of the astragalus has taken place.

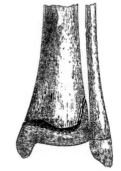

FIG. 266.—After Bruns, *Deutsche Chirurgie* ; *Die Lehre von den Knochenbrüchen*, 1886, S. 123

Separation with fracture of diaphysis. P. Bruns describes (Langenbeck's *Archiv für klin. Chirurg.* 1882, Bd. xxvii. S. 256) a case of separation of this epiphysis which occurred exactly through the epiphysial line, with the exception of the fracture of a small fragment of the outer edge of the diaphysis. Besides this there was a spiral fracture of the fibula and an oblique fracture of each thigh. Gangrene of both legs supervened, and death took place on the ninth day from pyæmia. The patient was a boy seventeen years old, whose legs had been caught between the spokes of a wagon-wheel (see fig. 266).

A more extensive fracture of the outer side of the diaphysis was found in a case reported and represented by Benjamin Anger (*Traité iconographique des Maladies Chirurgicales*, Paris, 1865, p. 18), whereas on the inner side the separation passed precisely through the epiphysial line. The accident occurred in a boy aged fifteen, whose leg was injured in a machine. The lower epiphysis of the fibula was also detached. The specimen is also figured by Nélaton in his *Éléments de Pathologie Chirurgicale.*

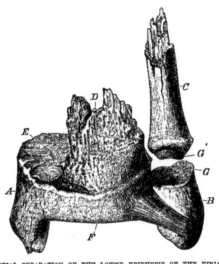

FIG. 267.—PARTIAL SEPARATION OF THE LOWER EPIPHYSIS OF THE TIBIA WITH FRAC-TURE OF THE DIAPHYSIS. SEPARATION OF THE LOWER EPIPHYSIS OF THE FIBULA

(After B. Anger) *A*, lower epiphysis of the tibia; *B*, lower epiphysis of the fibula; *C*, diaphysis of the fibula; *D*, portion of shaft of tibia; *E*, epiphysial separation at inner part; *F*, epiphysial line of tibia; *G*, epiphysial surface of the external malleolus; *G'*, end of the diaphysis of the fibula

E. E. Klein relates (Inaugural Dissertation, *Nonnulla de epiphysium dissolutione cum descriptione accuratiore casus ejus morbi in inferiori tibiæ epiphysi observati*, Gryphiæ, 1854) the case of a youth, aged thirteen years, who was injured by a threshing machine. There was complete separation of the lower epiphysis of the tibia, but this was accompanied by splintering and fracture of the lower end of the diaphysis, as well as by a fracture of the lower end of the fibula. Amputation of the thigh was performed on account of compound fracture of the upper part of the tibia, and was followed by death from collapse three-quarters of an hour afterwards.

In Dr. Wade's case, reported by R. W. Smith (*Dublin Quarterly Journal*, 1852, vol. xiii. p. 202), the fracture of the diaphysis was more complicated and somewhat comminuted. A large triangular portion of it was detached, and several fractures extended upwards for two or three inches. Into one of these longitudinal fractures some muscular fibres were found to be wedged. The separation of the lower epiphysis of the tibia was complete, and the fibula was fractured two inches from its lower extremity, but still retained its convexity outwards on account of the dovetailing of the extremities of the fragments. The patient, a boy, aged nine years, was injured by a portion of a wall falling on his left leg, producing a large wound of the front of the leg two inches above the ankle-joint, exposing the extensor tendons and severely injuring the soft parts. There was also free hæmorrhage; therefore primary amputation was performed. Shortening of the leg with inversion of the foot was noted at the time.

Fracture of the end of the shaft is noted in Hutchinson's case quoted below.

COMPOUND SEPARATIONS.—In eight out of thirteen cases of compound separation, the epiphysis was found on examination of the fragments to be completely and cleanly detached ; but five were combined with a fracture of the diaphysis of a greater or less extent, sometimes consisting merely of a thin flake of one or other edge of the diaphysial end.

Pure separation.—In other examples of compound separation the detachment has been found to be quite clean at the epiphysial line.

The protruded diaphysis, stripped of its periosteum for one or more inches, and devoid of cartilage, can in such cases be readily recognised by reason of the peculiar character of its rounded extremity—the stellate or radiating projections which have been already described.

Dr. Stephen C. Martin mentions (*Boston Medical and Surgical Journal*, September 27, 1877, p. 364) that he recognised this stellate radiation of the end of the diaphysis; which was perfect, after he had removed the dirt which was packed in between the irregularities of this surface. No portion whatever of the shaft was broken off ; the case was one of separation of the epiphysis purely. The case was that of a boy, aged eleven; who fell from the top of a telegraph pole, and produced a compound separation of the lower epiphysis of the tibia, with protrusion of the diaphysis through the wound on the inner side of the leg. It had been thrust into the hard frozen earth, and was much soiled with dirt. The periosteum was stripped from the shaft for a distance of about an inch and three-quarters on the outer side; and the fibula was fractured four inches above its lower end. After some difficulty reduction was effected by enlarging the wound. The wound healed slowly after ·three small pieces of bone had come away, and complete recovery took place in two months; with perfect restoration of the functions of the limb, so that the boy was about as usual.

Agnew (*Surgery*, 1878, vol. i. p. 991; vol. ii. p. 30, fig. 909)

3 II

figures and mentions a case of compound separation of the lower tibial epiphysis with displacement outwards of the foot, the diaphysis protruding some distance through the wound on the inner side of the leg. The patient, a lad ten years of age, was admitted into the Pennsylvania Hospital in 1876.

Spence figures (*Lectures on Surgery*, 2nd edit. 1875, vol. i. plate xiv. p. 288) a case sketched from nature of compound diastasis of the bones of the leg which was under his care at the Royal Infirmary, Edinburgh.

The tibia was separated from its lower epiphysis, stripped of its periosteum, and projected for the lower two-thirds of its extent, the soft parts being extensively lacerated. The posterior tibial vessels and nerve are seen torn and twisted. Primary amputation was performed.

Fracture of the fibula, or separation of the lower epiphysis of the same bone.—A more frequent complication of compound separation is that of fracture of the fibula an inch or more above the epiphysial line ; it has been noted in seven cases ; in three of these combined with displacement *outwards* of the tibial epiphysis. Outward displacement may occur, however, without fracture of the fibula, as in Clark's second case (just mentioned).

In Fischer and Hirschfeld's case of separation of the upper epiphysis of the tibia, the lower epiphyses of the tibia and fibula were found at the autopsy to be torn away close to the epiphysial line.

In Wade's and in Klein's cases the fibula was fractured at the lower end. In Bruns's case the fracture of the fibula was a spiral one, and accompanied by fracture of both femora. In Clark's case the patella was fractured two inches above the tip of the external malleolus. In Martin's case the fracture of the fibula was four inches from its lower end.

W. A. Albee reports a case in a boy, aged thirteen (*Transactions of the Maine Medical Association*, Portland, U.S.A. 1886, ix. pt. i. pp. 117–120) of compound separation of this epiphysis with fracture of the fibula. The author has, however, been unable to obtain the account of this case.

Separation of the lower fibular epiphysis was also found in Annandale's case. The injury in this instance was compound, the end of the diaphysis of the tibia protruding on the inner side.

Displacement of epiphysis outwards with fracture of the fibula.— Among compound separations displacement most frequently takes place outwards off the diaphysis. Its complete displacement in this direction can only be caused by great violence, producing severe injury to the soft parts.

Where the displacement outwards is not so complete, the diaphysis of the fibula is also fractured transversely from one to two inches above the tip of its malleolus. The fracture occurred in three out of four cases of this form of displacement. By reason of the lower part of the fibula below the fracture retaining its normal relation to the tibial epiphysis, the inferior tibio-fibular and ankle-joints escape injury. The anterior and posterior tibial vessels and nerves usually remain uninjured.

Fracture of the fibula is mentioned in Wade's and Kleiñ's cases of compound separation quoted above.

Mr. Bryant (*Practice of Surgery*, 4th edit. 1884, vol. ii. p. 354) mentions a case of compound separation of the lower epiphysis of the right tibia with outward displacement of the foot. William D., aged fifteen years, while getting into a van in motion, slipped and caught his leg between the spokes of the wheel. The leg was squeezed between these and the under part of the spring. He was able to withdraw the foot while the wheel was revolving, but could not stand. There was a transverse gaping wound five inches long on the inner side of the ankle, laceration of the deeper structures, and exposure of the tendons behind the internal malleolus. Through the wound the diaphysis protruded for over an inch, the epiphysis with the foot being displaced outwards. The fibula was fractured two inches above the malleolus, but the tibial vessels and nerves and ankle-joint were intact. The epiphysis was easily replaced under chloroform, and the foot and leg put up in splints. At the time of replacement it was thought that some flakes of the epiphysial cartilage were attached to the diaphysial end.

The author had the opportunity of seeing this case, and of observing the good recovery which followed; the patient left the hospital at the end of three months with good movement in the ankle-joint.

Mr. Cooper Forster had under his care at Guy's Hospital in January 1872 a boy (Robert F.), aged thirteen, who had been run over by a hansom cab, the wheel passing over his right ankle.

The lower end of the tibial diaphysis, torn from the epiphysis, projected for about one inch through a rent in the skin. The foot was much displaced and the fibula fractured one to two inches above the malleolus. The tibial arteries pulsated below. An inch of the lower end of the tibia had to be sawn off before reduction could be effected. He left the hospital at the end of six months with a perfectly sound limb.

Mr. H. E. Clark gives a detailed account (*Glasgow Medical Journal*, vol. xxvi. November 1886, p. 329) of a somewhat similar case. John McG., aged thirteen, was admitted into the Royal Infirmary on August 16, 1884, with what was at first supposed to be a compound dislocation of the left ankle. He stated that a sheet of iron fell forwards and struck him on the inner side of the leg. On examination there was found to be a wound, about two inches in diameter, and much lacerated, through which protruded the end of the shaft of the tibia. The end of the bone was rounded, and had the character of a diaphysis from which the epiphysis had been separated, but showed no appearance of fracture. The periosteum was completely stripped off the bone for about two inches from the end on the inner surface, and somewhat less on the outer. The ankle-joint was uninjured, as also were the tibial arteries and nerves. The fibula was fractured about two inches above the tip of the malleolus. It was found necessary to resect about three-quarters of an inch of the diaphysis before it was possible to reduce the deformity. The wound was dressed antiseptically, but suppuration ensued, and healing took place by granulation. The patient was discharged from the hospital on December 28, a sinus still remaining. The cicatrix broke down a little the following September, and again in July 1886. At the latter time the right tibia measured 30·5 centimetres, and the left 28·5, showing a shortening of two centimetres—about the amount of the resected diaphysis. It would appear, therefore, that there had been no arrest of growth of the limb during the year and ten months since the accident, and this was the more evident as the lad had himself grown considerably in height in the interval. The movements of the ankle-joint were perfect, and the patient could use the limb with every freedom, and could put all his weight on it.

In Martin's case the diaphysial end of the tibia protruded on the inner side and the foot was displaced outwards, the separation, which was entirely a pure one, being accompanied by fracture of the fibula about four inches from its lower extremity.

Displacement of epiphysis outwards with separation of the lower epiphysis of the fibula.—Dr. C. A. Sturrock says (*Edinburgh Hospital Reports*, vol. ii. 1894, p. 606) that Professor Annandale had had at least four cases under his care, two being simple and two compound. The following are the notes of one of these. The displacement of the epiphysis was outwards, and accompanied with separation of the lower fibular epiphysis.

A boy ten years of age, when climbing a railing, slipped, and was suspended from the railing by his left foot, remaining hanging in this position until removed. He was seen a few hours after the accident, when a lacerated wound, two inches in length, was observed over the internal malleolus, through which protruded (for two inches) the lower end of the shaft of the tibia partially stripped of periosteum; the epiphysis of the lower end of the fibula was also separated and the ankle-joint opened. A counter-opening was made over the outer ankle after the parts had been replaced in position, and a drainage tube was passed through the wounds. The patient made a good but tedious recovery. Eight years after the accident Dr. Sturrock found the ankle considerably thickened and two inches of shortening in the leg; but the movements at the ankle-joint were not impaired. The patient could walk eighteen miles, and had cycled fifty miles in a day without fatigue. The injured leg felt the stronger of the two.

Displacement of epiphysis outwards without fracture of fibula.—In other instances in which this form of displacement is not so marked the fibula is not broken.

Mr. H. E. Clark records a second case (*loc. cit. supra*, p. 330) of compound separation in which there was this absence of fracture of the fibula. J. W., aged thirteen years, was admitted on December 29, 1885, with what was believed to be a compound dislocation of the ankle. As he was standing on a tramway in a mine, with his foot resting on the sleeper and supporting the weight of his body, a truck came up and struck him on the outer side of his left leg about the middle. The diaphysial end was found to be forced through the skin, making a wound (two by one and a half inches) on the inner side of the leg just above the ankle. The periosteum was stripped off the diaphysis for about an inch and much lacerated. The ankle-joint was not implicated. The fibula was not broken, nor was there any separation of its lower epiphysis. Corrosive sublimate dressings were employed and side splints applied. The wound healed with a little suppuration, and the patient was dismissed on February 2 with an excellent limb. The movements of the ankle-joint were then perfect, and there was no measurable shortening.

Displacement of the epiphysis outwards with fracture of the diaphysis.—Mr. G. A. Wright, of Manchester (*Diseases of Children, Medical and Surgical*, Ashby and Wright, 2nd edit. 1892, p. 707) has seen a remarkable case of separation of the lower epiphysis of the tibia in a boy of about ten years, who was under the care of his colleague Mr. Hardie. The case was complicated by the presence of a vertical fracture running upwards from the epiphysial line. The foot and lower fragment were displaced outwards, and the deformity could not be reduced until some weeks after the accident, when the ends of the bone were exposed by operation and with some difficulty replaced. The case was still under treatment.

Displacement of epiphysis inwards.—Mr. Bryant had a boy (Chas. S.), aged fourteen, under his care at Guy's Hospital in September of 1887, in whom compound separation of this epiphysis was accompanied by great displacement of the foot inwards. The boy, in climbing over an iron fence, fell towards the opposite side; his left foot remained fixed between two rails, and received the whole weight of his body. The tibia protruded for nearly one inch through the wound on the inner side, which measured about two and a half inches transversely. The periosteum was stripped off the end of the tibia, and the lower epiphysis of the fibula was thought to have been separated. Reduction was easily accomplished by enlarging the wound. The wound rapidly healed with little suppuration, and the patient left the hospital in two months' time quite recovered.

The foot is described as *inverted* and the leg shortened in Wade's case (already described).

Displacement backwards of the lower epiphyses of the tibia and fibula.—A case of symmetrical separation of the lower epiphyses of the tibia and fibula is related by Mr. Jonathan Hutchinson (*Lancet*, 1875, vol. i. June 19, p. 857). A sailor, aged nineteen, was admitted into the London Hospital, having fallen a distance of twenty to thirty feet on to the ship's deck, alighting heavily on his feet. On examination there was a lacerated wound (three inches long) on the inner side of the right foot. The os calcis was comminuted, and the tibia and fibula fractured just above the ankle. On the left side there were similar fractures of the tibia and fibula, and the fracture of the os calcis was a simple one. Both feet were displaced backwards, carrying with them the lower ends of the tibia and fibula. Reduction was easily effected, and a good position was maintained by outside splints with foot pieces. On the sixth day erysipelas of the right leg set in, and on the eighth day a large slough was removed from the left leg. Death took place on the tenth day.

At the autopsy the right os calcis was comminuted, and the scaphoid fractured vertically. The lower epiphysis of the tibia was separated from the shaft and accompanied by a slightly irregular line of fracture. The fibula was fractured through the malleolus. On the left side the os calcis was even more comminuted than the right, and the lower epiphyses of the tibia and fibula were separated from their respective shafts exactly at the epiphysial line, but remained connected with one another. There was also considerable extravasation of blood in front of the spine and behind the peritoneum, extending along the left psoas muscle; but no fracture was found to account for this. The lungs were studded with tubercle, and completely adherent to the chest wall.

Besides the case just quoted, separation of the lower fibular epiphysis was found in one of Bryant's cases of displacement inwards, and in that of Anger mentioned above.

Articular lesions.—From the proximity of the synovial membrane of the ankle-joint to the epiphysial line, it would at first sight appear that the articular cavity will probably be opened. But it escapes any gross injury, even at the inferior tibio-fibular mortice, by reason of the periosteum attached to, and continuous with, the epiphysis.

This immunity of the ankle-joint has often been noted in cases of compound separation, but effusion of blood into its cavity is a constant sign from some minor lesion.

The joint was opened in Annandale's case of compound separation of the epiphyses of fibula and tibia.

Injury to vessels and nerves.—The anterior and posterior tibial vessels escape injury in a remarkable manner, even in the most complicated and compound cases.

In Wade's case, besides the severe injury to the soft parts, there was also free hæmorrhage, for which reason primary amputation was performed; but no mention is made of the vessels which were injured.

Detachment of periosteum.—Stripping off of the periosteum from the protruding diaphysis in cases of compound separation is a constant lesion; it occurs chiefly, but not exclusively, from the side of the diaphysis opposite to the displacement of the epiphysis.

In one of Clark's cases as well as in others already quoted, this detachment of the periosteum did not in any way interfere with the good result which followed.

Although in many of the examples related above there was more or less splintering or fracture of the diaphysis, the epiphysis seems to escape injury.

LATER COMPLICATIONS.—**Acute periostitis** need not necessarily follow, even though there be suppuration of the wound.

Necrosis.—In spite of the extensive separation of the periosteum in compound injuries, there does not appear to be much risk of subsequent necrosis, although Dr. Voss, of New York, relates a case (*New York Medical Journal*, vol. ii. 1865-6, p. 133) in which this is said to have taken place.

The separation of the lower end of the tibia occurred in a boy, about fourteen years of age, who fell down from the first story of a house, and caught his foot between two pieces of wood. The upper fragment, protruding through the skin, was reduced, and the limb was placed on a double-inclined plane. A portion of the epiphysis (?) became necrosed and was afterwards removed, but the boy finally recovered with a useful joint.

In Martin's case, also, of compound separation, three very small pieces of bone were discharged from the wound some weeks after the injury.

Gangrene.—Krackowizer reports (*American Medical Times*, November 7, 1863) a case of supposed traumatic separation of the lower epiphysis of the tibia in a boy, aged five. The limb became gangrenous from tight bandaging, and the lesion was detected only after amputation.

SYMPTOMS.—Professor R. W. Smith, in his address to the British Medical Association at Dublin in 1867 (*British Medical Journal*, 1867, vol. ii. p. 122), states that this is undoubtedly among the rarest of this class of epiphysial injuries.

The recorded cases of simple separation are certainly very few.

J. Hutchinson junior has collected seventeen recent cases.

In Champion's case (*loc. cit. supra*, p. 325) of separation of this epiphysis, brought about by violent traction by the midwife during delivery, no autopsy was made, and in other respects it is a very doubtful case. But few details are given, with the exception that the foot, with the epiphysis, was displaced forwards, and after reduction the thumb could be placed in a large gap at the seat of detachment.

Swelling.—If the patient be seen immediately after the accident, this sign may be but little marked; but soon considerable swelling about the ankle-joint will ensue from effusion of blood, caused by laceration of vessels by the edge of the diaphysis, and synovial effusion of blood into the joint cavity itself.

Crepitus is usually absent, especially in cases of displacement backwards where the lower epiphysis of the fibula is also separated, while the ankle-joint, when uninjured, may be moved freely and smoothly below this point.

Mobility about one inch above the flexure of the ankle-joint, in the neighbourhood of the epiphysial line, is a more trustworthy sign.

Mr. F. M. Corner relates (*Med. Times and Gazette*, vol. i. 1859, March 5, p. 239) a case which was diagnosed at the Poplar Hospital as one of separation of the lower epiphysis of the tibia and fibula. A boy, aged fourteen years and nine months, fell off the tail-board of a cart and alighted on his feet, the injured foot turning inwards.

The symptoms were great swelling about the ankle-joint and a deformity looking like dislocation of the foot backwards, the os calcis being drawn upwards and backwards. On tracing the spine of the tibia, a depression was felt for one inch to an inch and a half above the ankle-joint, and some motion at this part was noticed on pretty forcible manipulation, but no crepitus; the external malleolus pointed more posteriorly than on the opposite side. The displacement was reduced, and the limb placed in a suitable splint on the outer side in the flexed position.

Deformity is the most marked sign. Rognetta quotes M. A. Severino as having seen this injury in two boys, followed by extroversion of the foot, the foot being thus in the valgus position. The injuries were not verified by anatomical examination. It is remarkable that in all the four recorded cases of simple separation the displacement of the foot with the tibial epiphysis was *backwards*. The internal malleolus preserves its normal relations with the foot, but not with the rest of the leg or external malleolus. There is a depression just above the ankle-joint and below the projection forwards of the tibia.

In Dr. R. W. Smith's case (*British Medical Journal*, 1867, August 17; *Dublin Hospital Gazette*, vol. vii. 1860, October 1, p. 289; *Proceedings of the Pathological Society of Dublin*, N.S. vol. i. 1862, p. 130) the diagnosis made was that of separation of the lower epiphysis of the tibia and *partial displacement backwards* with the foot. The subject of it was a boy, aged about sixteen years, who fell, while leaping, with his right foot violently doubled under him and forcibly extended on the leg. He was admitted into the Richmond Hospital under the care of Mr. Adams. On examination six weeks after the accident it looked at first sight like a case of dislocation of the lower end of the tibia forwards. The curve of the tendo Achillis was greatly increased, and the lower end of the tibia seemed to form a considerable projection in front of the normal position of the ankle-joint. The foot was a little extended upon the leg when at rest, but the boy had the power of flexing it, and when standing up he was able to place the sole flat on the ground. The fibula was uninjured. Flexion and extension of the foot could be performed. A very short examination was sufficient to show that the injury was not a luxation of the tibia forwards at the ankle. The integrity of the fibula, the freedom with which the perfect application of the sole of the foot to the ground in walking was carried out, were both circumstances opposed to the idea of a true dislocation existing. The internal malleolus was placed further back than natural, being on a plane posterior to the margin of the projecting portion of the tibia, which was rough and unlike the sharpness of a fracture, or the smooth outline of the edge of the articular surface of the tibia. The distance between it and the tubercle of the tibia was a quarter of an inch or more shorter than that between the tubercle and the articular margin of the opposite tibia. From all these conditions, together with the age of the patient and the nature of the accident, it was inferred that the injury consisted in a separation of the lower epiphysis of the tibia, and partial displacement of this process backwards with the joint. The internal malleolus preserved its normal relations with the foot, but not with the leg or outer ankle ; whereas in the case of luxation of the lower end of the tibia the normal bearings of the inner ankle to the foot were lost, while those to the leg were preserved.

The parts had become so fixed in their abnormal position that no attempt was made to replace them. A cast of the injury was preserved in the Museum of the Richmond Hospital.

Mr. Richard Quain published a similar case (*British Medical Journal*, 1867, vol. ii. August 31, p. 180 ; *Biennial Retrospect of Medicine and Surgery*, 1867-8, p. 257), in which, however, the diagnosis was made soon after the accident. On October 22, 1851, a healthy-looking lad, seventeen years of age, was admitted into University College Hospital, having a short time before slipped in the street and fallen with his foot doubled under him. The tibia projected forwards below, and between the prominence and the foot there was a depression. This projection was one and a half inches higher than the lower margin of the fibula, and three-quarters of an inch above the lower edge of the malleolar process of the tibia. The distance between the prominent tibia and the end of the great toe was three-quarters of an inch less than on the sound side. The ankle-joint was uninjured. Two points were considered as diagnostic—viz. (1) the end of the displaced tibia was rounded, smooth, and, as it were, rugous, very unlike the hard, angular, almost sharp feel of actual broken bone, and corresponding to the line of the epiphysial junction ; and (2) there was an absence of the soft swelling which surrounds the broken ends of bone where any displacement exists. The deformity was easily reduced, and was maintained in position by means of a starch splint.

In many of the cases of backward displacement there is *separation of lower epiphysis of fibula* as well. The continuity of the diaphysis of the fibula is lost at the ankle-joint, and an irregularity or depression may be felt just above the extended malleolus.

An instance of separation of the lower epiphyses of the tibia and fibula was diagnosed by Mr. Adams at the London Hospital (*Med. Times and Gazette,* vol. i. 1859, p. 163).

The subject in this case was a boy, aged fourteen, who, when jumping off a bar of iron, caught his toes and fell forwards with great violence. The signs were well marked, as the boy was seen directly after the accident. The lower epiphyses of the tibia and fibula were displaced off their respective shafts and dragged *backwards* with the foot, the projection forwards of the lower end of the tibial shaft being considerable. Reduction was effected with some difficulty, and splints applied. Much swelling subsequently ensued, but recovery took place with firm union.

In Corner's case just quoted, and in Hutchinson's, of separations of both epiphyses the displacement was backwards.

The following cases were treated at Guy's Hospital, and appear to have been unaccompanied by much displacement, although there existed separation of both epiphyses.

No. 1. William W., aged eleven years, under the care of Mr. Durham, October 1874. Whilst riding behind a cart his right leg was caught in the spokes of the wheel, and the lower epiphyses of the tibia and fibula were separated. Treatment: posterior and lateral splints.

No. 2. Alice B., aged ten years, under the care of Mr. Durham, March 11, 1875. She caught her right foot in a step, and twisted her leg under her, separating the lower epiphyses of the tibia and fibula. There was some swelling about the ankle. Treatment: lateral splints. Discharged from hospital April 7, able to walk very well.

No. 3. George S., aged eleven years, under the care of Mr. Birkett, April 21, 1874. Fell from a cart, with his foot caught in the 'tail'-board. He was unable to walk after the accident. The ower epiphyses of the tibia and fibula were separated, with very slight displacement.

No. 4. Daniel R., aged five years, under the care of Mr. Birkett, April 21, 1873. A truck fell on his ankle, causing separation of lower epiphyses of the left tibia and fibula, and severe contusion of the ankle. Treatment: suspension of leg on an interrupted sling.

In other simple separations the fibula has given way in its lower third, somewhere above the epiphysial line.

Mr. Durham made the diagnosis of *fracture of the lower end of the fibula, with separation of the lower epiphysis of the tibia,* in two patients under his care at Guy's Hospital in 1885. Their ages were respectively thirteen and six years of age. In the former case the boy (David D.) fell towards the outer side of his leg, his foot being fixed among some timber. The lesion was accompanied by considerable contusion over the ankle and the lower end of fibula. There was but little deformity, the sole of the foot was everted, and there was no shortening. Under chloroform the foot was replaced in good position and fixed on a back splint reaching above the knee. Three weeks later a. 'Croft's' plaster dressing was applied, and a few days afterwards he was discharged with the foot in good position, and with very little callus to be felt at the seat of fracture. In the latter case the patient (Charles R.) had a truck fall on his right leg, causing considerable contusion about the malleoli and lower part of the leg, and a small wound one inch above the internal malleolus, which, however, did not apparently communicate with the separation. A back splint was applied, and he left the hospital a few weeks later without any deformity of the foot, with a 'Croft's' dressing.

Mr. Cooper Forster, at Guy's Hospital in January 1876, diagnosed a fracture of the *external malleolus and separation of the lower epiphysis of the tibia* in a boy (Henry W.), aged fourteen, who had his right foot caught between the spokes of a wheel in rapid motion. It was treated by posterior and lateral splints with a good result.

A case came under the author's care at the Miller Hospital, December 3, 1895, in a boy, aged eleven years, in which there was a partial separation of the lower tibial epiphysis with fracture of the diaphysis, with very little displacement, but accompanied by fracture of the fibula.

The accident happened while the patient was swinging on a gate. He slipped and fell with his foot under the gate, by which it was squeezed, and in trying to extricate his foot he twisted it. There was intense pain at the left ankle, with swelling and ecchymosis around it, extending halfway up the leg, and inability to use the leg. The fibula was fractured about two inches above the tip of the external malleolus without displacement. There was mobility and crepitus precisely at the level of the epiphysial line of the tibia, eleven-sixteenths of an inch above the apex of the malleolus. The crepitus was of a dry character on account of the separation of the lower epiphysis being a partial one, accompanied by a fracture of the outer part of the end of the diaphysis. There was very little displacement; a slight ridge of the lower tibial diaphysis only could be felt in front above the ankle at the epiphysial level. The slight displacement was reduced, and the leg kept for two weeks upon a posterior splint with a foot-piece. The patient left the hospital with a starch bandage. The fragments were in good position, swelling and deformity absent, and the movements of the ankle-joint perfectly free.

Displacement outwards of foot.— Separation at the epiphysial junction will allow but slight displacement of the fragment, indicated by some amount of eversion of the foot, unless the fibula be fractured or its lower epiphysis separated.

Some displacement outwards of the foot was noticed in a case at Guy's Hospital under the care of Mr. Cooper Forster in March 1879. James B., aged sixteen years, fell a height of five feet with his left foot under him. He was unable to walk after the accident. There was found a separation of the lower epiphysis of the tibia, with slight displacement outwards of the foot and much swelling about the ankle.

Eversion of the foot was marked in one of Mr. Durham's cases, associated with fracture of the fibula.

Displacement outwards of the foot has already been often alluded to among compound separations.

Mr. Bryant mentions that he had seen an example of this kind which was not compound.

SEPARATION WITHOUT DEFORMITY.—On the other hand, a large number of cases have been diagnosed as separations in which there was but little displacement ; in some there has been none at all.

Abnormal mobility above the ankle-joint and characteristic **soft crepitus**, together with the history of the injury and the age of the patient, are the chief points for guidance.

Mr. Birkett had the following case under his care at Guy's Hospital in July 1872.

Fred M., aged twelve, in endeavouring to walk along the top of a fence, fell, his left foot being caught between two of the rails. The separation of the lower epiphysis of the tibia which was found did not cause any deformity, but there was considerable contusion over the internal malleolus. The injury was treated by a long outside splint to the leg with a foot-piece, and the patient left the hospital between three and four weeks afterwards with a good limb.

Mr. Durham, in June 1873, had an almost similar case of separation with little or no displacement in a boy (Charles H.), aged six and a half, who had fallen whilst climbing on some palings. Posterior and lateral splints were used, and he left the hospital five weeks later able to walk well.

A third case was seen by Mr. Hilton in February 1869, in which the separation of the epiphysis of the right tibia was associated with very little displacement. The patient (Patrick G.) was aged five, and was treated by means of a starch bandage.

In other instances in infancy the separation is only partial, and more often of the nature described by Ollier under ' Juxta-epiphysial sprain.' For the symptoms associated with this the reader is referred to Part I. Chapter VII.

DIAGNOSIS. Compound dislocation.—It is quite possible that even compound separation may be mistaken for compound dislocation of the ankle, as indeed has happened in several cases—a mistake liable to be followed by very serious consequences if not detected. The somewhat rounded edge of the projecting diaphysis, with its mammillated surface and devoid of periosteum, should be sufficient to distinguish it from the cartilaginous articular surface of the tibia. Besides, in epiphysial separation the movements of the ankle-joint are free.

In Clark's case of compound separation accompanied by fracture of the fibula the injury was at first supposed to be a compound dislocation of the ankle.

Dislocation of the ankle.—Simple cases with displacement are easy of diagnosis when seen directly after the accident, before any great amount of swelling occurs, yet they ·may also be confounded with dislocation of the ankle.

We should always remember that in youths of from eleven to seventeen years of age separation is much more likely to happen than dislocation. In the former, the transverse ridge of the projecting end of the diaphysis is liable to be mistaken for the articular end of the bone; in these also the joint is usually intact and movable. In *displacement backwards* of the epiphysis with the foot, the distances between the malleolus and the various prominences of the foot remain normal, while that between the projecting end of the tibia and the great toe is shortened. .

In dislocation of the foot backwards the end of the tibia projects· forwards, and the distance between it and the toe or the base of the first metatarsal bone is likewise shortened; but its internal malleolus, while losing its relations with the foot, retains them with the rest of the leg; that is, there is no interruption in the line of the tibial crest about an inch or so above the ankle-joint, and the outline of the lower end of the fibula is also intact and regular. If there is a question of the lower end of the fibula being detached as well, the relation between the tip of external malleolus and projecting base of the fifth metatarsal bone will be also altered.

Dislocation of the tibia forwards at the ankle might at first sight much resemble an old separation which had not been detected for some weeks after the date of the accident.

The integrity of the fibula, the freedom with which the motions of flexion and extension of the foot can be performed, the perfect application of the sole of the foot to the ground in walking, are all signs opposed to the existence of a dislocation; whereas in the dislocation forwards the normal bearings of the inner ankle to the foot are lost, while those to the leg are preserved.

Pott's fracture.—When the foot is *displaced outwards*, and the lower epiphysis of the fibula is separated or the lower end of the bone fractured, the diagnosis from a *Pott's fracture* may at first sight appear very difficult. The latter is not a common injury in children.

If there be only a little swelling and the injury be seen soon after the accident, the prominent smooth and rounded edge of the diaphysial end may be recognised on the inner side, while the internal malleolus and the whole of the lower end of the tibia preserve their relations with the foot and ankle-joint. Muffled crepitus may also be detected during the reduction of the displaced epiphysis. In Pott's fracture the tip of the internal malleolus is usually broken off, and may be felt to move with crepitus on the inner side.

Fracture of shaft of tibia.—The rounded, more or less smooth end of the displaced diaphysis in epiphysial separation is quite unlike the pointed and sharp end of an ordinary fracture, with its dry crepitus.

PROGNOSIS, RESULTS, &c. Union.—The prognosis is not at all unfavourable. In Adams's and other cases firm union took place.

M. A. Severino, a Neapolitan surgeon, was the first, in 1632, to notice the deformities of the knee and foot which result from separation of the upper and lower epiphyses of the tibia.

Deformity.—Even in compound cases there will be, with care, but little subsequent deformity; in one of Clark's cases of compound diastasis of the lower tibial epiphysis, at the end of five weeks the patient left the hospital with an excellent limb, the movements of the ankle-joint being perfect, and no measurable shortening having resulted.

In R. W. Smith's case, however, which was not seen until six months after the accident, the displacement forwards of the diaphysis had not been reduced, and gave rise to marked deformity.

Suppuration and necrosis of diaphysis.— In the recorded examples, in spite of the extensive separation of the periosteum, necrosis has seldom resulted. This, however, occurred in Voss's case.

Mr. Hutchinson alludes (*London Hospital Reports*, vol. i. 1864, p. 89) to the case of a boy (G. A.) under his care in the London Hospital in which there was considerable displacement of the lower end of the right tibia though the skin was not injured. An abscess formed, however, round the lower end of the shaft, and free incisions were made, exposing the bone, which was perfectly bare over a large extent. The correctness of the diagnosis was confirmed by observing the end of the bone in the wound. The end of the shaft subsequently necrosed, became loose, and was removed.

Arrest of growth of the tibia, and subsequent shortening of the limb, with deformity, after epiphysial separation has not been of common occurrence.

For instance, in one of Mr. H. E. Clark's cases careful measurements were taken for two years with negative results; indeed, the loss of length at the end of this time was only about equal to the size of the portion sawn off.

Being one of the two parallel bones, the overgrowth of the fibula causes great deformity of the ankle and foot. The fibula appears to be lengthened, much increased in thickness, if the injury has occurred in early childhood, and becomes bowed outwards. The foot becomes much inverted and acquires the varus position, the child walking on the outer side of the foot, and in extreme cases even on the outer side of the ankle.

Mr. Wood exhibited before the Pathological Society of London (*Path. Soc. Trans.* vol. xxxi. p. 249) a specimen of dwarfing of the tibia after separation of the lower epiphysis.

Bouchut (*Traité pratique des maladies des nouveau-nés*, 5ème édit. Paris, 1867, p. 898) observed an arrest of growth in the bone after fracture of the lower epiphysis of the tibia, whilst the uninjured fibula continued to grow and produced a varus condition of the foot. M. Nélaton thought that the callus produced in the repair was the cause of the arrest of growth in length of the bone.

Mr. Davies-Colley showed before a meeting of the Medical Society (*Brit. Med. Journal,* vol. i. 1888) the case of a girl (Susan G.) who had come under his care on November 7, 1881. At ten years of age she was said to have fractured her left tibia and ruptured the internal lateral ligament. For this she was treated at St. Thomas's Hospital, and discharged as cured after forty-four days. When she first came under Mr. Davies-Colley's notice there was great prominence of the external malleolus, and the internal malleolus was small, flat, and high with respect to the external. There was one inch shortening, and the child suffered pain below the external malleolus and walked on the outer border of the foot. As the deformity was increasing, Mr. Davies-Colley on November 11 (under ether) removed one inch of the fibula, and divided the tibia subcutaneously. On April 4, 1884, he operated a second time, removing a wedge from the tibia. When seen on February 21, 1887, the patient could walk well, but still on the outer side of her boot.

At the same meeting Mr. William Rose alluded to another case of a boy with fracture of the leg above the internal malleolus. The boy subsequently returned to the hospital with marked deformity and inversion of the foot, in consequence of the growth of the fibula and the arrest of growth of the tibia. The surgeon removed an inch and a half of the fibula and thus restored the symmetry of the limb.

Mr. Jonathan Hutchinson alludes (*Med. Press and Circular,* November 18, 1885) to the case of a boy who attended occasionally at the Royal College of Surgeons for examination purposes, in whom the deformity existed in the ankle from unsymmetrical growth of one of the bones after epiphysial injury.

Mr. Edmund Owen describes (*Lancet,* October 3, 1891, p. 767) the following case of arrested development of tibia. L. B., aged fourteen, was admitted to St. Mary's Hospital at the beginning of July on account of lameness due to inversion of the left foot. The clinical history shows that five years previously she fell whilst climbing over a gate, and that, catching her foot between the bars, she broke her leg just above the ankle. The line of fracture passed, apparently, across the junction cartilage of the tibia, and detached the lower epiphysis. The effect of this injury was to check the due growth of the tibia. Careful measurement showed the left tibia to be an inch and three-quarters shorter than the right, whilst the left fibula was shorter than the right by only three-quarters of an inch. (This arrested development of the fibula may have been due to its epiphysis having been damaged by the hurt, or to the restraining influence of the short tibia. The latter explanation is probably the correct one, for the lower end of the fibula was not only much curved but also greatly thickened.) The bowing of the fibula was outwards, the tibia playing the part of the bow-string. As the presence of the strong interosseous ligaments between the lower ends of the tibia and fibula would have prevented any improvement in the position of the foot following resection of a piece of the shaft of the fibula, and as the girl walked with fair comfort, Mr. Owen thought that no speculative interference with the bone seemed justifiable. She was therefore discharged with a clumsy-looking but useful leg and foot.

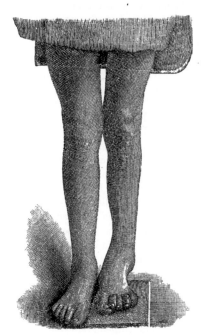

Fig. 268.—ARREST OF GROWTH OF TIBIA AND DEFORMITY (FIVE YEARS) AFTER INJURY TO THE LOWER TIBIAL EPIPHYSIS. PREVIOUS TO OPERATION

In the photograph from which the drawing was taken the shortened limb has been too much raised. (Author's case) .

The following most interesting case of deformity and arrest of growth following separation of the lower epiphysis of the tibia came under the author's care at the Miller Hospital in March 1891.

John M., aged thirteen years, had met with an injury to his leg five years previously, in 1886. He was climbing over some iron alings when he caught his foot in the top of the railings and fell over the opposite side, and hung by his foot. A lady passing released him and took him down. He was treated by wooden splints for some weeks, but did not bear any weight on that leg for four or five weeks. Some weeks after he had been walking about he felt the ankle weak, but it was not until some time later that the 'ankle began to grow out.' This steadily increased, getting much worse the last twelve months.

The boy now walked very lame, placing the outer margin of the left foot upon the ground, the foot being in a varus position. The whole leg was much wasted, the left calf being two and a quarter inches smaller in circumference than the right. The tibia was much smaller than that of the right leg, and measured exactly one inch less in length from the inner tuberosity to the internal malleolus than the right.

The fibula was much hypertrophied and uniformly enlarged, especially at the lower part, and very prominent, but with no sign of fracture. There was a very slight ridge and a concavity above the epiphysial line of the tibia, but no displacement. The patient complained of great weakness of the ankle without any particular pain. The movements of the ankle-joint were good.

In April, under chloroform, the author removed a wedge of bone from the fibula half an inch above the epiphysial line, and attempted to replace the foot in its normal attitude. The corrected position not being maintained, about a fortnight later the tibia was divided with a saw just above the epiphysial junction, and the deformity of the foot corrected by placing it in a valgus state and producing a depression at the seat of operation on the fibula. The limb was put in a Croft's splint. When seen some months later the position of the foot was much improved and the sole was flat on the ground. The patient was to wear a thick sole to his boot and a steel support to the inner side of his leg and ankle. Four years later, August 1895, the varus condition of the foot was almost corrected; but this was said to have increased slowly since the operation, and the statement was borne out by careful measurement, showing that the fibula had increased at a greater rate than the tibia. Notwithstanding the age of the patient, which was now nineteen years, it was proposed to remove the conjugal cartilage; therefore on August 1, 1895, the author operated upon the lower end of the fibula, and found only the remains of the conjugal disc twenty-five millimetres above the external malleolus as a very small nodule of cartilage at the anterior extremity of the line; the rest of the line could be traced as a thickened track in the cancellous tissue. The bone was very hard and sclerosed, as at the previous operation; it was then divided by a saw and a small piece removed. The gap left in the lower end of the bone permitted the external malleolus to be gradually everted.

Dr. H. E. Maberly, of Peckham, who saw the case immediately after the accident, kindly sent the author the following notes of the condition then present. 'The patient was brought to my house on November 29, 1886, directly after the accident. At the first glance I thought it was an ordinary case of fracture of the lower end of the fibula with very great displacement of the foot outwards, but on examination found that the displacement *was only apparent and not real*, the appearance being due to a very large effusion localised over the lower end of the tibia. There was no crepitus of any kind. The leg was put up in well-padded side splints, and when these

were removed on December 21 there was absolutely nothing to show
that he had ever met with any accident, and the boy soon began to
run about as usual.   It was only about a year ago (1890) I was told
that "his ankle was growing out." '

By a curious coincidence this patient's cousin, Thomas B., aged
ten, was in the Miller Hospital under the author's care two years
previously with simple separation of the lower tibial epiphysis, combined with fracture of the fibula, the injury having been caused in
precisely the same way—viz. climbing over a railing, getting his
foot fixed, and falling over.

An exactly similar deficiency of growth and deformity came
among the author's outpatients at the City Orthopædic Hospital in
March 1896.   In this case, however, the injury was to the diaphysis,
a transverse fracture above the epiphysial line.   The author's
colleague, Mr. Chas. Gordon Brodie, to whom he transferred the case,
showed it at the Clinical Society (*Lancet*, May 2, 1896, p. 1226 ;
Clinical Society's Transactions, vol. xxix. 1896, p. 252).   The
patient was a man, twenty-two years of age, who was admitted
into the Middlesex Hospital twelve years ago for a transverse
fracture of the tibia caused by the overturning of a hand-cart, which
snapped the bone above the ankle and caused a good deal of bruising
about the joint.   The patient was unable to recollect the precise
spot where the fracture occurred, but placed it well above the epiphysial line.   Examination showed that the end of the tibia was
dwarfed in its growth, with an inward curve of the lower fourth of
the bone, bringing the internal malleolus into strong relief, and
causing the tibio-fibular mortise to be inclined inwards slightly and
thus give the foot a list inwards.   No irregularity could be detected
along the anterior border of the tibia.   There was considerable
hypertrophy of the lower end of the fibula, while its subcutaneous
surface was marked by ridges, and projecting from the anterior
border of the malleolus was a large boss of bone, which made the
breadth one inch greater on this side than on the other.   In order
to compensate for the position the foot was thrown into by the
inclination of the mortise, there was well-marked valgus, the tubercle
of the scaphoid coming out strongly when the patient pressed his
foot on the ground.   Röntgen's rays revealed that there was
absolute continuity of the bone.

Mr. C. Mansell Moullin showed at the Clinical Society (*Lancet*,
February 1, 1896, p. 296 ; *Clinical Society's Transactions*, vol. xxix.
'1896' p. 235) a case in which impaired growth of the lower epiphysis and shaft of the tibia was consequent on a severe strain,
and was probably accompanied with the juxta-epiphysial lesions
described by Ollier.   Five years previously the lad (now seventeen) had caught his foot in a wheel and severely sprained it by
twisting.   After that he was in bed for some weeks without treatment, the case being deemed a simple sprain.   Since the accident
the lower end of the tibia had failed to grow, while the fibula had

grown at its normal rate; hence the external malleolus, by projecting extraordinarily downwards, had produced a spurious talipes varus. The internal malleolus was exceedingly small, but the lower end of the shaft of the tibia had also failed to grow, so that operative measures were required. The boy was unable to walk for more than half a mile, when he was prevented by severe pain in the shin. He (Mr. Moullin) proposed to resect a portion of bone (about an inch) from the fibula, dividing the tibia at the same time if necessary, and thus to bring the foot into its normal plane position.

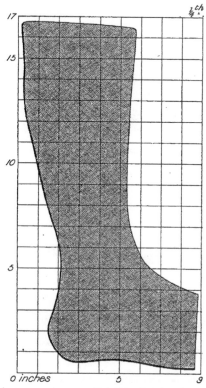

FIG. 269.—PATTERN OF LATERAL SPLINTS (CROFT'S) FOR LEG AND ANKLE WITH FOOT AT A RIGHT ANGLE. FOR A BOY OF FIFTEEN YEARS. REDUCED TO ONE QUARTER SIZE ON SCALE OF INCHES

The author has had under his observation during the last two years several examples of arrest of growth at the lower end of the tibia and curving of the bone after intra-uterine fracture. In one instance at birth the tibia was half an inch shorter than its fellow, and at one year and nine months one inch. These cases of intra-uterine injury and arrest of growth are not uncommon.

Besides the seventeen cases of recent separation alluded to above,

J. Hutchinson junior mentions two others of suppurative epiphysitis following a wrench or sprain, and eight cases of arrest of growth at this part after injury, with overgrowth of fibula and inversion of the foot (making a total of twenty-seven separations of the lower epiphysis of the tibia).

TREATMENT. Simple separation.—Replacement of the displaced bone in simple separation is generally effected with ease by extension

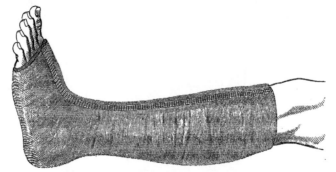

FIG. 270.—CROFT'S LATERAL SPLINT APPLIED TO LEG AND FOOT

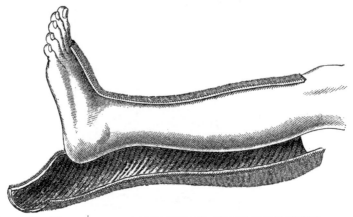

FIG. 271.—THE SAME WITH OUTER PIECE LAID ASIDE BY CUTTING THROUGH
THE GAP ALONG THE FOOT AND FRONT OF LEG

and counter-extension, for the almost flat separated surfaces do not offer the difficulty which is met with in some other separations. A starch or 'Croft's' plaster-of-Paris splint is then applied.

In separation with displacement backwards, and in separation or fracture of the lower end of the fibula, the thigh should be flexed towards the abdomen and the leg towards the thigh with the foot extended, on account of the action of the hamstring and leg muscles tending to keep up the displacement, when reduction may easily be effected with a little manipulation. The dorsum of the foot should be held with one hand and the heel with the other, while an assistant makes slight counter-extension by grasping the leg. A Croft's or other form of moulded splint should then be applied. Division of the tendo Achillis is rarely called for.

Compound separations.—*Amputation* should only rarely be resorted to—when there are most extensive injuries to the soft parts, the epiphysial separation being a small and unimportant element in the

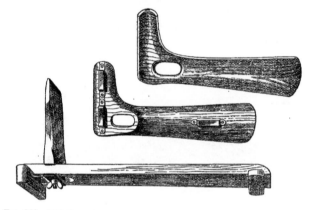

FIG. 272.—POSTERIOR AND LATERAL LEG SPLINTS WITH RECTANGULAR FOOT-PIECES AS USED AT GUY'S HOSPITAL

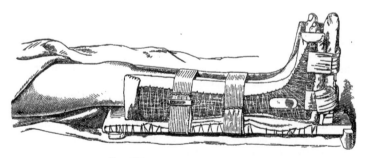

FIG. 273.—THE SAME APPLIED TO LEG

case. Lacerations of both the tibial vessels and even of the nerves, although serious lesions, do not of themselves demand amputation.

Resection of the exposed diaphysis should be performed when it is found to be impossible to otherwise reduce the deformity. There is every reason to save the limb when the damage to the soft structures is not too extensive. Good firm union may be expected with perfect use of the ankle-joint.

Erichsen performed resection of the displaced diaphysis of the tibia at the ankle, and reduced the protruding shaft, with an excellent result both as to union and freedom of movement of the articulation.

In compound separations, more especially where the violence has been direct and the fibula also injured, the greatest care should be taken to remove all soiled portions of the diaphysis and soft parts. The bone may be easily cut away by a short knife or chisel; and the wound having been in every angle carefully washed out with per-chloride of mercury or carbolic acid, so as to make it as aseptic as possible, should be dressed with some antiseptic gauze. The bone and soft parts must be carefully replaced in the position they were in before the accident.

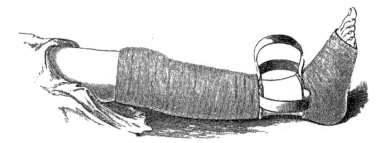

Fig. 274.—PLASTER-OF-PARIS SPLINT WITH INTERRUPTION AT ANKLE
FOR COMPOUND SEPARATIONS

Operations for deformity of ankle and foot due to arrest of growth of the tibia.—*Removal of osseous wedge from fibula*, with or without trans-verse division of the tibia, will meet with greater success than has hitherto been the case, if performed after the limit of the period of the growth in length is reached rather than when the fibula is in an active state of development.

This operation was performed in Mr. Davies-Colley's and in Mr. Rose's cases.

The simple operation of removal of the conjugal cartilages of the fibula may be practised under aseptic precautions, *conjugal chondrectomy* (Ollier), when the deformity has not existed any length of time, and the period of fusion of the epiphysis with the diaphysis is not a short distance off—before the eighteenth or nineteenth year.

M. Ollier has successfully corrected the varus condition produced by suppurative ostitis of the lower end of the tibia by chondrectomy (*Traité des résections*, 1891, p. 475, figs. 396, 397). He excised both epiphysial conjugal discs of the fibula and succeeded in arresting its growth, so that sixteen years after the operation the foot had lost its deformity and the lower ends of the tibia and fibula were in normal relationship.

Ollier says that the upper conjugal cartilages of the tibia and fibula are best accessible for chondrectomy—the former on its antero-internal aspect, the latter on its outer side.

The height of the end of the epiphysis from the epiphysial line at this point he gives as follows:

	Tibia	Fibula
At four years of age . .	12 millimetres	6 millimetres
At twelve years of age . .	16 millimetres	8 millimetres

He recommends a simple deep incision into the cartilage in the first instance, and if, after the lapse of three months, sufficient arrest of growth has not been produced, excision of the cartilage should be performed.

As an alternative operation for arrest of growth of the tibia he also suggests exciting the growth of the conjugal cartilage by indirectly irritating it—i.e. by irritation from a distance, such as by a nail penetrating the bone into the medullary canal or by successive cauterisations of the surface of the tibia, to produce more or less superficial necrosis. In both these conditions the irritation must be prolonged in order to produce the necessary hyperplasia of the cartilage, and consequently the operation must be repeated many times.

In some instances Ollier has combined the methods of excision of cartilage and of artificial irritation. In a case of deviation of the foot inwards following arrest of growth of the tibia, probably the result of an old juxta-epiphysial sprain, he inserted a leaden nail in the middle of the tibia, and

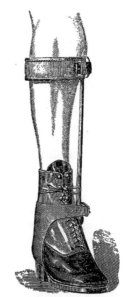

Fig. 275.— steel leg-iron with foot and t-strap for spurious talipes varus, the result of arrest of growth of the tibia, after epiphysial separation

excised the still growing epiphysial cartilage of the fibula. Although the patient, who was fifteen years of age, had not grown much since the operation, the deformity was completely rectified. The presence of the nail was well tolerated and affected the growth of the tibia, as four months afterwards it was more than three millimetres distant from the upper end, but continued the same distance from the lower end.

CHAPTER VIII

SEPARATION OF THE UPPER EPIPHYSIS OF THE FIBULA

ANATOMY.—At birth both ends of the fibula are cartilaginous ; soon after birth the diaphysis begins to take its characteristic prismatic shape.

The upper end has no trace of ossification until about four or four and a half years of age, when some osseous granules are distinguishable in the centre of the cartilage ; these rapidly coalesce and form a distinct centre between the fifth and sixth years. At the eighth year this centre is seen to be of an oval shape, rapidly extending in all directions, and by the eighteenth year the epiphysis is fully ossified.

The epiphysis includes the whole of the surface for the attachment of the tendon of the biceps femoris and external lateral ligaments. Its pointed styloid process behind gives attachment to the short external lateral ligament, while the rest of the head in front affords attachment to the biceps, long external lateral ligament, and anterior bands of the superior tibio-fibular joint. To its peroneal tubercle are connected some anterior fibres of the peroneus longus and extensor longus digitorum muscles. Behind, below the anterior tubercle, it gives attachment to the posterior bands of the superior tibio-fibular joint and the uppermost fibres of the outer head of the soleus.

Its outer aspect is prominent and subcutaneous, being covered only with some fibrous expansions of the muscles and ligaments to which the rest of the epiphysis gives attachment.

Its lower surface is almost flat, fitting upon the slightly convex end of the diaphysis, and is on a level with the lower end of the tonguelike process of the upper tibial epiphysis (forming the tubercle), that is, its most prominent part. Behind the conjugal line is a quarter to three-eighths of an inch below the oval articular surface for the outer tuberosity of the tibia, and more externally it passes directly below the surface for the biceps.

This epiphysis joins the diaphysis about the twentieth to the twenty-second year; its union may be delayed as late as the twenty-fifth year. Traces of the epiphysial line are often seen for some years beyond this date.

The articular tibial surface looks forwards, upwards, and inwards, and is an almost plane or slightly concave surface, covered with cartilage, and placed at an angle of 145° with the axis of the shaft.

The apex of the styloid process is three eighths of an inch below the level of the articular surface of the knee-joint in the fully developed epiphysis at about the twentieth year.

The epiphysial line at the eighteenth year is fifteen millimetres below the apex of the styloid process; at the fifteenth year it is twelve millimetres.

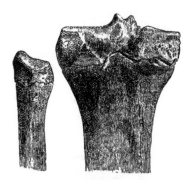

Fig. 276.—Posterior aspect of the fully formed upper epiphyses of the tibia and fibula, showing the fibular facet on the outer tibial tuberosity

The fibula has been rotated to show its articular surface

The synovial membrane of the superior tibio-fibular articulation is quite above the epiphysial line of cartilage of the fibula in childhood. Its nearest point is on the lower or inner side, where at eight years of age it is more than a quarter of an inch above it; but at the thirteenth year, from the upward growth of the diaphysis, the synovial membrane quite reaches the epiphysial disc on this side. The upper tibial disc of cartilage on the outer side approaches very intimately this joint, and its level is a short distance above the lower limit of the synovial membrane.

Very rarely the synovial membrane communicates with that of the knee-joint by means of a small opening at the posterior and upper part, where the articular capsule is always the thinnest. More frequently the author has found a communication with the large bursa beneath the tendon of the popliteus tendon, which always opens widely into the knee-joint, at the external semilunar cartilage of the joint.

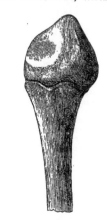

Fig. 277.—Epiphysis of the head of fibula at the nineteenth year, showing the facet for the outer tuberosity of the tibia

ETIOLOGY.—Were it not for the articulation of the fibular head with the inferior and outer aspect of the external tuberosity of the

tibia, its fixed-in position, and attachment to it by strong ligamentous bands (anterior and posterior ligaments of the superior
tibio-fibular joint), the action of the powerful external lateral ligaments and biceps tendon would prove a frequent cause of separation
of this epiphysis in lateral movements of adduction of the leg. In
the same way these peculiar anatomical safeguards may counter-
balance the tendency to which its prominent and subcutaneous position below the outer side of the knee exposes it in direct blows in this
situation. However, forcible inward
flexion of the leg upon the thigh by
violent overstretching of the external
lateral ligaments attached to the fibular
head may, under certain conditions,
cause the conjugal junction of the latter
with the diaphysis to be torn through.

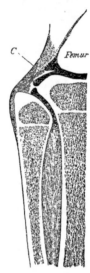

FIG. 278.—SECTION THROUGH SU-
PERIOR TIBIO-FIBULAR ARTICULA-
TION, SHOWING RELATION OF ITS
SYNOVIAL CAVITY TO THE CONJU-
GAL CARTILAGE OF THE TIBIA AND
FIBULA AND THE SMALL AMOUNT
OF TISSUE INTERVENING BETWEEN
IT AND THE ARTICULATION OF THE
KNEE. FROM A BOY AGED THIR-
TEEN AND A HALF YEARS

C, external semilunar cartilage on
section

Stanley Boyd states that strong
action of the biceps has occasionally
torn off the upper fibular epiphysis
(Treves, *System of Surgery*, vol. i. 1895).

AGE.—Of the three examples recorded here, one only was unassociated
with separation of the epiphyses of the
neighbouring femur or tibia—namely,
that of a child, aged eighteen months,
the injury being caused by direct crushing violence.

M. Delore, as stated later on, separated this epiphysis together with that
of the femur in a child aged seven.

In only one simple case has separation of the upper epiphysis of the fibula
been diagnosed during life, viz. at fourteen years of age.

PATHOLOGICAL ANATOMY.—Separation of this epiphysis alone can but
rarely be accomplished by any other
than direct violence. The close con-
nection of the fibula with the tibia in its whole length, and the
articulation with the outer tuberosity of the tibia above, prevent,
as stated just now, indirect violence having much effect upon the
upper epiphysial line.

It is remarkable that this epiphysis escapes injury in so large a
proportion of cases of separation of the upper epiphysis of the tibia ; it
was separated in Fischer and Hirschfeld's case and in Durham's case.

In the former instance both epiphyses of the fibula were completely detached.

The same lesions exist in the specimen in St. George's Hospital

Museum (see above), but here the lower epiphyses of the femur and tibia were separated as well as those of the fibula.

Dr. F. A. Stimson presented to the New York Surgical Society (*Medical Record,* New York, 1882, xxii. p. 77; *Treatise on Fractures,* London, 1883, p. 586) a specimen of separation of the upper end of the fibula by direct violence.

The child, aged eighteen months, was run over by a street car, and received injuries which caused its death a few hours afterwards. There was a lacerated wound on the outer side of the right leg, exposing the upper end of the fibula and opening the knee-joint.

The upper epiphysis of the fibula was completely and cleanly detached from the shaft and from the tibia, and remained attached to the external lateral ligament and the tendon of the biceps. There was also an incomplete fracture of the shaft of the fibula three-fourths of an inch below the epiphysial line, and the intermediate portion was denuded of its periosteum, which remained attached to the epiphysis.

M. Delore in straightening a case of knock-knee found on dissection that he had separated the upper epiphysis of the fibula as well as the lower epiphysis of the femur. The child, aged seven years, died of measles twenty-one days after the operation.

The proximity of the external popliteal nerve to the biceps tendon and upper fibular epiphysis is a constant source of danger.

SYMPTOMS.—The detached epiphysis may be felt as a hard fragment on the outer side of the knee, descending when the knee is extended. There may also exist some lateral mobility, especially inwards, of the knee, amounting in some instances almost to dislocation at the joint.

When displacement is absent, pain on pressure, localised to the conjugal cartilage, and slight mobility, combined with other signs of injury at this point, and the age of the patient, are the principal factors upon which a diagnosis can be made. Signs of a severe sprain to the knee and contusion on the outer side of the knee may throw the surgeon off his guard.

At Guy's Hospital in May 1868 Mr. Hilton is reported to have diagnosed a case of separation of the upper epiphysis of the left fibula in a boy (John M.), aged fourteen.

The patient was standing under an arch, which gave way and buried him in the bricks. There was effusion into the knee-joint as well as the epiphysial separation. The limb was put up in a posterior splint in a slightly flexed position, and the patient left the hospital four weeks later 'quite well,' without any impairment of movement of the limb.

TREATMENT.—After reduction of any displacement of the diaphysis that may exist, the knee should be kept flexed to a right angle by plaster of Paris or other immovable splint, to allow relaxation of the biceps muscle and secure apposition of the fragments.

SEPARATION OF THE LOWER EPIPHYSIS OF
THE FIBULA

ANATOMY.—Osseous particles are deposited in the centre of the lower epiphysis about the eighteenth to twentieth month after birth —during the second year according to Béclard—but this may occasionally be delayed till the end of the third year. This centre rapidly increases in all directions, so that between the eighth and ninth years this epiphysis is an almost osseous quadrilateral mass,

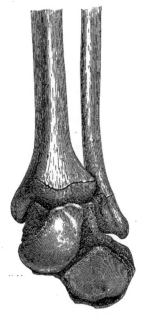

with the exception of the tip of the malleolus, which is still cartilaginous; but this too is soon invaded, and the whole is then quite ossified.

The lower epiphysis unites with the diaphysis from the nineteenth, twentieth, or twenty-second year— before the upper epiphysis.

It is interesting to remark that although the nutrient artery of the shaft runs downwards, the fibula is an exception to the general rule, inasmuch as the lower epiphysis, towards which it runs, is the first to appear instead of the last.

In a boy of eight years the epiphysial layer of cartilage will be found to lie eight millimetres below that of the tibia, and in a direct horizontal line with the opposed articular surfaces of the tibia and astragalus. It is separated from the synovial membrane of the ankle-joint by a small amount of connective tissue, which is readily torn through in epiphysial separations, and the articular cavity opened. It may

FIG. 279.—NORMAL RELATION OF THE EPIPHYSIAL LINES OF THE TIBIA AND FIBULA TO THE ANKLE-JOINT, FROM A SUBJECT AGED EIGHTEEN YEARS

therefore be said to be almost exactly on a level with the plane of the ankle-joint.

In the fully developed epiphysis at the eighteenth year, the epiphysial line on the outer side is twenty-two millimetres (seven-eighths of an inch) above the tip of the external malleolus; at about the fifteenth year it is rather less, about eighteen millimetres; at the eighth year sixteen millimetres.

On taking the section of the ankle-joint at thirteen years of age, the synovial membrane of the joint overlaps the diaphysis of the fibula for five millimetres (Sésary).

Mr. J. Bland Sutton has recently drawn attention to the comparative length of the external malleolus in man, which descends much lower in him than in the higher mammals—e.g. the ape.

ETIOLOGY. Indirect violence. The mechanism of this separation is more closely allied to that of Pott's fracture in the adult than to any form of injury about the ankle-joint.

In the author's case the twisting of the foot after a fall from a trapeze produced separation with displacement inwards of the foot, rather than outwards as in Pott's fracture.

It is probable that separation of this external malleolar epiphysis, with only slight displacement, is a frequent result of violent wrenches or twists of the foot, but are undetected.

The author is unable to refer to a single instance of simple separation with or without displacement which has been correctly diagnosed and described during life.

Direct violence.—Severe direct violence to the ankle generally produces separation of the outer malleolus combined with outer extensive lesions.

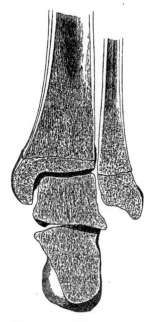

Fig. 280.—FRONTAL SECTION THROUGH BONES FORMING THE ANKLE-JOINT AT THE AGE OF SEVENTEEN AND A HALF YEARS. POSTERIOR HALF OF SECTION, SHOWING CANCELLOUS STRUCTURE OF THE EPIPHYSES AND THE RELATION OF THE CONJUGAL LINES TO THE ARTICULATIONS (⅔-size)

AGE.—Of the five recorded examples of separation of this epiphysis, uncomplicated with partial or complete separation of the lower tibial epiphysis, three were pathological specimens—two at 18 years of age and one at 6; while two were compound separations —one at 12 years of age, and one at an age not stated.

In three of the above five cases the lesion occurred in males; in the two others the sex was not given.

PATHOLOGICAL ANATOMY.—There are only two authentic specimens of this injury in the London museums, both compound and caused by very severe violence.

The first is in the Museum of the Middlesex Hospital, No. 115 (*Descriptive Catalogue of the Pathological Museum of the Middlesex*

Hospital, 1884, p. 14), and is described by Mr. Bland Sutton in the *Pathological Society's Transactions*, London, vol. xxv. 1884, p. 272.

It was taken from a lad, aged eighteen, whose left foot had been entangled in some machinery. There was such severe laceration of the structures about the ankle that it was found necessary to immediately amputate at the middle of the calf. The operation was followed by complete recovery. Besides severe injuries to the tendons and soft tissues about the joint, the deltoid ligament was torn through near the front of its attachment to the inner malleolus. The lower epiphysis of the fibula, completely freed from the diaphysis, remained attached to the astragalus and os calcis by means of the external lateral ligament. The anterior and posterior bands of the inferior tibio-fibular articulation were torn through at their attachment to the outer malleolus, the foot remaining connected with the leg by two or three tendons only.

In the second case, in the London Hospital Museum, the specimen (No. G. b. S. 37) was taken from a child, aged six, in whom also primary amputation was performed for severe compound injury to the foot.

The separation of the lower epiphysis of the fibula was complete, the epiphysial cartilage remaining attached to it, but being fissured at the posterior part. The diaphysis, which was stripped of its periosteum, was not fractured. The ligaments connecting the malleolus to the tarsus were uninjured, and the periosteum was still attached to this process. The internal malleolus was broken off by an obliquely vertical fracture. As in the case of the fibula, the ligaments below and the periosteum above were still connected with it. The diaphysis of the tibia was likewise devoid of its periosteum.[1]

The only other previously recorded specimen in London is that in the Museum of St. George's Hospital, and is described by Mr. Holmes in the *Transactions of the Pathological Society* (vol. xiii. p. 187). The condyloid epiphysis of the femur, the lower epiphysis of the tibia (compound), and both epiphyses of the fibula, were separated from the diaphysis. For the extensive injuries amputation was immediately performed, and the patient (aged eighteen) died of pyæmia on the thirteenth day. Mr. Holmes, however, adds, with regard to this specimen, in his *Surgical Treatment of the Diseases of Children*, 2nd edit. 1869, p. 237: 'Very unfortunately the bones have been macerated, so that it is impossible to see whether the separations, which do certainly exist in the specimen, are the result of injury or maceration.'

Nélaton, in his *Éléments de Pathologie Chirurgicale*, 2ème édit. tome 2ème, p. 234, gives an illustration of a specimen of pure separation of the lower epiphysis of the fibula. The lower epiphysis of the tibia was also separated in front on the inner side,

---

[1] This specimen, though in the old MS. catalogue, does not appear in the recent catalogue of the London Hospital Museum.

but on the outer side it was accompanied by a fracture of the shaft.

M. Anger's drawing (fig. 267) of the specimen has already been given (see under LOWER EPIPHYSIS OF THE TIBIA).

The only specimen known in London or elsewhere of this injury caused by indirect violence is one which the author dissected some years ago. Gangrene of the foot and part of the leg occurred on the third day after the application of a plaster dressing to the limb, and on the twenty-fifth day necessitated amputation, which was followed by recovery.

The lad, aged eighteen years, fell off a trapeze a distance of eight feet on to the outer side of his foot. There was thought to be a fracture of the fibula accompanied by displacement *inwards* of the foot. The foot was reduced soon after the accident.

The separation lay exactly and completely through the epiphysial cartilage, and was accompanied by stripping up of the periosteum from the lower end of the diaphysis, especially on the outer side. All the lateral ligaments were intact, as were also the inferior tibio-fibular ligaments, with the exception of a few of the anterior bands of the latter where they pass to the front of the malleolus. There was blood in the ankle-joint and beneath the separated periosteum, as well as around the detached epiphysis, which was only slightly displaced outwards.

Hamilton was 'unable to refer to any example of separation of the lower epiphysis of the fibula.'

COMPOUND SEPARATION.—Dr. O. H. Allis, of Philadelphia, has kindly sent the author the following note on an unpublished case of compound separation of the lower epiphysis of the fibula which proved fatal from tetanus.

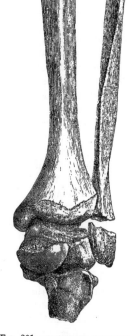

FIG. 281.—TRAUMATIC SEPARATION OF THE LOWER EPIPHYSIS OF THE LEFT FIBULA WITH DISPLACEMENT OF THE FOOT INWARDS

(Author's specimen)

' Compound separation of lower fibular epiphysis, never reported : R. S., about twelve years of age, fell between logs on which he was playing, and was brought to the Presbyterian Hospital immediately after. There was a transverse wound about an inch long that corresponded to the seat of separation at the lower epiphysis of the right fibula. The bone was in full view, and the separation was without splintering. The wound had probably been made from within outwards by the sharp edge of the diaphysis.

'When seen there was no displacement. The wound was dressed and recumbency enjoined. Both wound and separation did apparently well, but in about the third week symptoms of tetanus arose that proved fatal in a few days. Date about 1875.'

Mr. G. A. Wright (*Diseases of Children, Medical and Surgical,* Ashby and Wright, 3rd edit. 1896, p. 756) met with an instance of compound separation of the lower epiphysis of the fibula, in which the lower fragment became necrosed and was removed.

Mr. J. E. S. Barnett (*Lancet,* June 18, 1898, p. 1721) also briefly notes an instance of compound separation of the lower epiphysis of the fibula, with inversion of the foot and protrusion of the lower end of the diaphysis.

LATER COMPLICATIONS. **Suppuration and necrosis.**—As to these later complications, suppurative epiphysitis occurred in one instance. Necrosis may be expected in compound separations.

Tetanus resulted at the third week in Dr. Allis's case of compound separation.

Arrest of growth.—Should there be arrest of growth following injury to the lower epiphysis, which is the most important epiphysis of the fibula in this respect, there is little probability except in early childhood of its giving rise to any marked curving of the tibia, which is the main support of the lower extremity.

SYMPTOMS.—Although fracture of the fibula alone is rare in children, it is exceedingly probable that the majority of examples of supposed fracture of the lower end of the fibula occurring in youths from twelve to nineteen years of age are really separated epiphyses. The separation takes place, as in fracture, by lateral rotation of the astragalus and foot either inwards or outwards, from a fall, sudden twist, or adduction or abduction of the foot, but differs from it in that the solution of continuity is below the tibio-fibular interosseous ligaments. Although the anterior and posterior bands of the tibio-fibular articulation may be ruptured in separation, in the more common form of Pott's fracture this laceration often occurs.

In experiments upon the dead body the author found this to be one of the most readily separated epiphyses of the long bones, in the manner just mentioned, by violent adduction or abduction.

Without any marked displacement of the epiphysis and foot its detection cannot be easy. Mobility of the epiphysis is here difficult of recognition, and muffled crepitus may or may not be present. Pain on pressure over the epiphysial line, or some slight irregularity in the line of the fibula, is more likely to be present, and suggest a separation.

Displacement of epiphysis and foot.—If, however, the force applied has been such as to cause displacement of the foot, then the deformity should render the diagnosis a matter of comparative ease.

It may be *outwards*, as in a typical Pott's fracture, of a mild degree, and associated with more or less laceration of the internal lateral ligament or tearing away of the extreme tip of the internal malleolus.

The displacement may take place *inwards*, as in some rare forms of dislocation of the foot in adults, combined with fracture of the lower end of the fibula. This displacement existed in the author's case quoted above.

Probably in both forms of displacement some of the anterior or posterior fibres of the inferior tibio-fibular ligament will be lacerated.

Moreover, the articular cavity of the ankle-joint must necessarily be opened in all examples of severe separation with displacement.

In these instances the careful recognition of the exact point of mobility of the epiphysis at the epiphysial line is of the greatest importance, and in them muffled crepitus is more easily obtained than in others where no displacement has occurred.

Seeing that a separation of the lower fibular epiphysis will more probably involve the ankle-joint than a fracture of the lower end of the fibula just above the epiphysial line, it is for this reason alone of considerable importance to the surgeon.

TREATMENT.—Reduction should be at once carried out where there is displacement, and it will be found to be more easily effected than in the case of fracture in adults, where the displaced fibula has too often caused permanent deformity. A plaster-of-Paris splint, in the form of the Bavarian or, better, a 'Croft's,' splint, should then be applied. There need be no fear of applying this when there is but little swelling or extravasation of blood in the neighbourhood. The patient is kept in bed for ten to fourteen days to make sure that the plaster has not been applied too tightly; he may then get about on crutches for the following two or three weeks, when all apparatus should be discarded. Plaster-of-Paris bandages should never be employed in children on account of the danger attending them.

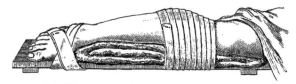

Fig. 282.—DUPUYTREN'S SPLINT FOR FRACTURE OF THE
EXTERNAL MALLEOLUS

In the more severe cases it may be found necessary to make use of wooden lateral and posterior splints with foot-pieces, while some may prefer a long internal splint to the leg and foot applied after the method of Dupuytren and with thick padding over the tibia.

It is improbable that any severe deformity or arrest of the proper growth of the limb will be likely to result from the separation if

3 K

properly reduced, inasmuch as the tibia is the principal bone upon which the leg depends for its increase in length, the fibula playing a subordinate part ; in fact, in man the upper part of the latter bone is in a comparatively rudimentary condition.

If arrest of growth of the lower end of the fibula ensue, it may, as it affects one of the parallel bones, be followed in after years by a talipes valgus condition of the foot.

Operation for deformity from arrest of growth.—If the valgus position be extreme from the continued growth of the tibia in *arrest of growth* of the fibula, it may be considered necessary to perform Ollier's simple operation of removal of the lower cartilage of union of tibia—conjugal chondrectomy (*chondrectomie conjugale*). The lower epiphysial cartilage of the tibia, being subcutaneous, is easily reached.

M. Ollier gives the approximate distance of the epiphysial lines of the tibia and fibula laterally from the point of the malleoli :

	Tibia	*Fibula*
At four years of age	14 millimetres	15 millimetres
At twelve years of age	17 millimetres	18 millimetres

CHAPTER IX

SEPARATION OF THE EPIPHYSES OF THE BONES OF THE FOOT

Separation of the epiphysis of the os calcis.—At birth the primary osseous nucleus of the os calcis, which appears about the centre of the cartilage at the fifth month of fœtal life, has already invaded much of it. By the tenth year nearly the whole bone is osseous, and at this period the cartilaginous epiphysis which caps the posterior extremity of the bone begins to ossify. Appearing just at the most convex part of the epiphysis, this centre spreads very rapidly throughout it, so that by the fourteenth year the epiphysis is entirely osseous. To its lower part behind is attached the tendo Achillis, and between its upper part and the tendon is situated a synovial bursa. The junction with the body of the bone begins about the

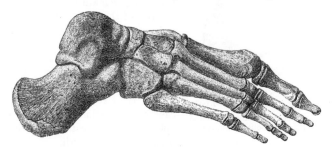

Fig. 283.—RIGHT FOOT SEEN FROM THE OUTER SIDE, SHOWING EPIPHYSES OF OS CALCIS, METATARSUS, AND PHALANGES AT THE AGE OF FIFTEEN AND A HALF YEARS ($\frac{1}{2}$-size)

sixteenth year at the lower part, and is usually completed by the eighteenth year. Traces, however, of the line of union are sometimes to be seen at the upper part as late as the twenty-third year.

Occasionally a separate centre appears in the outer calcanean tubercle at a somewhat later period than the centre for the main epiphysis, but more usually this process is formed and ossified from an extension forwards of the epiphysial plate behind. Even when this calcanean tubercle has a separate centre, it is joined to the epiphysis by a cartilaginous strip, by means of which it is soon ossified on. In rare cases this tubercle has been found as a detached process of bone.

It is possible that separation of this epiphysis may be produced by muscular action, and that cases which have been recorded of fracture of this process in youth produced by muscular action are really epiphysial detachments.

The author knows of no case where this separation has been diagnosed during life, but he has seen the epiphysis crushed off by the wheel of a tramcar in a case where other severe lesions from crushing of the foot necessitated amputation of the leg. He has also had to remove the epiphysis, which had become completely necrosed and loose, in a girl aged ten years.   Some weeks previously she had received a blow from a cricket-ball upon the heel.   This led to suppuration and exfoliation of this process, most probably from injury to the epiphysial line of junction, or from its partial detachment.

Perfect recovery of the use of the foot may result even if some displacement has occurred.

Separation of the occasional epiphysis of the astragalus.—The author reproduces one of four photographs given to him by Professor J. G. Adami of specimens from the McGill University Medical College Museum, which show a separate centre or ossification called the *os trigonum*, remaining isolated from the rest of the bone. This forms the outer posterior tubercle of the astragalus, for the attachment of the posterior astragalo-fibular ligament (posterior fasciculus of external lateral ligament of ankle-joint).

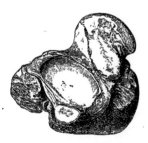

FIG. 284.—UNDER SURFACE OF ASTRAGALUS SHOWING OCCASIONAL EPIPHYSIS

(From a specimen in the Museum of McGill Medical College, Montreal)

E. H. Bennett has described a case of separation of the secondary epiphysis of the astragalus which is occasionally met with.

Separation of the epiphysis of the first metatarsal bone.—The first metatarsal bone is regarded by some anatomists as a phalanx, as it has its epiphysis at the proximal end or base. The centre for this is often found commencing as two osseous nuclei on either side of the middle axis of the bone at the third year. M. Mayet describes (*Bulletins de la Société anatomique*, Paris, Avril–Mai 1895, p. 384, ' Développement de l'extrémité postérieure du premier métatarsien ') one nucleus as forming the principal part of the epiphysis, and a small accessory one appearing about the same time—viz. from two to six years of age, and soon uniting with it. This epiphysis joins with the shaft a little earlier than the epiphysis of the other metatarsal bones, i.e. about the nineteenth year. .

There is very frequently found another distinct epiphysis at the head or distal extremity. A more common condition, however, is

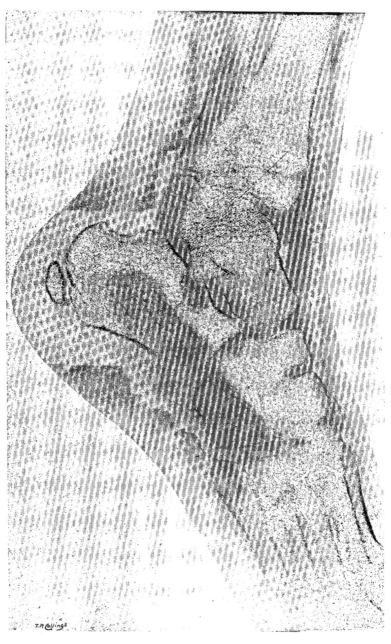

NORMAL EPIPHYSES OF ANKLE AND FOOT OF A FEMALE CHILD AGED SEVEN YE
Six seconds exposure.   Taken by Mr. W

to find the osseous nucleus of the epiphysis at this end extending forwards from the middle line of the diaphysis and then spreading out in a mushroom-like manner into the epiphysis, so that a section taken through either side at the middle line would represent the epiphysis ossified by a distinct centre and separated from the shaft by a complete layer of cartilage.

This anterior epiphysis (when present) is overlapped both above and below by the synovial membrane of the metatarso-phalangeal joint, and the latter is therefore likely to be opened in separation of this epiphysis.

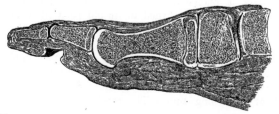

Fig. 285.—MEDIAN SAGITTAL SECTION THROUGH GREAT TOE AND INNER ROW OF TARSAL BONES IN A BOY AGED FOURTEEN YEARS .

Relation of synovial membranes of tarso-metarsal, metatarso-phalangeal, and interphalangeal joints to the epiphysial lines. None quite reach the epiphysial boundary. If an anterior epiphysis exists to the first metatarsal bone, it will be overlapped above and below by the synovial membrane ' (⅔-size)

Separation of the epiphyses of the four outer metatarsal bones.—The shafts of the metatarsal bones are advanced in the process of ossification at the time of birth, the ends being still cartilaginous.

In the four outer metatarsal bones a separate osseous centre appears in the distal end or head between the third and the fifth or even the eighth year. This head is entirely osseous by the tenth to the twelfth year, and is separated from the shaft only by the thin layer of epiphysial cartilage. These epiphyses unite with the shafts from the eighteenth to twentieth year.

Occasionally the tuberosity of the fifth metatarsal bone is developed, according to Gruber, by a separate epiphysis. On the upper and under aspects the synovial membrane of the metatarso-phalangeal joint overlaps the epiphysial cartilage line (especially on the plantar aspect), whereas on the lateral aspects it extends only as high as the attachment of the lateral ligaments, and hence it is at these points below the level of the epiphysial junction. On the plantar aspect there is a considerable amount of dense connective tissue separating the latter from the synovial cavity of the joint, as well as from the sheath of the flexor tendons lying more superficially.

In the London Hospital Museum Mr. Holmes states (*Surgical Treatment of Diseases of Children*, 2nd edit. 1869, p. 238) that there are two specimens of separation of the metatarsus associated with slight fracture. The author has been unable to find these, and they are not contained in the recent catalogue of the museum of that hospital (*loc. cit. supra*).

The following case is recorded by Mr. James Mason (*Lancet*, September 24, 1887) as a case of separation of the epiphysis of the *second metatarsal bone*, but from the report it appears that it was probably due to some disease at the epiphysial line.

A girl, aged seventeen years, complained of pain and swelling over the root of the second toe of the left foot. She stated that the 'lump' had been there for some time; it occasionally disappeared when she put her foot in a certain position, but immediately she tried to walk it reappeared. On examination it could be easily reduced, but as readily returned to its old position when pressure was removed. The movement at the joint was perfect. Well-marked crepitus could be felt about a quarter of an inch behind the joint. The fragments were put in apposition, and a pad applied. She could not remember having received any injury or twist, and considered it simply an 'enlarged joint.' She had been able to walk about for a long time. The result of the treatment is not recorded.

The author has seen a similar case of painless displacement, due to disease, of the second metatarsal diaphysis of the left foot in a boy, aged seven years.

Separation of the epiphyses of the phalanges of the toes.—At birth the shafts of all the phalanges are well advanced in ossification, their ends being cartilaginous.

The epiphysial ends of all the phalanges are formed at the proximal extremity, and their ossific nuclei, often two in number on either side of the middle line, appear about the fourth to the sixth year, and form flattened plates about the tenth year, concave on their articular aspect, and separated from the shafts by a layer of cartilage.

These epiphyses join the shaft from the seventeenth to the twentieth year, and ossification usually takes place in these phalanges, like the metatarsal bones, from the first to the fifth toe. Béclard gives the appearance of the ossification of the epiphyses of the first row of phalanges as about the fourth year, and union with the shaft at the eighteenth year; that of the second row about the sixth year, and union about the seventeenth year; that of the third row about the seventh year, and union about the seventeenth year.

The synovial cavity in none of the corresponding articulations comes in contact with the epiphysial lines.

L. A. Stimson (*Treatise on Fractures*, London, 1883, p. 51) relates a case of compound separation of the first phalanx of the great toe.

A boy, aged thirteen years, caught his foot in machinery, and received a compound comminuted fracture of the proximal phalanx of the great toe. The smooth cartilaginous disc limiting the epiphysis could be seen and felt through the wound. The patient made a good recovery, and had a movable joint.

Mr. Gascoyen relates (*British Med. Journal*, April 1871, vol. i. p. 338) the case of a child, eight years of age, who was under his care at St. Mary's Hospital. The case at first sight might have been mistaken for one of talipes equinus, as the child walked on the outer side of the foot; but on further examination it was found that the head of the metatarsal bone of the great toe was unnaturally prominent, and the extensor longus pollicis extremely tense, the end of the toe being raised. All these appearances passed away when the heel was put to the ground. There was a little pain on manipulation, but no grating. The head of the metatarsal bone could be felt intact, with a rounded movable piece adherent to it, upon which the toe appeared to play. Extension completely reduced the distortion, which, however, returned when the extension was removed. Mr. Gascoyen accordingly thought that the case was an example of separation of the epiphysis of the first phalanx of the toe. The injury was produced by the child getting the toe under a door whilst at play, and struggling to release herself. This was three months previous to admission into hospital. Mr. Gascoyen divided the extensor longus pollicis, and, after the wound had healed, put the foot in a gutta-percha splint, which was firmly moulded to the toe. The patient did well, and in about three weeks was able to walk about almost naturally.

PART IV

SEPARATION OF THE EPIPHYSES OF THE VERTEBRÆ AND RIBS

———•◦•———

CHAPTER I

SEPARATION OF THE EPIPHYSES OF THE VERTEBRÆ GENERALLY

MOST of the vertebræ at the time of birth consist of three separate osseous pieces, one for the body and one for each lamina, corresponding to the *three primary centres*. During the first year of life the laminæ become united behind in the cartilage of the spinous process, which remains cartilaginous for some time, usually till the age of puberty. Between the third and fourth years the body is joined to the arch on each side; first in the third cervical vertebra about the third year, and last in that of the fourth lumbar vertebra about the sixth year.

Five secondary epiphyses are formed as follows:

One or two for the tips of the *spinous processes* at sixteen years of age.

One for the end of each *transverse process* at sixteen to eighteen years of age.

Two thin *circular plates*, or, more often, irregular rims of bone, one on the upper, and the other on the lower surface of the body of the vertebra; the former piece being usually the thicker and appearing from the eighteenth to the twentieth year, but showing itself first in the lumbar region somewhat earlier, viz. at the seventeenth year. They are present in all the vertebræ except the atlas and the last three coccygeal vertebræ.

These epiphyses unite at the twenty-fifth year or even later.

Two specimens in the London hospital museums show the ease with which the epiphysial discs of the bodies of the vertebræ may be detached by severe crushing violence. As shown however by the following example, the intervertebral cartilage may give way at the junction with the epiphysis of the body of the vertebra rather than the epiphysis at its line of union with the body.

Before the Pathological Society in March 1886 (*Transactions of the Pathological Society*, London, vol. xxxvii. 1886, p. 385) Mr. G. H. Makins showed a specimen of diastasis of the cervical spine taken from the body of a male patient, aged twenty. Knocked down in a street brawl, twenty-four hours before death, he had struck his head on the paved tram-line and become unconscious. He was subsequently severely kicked. No more precise details could be obtained.

When admitted he was conscious, but there was entire loss of motive power from the neck downwards, and of sensation below the third rib. Respiration was entirely diaphragmatic; pulse 60, regular; temperature in axilla, 95·0°; semi-erect condition of

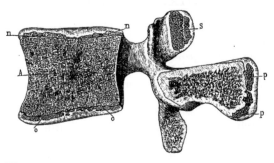

FIG. 286.—LUMBAR VERTEBRA ABOUT THE NINETEENTH YEAR.   VERTICAL SECTION

A, body of vertebra; on its upper and lower surfaces osseous granules (n n, o o) appear in the cartilaginous plates and are most numerous and thick towards the circumference; p p, osseous centres, upper and lower, for the apex of the spinous process; S, additional centre in lumbar vertebræ for the back part of the superior articular process (mammillary process)   (Rambaud and Renault)

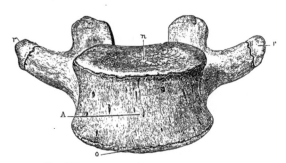

FIG. 287.—ANTERIOR VIEW OF LUMBAR VERTEBRA

A, body; o, lower epiphysial plate; n, upper epiphysial plate, thicker in circumference than in centre; r, epiphysis for apex of transverse process   (Rambaud and Renault)

penis. He complained of tenderness over the mid-region of the cervical spine when the fingers were passed along the processes, but there was no deformity. He vomited occasionally, and had a catch in the breath. The temperature began to rise eight hours after admission, and rose to 106° shortly before death. At the autopsy a considerable amount of dark blood was seen effused into the muscles and coverings of the spine in the neck and upper dorsal region of the spine. On examining the bodies of the vertebræ, there was distinct gaping between the bodies of the fifth and sixth cervical ; they were still attached, however, by a portion of the anterior common ligament. When this was divided the head at once fell back, the bodies gaping widely, the intervertebral disc remaining attached to the under surface of the fifth vertebra. There was some effusion of blood between the bones and the dura mater, but the sheath was untorn.

In the London Hospital Museum, No. 218, there is a specimen of part of the spinal column of a young child in which the upper epiphysis of the fourth dorsal vertebra has been torn off, and the third dorsal, to which it is attached, is displaced backwards. The child was brought to the hospital dead, having sustained fracture of several ribs and laceration of the left lung by being run over.

Mr. J. Jackson Clarke kindly drew the author's attention to the following specimen which he had placed in St. Mary's Hospital Museum, No. 196. Dislocation forwards of the twelfth dorsal vertebra had occurred, with complete dislocation of the last three ribs on the left and partial dislocation of those on the right side. The intervertebral disc and the lower epiphysial plate of the twelfth dorsal vertebra remained attached to the first lumbar vertebra. The cord was completely crushed. On section the other epiphysial plates of the bodies appeared to be just uniting. The specimen was taken from a man, aged about twenty-three, who was caught between the buffers of two railway trucks.

The author has already drawn attention in this volume to the probable origin of many cases of tuberculous disease of the spine, viz. a partial separation or sprain of the upper or lower laminar plate, giving rise in a tuberculous patient to caries and abscess.

Mr. Howse, at Guy's Hospital in 1887, removed a small nodule of bone from an abscess cavity situated over the eighth to eleventh dorsal spines in a boy (Thos. K.), aged thirteen years. He believed it to be a separation of the epiphysis of the dorsal spinous process. The abscess had developed after the use of the horizontal bar eighteen months previously. There was no evidence of other disease of the spine. Complete recovery ensued.

SEPARATION OF THE EPIPHYSES OF THE DIFFERENT VERTEBRÆ

Separation of the epiphyses of the cervical vertebræ.—In addition to the centres common to the vertebræ generally, the anterior or costiform parts of the transverse processes of the seventh, sixth, and sometimes the fifth and second cervical vertebræ are developed from separate osseous centres. They appear before birth (sixth month of fœtal life), and join at the fifth or sixth year, and are analogous to the ribs in the dorsal region.

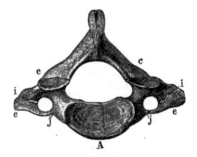

Fig. 288.—A CERVICAL VERTEBRA. THE EPIPHYSIAL PLATE ON THE UPPER SURFACE OF THE BODY CONCEALS THE JUNCTION OF THE BODY WITH THE LATERAL MASS ON EITHER SIDE

A, body of vertebra ; c, laminæ ; e, e, costiform epiphyses of transverse processes joining at j with the lateral mass and at i with the extremity of the transverse process. (After Rambaud and Renault)

The spinous processes usually develop by two well-marked epiphysial centres.

Rambaud and Renault figure (*Origine et développement des os*, 1864, p. 97, 'Atlas,' Plate VI., fig. 13) and describe a specimen of an axis, communicated to them by M. Faucher, in which the right epiphysial tubercle of the spine of the axis is believed to have been separated by muscular action.

This portion of the spinous process has been displaced outwards, but is still held to the bone by a well-marked ligamentous bundle, and to its apex the rectus capitis posticus major and inferior oblique muscle are still attached. It is, moreover, connected by fibrous bands to the inferior articular process of the axis, and to the corresponding bifurcation of the spinous process of the third cervical vertebra.

Separation of the epiphysial parts of the atlas.—The atlas at the time of birth consists of two lateral portions of bone, comprising the posterior arches and the greater part of the articular processes. These two lateral pieces are separated behind by a small cartilaginous interval and in front by the cartilaginous anterior arch. Ossification commences in the anterior arch of the atlas at the end of the first year, and consolidation with the lateral portions does not take place till the fifth or sixth year. The posterior arches unite about the third year.

For a detailed account of the development of the atlas the reader is referred to Professor A. Macalister's article, ' Note on the Development and Variation of the Atlas,' *Journal of Anatomy and Physiology*, N.S. 7, 1892–93, p. 519.

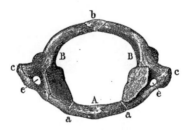

FIG. 289.—ATLAS AT THE END OF THE FIRST YEAR OF LIFE, THE CENTRES OF OSSIFICATION
ALREADY GREATLY DEVELOPED

A, median centre; B, B, lateral arches; a, a, cartilage between the body and the lateral masses, the last vestige of the cartilaginous body; b, cartilage separating the arches behind; c, c, transverse process; e, e, foramen for vertebral artery. (After Rambaud and Renault)

J. Macdonnell mentions (*Cyclopædia of Practical Surgery*, vol. ii., article on ' Fracture ') that cases are recorded of rupture of the atlas into its two lateral halves and of the odontoid process from the axis ; but of these the author has been unable to obtain any account.

They will be exceedingly difficult to diagnose from external symptoms, while as regards treatment every care should be taken to prevent movement of the head or spine.

Separation of the epiphyses of the axis.—At birth the axis is composed of four pieces of bone—one for the odontoid process (originally formed of two nuclei before birth), another for the lower part of the body and base of the odontoid process, and one for each arch and lateral process.

The base of the odontoid process joins the body of the bone and the neural arches on each side between the third and fourth year. Soon after this time the lateral portions of bone join in front and behind, completing the neural arch. Traces of the intervertebral cartilaginous disc between the odontoid process and the body of the bone are clearly to be seen at the twelfth year in a vertical section, and traces may even persist throughout life.

The apex of the odontoid process is often formed by a distinct centre of ossification appearing at the beginning of the second year, and joining from the fourth to the twelfth year.

The centres for the spinous and transverse processes appear about the seventeenth year.

There is a circular lamellar epiphysis as in the other vertebræ on the lower aspect of the body.

For a minute account of the development of the axis see an article by Professor A. Macalister, 'The Development and Varieties of the Second Cervical Vertebra,' *Journal of Anatomy and Physiology*, N.S. 8, Jan. 1894, p. 257.

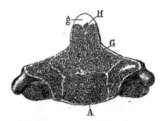

Fig. 290.—AXIS TOWARDS THE MIDDLE OF THE SECOND YEAR.   VERTICAL SECTION
THROUGH ODONTOID PROCESS, EXPOSING FIVE CARTILAGINOUS LINES

The pedicle on each side is received into the retiring angle formed by the body, A, and odontoid process, G.   These two parts are separated by a cartilaginous layer, thicker in centre than at either extremity, where it meets the apex of the angles.   An osseous centre, H, at this period appears in the cartilaginous apex, g, of the odontoid process, which is soon invaded by it (Rambaud and Renault)

The examples of separation of the odontoid process of the axis and of other parts of the cervical vertebræ given by Rognetta and other writers are untrustworthy, and were in all probability due to caries or other disease.

Separation of the epiphyses of the lumbar vertebræ.—In addition to the centres common to the other vertebræ, the lumbar vertebræ have separate centres of ossification for the mammillary processes which are placed upon the superior articular processes.   These small epiphyses appear from the sixteenth to the twentieth year, and unite, like the rest of the secondary epiphyses, about the twenty-fifth year.

The whole of the transverse process of the first lumbar vertebra is sometimes developed as a separate process.

SEPARATION OF THE EPIPHYSES OF THE SACRUM

Besides the lamellar plates on the upper and inferior surfaces of the bodies of the sacral vertebræ (especially marked in the first three), and the centres for each lamina and spinous tubercle, several centres appear at the twentieth year in the lateral cartilages at the level of each vertebra, which coalesce to form three epiphysial laminæ, while

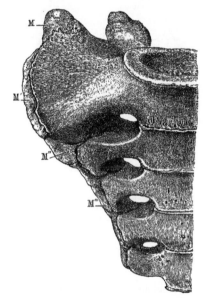

FIG. 291.—ANTERIOR SURFACE OF THE SACRUM AT THE TWENTY-THIRD YEAR

M, epiphysis of the transverse process of the first sacral vertebra; M', M'', M''', centres in the epiphysial plate of the lateral masses constituting three epiphysial centres, which unite to one another and with the rest of the bone at the twenty-eighth year   (Rambaud and Renault)

the epiphysis of the transverse process of the first sacral vertebra remains also distinct.

The three masses just mentioned often join to form a single plate; other anatomists describe them as two plates, one at the annular surface, the other for the rest, or thinner portion of the lateral margin below.

SEPARATION OF THE EPIPHYSES OF THE RIBS

Separation of the epiphysis of the head of the rib.—Towards the end of puberty (about the eighteenth year) an osseous centre appears in the cartilaginous head of the rib. This soon assumes the form of a small osseous plate, extends to the peripheral border of the cartilage, and blends with the body of the bone about the twenty-fourth or twenty-fifth year.

No instance has been recorded from injury.

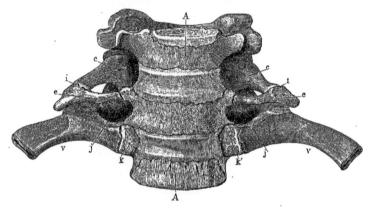

Fig. 292.—Last two cervical and first dorsal vertebræ, between the eighteenth and nineteenth year

A A, bodies of vertebræ; e, cervical rib articulating at ·j with the lateral part of seventh cervical body, and at i with the apex of the transverse process, c, of the same vertebra. This represents the costiform centre so often seen in this and occasionally in other lower cervical vertebræ, forming the front part of the foramen for the vertebral artery. V, first rib; K, epiphysis of head of first rib (Rambaud and Renault)

Separation of the epiphysis of the tuberosity of the rib.—About the same time as the centre of the head there appears an epiphysis for the articular portion of the tuberosity (corresponding to the transverse process of vertebræ). MM. Rambaud and Renault have also found in subjects of twenty-five years another osseous centre for the non-articular portion for the posterior costo-transverse ligament.

The articular epiphyses of the tuberosities of the eleventh and twelfth ribs are either very slightly developed or, more usually, quite absent.

These epiphyses unite with the body of the ribs at the twenty-fifth or twenty-sixth year.

No instance of traumatic separation has been recorded.

[Separation of the three pieces of which the *sternum* is composed is not considered in this volume.]

APPENDIX

—◆◇◆—

LITERATURE INACCESSIBLE TO THE AUTHOR

SCHNIEBS (R. H.), *Einiges über Epiphysenlösung.* 8°. Leipzig 1869.

BARTH (O.), 'Ueber Epiphysenlösung und deren Heilung,' *Arch. d. Heilk.* Leipz. 1870, xi. 263–571, 1 pl.

BARTH (O.), 'Epiphysenlösung im späteren Alter; hochgradige Arthritis deformans,' *ibid.* 1872, xiii. 477–79.

FISCHER (G.), 'Epiphysentrennung,' *Mitth. a. d. chir. Univ. Klin. zu Göttingen,* 1861, 82–107.

VON GERICHTEN (C. E.), *Ueber die Abtrennung der Knochenansätze,* Inaug.-Dissert. 8°. Erlangen 1841.

KLOSE (C. W.), 'Die Epiphysentrennung, eine Krankheit der Entwickelungszeit,' *Prager Vierteljahrsschrift,* 1858. Bd. 57, 97–124. For abstract see *Archiv. gén. de Méd.* 1858, 5. 2ème série 146–55.

BAYER (G.), *Ueber entzündliche Epiphysenablösung.* 8°. Tübingen 1877.

SCHLICHTING (W.), *Ein Fall von Epiphysentrennung.* 8°. Rostock 1863.

MICHNIOVSKI (S.), *Izsliedovanija zajivlenija otorvannich epiphezov* ('On the Separation of the Epiphysis'). St. Petersburg 1864.

MAZZIOTTI (G.), 'Del distacco delle epifise, e sue differenze dalle fratture,' *Gior. internaz. d. sc. med.* Napoli 1880, ii. 957–72.

GUIDONE (P.), 'Contributo alla etiologia e patogenesi del distacco epifisario,' *Riforma med.* Napoli 1891, vii. 579–83.

ZAPPALÀ (C.), 'Contributo alla patologia ed alla clinica del distacco epifisario,' *Raccoglito remed.* Forli 1885, 4 s. xxiii. 187, 217.

Upper Epiphysis of the Humerus

HARRIS (E.), 'Case of Fracture through the Articulation of the Epiphysis with the Shaft of the Humerus, with impaction and remarkably speedy recovery.' *New York Medical Times,* 1852–3, ii. 379–82.

PETERSON (F.), 'A Case of Epiphysial Fracture of the Humerus, with dislocation.' *Buffalo M. and S. Journal.* 1877–8, xvii. p. 449.

NOVARO (G. F.), 'Divulsione traumatica dell' epifisi superiore dell' omero destro,' *Osservatore.* Torino 1875, xi. 785, 801, 818.

FUQUA (W. M.), 'Epiphysial Fracture of the Superior Extremity of the Humerus,' *Medical Herald.* Louisville 1881–2, iii. 420.

Lower Epiphysis of the Humerus

BOTTINI (E.), 'Distacco traumatico dell' epifisi inferiore dell' omero sinistro,' *Osservatore.* Torino 1880, xvi. p. 296.

BOTTINI (E.), *Bulletin Gén. de Thérapeut.* Paris 1850, xxxix. pp. 167-170.

McDiarmid (J. L.), 'Case of Separation of the Lower Epiphysis of the Humerus,' *Canada Lancet.* Toronto 1875–6, viii. p. 63.

Stuart (A. B.), 'A Case of Supposed Separation of the Lower Epiphysis of the Humerus,' *Trans. Minnesota Med. Soc.* St. Paul 1876, p. 49.

Werner, 'Diductio epiphyseos inferioris humeri,' *Ztsch. f. Wundärzte u. Geburtsh.* Stuttg. 1865, xviii. p. 89.

Wight (J. S.), 'Partial Fracture of both Bones of the Forearm near the wrist-joint and Separation of the distal Epiphysis of the Humerus from a fall on the palm of the hand,' *Med. and Surg. Reporter.* Phila. 1880, xliii. 141.

Upper Epiphysis of the Radius

Stuart (A. B.), 'Separation of the Upper Epiphysis of the Radius,' *Pacific M. and S. Journal.* San Fran. 1878-9, xxi. 164–166.

Lower Epiphysis of the Ulna

Tuckerman (L. B.), 'Separation of the Lower Epiphysis of the Ulna,' *The Transactions.* Youngstown. Ohio 1879–80, i. 101.

Anterior Superior Spine of the Ilium

Albertin, 'Note sur un cas d'arrachement de l'épine iliaque antéro-supérieure par la contraction musculaire du couturier,' *Province Méd.* Lyon 1887, ii. 741.

Upper Epiphysis of the Tibia

Watson (J.), *N. York Med. Times.* 1853–4, iii. 187.

Powell (N. A.), 'Bilateral Diastasis at the Superior Tibial Epiphyses,' *Canada Lancet.* 1880–81, xiii. 324.

Poucel, *Marseille Méd.* 1869, vi. 847–58.

Tubercle of the Tibia

Mazzoni (G.), 'Un caso di distacco della tuberosità della tibia per avulsione (arrachement), *Bull. d. Soc. Lancisiana d' osp. di Roma.* 1882, ii. 71–74.

Lower Epiphysis of the Tibia

Albee (W. A.), 'Compound Separation of the Lower Epiphysis with Fracture of the Fibula,' *Tr. Maine Med. Assoc.* Portland 1886, ix. pt. i. 117-20.

INDEX OF NAMES

simple separation of upper epiphysis of tibia, 815; cases of simple separation of lower epiphysis of tibia and fibula, 842, 844

BIRMINGHAM, A. (Dublin), anatomy of epiphysis of third trochanter, 677

BITOT, specimen of separation of upper end of humerus produced during delivery, 43, 175

BLASIUS, specimen of separation of upper epiphysis of tibia, 806

BLOT, opinion as to occurrence of epiphysial separation (1865), 10

BŒCKEL, E., case of compound separation of lower epiphysis of radius, 513

BOERHAAVE, detachment of head of femur, 621, 652

BONAMY, experiments in pathological anatomy, 59

BOND, C. J. (Leicester), case of separation of lower epiphysis of humerus with dislocation of elbow-joint, 284

BORCK, EDWARD, erroneous views as to union after epiphysial separation, 98

BOTTINI, E., views upon separation of lower epiphysis of humerus, 335

BOUCHUT, description in 1867 of separation of the epiphyses, 10; muscular violence a cause of separation of the upper humeral epiphysis, 42; several epiphyses separated from syphilis, 85; dull crepitus in epiphysial separation, 92; case of separation of upper epiphysis of humerus by muscular action, 174; case of arrest of growth of tibia after fracture of lower epiphysis, 847

BOURGUET, painful pronation of the arm in young children, 95

BOUSSEAU, specimen of separation of anterior spines of ilium, 608; specimen of separation of epiphysial head of femur, 625

BOYD, STANLEY, muscular action causing detachment of upper epiphysis of fibula, 42, 858

BOYER, possibility of epiphysial separation at upper end of femur and humerus (1815), 4; causes sufficient to produce separation of the neck of the humerus, 38; rarity of separation of upper epiphysis of humerus, 176; symptoms of separation of epiphysial head of femur, 632

BRADFORD, E. H. (Boston, U.S.A.), cases of separation of epiphysial head of femur, 637, 650, 660

BRET, J., histological features of epiphysial separations, 60

BRINTON, JOHN H., specimen of separation of lower epiphysis of femur, 734

BRISTOW, compression of brachial artery in simple separation of lower end of humerus, 294

BROCA, A., epiphysial separation easily produced on the dead subject (1865), 10; difference in the growth of the ends of the bones (1852), 18, 104; growth in length of long bones due to greater thickness of chondroid layer of conjugal cartilage, 28; anatomy of the conjugal cartilage, 32, 33; experiments in pathological anatomy of epiphysial separations, 60; case of compound separation of the

lower end of femur through the conjugal cartilage, 73, 698; epiphysial cartilage remains with the epiphysis, 76; specimen of separation of lower epiphysis of femur, 708

BRODIE, CHAS. GORDON, case of arrest of growth of tibia after transverse fracture, 850

BROOKES, W. P. (Cheltenham), case of compound fracture of external condyle of femur, 723, 793

BROWN, C. HAIG, case of separation of anterior superior spine of ilium, 607

BROWN, W. H., case of arrest of growth of radius after separation of lower epiphysis, 568

BRUCE, W. (Dingwall), treatment of fractures of the elbow-joint, 326

BRUN-BOURGERET, osteotomy for deformity after fractures of external epicondyle of humerus, 404

BRUNN, A. V., relation of synovial membranes of joints to conjugal cartilages, 37; anatomy of epiphyses of phalanges of digits (fig. 180), 600

BRUNNER, CONRAD (Zürich), case of tetanus from pressure of callus in simple separation of lower epiphysis of radius, 121, 518

BRUNS, PAUL (Tübingen), monograph in 1882 on cases of epiphysial separation verified by an autopsy, 14; statistics as regards age in epiphysial separation, 48; frequency of the various separations, 52; seventy-eight cases in 1882 verified by direct examination, 54; pure separations, 73; number of instances of pure separations, 74; statistics of separation with fracture of the diaphysis, 81; compound separations, 86; union after separation of the epiphyses, 98; non-union after separation, 100; statistics of arrest of growth in one hundred cases, 106; arrest of growth of humerus after separation of upper epiphysis, 106; lengthening of femur after fracture, 116; arrest of growth due to inflammatory affections near the epiphysial cartilage, 120; complications in epiphysial separations, 121; replacement of diaphysis by operation in simple cases, 130; resection of diaphysial end in old separations, 132; case of separation of the upper epiphysis of the humerus, 171; statistics of specimen of separation of upper epiphysis of humerus, 177, 193; statistics of compound separation of upper epiphysis of humerus, 185; necrosis following compound separation of upper epiphysis of humerus, 187; symptoms in separation of upper epiphysis of humerus, 196, 203; case of separation of upper epiphysis of humerus, 207; operative treatment of recent separation of upper epiphysis of humerus, 226; operative treatment of old separation of upper epiphysis of humerus, 233; cases of arrest of growth of humerus after separation of upper epiphysis, 256; etiology of separation of lower epiphysis of radius, 483; statistics of separation of lower epiphysis of

DOWD, C. N., dislocation of humerus with fracture of surgical neck, 186 .

DUBROCA, epiphysial separation of upper end of humerus during childbirth, 43, 175

DUGAS, L. A., test for dislocation of head of humerus, 216

DUHAMEL, anatomy and physiology of the ends of the bones, 17, 18, 104; intimate connection of the epiphyses with the periosteum, 35

DUKES, CLEMENT (Rugby), case of separation of internal epicondyle of humerus, 349; case of simple separation of lower epiphysis of femur, 762

DUMONT-PALLIER, articular epiphyses separated in scurvy, 86

DUNN, L. A., case of separation of capitellum of humerus, 454

DUPLAY, case of separation of upper epiphysis of humerus by indirect violence, 173

DUPUY, case of suppuration following compound separation of upper epiphysis of humerus, 188

DUPUYTREN, dismissal of subject of epiphysial injuries in 1815, 4; case of simple separation of lower end of humerus mistaken for dislocation, 287, 301; treatment of fractured olecranon, 467; separation of lower epiphysis of radius, 487, 526; specimen of dwarfed radius with displacement forwards of its lower epiphysis, 521; case of separation of os innominatum into its original parts, 605; separation of epiphysial head of femur, 625

DURHAM, A. E., case of simple separation of upper epiphysis of humerus, 191; cases of separation of upper epiphysis of humerus, 213, 220, 223; case of separation of lower end of humerus, 296; case of condylo-trochlear fracture of humerus, 411; case of simple separation of lower epiphysis of radius, 530; specimen of separation of lower epiphysis of femur, 712; cases of simple separation of lower epiphysis of femur, 762, 775; specimen of separation of upper epiphysis of tibia, 803, 808; case of simple separation of upper epiphysis of tibia, 812; case of separation of lower epiphysis of tibia, 829; cases of simple separation of lower epiphyses of tibia and fibula, 842, 844

DUROCHER, CHAPELAIN, separation of humeral epiphysis at birth, 41; separation of upper end of humerus in the newly born, 176; non-union after separation of upper epiphysis of humerus, 100, 253

DUVAL, ANGE, case of compound separation of lower epiphysis of femur, 723

DUVERNEY, G. J., fractures and separations of the neck of the femur, 1751, 3; separation of epiphysial head of femur, 624, 632

DWIGHT, times of union of epiphyses, 25, 27, 28

EAMES, WILLIAM, case of fracture of olecranon epiphysis, 462

ELDER, J. M. (Montreal), etiology of separation of lower epiphysis of femur, 691;

case of compound separation of lower epiphysis of femur, 700

ELSNER, F. W., case of simple separation of lower epiphysis of femur, 760; case of separation of lower epiphysis of femur treated by operation, 788

ERDMANN, J. F. (New York), case of separation of upper epiphysis of humerus mistaken for dislocation, 214; case of impaired growth of humerus after separation of upper epiphysis, 256; case of simple separation of lower epiphyses of radius and ulna, 540

ERICHSEN, Sir JOHN E., articular lesions often absent in epiphysial separations, 84; resection of diaphysial end in compound separations, 128; erroneous view of anatomy of lower epiphysis of humerus, 265; case of compound separation of lower end of humerus, 329

ESMARCH, case of separation of the upper end of the humerus through the conjugal cartilage, 73; suppuration after epiphysial separation, 118; resection of diaphysial end in compound separation, 128; case of compound separation of upper epiphysis of humerus, 178, 241; suppuration following separation of upper epiphysis of humerus, 186

EVE, F. S., specimen of compound separation of lower epiphysis of femur, 704

EYSSONIUS, H., diseases and separations of the bones in children (1625), 2

FABRICE DE HILDEN, allusion in 1646 to separation of the upper epiphysis of the femur, 2; case of separation of epiphysial head of femur, 624, 642

FALLIER, age and sex in separation of external epicondyle of humerus, 352; detachment of internal epicondyle with dislocation of elbow, 358, 361, 362, 368; cases of dislocation of ulna with fracture of internal epicondyle, 370, 371, 372, 382

FARABEUF, article on separation of the lower epiphysis of the humerus (1886), 14, 270; views upon separation of lower epiphysis of humerus, 335, 341; etiology of separation of lower epiphysis of humerus, 339; epicondylo-capitellar separation of humerus, 422

FAUCHER, specimen of separation of epiphysis of spine of axis, 876

FENWICK (Montreal), specimen of separation of epiphysis of lesser trochanter, 675

FERGUSSON, Sir WILLIAM, epiphysial separation the same as fracture, 1846, 12; diagnosis of separation of the epiphyses, 95; non-union of acromion process, 149

FINLEY, HARRY, case of compound separation of lower epiphysis of humerus, 279

FISCHER, F., resection in old condylo-capitellar fractures of humerus, 446

FISCHER, H., suppuration of joint following epiphysial separation, 103; necrosis of epiphyses of fibula after separation, 120; arrest of growth due to inflammatory affections near the epiphysial cartilage, 120; case of separation of lower epiphysis

INDEX OF SUBJECTS

MASSAGE, treatment by, 126
    immediate treatment by, 127
    in loss of function of limb, 131
    in separation of upper epiphysis of humerus, 244
    immediate treatment by, in separation of lower epiphysis of radius, 576
    and passive motion in separation of epiphysial head of femur, 659
    in separation of lower epiphysis of femur, 792
Measurements of epiphysis of clavicle, 135
    upper epiphysis of humerus, 165
    lower epiphysis of humerus, 264
    internal epicondyle, 348
    external epicondyle, 392
    lower epiphysis of radius, 479
    lower epiphysis of ulna, 580
    epiphysial head of femur, 618
    great trochanter of femur, 662
    lower epiphysis of femur, 679
    upper epiphysis of tibia, 799
    lower epiphysis of tibia, 825
    upper epiphysis of fibula, 857
    lower epiphysis of fibula, 860
Mechanism of traumatic separation of the epiphyses, 58
Mechanism, and experiments, in epiphysial separations, 63, 64
Metacarpal bone of thumb, anatomy of, 588 ; separation of, 588 :—etiology, 588 : – age, 589 :—pathological anatomy and symptoms, 589 :—complications, 590 ; diagnosis, 590 ; treatment, 590
    bones, true epiphyses of, anatomy of, 591 ; separation of, 591 :—etiology, 591 : —age, 592 :—pathological anatomy and symptoms, 592 :—clinical cases of, 593 :—diagnosis, 596 :—prognosis, 597 :—treatment, 598
Metatarsal bone, first, anatomy, 868
    bones, outer, anatomy of, 869 ; separation of, specimens of, 869 :—case of, 870
Mobility of fragments, cause of arrest of growth, 112
    in separation of upper epiphysis of humerus, 202
    lower epiphysis of radius, 535
    epiphysial head of femur, 642
    lower epiphysis of femur, 777
    upper epiphysis of tibia, 813
    lower epiphysis of tibia, 840, 844
Morton's method of reduction of fracture of lower end of radius, 576
Multiple separation of epiphyses, 83
Muscular action in epiphysial separations, 42
    in separation of upper epiphysis of humerus, 174
    epiphysis of great trochanter of femur, 663
    epiphysial head of femur, 621
Muscular atrophy, after epiphysial separations, 103

NECROSIS, after separation of upper epiphysis of humerus, 186, 260
    lower epiphysis of femur, 738
    tibia, 839, 846
    fibula, 864
Nerve lesions, in separation of upper epiphysis of humerus, 212
    lower end of humerus, 294, 309
    internal epicondyle of humerus, 359, 365, 380
    condylo-trochlear and epicondylo-trochlear fractures of humerus, 409, 413
    separation of lower epiphysis of radius, 516, 518
    femur, 731, 782
    tibia, 838
Newly born infants, first allusion to separation in, 1
    experiments on, by Ruysch, 2
    separation of upper epiphysis of humerus in, 175, 176
Non-union, after epiphysial separations, 100
    due to mobility, 101
    of acromion process, 149
    after separation of upper epiphysis of humerus, 253
    internal epicondyle of humerus, 353, 354
    condylo-trochlear fracture of humerus, 427
    separation of lower epiphysis of radius, 561
    epiphysial head of femur, 652
Nutrient canals, relation with union of epiphysis to diaphysis (Bérard's law), 22
    influence on union of fractures, 22
    direction in long bones, 22

PRINTED BY
SPOTTISWOODE AND CO., NEW-STREET SQUARE
LONDON